HUMAN HEMOGLOBINS

H. FRANKLIN BUNN, M.D.
Associate Professor of Medicine,
Harvard Medical School;
Chief of Hematology Section,
Peter Bent Brigham Hospital, Boston

BERNARD G. FORGET, M.D.
Associate Professor of Medicine,
Chief of Hematology Section,
Yale University School of Medicine, New Haven

HELEN M. RANNEY, M.D.
Professor and Chairman Department of Medicine,
University of California, San Diego

1977

W. B. SAUNDERS COMPANY
Philadelphia / London / Toronto

W. B. Saunders Company: West Washington Square
Philadelphia, PA 19105

1 St. Anne's Road
Eastbourne, East Sussex BN21 3UN, England

1 Goldthorne Avenue
Toronto, Ontario M8Z 5T9, Canada

Library of Congress Cataloging in Publication Data

Bunn, Howard Franklin,

Human hemoglobins.

Includes index.

1. Hemoglobinopathy. 2. Hemoglobin. I. Forget, Bernard G., joint author. II. Ranney, Helen M., joint author. III. Title. [DNLM: 1. Hemoglobinopathies. 2. Hemoglobins. WH150 B942ha]

RC641.7.H35B87 612′.1111 76–14677

ISBN 0–7216–2178–3

Human Hemoglobins ISBN 0-7216-2178-3

Last digit is the print number: 9 8 7 6 5 4 3 2 1

ACKNOWLEDGMENTS

We are indebted to many individuals for their valuable help at all stages of this project.

Individual chapters were thoroughly reviewed by the following colleagues: Arthur Arnone, Philip Bromberg, George Buchanan, William Eaton, Stuart Edelstein, Alan Keitt, Philip Pulsinelli, Ronald Rieder and Vijay Sharma.

Edward Benz contributed immensely to the literature search and organization of material related to the sections on the biosynthesis of hemoglobin and the molecular genetics of the thalassemias.

Philomena Burkhardt and Kathy Strutz provided expert secretarial assistance. Their patience, good humor and conscientious attention to detail continued throughout the book's long gestation. We are also indebted to the library staff at UCSD School of Medicine for their painstaking check of all the references, and to Betsy Bunn for extensive proofreading of both typescript and page proofs.

Diane Forti has been an exceptionally able copy editor, providing invaluable advice on style, usage and organization as well as an unfailing eye for inconsistencies, omissions, redundancies, etc. We also thank the senior editors at Saunders, John Dusseau and Jack Hanley, for their sound advice and enthusiastic cooperation.

Finally, we thank those friends and colleagues with whom our interest in hemoglobin began:

The Benesches	Irving London
Robin Briehl	David Nathan
James Jandl	Sherman Weissman

CONTENTS

Chapter 1

HEMOGLOBIN STRUCTURE

HISTORICAL BACKGROUND[1]

The term "hemoglobin" was first used by Hoppe-Seyler (1864) to describe the red pigment in erythrocytes. Hoppe-Seyler observed the characteristic optical absorption of oxygenated hemoglobin, and Stokes (1864) noted the change in the spectrum on deoxygenation. The reversible binding of oxygen by hemoglobin was analyzed quantitatively at the turn of the century by a group of distinguished physiologists, including Bohr and Krogh in Denmark and Barcroft and the elder Haldane in England (see Chapter 2). In 1852 the chromophore of hemoglobin had been isolated in the form of hemin chloride (Teichman, 1853). During the 1920's this iron-containing prosthetic group was exhaustively investigated. The structure of heme was worked out by Küster (1912). Several years later heme was synthesized in the laboratory of Dr. Hans Fischer (1929). This remarkable achievement permitted a detailed comparison of the natural and synthetic compounds, which were shown to be functionally identical. It soon became apparent that this particular porphyrin was the prosthetic group not only of hemoglobins of a wide variety of species, but also of other respiratory proteins such as myoglobins and some of the cytochrome enzymes (Haurowitz, 1928).

Once the nature of the prosthetic group of hemoglobin was known, a more complete understanding of its interrelationship with the protein globin was possible. Englehardt (1825) had found that the iron content of hemoglobin was 0.35 per cent of the total weight of

[1]Edsall (1972) has recently completed a richly detailed history on the chemistry and physiology of hemoglobin.

the protein. This value is identical to the correct one (0.346 per cent) determined from the known structure of hemoglobin. From this figure a minimum molecular weight of 16,000 Daltons could be calculated. However, accurate determinations of hemoglobin's molecular weight made in the 1920's both by measurement of osmotic pressure (Adair, 1925) and by analytical ultracentrifugation (Svedberg, 1926) gave values of 64,000 to 68,000 Daltons. Therefore it seemed likely that the hemoglobin molecule contained four heme-containing subunits.

Since hemoglobin is a highly colored substance, its various forms were found to have strong and specific absorption bands in the visible spectra. The development of adequate monochromators and photomultiplier tubes for the measurement of small differences in absorbed light permitted the detailed determination of spectral properties of hemoglobin (Drabkin, 1949; Heilmeyer, 1943). The absorption spectra in the visible region were shown to be the most accurate and convenient measure of the binding of oxygen to hemoglobin. There was excellent agreement between spectrophotometric and gasometric measurements of oxygen binding to hemoglobin. The oxidation of hemoglobin to methemoglobin and the interaction of hemoglobin with various other heme ligands such as carbon monoxide and nitric oxide were also shown to result in characteristic alterations in the visible absorption spectra. Some of these are shown in Figure 1–1.

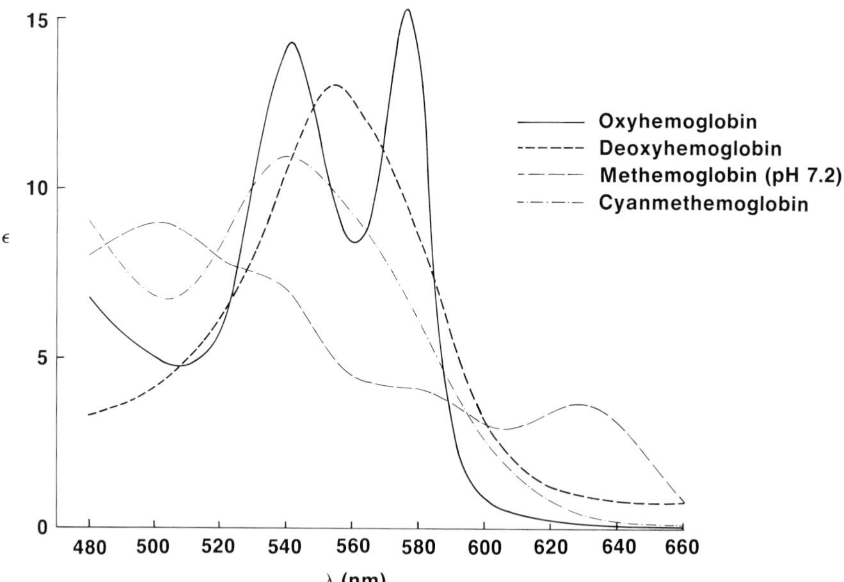

Figure 1–1. Absorption spectra of oxyhemoglobin (Fe^{++}-O_2), deoxyhemoglobin (Fe^{++}), methemoglobin (Fe^{+++}), and cyanmethemoglobin (Fe^{+++}-CN).

In contrast to the uniformity of the heme in vertebrate hemoglobins, comparisons of physical and chemical properties pointed to differences in the globin. Although hemoglobins in general were found to have identical absorption spectra in visible light, many differed in functional properties such as oxygen affinity. In 1866, Körber had noted that hemoglobins differed markedly in their rates of denaturation in strong acid and alkali. His observation that the hemoglobin of human newborns is remarkably resistant to alkali denaturation provided the basis for the method of estimating fetal hemoglobin which is still widely used in clinical laboratories. Differences in the solubilities (Jope and O'Brien, 1949) and crystalline forms (Reichert and Brown, 1909) of various mammalian hemoglobins were also noted. Titration of sulfhydryl groups showed that mammalian hemoglobins differed considerably in cysteine content (Ingram, 1955; Allison and Cecil, 1958). From these considerations it was anticipated that considerable heterogeneity existed among globins of various species.

From the molecular weight of hemoglobin and its amino acid composition, it was apparent that the globin moiety contained approximately 580 residues. The presence of subunits was suspected because of the existence of four heme groups per molecule. A major breakthrough occurred when Ingram (1956) separated the peptides produced after globin had been hydrolyzed with the proteolytic enzyme trypsin, which cleaves polypeptides only at lysine and arginine residues. Although arginine and lysine account for 60 amino acid residues per mole of hemoglobin, only 30 tryptic peptides were obtained, strongly suggesting that hemoglobin consisted of two identical half molecules. Careful re-examination of N-terminal sequences of human globin by Rhinesmith et al. (1957) and Braunitzer (1958) revealed 2 moles of Val-Leu and 2 moles of Val-His-Leu per mole of globin. Taken together, the evidence thus indicated that hemoglobin was a tetramer composed of two pairs of unlike polypeptide chains which were designated α and β. It seemed reasonable to assume that each globin chain was attached to a heme group.

The advent of new and powerful methods for the determination of protein structure in the early 1960's allowed the structure of hemoglobin to be worked out over a very few years. Rapid progress was made on two fronts. Techniques became available for the determination of primary amino acid sequences of the subunits of human hemoglobin. At the time of this writing, the primary structure has been determined for hemoglobins of 26 mammalian and 6 nonmammalian species (Dayhoff, 1972). Secondly, Perutz and his associates at Cambridge, England, have successfully determined the three-dimensional structure of oxy- and deoxyhemoglobin. This contribution earned Perutz a Nobel Prize in 1962. During the last decade his laboratory has continued to define hemoglobin structure in greater detail. As we shall discuss in Chapter 2, these studies have permitted considerable progress in correlating hemoglobin structure and function.

NORMAL HUMAN HEMOGLOBINS

The identification of different hemoglobin species in normal man depended on the introduction of analytical techniques that could separate structurally different proteins. Examination of a normal hemolysate by moving-boundary (Tiselius) electrophoresis revealed only a single monodisperse component. The development of zone electrophoresis in various solid or semisolid media permitted much greater resolution. Kunkel and Wallenius (1955) demonstrated by electrophoresis on starch granules that normal human hemolysate consisted of three components, which they called A_1, A_2, and A_3. These components are listed in Table 1–1.

Hemoglobin A (A_1)

Hemoglobin A (A_1) makes up about 95 per cent of the total hemoglobin of normal adults. The structure and function of this hemoglobin will be considered in detail in this and the following chapter.

Hemoglobin A_2

A minor component having a higher isoelectric point and making up about 2.5 per cent of the total was designated as hemoglobin A_2 (see Figure 1–2). Later studies showed that increased amounts of this hemoglobin are found in individuals with homozygous and heterozygous β thalassemia (Kunkel et al., 1957) (see Chapter 5). In addition, hemoglobin A_2 may be increased in megaloblastic anemia (Josephson et al., 1958). In contrast, in iron deficiency (Chernoff, 1964) and sideroblastic anemias (Reed and Mollin, 1968; White et al., 1971) it is decreased. The marked differences in the proportion of hemoglobin A_2 in these disorders of red cell maturation may be related to the fact that the relative rate of synthesis of this minor component is markedly curtailed in the final stages of erythroid development (Rieder and Weatherall, 1965). Hemoglobin A_2 has been shown to be evenly distributed in red cells (Heller and Yakulis, 1969).

Ingram and Stretton (1961) analyzed the globin of hemoglobin A_2 and demonstrated the presence of normal α chains and chains which differed structurally (in 10 of 146 residues) from normal β chains (see section on primary structure).

TABLE 1–1. *Human Hemoglobins*

Hemoglobin	Structure	% of Normal Adult Hemolysate	Increased In	Decreased In
A	$\alpha_2\beta_2$	92		
A_2	$\alpha_2\delta_2$	2.5	β thalassemia Megaloblastic anemia	Iron deficiency Sideroblastic anemia
A_{Ia}	Not known	< 1	Diabetes mellitus (applies to A_{Ia}, A_{Ib}, A_{Ic})	Hemolytic anemia
A_{Ib}	" "	2		
A_{Ic}	$\alpha_2(\beta\text{-N-glucose})_2$	5		
F	$\alpha_2\gamma_2$	< 1	Fetal red cells β thalassemia Marrow "stress": Sickle cell anemia, pernicious anemia, etc. (applies to F, F_I)	
F_I	$\alpha_2(\gamma\text{-N-acetyl})_2$	< 1		
Gower 1	$\zeta_2\epsilon_2$	0	Early embryo (applies to Gower 1, Gower 2, Portland)	
Gower 2	$\alpha_2\epsilon_2$	0		
Portland	$\zeta_2\gamma_2$	0		
H	β_4	0	α thalassemias (applies to H, Bart's)	
Bart's	γ_4	0		

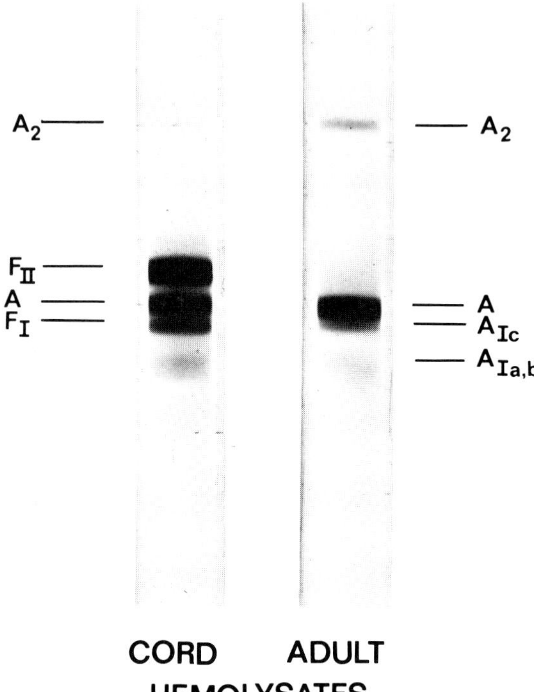

Figure 1–2. Analysis of human cord and adult blood hemolysate by gel electrofocusing.

Hemoglobin A_3

On starch-gel electrophoresis at alkaline pH, there is a third component which migrates anodally to the main component but is not clearly separated from it. This "spearhead" of the main component was designated by Kunkel and Wallenius (1955) as hemoglobin A_3. Subsequently, Allen, Schroeder, and Balog (1958) and Huisman and his associates (1958a) used chromatography on cation-exchange resins to separate hemoglobins. They showed that hemoglobin A_3 consisted of several minor components which were designated by Schroeder as hemoglobins A_{Ia}, A_{Ib}, and A_{Ic}. Very little is known about the structure or function of hemoglobins A_{Ia} and A_{Ib}. An additional minor fast-moving peak appears to be a complex of normal hemoglobin A with pyridoxal phosphate (Srivastava et al., 1972). This component is present in only trace amounts in normal red cells.

Hemoglobin A_{Ic}

Hb A_{Ic} is the "major" minor component of human hemolysate, making up about five per cent of the total. This hemoglobin differs from hemoglobin A only at the N terminus of the β chain, where in A_{Ic} glucose is linked by means of a Schiff base (Bookchin and Gallop, 1968; Holmquist and Schroeder, 1966). Upon acid hydrolysis, glucose and mannose can be recovered from Hb A_{Ic} in a ratio of approximately 3:1 (Bunn et al., 1975a). Hb A_{Ic} appears to be formed by the condensation of glucose and hemoglobin, reactants that are present in high concentrations within the red cell. The initial β-chain–glucose-Schiff base (aldimine) linkage probably rearranges to form a more stable ketoamine attachment (Bunn et al., 1975a):

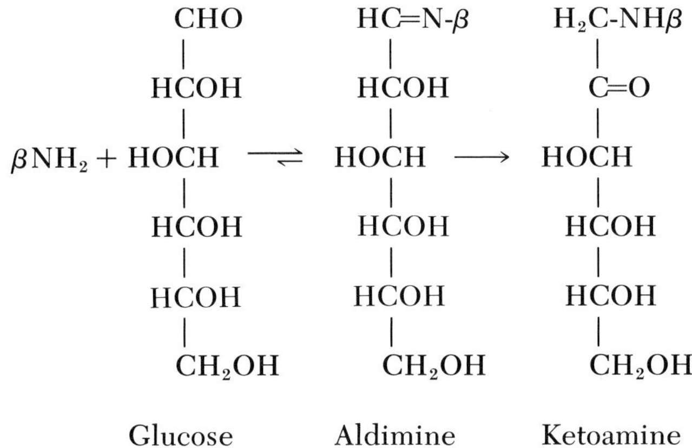

When the ketoamine is subjected to acid hydrolysis, there is racemization at the C2 atom, resulting in the formation of glucose and its C2 epimer, mannose. Hb A is converted to Hb A_{Ic} slowly and continuously throughout the life span of the red cell (Bunn et al., 1976; Ranney, unpublished observation). It is likely that this reaction is nonenzymatic. Accordingly, the percentage of Hb A_{Ic} in red cells is a function of the glucose concentration within the cell and of the red cell life span.

Interest in Hb A_{Ic} has been considerably enhanced by the fact that this glycoprotein is increased about twofold in patients with diabetes mellitus (Paulsen, 1973; Rahbar, 1968; Rahbar et al., 1969; Trivelli et al., 1971). The level of Hb A_{Ic} does not appear to correlate with the duration or severity of the diabetes. From the biosynthesis studies described above, Hb A_{Ic} in the diabetic should be proportional to the time-averaged concentration of glucose within the red cell. Thus the level of Hb A_{Ic} should be a reflection of the adequacy of control over a sustained time period. Tattersall et al. (1975) showed that the monozygotic twin of a diabetic has normal levels of Hb A_{Ic}. This study provides independent evidence that increased Hb A_{Ic} in diabetes is not a genetic phenomenon but depends upon the presence of clinically apparent diabetes. Recently, Koenig and Cerami (1975) found an increase in a minor hemoglobin component in a strain of diabetic mice. Labeling experiments indicate that the formation of this minor hemoglobin component, like human Hb A_{Ic}, is a post-translational event. The glycosylation of hemoglobin in diabetics raises the question of what other proteins may be similarly modified during sustained periods of hyperglycemia. Such alterations in protein structure may be important in the pathogenesis of diabetes and its complications.

Hemoglobin F

It was long suspected that the red cells of newborns contained structurally distinct hemoglobin in view of the marked resistance of hemoglobin from cord blood to denaturation in alkaline solutions. Fetal hemoglobin (Hb F) can be identified both electrophoretically (see Figure 1–2) and chromatographically. In many mammalian species which have been tested, the hemoglobin of the newborn differs from that of the adult. (Exceptions include the horse [Stockell et al., 1961], the pig [Tautz and Kleihauer, 1972], and the dog [LeCrone, 1970].) During early development, the fetus may have one or more embryonic hemoglobins that cannot be detected at birth (see Chapter 4 and Table 1–1).

The hemolysate of the human newborn contains three main components: hemoglobin F (60 per cent), F_I (15 per cent), and A (15 per cent). Analyses of the globins indicate that hemoglobin F consists of normal α chains and a structurally distinct non-α chain, designated γ (Schroeder et al., 1963). Hemoglobin F_I differs from F only at the N terminus of the γ chain, where it is acetylated (Schroeder et al., 1962; Huehns and Shooter, 1966). During the first 6 months of postnatal life, the F hemoglobins decrease steadily, so that this hemoglobin is barely detectable in the red cells of older children and adults. Chapter 4 contains a more complete discussion of the alterations in hemoglobin synthesis during embryonic and fetal development.

Hemoglobin F can be quantitated by a number of approaches: alkali denaturation, electrophoresis, chromatography, and analysis of isoleucine (absent in α, β, and δ chains). In addition, it can be detected by immunological techniques or by the increased absorption at 294 nm, related to its increased tryptophan content. The proportion of Hb F in a hemolysate is usually measured by its resistance to alkali, but this method cannot accurately detect small amounts.

The red cells of adults contain very small amounts of hemoglobin F. This minor component is difficult to detect by either electrophoresis or column chromatography but has been demonstrated by immunofluorescent techniques using a fluorescent labeled antibody to hemoglobin (Hosoi, 1965). By this technique hemoglobin F appears to be confined to only a few erythrocytes (Boyer et al., 1975).

Hemoglobin F is increased to a variable extent in several hereditary disorders, including β thalassemia, hereditary persistence of fetal hemoglobin, and sickle cell anemia (see Chapters 5 and 7). In addition, increased levels of hemoglobin F of up to 10 per cent may be seen in a variety of acquired hematologic disorders, including megaloblastic anemia, aplastic anemia, and leukemias (see Chapter 4) (Newman et al., 1973). Children with chronic myelocytic leukemia may have marked elevations in Hb F. In these acquired disorders, the Hb F is distributed unevenly among red cells. The mechanism underlying this return to γ-chain synthesis is unknown. The regulation of Hb F synthesis is discussed in more detail in Chapter 4.

Other Hemoglobins

Hemoglobin H and hemoglobin Bart's are tetramers of β chains and γ chains, respectively. For physiologic oxygen transport, a hemoglobin tetramer consisting of pairs of α and non-α (β, γ, or δ) chains appears to be necessary. In contrast, hemoglobins H and Bart's have very high oxygen affinity and absent heme-heme interaction and Bohr effect. These hemoglobins are found to a variable extent in patients with different types of α thalassemia. The thalassemias are discussed in detail in Chapter 5.

The Gower hemoglobins ($\alpha_2\epsilon_2$, and $\zeta_2\epsilon_2$) are detectable only in the first three months of fetal development. Epsilon chains are probably synthesized in the yolk sac. Only minute amounts of these hemoglobins can be obtained, and their structural properties have not been studied.

PRIMARY STRUCTURE

Proteins are polymers consisting of amino acids arranged in specific linear sequence and linked by peptide bonds. The general structure of such a polypeptide polymer would be

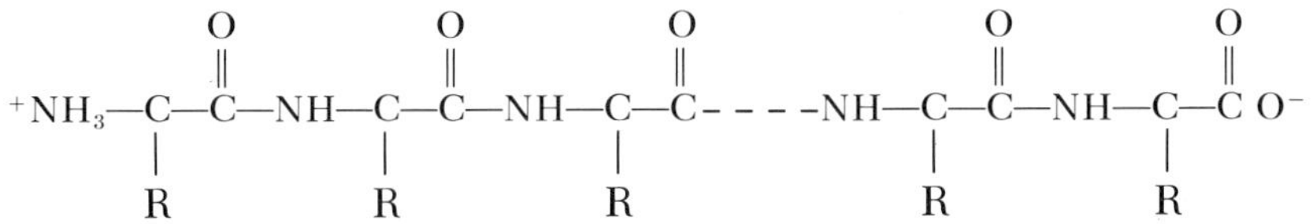

```
          O           O           O              O           O
          ‖           ‖           ‖              ‖           ‖
+NH3—C—C—NH—C—C—NH—C—C- - - -NH—C—C—NH—C—C O⁻
     |           |           |              |           |
     R           R           R              R           R
```

The "R" radicals represent the side groups of the 20 amino acid residues which are used as the building blocks in the construction of proteins. There is convincing evidence that the primary amino acid sequence is the important determinant of the folding of the protein in three-dimensional space (Anfinsen, 1973). Proteins may be linked to carbohydrates (glycoproteins), lipids (lipoproteins), and specific functional prosthetic groups such as heme. The presence of groups such as these has an additional influence in determining the tertiary (and quaternary) structure of the protein and its functional properties.

METHODS FOR DETERMINATION OF PRIMARY SEQUENCE

Before the detailed studies on the structure of hemoglobin could be undertaken, it was necessary to isolate the constituent polypeptide chains. The structure of hemoglobin A is commonly designated $\alpha_2{}^A\beta_2{}^A$. The human α chain also forms stable tetramers with other gene products differing in structure from the β chain. Hemoglobin F is designated $\alpha_2\gamma_2$, while hemoglobin A_2 is designated $\alpha_2\delta_2$. Fortunately, the human α and non-α chains differ widely in their isoelectric points and therefore can be readily separated by methods dependent on differences in the overall surface charge of the protein. For initial structural work, human α and β chains were separated by countercurrent distribution (Hill and Craig, 1959). However, a much more convenient and effective method of chain separation was developed (Chernoff, 1961; Clegg et al., 1966) using ion-exchange chromatography in the presence of high concentrations of urea.

Establishment of the primary sequence of normal human globin chains was due in large part to contributions from the laboratories of Braunitzer in Munich, Konigsberg and Hill in New York, and Schroeder in Pasadena. Their basic methodological approach, outlined here, is still employed in the determination of the primary structure of protein subunits. Isolated chains are digested with an enzyme to break them up into smaller peptides. Trypsin, the most generally used of these enzymes, cleaves the polypeptide chain specifically on the carbonyl side of lysine and arginine residues. Thus, the number of peptides obtained is determined by the number of lysine and arginine residues in the chain. Except for the C-terminal peptide, the other peptides will have one of these two residues at their C terminus. The peptides of a globin chain are then analyzed.

Ingram approached this by the use of *fingerprinting* (Ingram, 1956). The enzyme digest is spotted on filter paper and separated by high-voltage electrophoresis. Then the peptides are further separated from one another by paper chromatography done at a 90-degree angle to the electrophoresis. After appropriate staining, a two-dimensional pattern appears, consisting of a spot for each peptide. This pattern is reproducible for a given globin chain under defined experimental conditions, hence the term "fingerprint." A fingerprint of a tryptic digest of the β chain of human hemoglobin is shown in Figure 1–3. Alternatively, peptides can be separated by ion-exchange column chromatography (Jones, 1964). Individual peptides are then eluted from the fingerprint (or the column). The total amino acid composition (but not the sequence) is determined following hydrolysis of the peptide bonds in strong acid.

The amino acid sequence of individual peptides can be determined by Edman analysis, which removes residues in order, beginning at the N terminus. Recently, this analytical approach has been

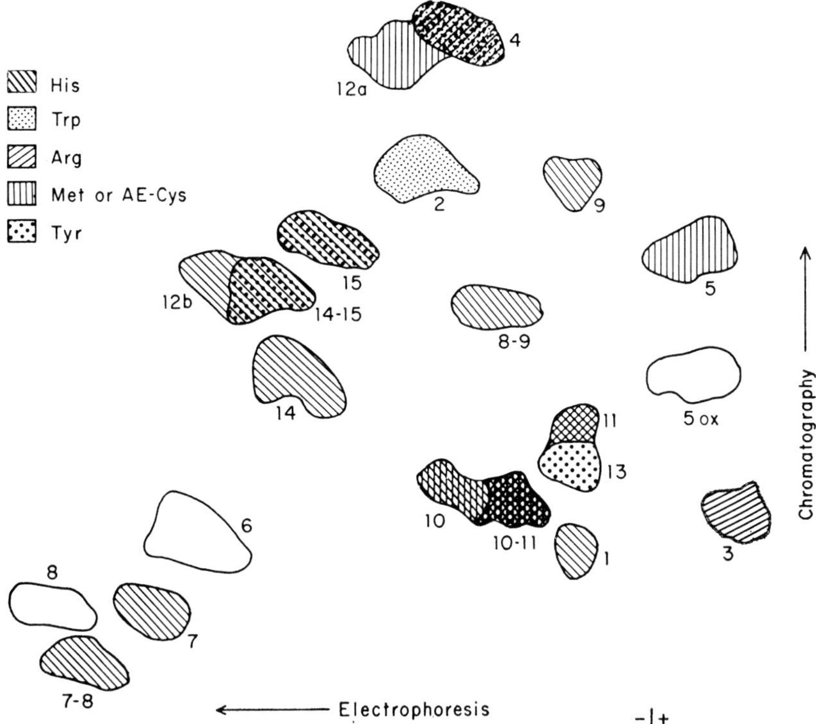

Figure 1–3. Two-dimensional peptide map (fingerprint) of normal human β chain. (From Stamatoyannopoulos, G., et al.: J. Clin. Invest. 52:342, 1973.)

completely automated and permits sequencing of polypeptide chains up to 60 residues in length. Alternatively, the structure of peptides can be partially or completely established by digestion with carboxypeptidase, which cleaves amino acid residues sequentially at the C terminus. Finally, the order of the peptides in the chain must be determined. This can be done by structural analyses of peptides formed by other enzymes which attack the protein at alternate sites. For example, the overlapping peptides formed by pepsin and chymotrypsin, as well as trypsin, were analyzed in working out the structure of human α and β chains.

The determination of the primary amino acid sequence of proteins resembles the challenge of solving a complex but ultimately logical jigsaw puzzle. Once the structure of normal human α and β chains was established the analysis of hemoglobin variants became much less formidable, since these generally represent single amino acid substitutions. Therefore, a fingerprint of the variant subunit usually reveals the displacement of only one of the tryptic peptides, and attention is directed to this peptide.

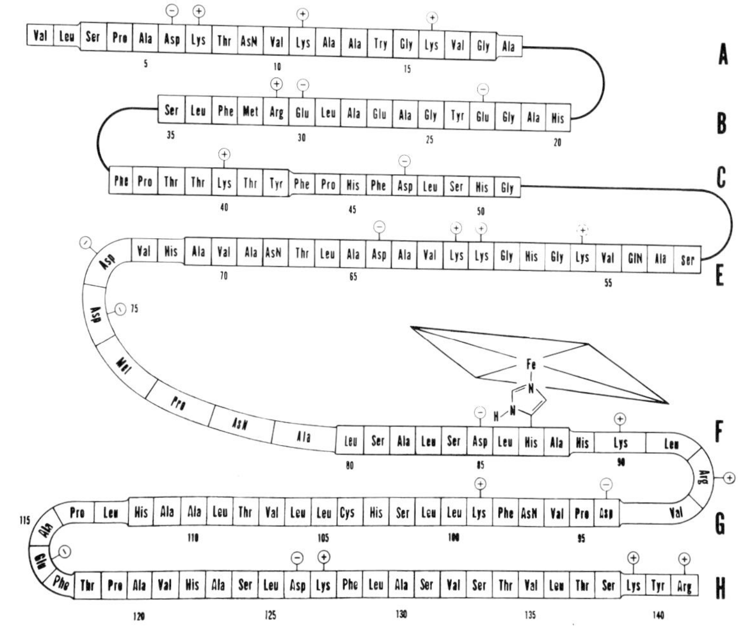

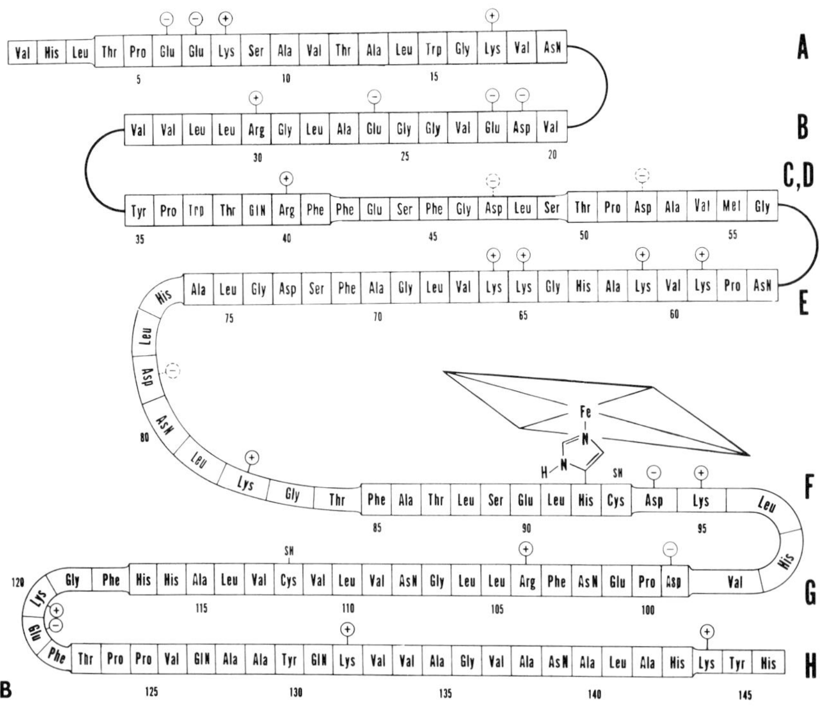

Figure 1–4. *See legend on the opposite page.*

Primary Structure of Human Globin Subunits

α Chain

The human α chain consists of 141 amino acids in linear sequence. The primary structure is shown in Figure 1–4*A*. As this figure indicates diagrammatically, the heme group is bound covalently by a linkage between the heme iron and the imidazole of a histidine residue at position 87 (counting from the N-terminal end of the polypeptide). This is the so-called proximal histidine. A more detailed treatment of the heme-globin linkage will be presented at the end of this chapter.

β Chain

The β chain is slightly longer than the α chain (146 residues). Its primary structure is shown in Figure 1–4*B*. Unlike many other proteins including such diverse examples as gamma globulin, ribonuclease, or insulin, there are no disulfide bridges (cystine residues) either within or between hemoglobin subunits. The cysteine residue at position 93 of the β chain is highly reactive and readily undergoes oxidation to form mixed disulfides and other thio ethers. This phenomenon may be involved in hemoglobin catabolism and will be discussed in Chapter 8, Unstable Hemoglobin Variants.

δ Chain

Hemoglobin A_2 is an electrophoretically distinct minor component making up about 2.5 per cent of the total hemoglobin in normal individuals. Ingram and Stretton (1961) showed that this hemoglobin is a tetramer consisting of α chains and a different type of subunit, which they designated δ chain. As shown in Table 1–2, the amino acid sequence of the δ chain is very similar to that of the β chain, differing only in 10 of 146 amino acids. Hemoglobin A_2 is identical in function to hemoglobin A. The two have the same oxygen affinity (Bunn and Briehl, 1970; DeBruin and Janssen, 1973; Eddison et al., 1964), Bohr effect (DeBruin and Janssen, 1973; Eddison et al., 1964), and reactivity to 2,3-DPG (Bunn and Briehl, 1970; DeBruin and Jans-

---

Figure 1–4. The primary structure of the α chain (*A*) and β chain (*B*) of human hemoglobin A. Those residues which are oriented in the form of an α helix are depicted by squares; nonhelical residues are depicted by rectangles. The site for heme attachment is shown. (From Murayama, M., in Nalbandian, R. M. (ed.): Molecular Aspects of Sickle Cell Hemoglobin, 1971. Courtesy of Charles C Thomas, Publisher, Springfield, Illinois.)

sen, 1973). Thus, it is unlikely that the residues that differ between the β and δ chains are crucial to the maintenance of normal hemoglobin function.

γ *Chain*

The structure of the γ chain of hemoglobin F is also strongly analogous to that of the β chain. The amino acid sequences of the two proteins differ in 39 of 146 residues (Table 1–2). In addition, at the 136th residue, γ chains may contain either glycine or alanine, evidently reflecting the presence of multiple genetic loci responsible for γ-chain synthesis (see Chapter 4). The differences between the γ and β chains must be sufficient to account for significant differences in the functional properties of hemoglobins F and A. These are discussed in the following chapter on hemoglobin function. Structural differences between the γ and β chains must also account for the relative resistance of hemoglobin F to alkali denaturation. Perutz (1974) has pointed out that there are two residues buried within the β chain of hemoglobin A (112 Cys and 130 Tyr) which may become ionized by alkali and hydrated, favoring the formation of readily denatured hemoglobin monomers. In contrast, on the γ chain, threonine is at position 112 and tryptophan is at position 130, thereby conferring relative protection from attack.

NONHUMAN HEMOGLOBINS

At the time this chapter was written, the complete primary structure has been determined for α chains of 20 mammalian species and for β chains of 26 mammalian species (Dayhoff, 1972). In addition, globins from the chicken, carp, frog, and lamprey have been sequenced (Dayhoff, 1972). This prodigious accumulation of data has been of great value in several respects. The chains from different species can be aligned in such a way that structural homology is maximized. It can be readily seen that at certain sites in the primary sequence there is a single amino acid common to most, if not all, species. These so-called invariant residues indicate a structural site in the molecule crucial to hemoglobin function. Examples include the histidine to which the heme group is covalently linked and the tyrosines which make up the penultimate residues of both the α and β chains. Amino acids at the interface or contact points between hemoglobin subunits also tend to be invariant. The functional significance of these sites will be discussed in detail in the next chapter.

A close comparison of the structural differences between aligned globin subunits has provided valuable information about evolutionary divergence. If it is assumed that accepted mutations occur in a

TABLE 1–2. *Primary Structure of Human Globin Subunits*

Helix*	α	ζ	Helix*	β	δ	γ
NA1	1 Val		NA1	1 Val	Val	Gly
			NA2	2 His	His	His
NA2	2 Leu		NA3	3 Leu	Leu	Phe
A1	3 Ser		A1	4 Thr	Thr	Thr
A2	4 Pro		A2	5 Pro	Pro	Glu
A3	5 Ala		A3	6 Glu	Glu	Glu
A4	6 Asp		A4	7 Glu	Glu	Asp
A5	7 Lys		A5	8 Lys	Lys	Lys
A6	8 Thr	(Thr	A6	9 Ser	Thr	Ala
A7	9 Asn	Ser	A7	10 Ala	Ala	Thr
A8	10 Val	Leu	A8	11 Val	Val	Ile
A9	11 Lys	Lys)	A9	12 Thr	Asn	Thr
A10	12 Ala	(Asn	A10	13 Ala	Ala	Ser
A11	13 Ala	Ala	A11	14 Leu	Leu	Leu
A12	14 Try	Try	A12	15 Try	Try	Try
A13	15 Gly	Gly	A13	16 Gly	Gly	Gly
A14	16 Lys	Lys)	A14	17 Lys	Lys	Lys
A15	17 Val	(Ile	A15	18 Val	Val	Val
A16	18 Gly	Ser				
AB1	19 Ala	Thr				
B1	20 His	Asp	B1	19 Asn	Asn	Asn
B2	21 Ala	Thr	B2	20 Val	Val	Val
B3	22 Gly	Thr	B3	21 Asp	Asp	Glu
B4	23 Glu	Glu	B4	22 Glu	Ala	Asp
B5	24 Tyr	Ile	B5	23 Val	Val	Ala
B6	25 Gly	Gly	B6	24 Gly	Gly	Gly
B7	26 Ala	Thr	B7	25 Gly	Gly	Gly
B8	27 Glu	Glu	B8	26 Glu	Glu	Glu
B9	28 Ala	Ala	B9	27 Ala	Ala	Thr
B10	29 Leu	Leu	B10	28 Leu	Leu	Leu
B11	30 Glu	Glu	B11	29 Gly	Gly	Gly
B12	31 Arg	Arg)	B12	30 Arg	Arg	Arg
B13	32 Met	(Leu	B13	31 Leu	Leu	Leu
B14	33 Phe	His	B14	32 Leu	Leu	Leu
B15	34 Leu	Leu	B15	33 Val	Val	Val
B16	35 Ser	Ser	B16	34 Val	Val	Val
C1	36 Phe	Phe	C1	35 Tyr	Tyr	Tyr
C2	37 Pro	Pro	C2	36 Pro	Pro	Pro
C3	38 Thr	Thr	C3	37 Try	Try	Try
C4	39 Thr	Gln	C4	38 Thr	Thr	Thr
C5	40 Lys	Lys)	C5	39 Gln	Gln	Gln
C6	41 Thr		C6	40 Arg	Arg	Arg
C7	42 Tyr		C7	41 Phe	Phe	Phe
CE1	43 Phe		CD1	42 Phe	Phe	Phe
CE2	44 Pro		CD2	43 Glu	Glu	Asp
CE3	45 His		CD3	44 Ser	Ser	Ser
CE4	46 Phe		CD4	45 Phe	Phe	Phe
			CD5	46 Gly	Gly	Gly
CE5	47 Asp	(Leu	CD6	47 Asp	Asp	Asn
CE6	48 Leu	Leu	CD7	48 Leu	Leu	Leu
CE7	49 Ser	Ser	CD8	49 Ser	Ser	Ser
CE8	50 His	His	D1	50 Thr	Ser	Ser
			D2	51 Pro	Pro	Ala
			D3	52 Asp	Asp	Ser
			D4	53 Ala	Ala	Ala

*The residues have been aligned to demonstrate homology between subunits.

Table 1–2 continued on the following page.

TABLE 1–2. Primary Structure of Human Globin Subunits (Continued)

HELIX*	α	ζ	HELIX*	β	δ	γ
			D5	54 Val	Val	Ile
			D6	55 Met	Met	Met
CE9	51 Gly	Gly	D7	56 Gly	Gly	Gly
E1	52 Ser	Phe	E1	57 Asn	Asn	Asn
E2	53 Ala	Ala	E2	58 Pro	Pro	Pro
E3	54 Gln	His	E3	59 Lys	Lys	Lys
E4	55 Val	Val	E4	60 Val	Val	Val
E5	56 Lys	Lys)	E5	61 Lys	Lys	Lys
E6	57 Gly	(Ala	E6	62 Ala	Ala	Ala
E7	58 His	His	E7	63 His	His	His
E8	59 Gly	Gly	E8	64 Gly	Gly	Gly
E9	60 Lys	Ser	E9	65 Lys	Lys	Lys
E10	61 Lys	Lys)	E10	66 Lys	Lys	Lys
E11	62 Val	(Val	E11	67 Val	Val	Val
E12	63 Ala	Ala	E12	68 Leu	Leu	Leu
E13	64 Asp	Glu	E13	69 Gly	Gly	Thr
E14	65 Ala	Ala	E14	70 Ala	Ala	Ser
E15	66 Leu	Leu	E15	71 Phe	Phe	Leu
E16	67 Thr	Thr	E16	72 Ser	Ser	Gly
E17	68 Asn	Ser	E17	73 Asp	Asp	Asp
E18	69 Ala	Ile	E18	74 Gly	Gly	Ala
E19	70 Val	Leu	E19	75 Leu	Leu	Ile
E20	71 Ala	Gly	E20	76 Ala	Ala	Lys
EF1	72 His	Pro	EF1	77 His	His	His
EF2	73 Val	Val	EF2	78 Leu	Leu	Leu
EF3	74 Asp	Asp	EF3	79Asp	Asp	Asp
EF4	75 Asp	Ser	EF4	80Asn	Asn	Asp
EF5	76 Met	Phe	EF5	81 Leu	Leu	Leu
EF6	77 Pro	Lys)	EF6	82 Lys	Lys	Lys
EF7	78 Asn	(Asn	EF7	83 Gly	Gly	Gly
EF8	79 Ala	Ala	EF8	84 Thr	Thr	Thr
F1	80 Leu	Val	F1	85 Phe	Phe	Phe
F2	81 Ser	Gly	F2	86 Ala	Ser	Ala
F3	82 Ala	Ala	F3	87 Thr	Gln	Gln
F4	83 Leu	Leu	F4	88 Leu	Leu	Leu
F5	84 Ser	Ser	F5	89 Ser	Ser	Ser
F6	85 Asp	Glu	F6	90 Glu	Glu	Glu
F7	86 Leu	Val	F7	91 Leu	Leu	Leu
F8	87 His	His	F8	92 His	His	His
F9	88 Ala	Ala	F9	93 Cys	Cys	Cys
FG1	89 His	Lys)	FG1	94 Asp	Asp	Asp
FG2	90 Lys	(Ile	FG2	95 Lys	Lys	Lys
FG3	91 Leu	Leu	FG3	96 Leu	Leu	Leu
FG4	92 Arg	Arg)	FG4	97 His	His	His
FG5	93 Val		FG5	98 Val	Val	Val
G1	94 Asp		G1	99 Asp	Asp	Asp
G2	95 Pro		G2	100 Pro	Pro	Pro

*The residues have been aligned to demonstrate homology between subunits.

***TABLE 1–2.** Primary Structure of Human Globin Subunits (Continued)*

HELIX*	α	ζ	HELIX*	β	δ	γ
G3	96 Val		G3	101 Glu	Glu	Glu
G4	97 Asn		G4	102 Asn	Asn	Asn
G5	98 Phe		G5	103 Phe	Phe	Phe
G6	99 Lys		G6	104 Arg	Arg	Lys
G7	100 Leu	(Ala	G7	105 Leu	Leu	Leu
G8	101 Leu	Leu	G8	106 Leu	Leu	Leu
G9	102 Ser	Ser	G9	107 Gly	Gly	Gly
G10	103 His	His	G10	108 Asn	Asn	Asn
G11	104 Cys	Cys	G11	109 Val	Val	Val
G12	105 Leu	Leu	G12	110 Leu	Leu	Leu
G13	106 Leu	Gly	G13	111 Val	Val	Val
G14	107 Val	Lys)	G14	112 Cys	Cys	Thr
G15	108 Thr	(Ser	G15	113 Val	Val	Val
G16	109 Leu	Leu	G16	114 Leu	Leu	Leu
G17	110 Ala	Glx	G17	115 Ala	Ala	Ala
G18	111 Ala	Ala	G18	116 His	Arg	Ile
G19	112 His	His	G19	117 His	Asn	His
GH1	113 Leu	Leu	GH1	118 Phe	Phe	Phe
GH2	114 Pro	Tyr)	GH2	119 Gly	Gly	Gly
GH3	115 Ala	(Ala	GH3	120 Lys	Lys	Lys
GH4	116 Glu	Glx	GH4	121 Glu	Glu	Glu
GH5	117 Phe	Phe	GH5	122 Phe	Phe	Phe
H1	118 Thr	Thr	H1	123 Thr	Thr	Thr
H2	119 Pro	Ile	H2	124 Pro	Pro	Pro
H3	120 Ala	Gly	H3	125 Pro	Gln	Glu
H4	121 Val	Val	H4	126 Val	Met	Val
H5	122 His	Asx	H5	127 Gln	Gln	Gln
H6	123 Ala	Ala	H6	128 Ala	Ala	Ala
H7	124 Ser	Ser	H7	129 Ala	Ala	Ser
H8	125 Leu	Leu	H8	130 Tyr	Tyr	Try
H9	126 Asp	Asp	H9	131 Gln	Gln	Gln
H10	127 Lys	Lys)	H10	132 Lys	Lys	Lys
H11	128 Phe	(Phe	H11	133 Val	Val	Met
H12	129 Leu	Leu	H12	134 Val	Val	Val
H13	130 Ala	Ala	H13	135 Ala	Ala	Thr
H14	131 Ser	Ser	H14	136 Gly	Gly	Gly, Ala
H15	132 Val	Val	H15	137 Val	Val	Val
H16	133 Ser	Ser	H16	138 Ala	Ala	Ala
H17	134 Thr	Thr	H17	139 Asn	Asn	Ser
H18	135 Val	Val	H18	140 Ala	Ala	Ala
H19	136 Leu	Leu	H19	141 Leu	Leu	Leu
H20	137 Thr	Glx	H20	142 Ala	Ala	Ser
H21	138 Ser	Ser	H21	143 His	His	Ser
HC1	139 Lys	Lys)	HC1	144 Lys	Lys	Arg
HC2	140 Tyr	(Tyr	HC2	145 Tyr	Tyr	Tyr
HC3	141 Arg	Arg)	HC3	146 His	His	His

*The residues have been aligned to demonstrate homology between subunits.

random fashion over a prolonged time frame, then greater differences in primary sequence between species indicate a more distant time at which the two species had common ancestors. Furthermore, species can be grouped so that a minimum number of mutations from common ancestors will produce the observed primary sequences. Using such approaches, evolutionary trees can be constructed which provide independent evidence for the origins and interrelationships of various organisms. Figure 1–5 shows phylogenetic trees derived from structural studies of α chains. Comparative studies on the structure of cytochrome C have also been particularly valuable in developing phylogenetic relationships. These results are in excellent agreement with conclusions reached by studies of taxonomy and phenotypic differences between species.

SECONDARY STRUCTURE

The amino acid sequence is the primary determinant of how a protein is arranged in three-dimensional space. Secondary structure refers to the spatial relationship between adjacent residues along the chain. Segments of polypeptide chains can be stabilized by orientation into one of two basic configurations: the α helix and the β pleated

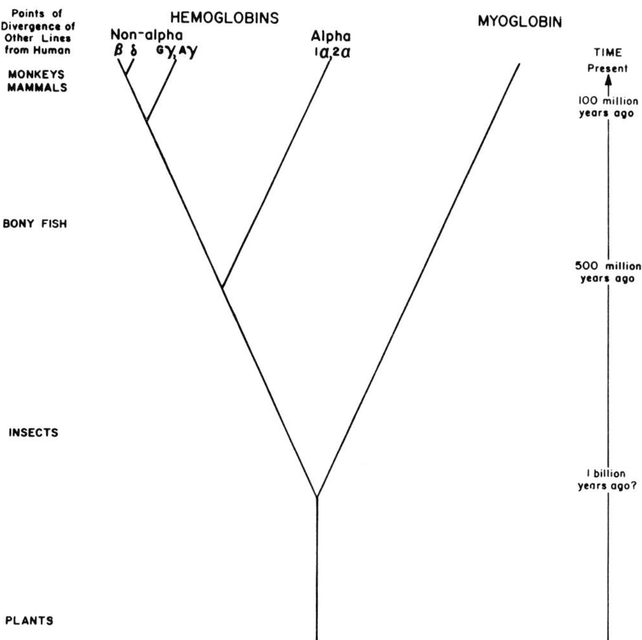

Figure 1–5. Molecular evolution of heme proteins. A, Myoglobin and the subunits of hemoglobin.

sheet. Some insoluble and fibrous proteins such as keratin or myosin are in the form of an α helix, while others such as silk fibroin are in the form of a β pleated sheet. Collagen, which is rich in proline and hydroxyproline, cannot form either structure and has its own unique spatial configuration. Most soluble and globular proteins are to varying degrees in the form of an α helix. This configuration, first worked out by Pauling and Corey (1951), involves the orientation of the polymer into a single-stranded helix, or coil, with 3.6 amino acid residues per turn (Fig. 1–6). The side groups of the residues are oriented externally in a radial fashion. The helix is stabilized by hydrogen bonding between the carbonyl group of each residue and the amino group four residues away.

In its native state about 75 per cent of hemoglobin is in the form of an α helix, as measured by physical techniques such as optical rotary dispersion. This relatively high helical content in comparison to other globular proteins simplified the solution of the three-dimensional structure of hemoglobin. Upon the removal of heme, the helical content of globin decreases to about 50 per cent (Beychok et al., 1967). At specific locations in the hemoglobin subunits, the α helix is interrupted by segments which lack a helical conformation. At these sites

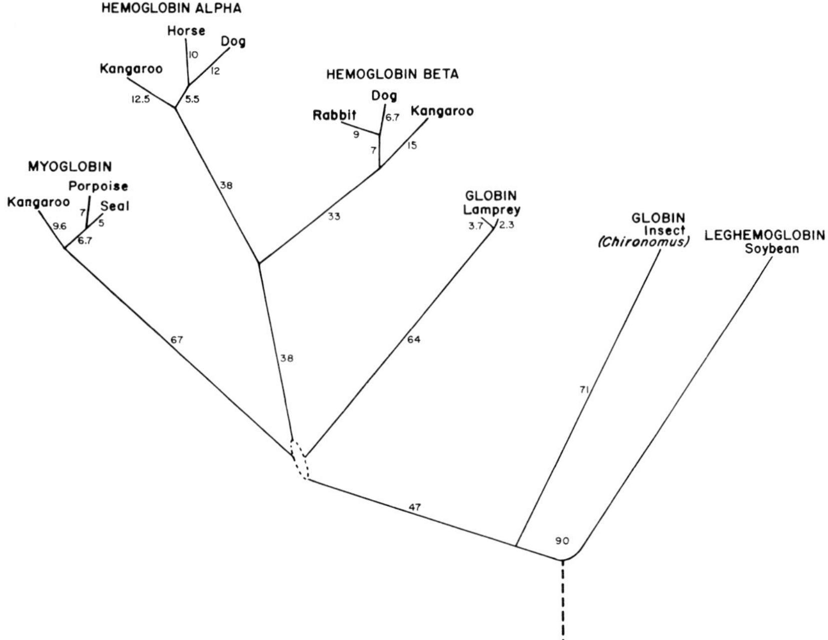

Figure 1–5. Continued. *B*, Alpha chains of hemoglobin. (From Dayhoff, M. O.: Atlas of Protein Sequence and Structure, Vol. 5, 1972. National Biomedical Research Foundation, Washington, D.C.)

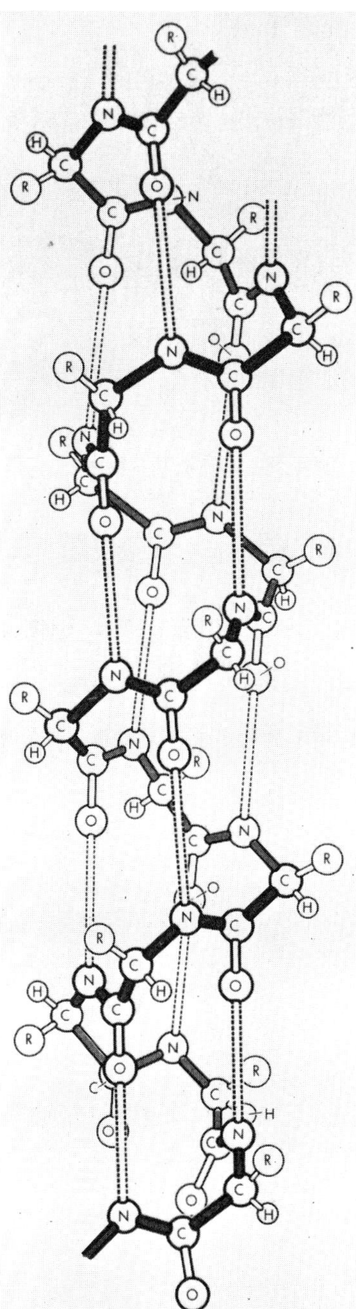

Figure 1–6. Right-handed α helix showing hydrogen bonds between carbonyl groups and amino groups (::::::::). (From Kendrew, J. C.: Scientific American *205*:104, 1961. Copyright © 1961 by Scientific American, Inc. All rights reserved.)

the polypeptide chain can turn corners, accounting for the complex convoluted three-dimensional structures of hemoglobin and myoglobin. In some segments of the polypeptide chains the interruption of the α helix is due to the presence of proline, which is unable to participate in this configuration except at the first three residues from the N-terminal end.

During the investigation of the three-dimensional structures of hemoglobin and myoglobin by x-ray crystallography, Perutz and his associates realized that the individual subunits of hemoglobin and myoglobin showed striking conformational similarities. They concluded that these protein subunits probably had analogous helical segments. The β subunit was shown to have 8 helical segments, lettered A through H. The helical segments of the α chain are closely comparable to those of the β chain, but the residues making up the D helix of the β chain are absent in the α chain. Accordingly, amino acid residues in these subunits can be assigned helical designations. For example, the "proximal" or heme-linked histidine is F8 (see Figs. 1–4*A* and 1–4*B*). When these chains are aligned according to their helical designations, maximal homology between subunits is apparent. This is illustrated in Table 1–2. From a comparison of the structures of globin chains, Dayhoff (1972) has concluded that the α chain and the β chain diverged from a common precursor about 500 million years ago (Fig. 1–5). This antedated the differentiation of vertebrates into various orders. About 1 billion years ago, prior to the development of vertebrates, the hemoglobin precursor and myoglobin diverged from a common heme protein. During the eons that have elapsed since hemoglobin has been in existence, it has evolved into a molecule well designed for its physiological functions.

TERTIARY AND QUATERNARY STRUCTURE

X-RAY CRYSTALLOGRAPHY

Tertiary structure refers to the configuration of a protein subunit in three-dimensional space. The spatial relationships of each of the four subunits of hemoglobin to the others determine the quaternary structure. The three-dimensional structure of various molecules can be determined from studying the x-ray diffraction patterns of their crystals. At the present time the tertiary and quaternary structures of hemoglobin have been worked out through x-ray crystallography with such a high degree of resolution (~2.5 Å) that each of the many atoms of this complex molecule can be spatially oriented with respect to one another. This remarkable achievement can be attributed entirely to Dr. Max Perutz and his associates at the Medical Research Council Laboratory in Cambridge, England.

Many relevant observations preceded the elegant studies of

Perutz. The crystalline forms of a variety of mammalian hemoglobins had been thoroughly catalogued (Reichert and Brown, 1909). Furthermore, it was known that the oxy and deoxy forms of horse hemoglobin differed in crystalline structure. Haurowitz (1938) observed that when crystals of horse deoxyhemoglobin were exposed to oxygen, extensive disintegration (crazing) took place. These observations provided the first evidence that oxygenation results in a marked change in the conformation of hemoglobin.

In 1935 Perutz left his native country, Austria, to join Dr. Lawrence Bragg at the Cavendish Laboratories in Cambridge. Bragg and his father, W. H. Bragg, were pioneers in developing the science of x-ray crystallography. In 1915 they determined the structure of crystalline sodium chloride. Subsequently, crystals of other molecules were successfully analyzed, including inorganic salts, minerals, and relatively simple organic compounds. The analysis of molecules as complex as proteins proved to be much more formidable. In the 1920's and 30's, x-ray diffraction patterns were observed on fibrous proteins such as keratin, collagens, and silk fibers. Despite the poor quality of the patterns, the structures of fibrous proteins were approachable because they are ordered along a long central axis with repeating segments of identical structure. Although the single crystals of globular proteins could be studied at much higher resolution, analysis of the complicated diffraction patterns presented enormous theoretical and technical problems. In 1934 Bernal and Crowfoot obtained x-ray diffraction photographs of pepsin crystals. The following year Dr. Crowfoot initiated studies on insulin crystals. (Twenty years later her determination of the structure of vitamin B_{12} by x-ray crystallography earned her a Nobel Prize, but it wasn't until 1968 that she and her colleagues succeeded in elucidating the structure of insulin.) Perutz and Bragg, along with J. D. Bernal, became intrigued by the prospect of determining the structure of another large globular protein, hemoglobin. The attempt to study hemoglobin seemed worthwhile for three reasons: it could be purified and crystallized, the electron-rich heme groups would be useful in interpreting x-ray diffraction patterns, and the molecule was of obvious biological importance. Studies of other large biological molecules were initiated, including bushy stunt and tobacco mosaic viruses, by Bernal and his associates.

The theoretical resolution limit of a microscope is approximately equal to the wavelength of the radiation used to illuminate the object. Therefore, in order to resolve the distances between atoms using electromagnetic radiation, x-rays must be used with a wavelength of about 1 Å. In theory, x-ray crystallography is a form of microscopy, but in practice the method is difficult to apply because no one has yet devised a lens for x-rays. Instead, one proceeds as follows: A well-formed crystal suspended in its mother liquor is placed on a turntable. The crystal is rotated in a beam consisting of parallel monochromatic x-rays. The rays are diffracted by the crystal in the same way as an optical grating diffracts visible light. The diffracted rays are collected on a photographic plate, giving a geometric pattern of spots of varying intensities. At certain angles, x-rays penetrating planes of the crystal are mutally reinforced and result in geometrically ordered spots radiating from the x-ray beam. This phenomenon is expressed quantitatively by Bragg's law: $\lambda = 2d \sin \theta$, where θ is the angle of the incident rays, d is the distance between planes, and λ is the wavelength. The amount of scattering of the x-rays depends on the number of electrons encountered by the beam. Accordingly, the relative intensity of the spots is a function of electron density within the unit cell of the crystal. From the amplitudes and phase angles of all diffracted rays, the coordinates of the atoms in the unit cell can be calculated by means of a mathematical operation known as a Fourier summation, the solution of which is greatly facilitated by the use of a computer. The computer is in effect the lens of the "x-ray microscope." The results generated from Fourier summations can be expressed in terms of contour maps which reflect electron density in a given plane. An example is shown in Figure 1–9.

The central problem in this procedure is the determination of the phase angles of the diffracted x-rays. Perutz and his colleagues solved this problem by the elegant application of the method of isomorphous replacement. This method requires that the protein be labeled with an electron-rich ligand, such as a heavy metal, at a specific site (or sites) on the molecule. If the crystalline structure of the chemically modified hemoglobin is isomorphous with that of the protein, its x-ray diffraction pattern can be used to determine the phases of the x-rays scattered from the native (unlabeled) protein. Paramercuribenzoate and silver ions were shown to interact specifically with the β93 sulfhydryl group of hemoglobin (Green et al., 1954), and these derivatives provided the first test of the isomorphous replacement as applied to protein structure. This approach was also used in the x-ray analysis of sperm whale myoglobin in Dr. John Kendrew's laboratory, and by 1963 the three-dimensional structure of myoglobin had been determined at a very high degree of resolution (1.4 Å). During this time Perutz and his colleagues had worked out a 5.5 Å resolution Fourier synthesis of horse oxyhemoglobin and human deoxyhemoglobin. Their results indicated that the subunits in the hemoglobin tetramer had a tertiary configuration very similar to that of myoglobin. Perutz and his associates also took advantage of the growing body of information on the amino acid sequences of hemoglobin subunits. Knowledge of the primary structure was very useful in interpreting the computer-generated electron-density maps.

Conformational Isomerization and Subunit Interactions

The subunits of hemoglobin were shown to be oriented in a globular unit having a twofold dyad axis of symmetry. This means that if any part of the molecule is rotated 180 degrees on this axis it will coincide with a segment of identical structure. This axis runs down a water-filled cavity in the center of the molecule. One particularly provocative finding was the marked difference found in the *quaternary* structures of horse oxyhemoglobin and human deoxyhemoglobin. Following deoxygenation, the β chains move apart by about 7 Å, a relatively large distance compared to the overall dimensions of the hemoglobin tetramer (an ellipsoid measuring approximately $64 \times 55 \times 50$ Å). Subsequently the oxygenation-dependent conformational isomerization was confirmed in a comparison of the oxy and deoxy forms of the same species (human hemoglobin [Fig. 1–7]). As this model shows, the heme groups were found to be approximately equidistant from one another on the surface of the molecule. Thus the "heme-heme interaction" encountered in the cooperative binding of oxygen to hemoglobin could not be explained on the basis of direct contact between heme groups. The distances between the iron atoms of the four hemes of oxy- and deoxyhemoglobin are shown in Table 1–3.

The change in quaternary structure upon oxygenation is quite compatible with the large number of physical and chemical differences known to exist between oxyhemoglobin and deoxyhemoglobin. This conformational isomerization must involve movement of hemoglobin subunits relative to one another. From inspection of a three-dimensional model of hemoglobin, such as depicted in Figure 1–7, it is apparent that each α chain impinges upon the two β chains along two different surfaces. Hence, if the subunits are designated α_1, α_2, β_1, and β_2, two interfaces between unlike subunits can be defined as $\alpha_1\beta_1$ and $\alpha_1\beta_2$. From considerations of symmetry the $\alpha_1\beta_1$ interface is structurally identical to $\alpha_2\beta_2$ and the $\alpha_1\beta_2$ interface is identical to $\alpha_2\beta_1$. The high-resolution (2.8 Å) models indicated that during oxygenation there is considerable movement at the $\alpha_1\beta_2$ interface. In contrast, the $\alpha_1\beta_1$ interface remains relatively fixed.

The subunits of hemoglobin interact with one another by means of relatively weak, noncovalent bonds such as Van der Waals forces and hydrogen bonds. In addition, as discussed below, deoxyhemoglobin is stabilized by both intra- and inter-subunit salt bonds. The interactions between the amino acid residues at the $\alpha_1\beta_1$ and $\alpha_1\beta_2$ interfaces are shown in Figure 1–7. In oxyhemoglobin there are 31 Van der Waals contacts and 3 hydrogen bonds between residues at the $\alpha_1\beta_1$ interface. In contrast, the overall bonding at the $\alpha_1\beta_2$ interface is considerably weaker, with only 15 Van der Waals interactions and 2 hydrogen bonds. Under physiologic conditions oxyhemoglobin is

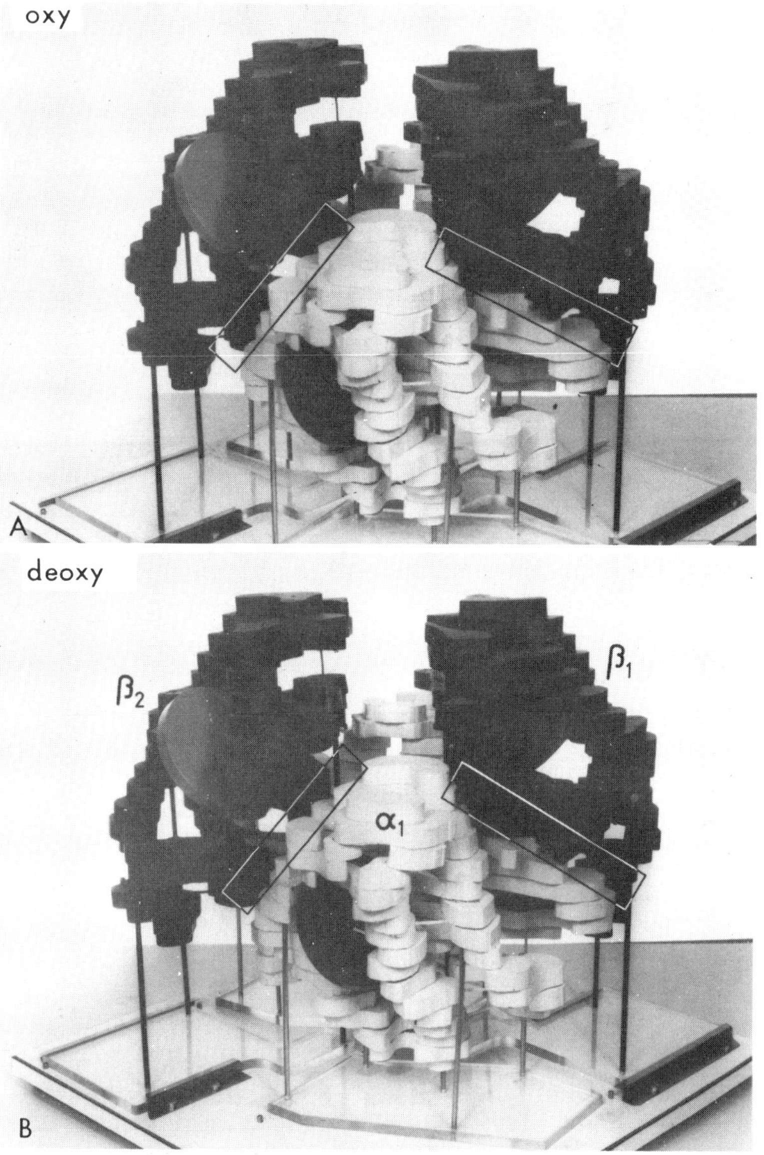

Figure 1-7. A three-dimensional model of hemoglobin, based on x-ray crystallographic analysis (*A*, oxy; *B*, deoxy). The α chains are shown in white, the β chains in black; the boxed areas are the $\alpha_1\beta_2$ contact areas. The heme groups are depicted as disks inserted into each subunit. There is an axis of symmetry which is parallel to the plane of the paper. Note the difference in conformation between oxy- and deoxyhemoglobin. (From Muirhead, H., Cox, J. M., et al.: J. Molec. Biol. *28*:117, 1967.)

TABLE 1–3. Distances Between Heme Iron Atoms

	OXY	DEOXY
	(Å)	
α_1–α_2	36.0	34.9
α_1–β_2 (α_2–β_1)	25.0	24.6
α_1–β_1 (α_2–β_2)	35.0	36.9
β_1–β_2	33.4	39.9

known to dissociate reversibly into like dimers: $\alpha_2\beta_2 \rightleftharpoons 2\alpha\beta$ The above stereochemical considerations strongly suggest that the symmetrical dissociation of hemoglobin occurs at the $\alpha_1\beta_2$ interface, giving two identical dimers, $\alpha_1\beta_1$ (and $\alpha_2\beta_2$). Independent evidence for this has been provided (Rosenmeyer and Huehns, 1967). From inspection of the contact points of deoxyhemoglobin, it appears as if little or no conformational change has occurred at the $\alpha_1\beta_1$ interface as a result of deoxygenation. In contrast, at the $\alpha_1\beta_2$ interface the residues are differently aligned. During conformational isomerization the two subunits slip over one another in a tongue and groove fashion (Fig. 9–1). It is not surprising that amino acid residues at the $\alpha_1\beta_2$ interface are "invariant" residues. Furthermore, those human hemoglobin variants having substitutions at the $\alpha_1\beta_2$ interface may have drastic alterations in function (see Chapter 9).

The extent to which hemoglobin dissociates symmetrically into dimers depends markedly on whether it is oxygenated. The reaction occurs about 10^6 times more readily in oxyhemoglobin than in deoxyhemoglobin. Thus the binding energy between $\alpha\beta$ dimers must be considerably greater in the deoxygenated form. However, a comparison of the number of Van der Waals contacts and hydrogen bonds at the $\alpha_1\beta_2$ interface reveals very little difference between oxyhemoglobin and deoxyhemoglobin. Recently, Perutz and his associates have shown that the increased stability of deoxyhemoglobin (and the corresponding reduction in symmetrical dissociation into dimers) is related to the presence of inter- (and intra-) subunit salt bonds. For example, the C-terminal carboxyl of each β chain forms a salt bridge with the ϵ-amino group of α40 Lys while the imidazole of the C-terminal histidine of each β chain is linked to an aspartate residue at position 94 of the same chain. This is shown diagrammatically in Figure 1–8. The increased affinity of protons at this site following deoxygenation accounts for about 50 per cent of the Bohr effect. Earlier x-ray data indicating that the N-terminal amino group of each α chain is linked to the C-terminal carboxyl of the other are probably not correct (Fermi, 1975).

In deoxyhemoglobin, the penultimate tyrosine residue of each of the four subunits is firmly anchored in a pocket between the F and H helices. This is illustrated in Figure 1–8. This interaction contributes to the stabilization of the deoxy conformation. Upon oxygenation, these tyrosines are evicted, freeing up the C-terminal portion of each subunit.

Organic phosphates also enhance the stability of the deoxy conformation. In mammals, 2,3-diphosphoglycerate (2,3-DPG) has been shown to mediate hemoglobin function within the red cell. The physiological importance of this cofactor will be discussed in detail in the next two chapters. Recent x-ray diffraction studies of Arnone (1972) indicate that 2,3-DPG binds electrostatically to the β chains of deoxyhemoglobin at a specific site on the molecule on the dyad axis of symmetry at the entrance to the central cavity. The phosphate groups of 2,3-DPG form salt bonds with the β N-terminal amino groups and the imidazoles of β143-histidine. The carboxyl group of

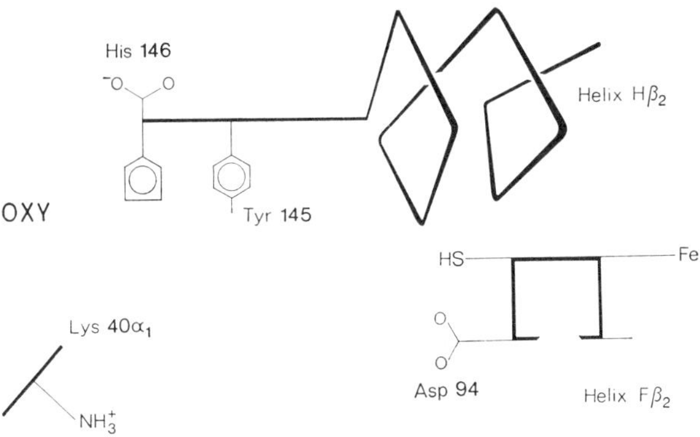

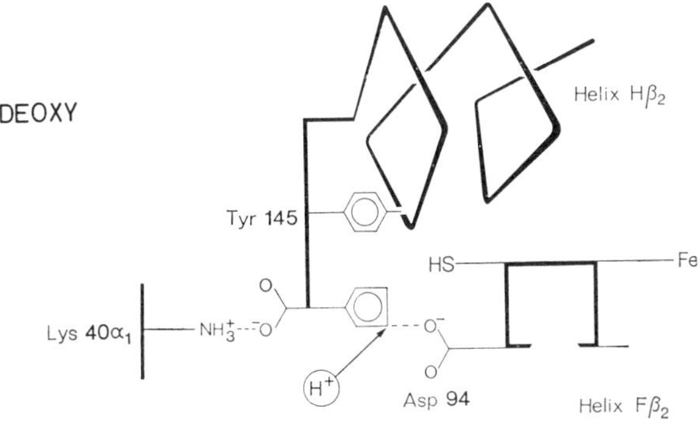

Figure 1–8. Change in conformation of C-terminal residues of β chain. The salt bridges of β146 His probably break when the quaternary structure changes from T to R or when the β chain hemes take up oxygen, whichever comes first. (From Perutz, M.: Nature 228:734, 1970.)

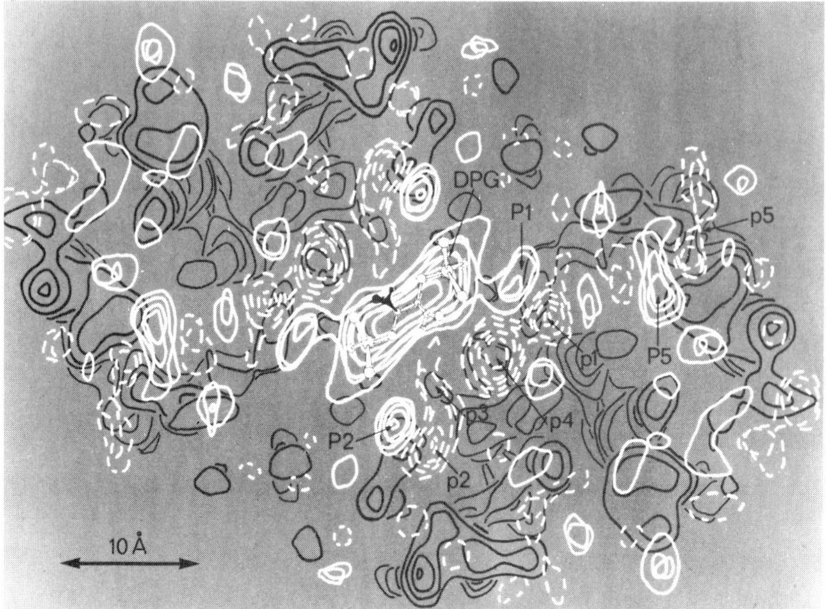

Figure 1–9. Electron-density map of human deoxyhemoglobin, showing the same parts of the molecule sketched in Figure 1–10. Sections are perpendicular to the two-fold axis of symmetry. The effect of 2,3-DPG on the tertiary structure of the β chain is shown. White lines show difference electron-density map $\pm$ 2,3-DPG. Solid contours and upper case letters mark positive difference density; broken contours and lower case letters mark negative difference density. (From Arnone, A.: Nature *237*:146, 1972.)

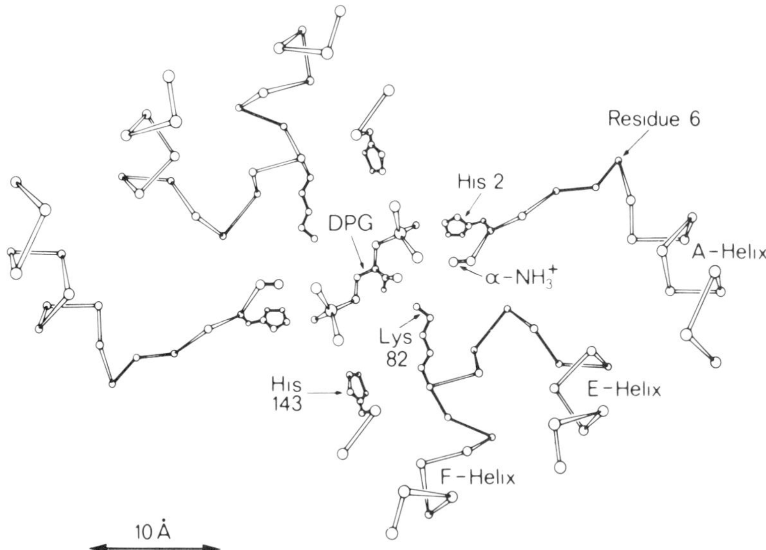

Figure 1–10. The binding of DPG to human deoxyhemoglobin. The stereochemistry of DPG complements the basic residues of the central cavity to form salt bridges with N-terminal valines and histidines 2 and 143 of both β chains and with lysine 82 of one β chain. (From Arnone, A.: Nature *249*:34, 1974.)

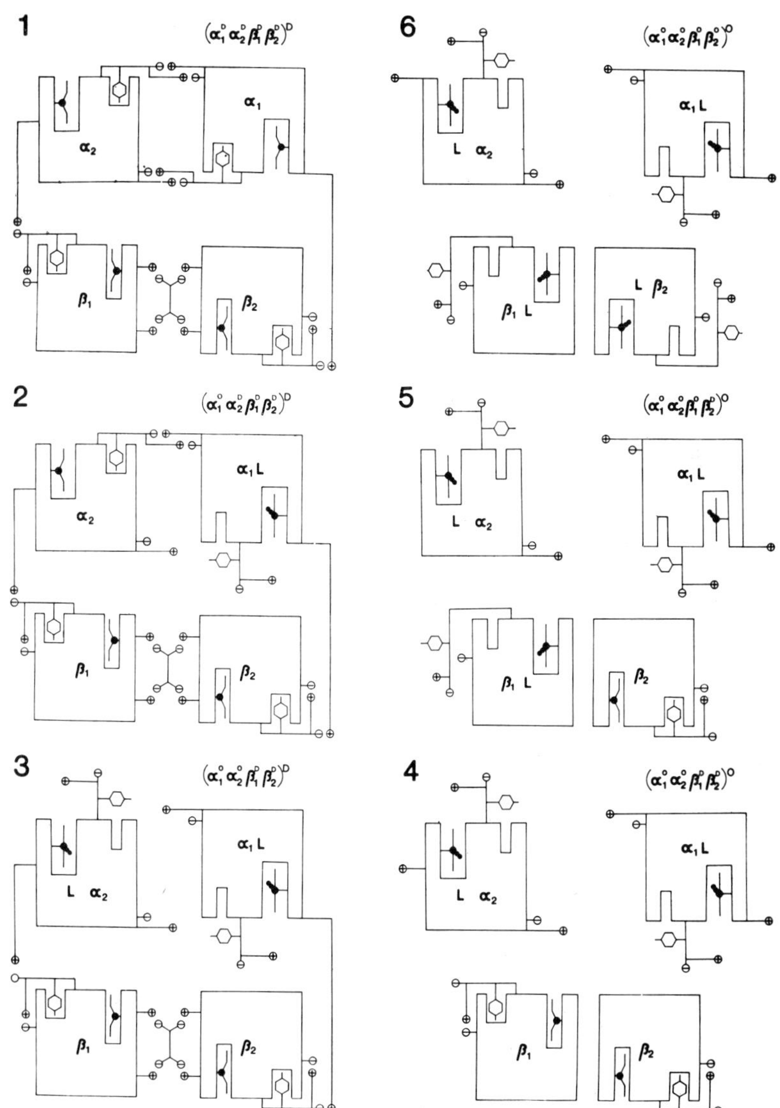

Figure 1–11. Diagrammatic representation of the quaternary configuration of deoxy (1), oxy (6) and partially liganded hemoglobins (2 to 5). The salt bonds are sequentially broken upon oxygenation of the molecule. (From Perutz, M.: Nature 228: 734, 1970.)

2,3-DPG is bonded to the ϵ-amino group of β82-lysine. Figure 1–9 is an electron-density map showing 2,3-DPG situated at this site. A more diagrammatic representation is shown in Figure 1–10. The plane of these figures is perpendicular to the three-dimensional model shown in Figure 1–7. The x-ray data indicate that the binding of 2,3-DPG results in a small but significant change in the tertiary structure of the β subunits (Arnone, 1972).

The change in quaternary configuration with oxygenation is shown diagrammatically in Figure 1–11. As the four heme groups are successively oxygenated, the inter- and intra-subunit salt bonds are successively broken. The 2,3-DPG molecule and protons are rejected. Fully oxygenated hemoglobin has fewer constraints, enabling it to dissociate along the $\alpha_1\beta_2$ interface more readily than deoxyhemoglobin. The change in tertiary and quaternary conformation during oxygen binding is the basis for heme-heme interaction, a subject which will be discussed in Chapter 2, Functional Properties of Hemoglobin.

Heme and the Heme-Globin Linkage

Heme, the prosthetic group of hemoglobin, is ferroprotoporphyrin IX. Its structure is shown in Figure 1–12. Heme is also the prosthetic group of myoglobin, erythrocruorin, catalase, peroxidase, and cytochromes of class *b*. Heme has a molecular weight of 614. The four heme groups therefore account for 2.6 per cent of the mass of the hemoglobin molecule (M.W. = 64,400). Heme can be prepared by diluting hemoglobin in cold acid acetone which precipitates the globin, leaving the heme in solution. During this extraction the iron is completely oxidized. In alkaline solution this brown pigment is called hematin. At lower pH it is called hemin. The biosynthesis of heme is described in Chapter 4. Asymmetry is introduced into the molecule at two steps in the synthesis. Uroporphyrin isomerase enables uroporphyrinogen III to be formed in preference to the symmetrical uroporphyrinogen I. Protoporphyrinogen IX is formed from coproporphyrinogen III by the selective oxidation of two of the four propionic acid groups, located on adjacent pyrroles. It is likely that the final product, ferroprotoporphyrin IX, has been "engineered" during the evolutionary development to provide optimal fit with the apoprotein globin. Indeed, the interactions of globin with a variety of other synthetic protoporphyrins are less stable.

The high-resolution x-ray studies have provided precise information on the details of the heme-globin linkage. The heme is inserted in a cleft between the E and F helices. The iron is linked covalently

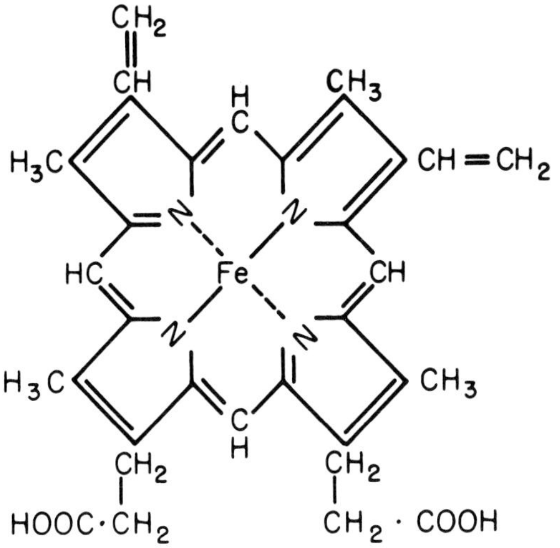

Figure 1–12. Structure of heme (ferroprotoporphyrin IX).

to the imidazole nitrogen of the "proximal" F8 histidine at position E7. Residue E11 of the β-chain valine appears to "guard" the access of oxygen to the heme pocket. This is also an invariant residue which is substituted in three of the unstable hemoglobin variants discussed in Chapter 8. The heme is so oriented that the asymmetrically placed nonpolar vinyl groups are buried deep in the hydrophobic interior of the cleft, while on the other side of the porphyrin the charged propionic acid groups are oriented toward the hydrophilic surface of the subunit. The heme is stabilized by a large number of interatomic contacts. There is a high degree of complementariness between heme and globin structure.

In heme the iron atom occupies the center of the porphyrin ring. Iron is a transition metal having an atomic number of 26. Its electronic configuration depends on its ionic state:

Elemental iron	$1s^2$	$2s^2$	$2p^6$	$3s^2$	$3p^6$	$3d^6$	$4s^2$
Ferrous iron (Fe^{++})	$1s^2$	$2s^2$	$2p^6$	$3s^2$	$3p^6$	$3d^6$	
Ferric iron (Fe^{+++})	$1s^2$	$2s^2$	$2p^6$	$3s^2$	$3p^6$	$3d^5$	

In general, the electrons of the outermost 3d orbitals of transition metals are involved in the formation of coordination compounds. The physicochemical properties (such as visible spectra, ionic radii, magnetic moments, and so on) of these compounds depend on the detailed electronic configuration of 3d electrons. In the absence of ligands the five d orbitals are energetically equivalent, and the first five d electrons occupy these orbitals singly (Fig. 1-13*A*). The last electron, however, has no vacant orbital available to it and therefore is forced to couple with one of the other five electrons. As we can see, in this state there are four unpaired electrons in the d orbitals of the metal ion. However, in the presence of ligands* the five d orbitals are not equivalent. This is because electrons on the donor atoms of a ligand exert repulsion on d-orbital electrons. Two of the orbitals face ligands directly and therefore experience the repulsive force most. They become high-energy orbitals (Fig. 1–13*B*), not favored by the electrons. The remaining three d orbitals are at relatively lower energy because they are oriented away from the ligands. If the ligand (or a group of ligands) exerts only a small repulsive force (i.e., weak field ligands), the energy separating t_{2g} and e_g orbitals is small; then the first five electrons are able to occupy the five d orbitals just as they do in the absence of ligands, and only the sixth electron is forced to couple.

Iron in deoxyhemoglobin is five-coordinated, with the four pyrrole→nitrogens of the porphyrin and the imidazole nitrogen of the proximal histidine (F8). Accordingly, the field due to the ligands is a relatively weak one. The distribution of electrons in deoxyhemoglobin is represented in Figure 1–13*C*.

In contrast, the iron in oxyhemoglobin is six-coordinated. As an

*In the context of this discussion, the term "ligand" refers to any atom that forms a bond with the iron atom.

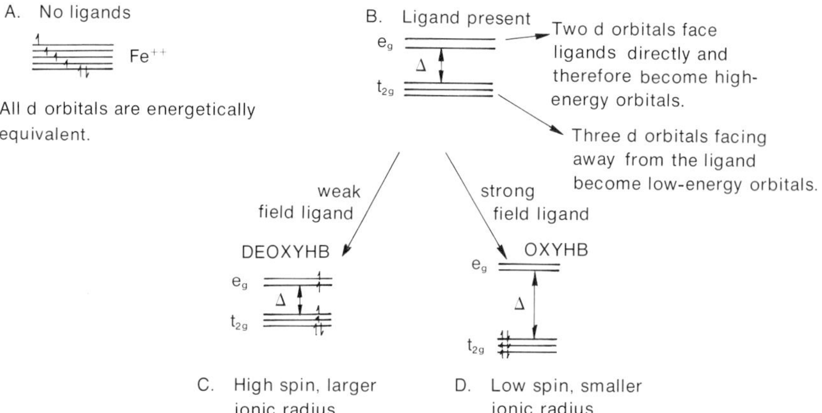

Figure 1–13. State of d orbitals of ferrous iron (Fe^{++}) and the effect of ligand. (Courtesy of Dr. V. S. Sharma.)

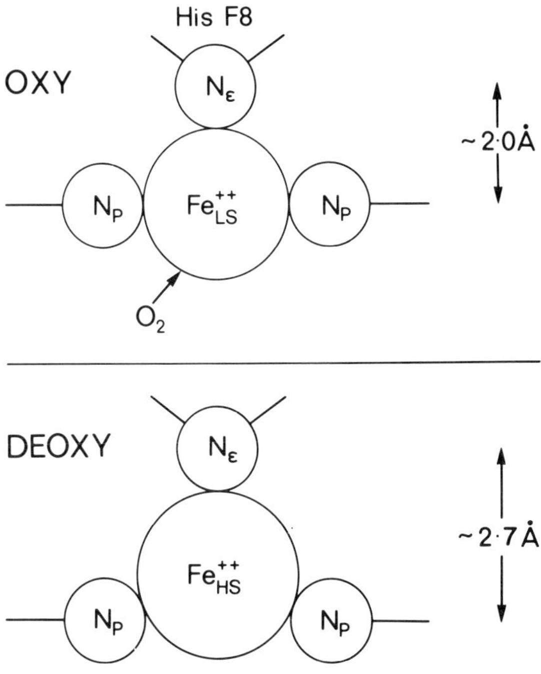

Figure 1–14. Comparison of atomic radius of iron in oxyhemoglobin and deoxyhemoglobin. (Courtesy of Dr. M. F. Perutz.)

additional ligand, oxygen enhances the overall ligand field strength. This is due in part to the increased number of ligands around the metal ion and in part to the distance between the metal ion and the four porphyrin nitrogen donors. As a result, the energy separation between t_{2g} and e_g orbitals is much larger. As electrons prefer to occupy lower-energy orbitals, the first three electrons go in the t_{2g} orbitals. The fourth, fifth, and sixth electrons find the energy difference between t_{2g} and e_g orbitals too great to transfer up into the e_g orbitals and therefore are forced to couple with electrons already in the t_{2g} orbitals (Fig. 1–13*D*). As a result, there are no unpaired electrons in oxyhemoglobin. As we can see from Figures 1–13*C* and 1–13*D*, the number of electrons in the orbitals facing the ligands (i.e., e_g orbitals) has also decreased from two to zero. As a result, the ligands are able to come closer to the iron. This is an oversimplified way of saying that in oxyhemoglobin the "effective" ionic radius of iron has decreased, as shown schematically in Figure 1–14.

No doubt the picture given above is oversimplified and inadequate to explain some of the more complex phenomena associated with hemoglobin chemistry. Yet it is good enough to explain two frequently discussed differences between deoxy- and oxyhemoglobin—namely, reduced ionic radius and reduced magnetic moment or spin state of oxyhemoglobin. Thus, in deoxyhemoglobin, iron is displaced about 0.6 Å from the plane of the porphyrin ring (Fig. 1–14). Upon oxygenation the electrons become paired, resulting in a low spin state and a reduction of magnetic moment. There is a corresponding decrease in the atomic radius of the iron, so that it is now able to sit flush in the plane of the porphyrin ring. This is shown diagrammatically in Figure 1–14. In like manner, methemoglobin (Fe^{+++}) at neutral or acid pH has a high spin state. The iron atom is sufficiently enlarged so that it is displaced from the plane of the porphyrin ring (although to a lesser degree than in deoxyhemoglobin). Upon the addition of negatively charged ligands such as OH^-, cyanide (CN^-), or azide (N_3^-), the heme iron becomes low spin and enters the porphyrin plane.

These considerations have led Perutz to conclude that the shift of iron in and out of the plane of the porphyrin ring with oxygenation and deoxygenation is the "trigger" which results finally in the marked alteration in quaternary structure described above (and shown in Figure 1–7). Deoxyhemoglobin may be considered a set trap. The salt bonds holding the molecule in its tense conformation represent a considerable amount of potential energy. With oxygen binding to successive heme groups, the small (0.6 Å) shift in the heme iron is amplified into much larger conformational changes as the salt bonds are ruptured. The changes in the structure on ligand binding involve large rotations of the subunits combined with small translations, relative to each other. Addition of each oxygen molecule is thus accompanied by reduced constraints on the subunits still in unliganded form. As the successive ligands bind to the hemoglobin molecule at one stage, depending on experimental conditions such as pH, concentration of organic phosphates, etc., the hemoglobin molecule snaps into the relaxed or "oxy" conformation. The remaining heme groups of this postulated intermediate would have an increased affinity for oxygen. Here then is a stereochemical explanation for "heme-heme" interaction. This phenomenon will be explored in more detail in the next chapter.

The x-ray studies on human oxy- and deoxyhemoglobins have progressed to the point where the three-dimensional coordinates of all of their many atoms are established with a fair degree of certainty. This information—the cumulation of 35 years of dedication to this project—permits a deeper understanding of the way in which hemoglobin functions. Once on a recent television broadcast, Perutz was asked what he thought was the essence of scientific creativity. He paraphrased an admonition of Sir Isaac Newton: ". . . always keep the problem foremost in your mind."

Chapter 2

FUNCTIONAL PROPERTIES OF HEMOGLOBIN

At the turn of the century a number of distinguished physiologists began to study hemoglobin in order to gain a better understanding of oxygen transport. They developed a sophisticated conception of hemoglobin function at a time when knowledge of the structure of hemoglobin was rather primitive. It is difficult to improve on Barcroft's assessment (1928) of the important physiological requisites of a respiratory pigment:

1. "Capability of transporting a large quantity of oxygen."
2. "Great solubility."
3. The uptake and release of oxygen at "appropriate pressures."
4. "Power of buffering a bicarbonate solution."

For a while the nature of the interaction of hemoglobin with oxygen was a subject of lively debate. In 1908, Wolfgang Ostwald advanced the hypothesis that the small oxygen molecules became adherent to the surface of the large hemoglobin molecule by some type of electrical attraction. About this time Peters (1912) (later Professor of Biochemistry at Oxford) began to make painstaking measurements of the oxygen and iron content of red cells. According to a method devised by J. S. Haldane, heme iron was oxidized by the addition of an excess of ferricyanide. The oxygen which was quantitatively liberated could then be measured manometrically. A refinement of this technique developed by Van Slyke is still widely used for the precise measurement of oxygen content in blood. Elemental iron was measured after red cells had been carefully ashed. Peters obtained a mean value of 0.975 mole of O_2 per mole of iron. This stoichiometric relationship indicated that oxygen reacted with hemoglobin at specific sites on that molecule rather than through non-specific absorption. Thus, it was readily apparent that hemoglobin satisfied the first two of Barcroft's criteria: it was a highly soluble protein capable of specifically binding large quantities of oxygen (1.34 ml O_2 per gram of hemoglobin).

Demonstration of the ability of hemoglobin to load and unload oxygen at physiologic oxygen tensions depended on the development of suitable methods for determining the equilibrium between hemoglobin and oxygen, the so-called oxygen dissociation curve. Initially, there was considerable uncertainty in these measurements. However, by 1930, the classic sigmoid shape of the oxygen dissociation curve was well established for both whole blood and hemoglobin in solution (Fig. 2–1). The physiological significance of this phenomenon was readily appreciated. At the oxygen tension found in the air sacs of the lung, the hemoglobin in red cells becomes 97 per cent saturated with oxygen. Thus, normal blood, having a hemoglobin concentration of 15 g/100 ml, would carry 1.34 × 15 or 20 ml O_2 per 100 ml blood (20 volumes/100 ml). Following circulation through the capillary bed,

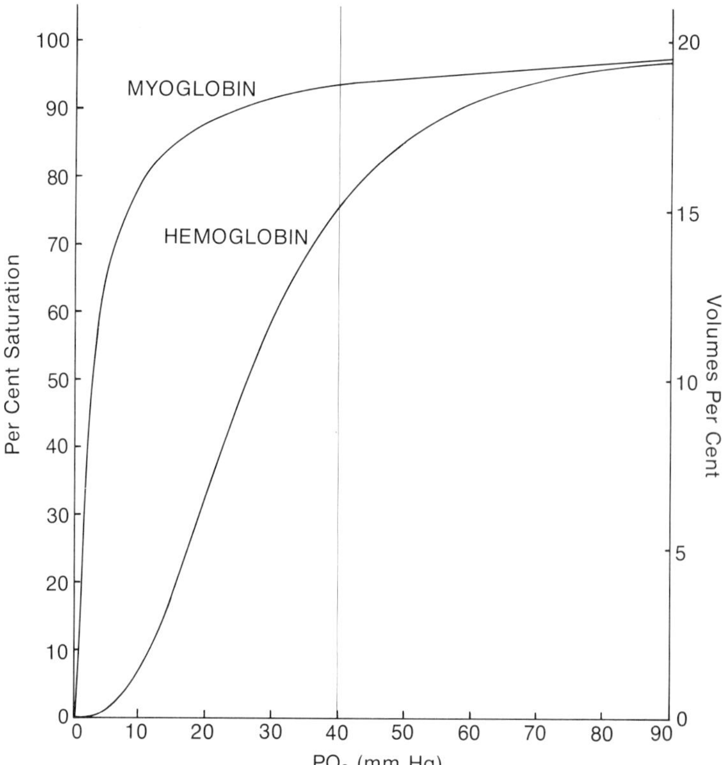

Figure 2–1. Oxygen binding curves of hemoglobin (whole blood) and myoglobin at 37° C and pH 7.4.

the mixed venous oxygen tension is normally about 40 mm Hg. As shown by the oxygen dissociation curve for whole blood of normal individuals (Fig. 2–1), at a PO_2 of 40 mm Hg, hemoglobin is about 75 per cent saturated with oxygen. Thus, blood normally gives up an average of $1.34 \times 15 \times (0.97–0.75)$ or 4.5 volumes of oxygen per 100 ml, during its circulation through the tissues. Oxygen is released at a high enough PO_2 to maintain an adequate supply for intracellular utilization. Such an efficient mechanism for oxygen transport would not be possible were it not for the sigmoid shape of the oxygen dissociation curve. This sigmoid curve reflects the fact that oxygenation of each heme increases the oxygen affinity of the others, so-called heme-heme interaction (or subunit cooperativity). If each of the four heme groups of the hemoglobin molecule bound oxygen independently of the others, the oxygen dissociation curve would have a hyperbolic shape, like that of myoglobin. As shown in Figure 2–1, such a curve would be most unsuitable for oxygen transport. In going from an arterial PO_2 of 95 mm Hg to a mixed venous PO_2 of 40 mm Hg only 0.8 vol/100 ml O_2 would be unloaded. Further release of oxygen would be possible only at considerably lower oxygen tension.

In summary, in order to satisfy the third of Barcroft's criteria, the loading and unloading of oxygen at physiologic oxygen tensions, hemoglobin must have an appropriate affinity for oxygen and heme-heme interaction. The stereochemical bases for these phenomena will be considered in this chapter. In addition, we will discuss the buffering power of hemoglobin (Barcroft's fourth criterion) as part of a detailed consideration of the Bohr effect. Chapter 3 will be concerned with the control of hemoglobin function by intracellular constituents, particularly 2,3-diphosphoglycerate, under normal and pathologic circumstances.

OXYGEN AFFINITY

As mentioned above, in order for hemoglobin to fulfill its physiologic role it must bind to oxygen with an appropriate degree of affinity. If the hemoglobin-oxygen bond were too weak, blood would not become oxygenated in the pulmonary circulation. If it were too strong, insufficient oxygen would be unloaded to tissues. The affinity of oxygen for hemoglobin can be conveniently expressed by the term P_{50}, the oxygen tension at which hemoglobin is half saturated. The higher the affinity of hemoglobin for oxygen, the lower the P_{50} and vice versa (Fig. 2–2). Thus, P_{50} is inversely related to oxygen affinity.

The P_{50} for human blood at physiologic pH (7.4) and temperature (37° C) is 26 ± 1 mm Hg. However, a number of genetic and environmental factors can alter the oxygen affinity of human blood. (The latter will be considered in detail in Chapter 3.) From a comparison of oxy-

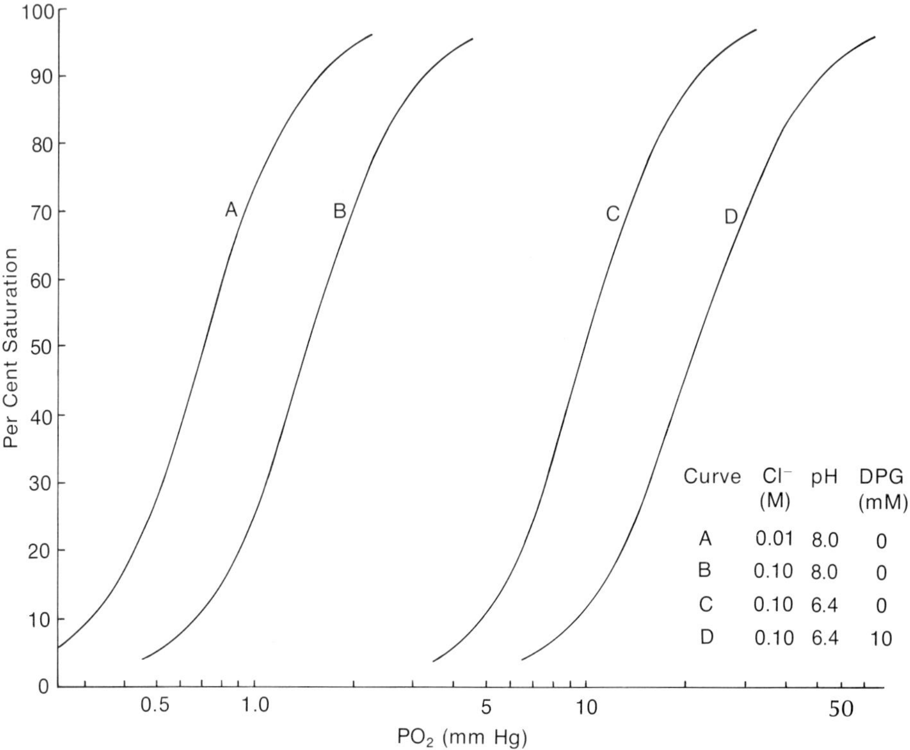

Figure 2–2. Effect of ionic strength, pH, and 2,3-DPG on oxygen affinity of human hemoglobin A at 20° C.

gen binding curves of blood from several different mammals, it is apparent that P_{50} values vary widely (from 18 mm Hg to 50 mm Hg)[1] (Bartels and Harms, 1959; Schmidt-Nielson, 1972). P_{50} tends to be inversely proportional to the size of the animal (Schmidt-Nielson, 1972). The variability in P_{50} is due in part to the intrinsic structural differences between mammalian hemoglobins and in part to differences in the intracellular milieu (Bunn, 1971). The oxygen affinity of hemoglobin can be markedly influenced by alterations in solvent conditions. Figure 2–2 shows how the P_{50} of human hemoglobin can vary over a 100 fold range owing to changes in pH, ionic strength, and, in particular, organic phosphates. In addition, oxygen affinity is inversely related to temperature (see section at end of this chapter). As discussed in Chapter 1, hemoglobin exists in two quaternary forms: oxy (or R) and deoxy (or T). The T structure has a relatively low affinity for heme ligands such as oxygen and carbon monoxide. Environmental factors such as protons and organic phosphates which stabilize the T structure will lower oxygen affinity. Conversely, many chemical

[1] pH 7.4, 37° C.

and genetic modifications of hemoglobin impair its ability to assume a stable deoxy conformation. As a result, these modified hemoglobins have increased oxygen affinity. One of the prime results of the evolutionary "engineering" of hemoglobin has been the development of a molecule with a sufficiently low ligand affinity so that it can unload oxygen at a physiologic range of PO_2.

HEME-HEME INTERACTION

The sigmoid shape of the oxyhemoglobin dissociation curve reflects heme-heme or subunit interaction. The oxygenation of each heme in the tetramer increases the affinity of the remaining (unoxygenated) hemes for oxygen. This implies that there is cooperativity between the subunits of hemoglobin. Before the tetrameric structure of hemoglobin had been established, A. V. Hill (1910) devised an empirical expression for the equilibrium of hemoglobin with oxygen. This equation was derived before it was established that one molecule of hemoglobin binds four molecules of oxygen. Therefore, it is without apparent physical basis. Nevertheless, the Hill equation has proved useful in expressing oxygen binding data. If hemoglobin binds oxygen according to the reaction

$$Hb + nO_2 \rightleftharpoons Hb(O_2)_n,$$

the dissociation equilibrium constant is

$$K_d = \frac{[Hb]\ [PO_2]^n}{[Hb] + [Hb(O_2)_n]},$$

and the fractional saturation of hemoglobin with oxygen is

$$Y = \frac{[Hb(O_2)_n]}{[Hb] + [Hb(O_2)_n]}.$$

Therefore

$$\frac{Y}{1-Y} = \frac{[PO_2]^n}{K_d}.$$

At $Y = 0.5$,

$$PO_2 = P_{50}$$
$$K_d = (P_{50})^n.$$

Thus

$$\log \frac{Y}{1-Y} = n \log\left(\frac{PO_2}{P_{50}}\right) \quad \text{(Hill equation).}$$

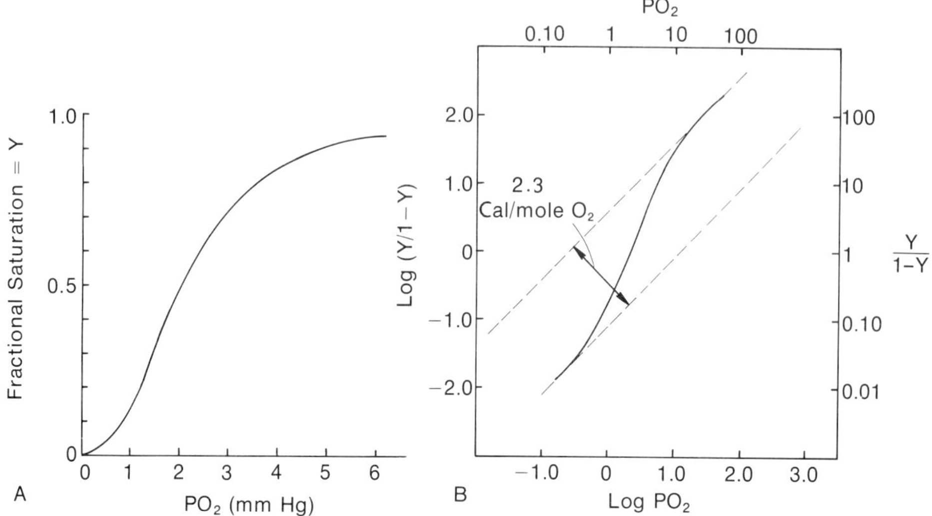

Figure 2–3. Oxygen binding curve of human hemoglobin A at 25° C and pH 7.4. *A*, Arithmetic plot. *B*, Hill plot. (This figure was constructed from data of Tyuma, I., Shimizu, K., and Imai, K.: Biochem. Biophys. Res. Commun. *43*:423, 1971.

If measurements of oxygen equilibria are plotted according to the Hill equation with log Y/1-Y on the ordinate and log PO_2 on the abscissa, a linear plot would be expected. As shown in Figure 2–3, a Hill plot of oxygen binding data is generally linear for values of Y between 0.1 and 0.9 (10 to 90% saturation). The x intercept of this line at Y = 0.5 gives the P_{50} value. The slope of this line, *n*, is a measure of subunit cooperativity. The Hill plots of normal human hemoglobin (and those of most other mammalian hemoglobins) reveal *n* values of 2.8 to 3.0. This number is without direct physical meaning. Heme proteins which have a single subunit, such as isolated α chains or myoglobin, have *n* values of 1.0. Thus, their oxygen binding curves have the form of a rectangular hyperbola. Likewise, tetrameric hemoglobins which fail to change conformation on oxygenation have an absence of subunit cooperativity and Hill plots in which $n = 1.0$. Examples include hemoglobin H (β_4) (Benesch et al., 1961), certain high-affinity variants such as hemoglobins Bethesda and Kempsey (see Chapter 9), and certain chemically modified hemoglobins (Simon and Konigsberg, 1966; Antonini et al., 1961; and Neer and Konigsberg, 1968).[2] In contrast, if the oxygenation of one subunit of hemoglobin resulted in an infinite increase in the affinity of the other three hemes

---

[2]Hemoglobin may lose all subunit cooperativity following structural modification with a number of chemical reagents including bis maleimidomethyl ether (BME) (Simon and Konigsberg, 1966), carboxypeptidase (Antonini et al., 1961), and 1 fluoro-2,4-dinitrobenzene (Neer and Konigsberg, 1968).

for oxygen, then the partially oxygenated intermediate would not exist and the slope of the Hill plot would be 4.0. Thus, the Hill plots of normal (native) hemoglobins indicate that there is a strong but not infinite degree of cooperativity between subunits. This phenomenon depends on the change in conformation induced by oxygen binding.

In the initial stages of ligand binding, no significant conformational isomerization occurs, and evidence of subunit cooperativity is lacking ($n = 1.0$). Likewise, when all hemoglobin molecules are at least 75 per cent saturated (at values of $Y > 0.9$), hemoglobin is exclusively in the oxy or R conformation, and no further cooperativity between subunits is demonstrable. Thus, the extremes of the Hill plot for normal hemoglobin approach $n = 1$. As shown by Wyman (1964), the energy of interaction between hemoglobin subunits can be determined from the distance (D) between these asymptotes. The minimum interaction is equal to D RT $\sqrt{2}$ (Wyman, 1964). Thus, in Figure 2–3 precise measurements of oxygen equilibrium of human hemoglobin indicate that the free energy change in going from deoxy (T) to oxy (R) conformation is about 10 to 12 Cal/mole tetramer. From the invariance of the shape of the oxygen binding curve with temperature, Wyman and Allen (1951) concluded that heme-heme interaction was due primarily to changes in entropy upon oxygenation of hemoglobin.[3] This observation is in complete accord with the marked conformation differences between oxy- and deoxyhemoglobin demonstrated by x-ray crystallography. Perutz (1970a, 1970b) has presented convincing structural evidence that deoxyhemoglobin is held in a tense (T) conformation by virtue of 6 intra- and inter-subunit salt bonds. A typical electrostatic (salt) bond carries about 1 to 2 Cal of energy. Thus, the total amount of energy due to these salt bonds stabilizing the T structure (6 to 12 Cal) agrees quite well with the 10 to 12 Cal of interaction energy estimated from the oxygen binding curves.

Recently, Perutz (1970a, 1970b, 1972) has proposed a detailed structural mechanism for heme-heme interaction. The combination of recent high-resolution x-ray data with optical, electron spin resonance, and nuclear magnetic resonance measurements provides strong support for this formulation. When no oxygen is bound to heme, the iron is in a state of high spin (see Chapter 1). In the high spin state the atomic diameter of the heme iron is too large to allow it to sit in the plane of the porphyrin ring, and it is displaced 0.6 Å out of the plane toward the proximal F8 histidine. Upon oxygenation, the outermost electrons of the iron atom fill up the shell with nonbonding orbitals, putting it into a low spin state and reducing its atomic

[3]Thermodynamic analyses of more recent and precise oxygen binding curves of Imai and Tyuma (1973) indicate that hemoglobin subunit interaction also involves changes in enthalpy.

radius, so that it can snap flush into the plane of the porphyrin ring. In deoxyhemoglobin, the distal βE7-histidine and βE11-valine block the ready access of O_2 to the heme iron. In comparison, the heme pocket of the deoxygenated α chain is more open, allowing adequate space for oxygen binding. From this structural evidence, Perutz has suggested that the α chains of deoxyhemoglobin are oxygenated preferentially. Some functional studies support this proposal (Lindstrom and Ho, 1972; Henry and Cassoly, 1973). Huestis and Raftery (1973) have presented evidence that both α chains are bound to CO before the β chains react. The movement of the heme iron back into the plane of the porphyrin ring results in a tilt of the heme in its pocket. The resulting perturbation is amplified to the extent that the tertiary structure of the subunit changes from t to r.[4] The transition in quaternary structure from T to R probably occurs abruptly, as a result of successive rupture of the salt bonds which stabilize the deoxy structure and, secondly, constraints imposed at the interface between α_1 and β_2 subunits. There is some experimental evidence that this "click" in quaternary structure occurs after the third O_2 has been bound (Gibson and Parkhurst, 1968; Caldwell et al., 1971; Salhany et al., 1972). It is more generally correct to say that the point in ligation at which the transition occurs is dependent on the solvent conditions which affect the relative stability of the R and T structures.

Just as a perturbation in the local structure of the heme group by oxygenation results in an alteration in tertiary structure of the subunit, the shift in quaternary structure can be reflected in the local environment of heme groups. Perutz and his associates (1972, 1974a, 1974b) have presented optical data indicating that the binding of ligands to hemoglobin results in a lowering in the spin state of the unliganded heme groups. The shift from T to R opens up the pockets of the unliganded hemes, greatly increasing their affinity for oxygen. However, Hensley et al. (1975) have not found such a clear-cut relationship between hemoglobin conformation and the spin state of heme iron.

THE BOHR EFFECT

In 1904, Christian Bohr wrote two important papers. In one (Bohr, 1904) he presented the first data demonstrating the sigmoid shape of the oxyhemoglobin dissociation curve. In the other (Bohr et al., 1904) he showed that the position of the curve was sensitive to changes in carbon dioxide pressure. It was later realized that CO_2 has a dual effect on the oxygen affinity of hemoglobin. First, CO_2

[4]The tertiary conformations of subunits are designated by the lower case letters t and r, while the capital letters T and R refer to quaternary conformations.

binds directly to hemoglobin, forming carbamino compounds (see below). Second, there is the indirect but quantitatively more important effect of PCO_2 on pH. Thus, Bohr and his associates are credited with establishing the relationship between pH and the oxygen affinity of hemoglobin. In addition, Bohr was the father of Niels Bohr, a pioneer in nuclear physics who first conceived of the planetary atom, and a grandfather of Aage Bohr, a recent Nobel laureate in physics. One wonders which of these achievements constitutes Christian Bohr's most important legacy!

Physiologists were quick to grasp the significance of the Bohr effect. An organism can be considered to bind and unload oxygen and CO_2 reciprocally: oxygen is picked up by the lungs as CO_2 is expelled. In the tissues, the reverse process occurs. Because of the Bohr effect, CO_2 exchange *facilitates* oxygen exchange and vice versa. As shown in Figure 2–4, over a physiologic pH range, P_{50} varies inversely with pH. This is the so-called alkaline Bohr effect. As CO_2 is expelled during circulation through the lungs there is a corresponding increase in pH and thus a shift to the left in the oxygen dissociation curve. Thus, the relative increase in oxygen affinity favors the binding of oxygen to hemoglobin. Conversely, as blood circulates through capillaries, CO_2 enters the plasma and red cells. Because of the abundance of carbonic anhydrase in red cells, carbonic acid is readily formed: $CO_2 + H_2O \rightleftharpoons H_2CO_3$. The ionization of this weak acid ($H_2CO_3 \rightleftharpoons H^+ + HCO_3^-$) results in a decrease in intracellular pH. Because of the Bohr effect, hemoglobin's oxygen affinity is now relatively decreased, resulting in enhanced unloading of oxygen to the respiring tissues. Thus, the Bohr effect permits a physiologically appropriate cycle for the transport of oxygen and CO_2 by the organism (Fig. 2–5).

As a result of the influx of CO_2 into red cells traversing the capillary circulation, there is an increase in intracellular H^+ and HCO_3^- concentrations. The binding of protons to hemoglobin represents the most important buffer system for maintaining intracellular pH at neutrality. As we shall discuss below, this phenomenon is directly dependent upon the Bohr effect. The bicarbonate ion diffuses out of the

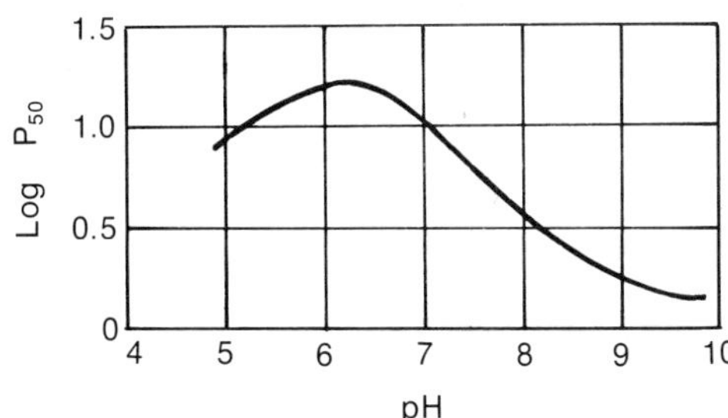

Figure 2–4. The effect of pH on oxygen affinity of human hemoglobin. The slope of the curve between pH 6.5 and 7.5 is a measure of the alkaline Bohr effect.

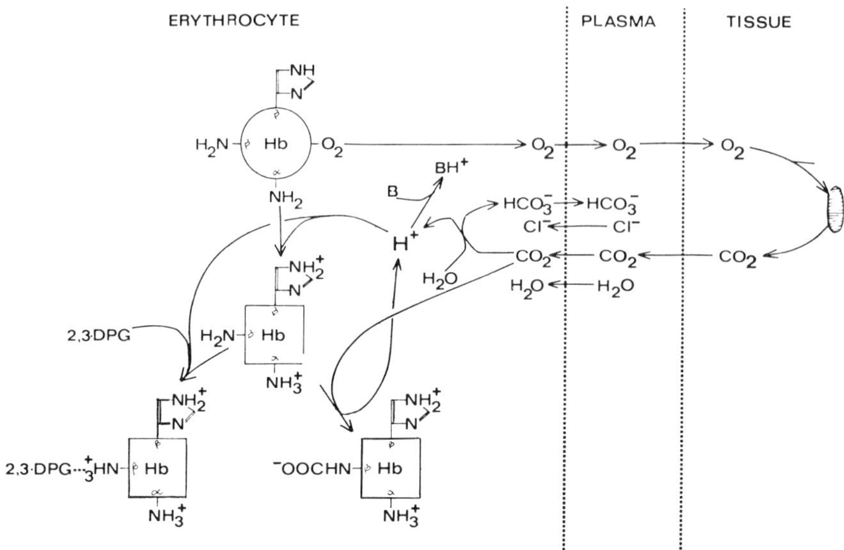

Figure 2–5. The unloading of oxygen and the uptake of protons and CO_2 during the circulation of the red cell through tissues. (From Rørth, M.: Series Haemat. 5:1, 1972.)

red cell and is replaced by chloride ion, thus preserving electrical neutrality. This anion exchange, the so-called Hamburger effect, is depicted in Figure 2–5. Finally, a minor proportion of the CO_2 which enters the red cell becomes covalently bound to hemoglobin as a carbamino complex. This phenomenon will be covered in the next section of this chapter.

In view of the physiological considerations mentioned above, it is not surprising that direct titrations revealed oxyhemoglobin to be a stronger acid than deoxyhemoglobin. This phenomenon is a direct corollary of the dependence of oxygen affinity on pH. The Bohr effect can be considered an example of a linked function:

$$\begin{array}{ccc} \mathrm{Hb} + 4\mathrm{O_2} & \rightleftharpoons & \mathrm{Hb(O_2)_4} \\ + & & + \\ \mathrm{H^+} & & \mathrm{H^+} \\ \downarrow\uparrow & & \downarrow\uparrow \\ \mathrm{HbH} + 4\mathrm{O_2} & \rightleftharpoons & \mathrm{HbH(O_2)_4} \end{array}$$

The equilibria shown horizontally represent the oxygenation of hemoglobin and can readily be demonstrated experimentally by measuring oxygen dissociation curves at different pH's. The reactions shown vertically represent protonation of deoxy- and oxyhemoglobins. These equilibria can be measured directly by following pH during the stepwise addition of alkali. A fundamental thermodynamic principle states that the state of a chemical reaction at equilibrium is independent of the path taken. Thus, these two experimental approaches are really measuring the same phenomenon. These relationships were expressed quantitatively by Wyman (1964) in terms of linkage equations:

$$\left(\frac{\partial H^+}{\partial Y}\right)_{pH} = \left(\frac{\partial (\log p)}{\partial pH}\right)_{\overline{Y}}$$

where Y is the fractional saturation of hemoglobin with oxygen and p is oxygen tension. The right-hand expression can be measured by oxygen equilibria, whereas the expression on the left can be determined by titration experiments. These two methods for measuring the Bohr effect are in excellent agreement. In the physiologic pH range (6.6 to 7.6), $\Delta \log P_{50}/\Delta pH$ is about −0.6 for normal human hemoglobin. According to the preceding equation, with the binding of 4 moles O_2 to deoxyhemoglobin, 4 × 0.6 or 2.4 protons would be released. Thus, the cycle of reactions shown above can be simplified as follows:

$$Hb(H) + 4O_2 \rightleftharpoons Hb(O_2)_4 + 2.4\ H^+$$

As this equation indicates, deoxyhemoglobin has a higher affinity for protons than has oxyhemoglobin. The recent model of Perutz (1970a) provides a stereochemical basis to account for most of the (alkaline) Bohr effect. In essence, the model identifies four specific acid groups of hemoglobin which are more readily protonated in the deoxy form. They make up some of the important salt bonds which stabilize the T structure. About 50 per cent of the Bohr effect is due to the salt bond between the protonated imidazole of β146-histidine and the negatively charged β94-aspartate on the same chain (Kilmartin and Rossi-Bernardi, 1969). Another 25 per cent may be attributed to salt bonds between the protonated N-terminal amino of one α chain and the terminal carboxyl group of the other (Kilmartin and Rossi-Bernardi, 1969), although x-ray evidence for these bonds is lacking (Fermi, 1975).

CARBAMINO FORMATION

Early gasometric measurements established the reciprocal relationship between the oxygen and carbon dioxide content of blood. As explained in the previous section, carbon dioxide is transported primarily as bicarbonate, following its hydration and ionization within the red cell. In addition, in 1934 Ferguson and Roughton presented evidence that a portion of carbon dioxide is bound chemically to hemoglobin. They showed that hemoglobin solutions contained more total analyzable CO_2 than a protein-free solution of comparable pH and PCO_2. From a consideration of the structure of carbon dioxide

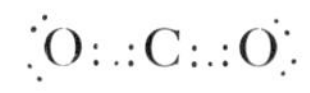

$$\ddot{\text{O}}::\text{C}::\ddot{\text{O}}$$

it can be seen that its electron-poor carbon atom is capable of attack on nucleophiles such as electron-rich amino groups

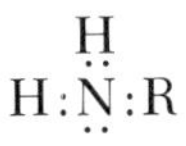

$$\begin{array}{c}\text{H}\\ \text{H}:\ddot{\text{N}}:\text{R}\end{array}$$

to form a carbamino complex

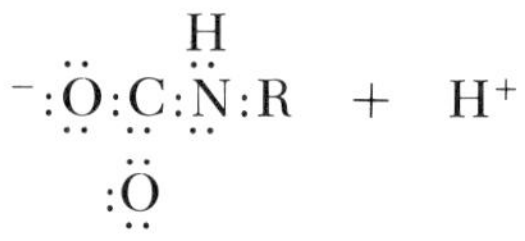

$$\begin{array}{l}{}^{-}:\ddot{\text{O}}:\text{C}:\ddot{\text{N}}:\text{R} \quad + \quad \text{H}^{+}\\ \qquad :\ddot{\text{O}}\end{array}$$

This reaction depends on the existence of free primary amino groups in the protein. If an amino group is protonated (H_3^+NR), the reaction will not occur. In proteins, free (primary) amino groups occur in two forms: the N-terminal amino group of each polypeptide chain and the ϵ amino group of lysine residues

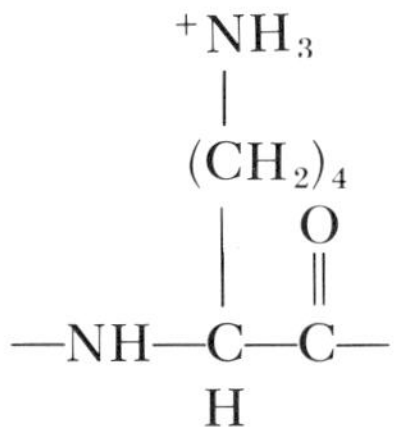

$$\begin{array}{c}{}^{+}\text{NH}_3\\ |\\ (\text{CH}_2)_4\quad \text{O}\\ |\qquad \|\\ \text{—NH—C—C—}\\ \text{H}\end{array}$$

The latter amino groups have a pK of about 9. Thus, at neutral (physiologic) pH they are 99 per cent protonated and unable to bind CO_2. In contrast, the pK of N-terminal amino groups is close to neutrality (Garner et al., 1975). On chemical grounds, it seems reasonable that CO_2 can combine nonenzymatically with the N-terminal amino groups of hemoglobin. Experimental verification has been provided by Kilmartin and Rossi-Bernardi (1969, 1971), who measured CO_2 binding to hemoglobins which had been modified by selective blocking of the N termini of the α and β chains. From these considerations, one would expect that carbamino formation would vary directly with pH. As Figure 2–7 shows, this was demonstrated experimentally by Rossi-Bernardi and Roughton (1967). Morever, these investigators showed that at a given pH, deoxyhemoglobin bound CO_2 more readily than did oxyhemoglobin (Fig. 2–6). Thus, the com-

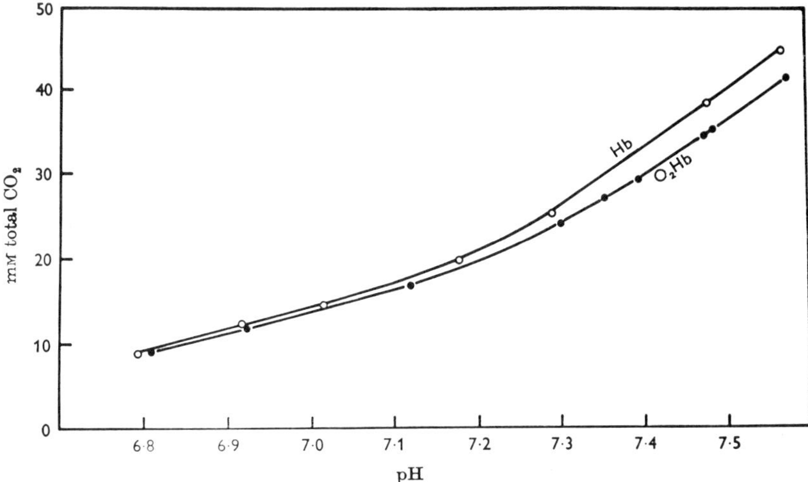

Figure 2–6. The effect of pH and oxygenation on the binding of carbon dioxide to a concentrated solution of hemoglobin at 37° C, PCO_2=42 mm Hg. (From Kilmartin, J. V., and Rossi-Bernardi, L.: Physiol. Rev. *53*:836, 1973.)

bination of CO_2 and hemoglobin to form a carbamino complex is an example of an oxygen-linked reaction. Other oxygen-linked functions include the interaction of protons and organic phosphates with hemoglobin. Similar linkage equations can be written for all these interactions (Garby et al., 1972). In the case of CO_2, the following equilibrium applies:

$$Hb(CO_2)_n + 4O_2 \rightleftharpoons Hb(O_2)_4 + nCO_2$$

This reaction is identical in form to that shown in the previous section on the Bohr effect, except that the H^+ ion is replaced by CO_2. Analogous to the binding of protons to hemoglobin, the above reaction implies that, at a given pH, carbamino hemoglobin has a lower affinity for oxygen than has hemoglobin in the absence of CO_2. This relationship can readily be demonstrated by measuring the oxygen dissociation curves at various pH's in the presence and absence of CO_2. As Figure 2–7 shows, CO_2 has a minimal effect on P_{50} at pH of less than 6.8 because the N-terminal amino groups are now predominantly in the protonated form. The stereochemical basis for the interaction of CO_2 and hemoglobin is less well understood than that of the Bohr effect. It seems likely that CO_2, like protons, stabilizes the deoxy conformation. Rossi-Bernardi and his associates (1972; Perella et al., 1975) have demonstrated heterogeneity in the binding of CO_2 to human deoxyhemoglobin. With oxygenation, relatively more

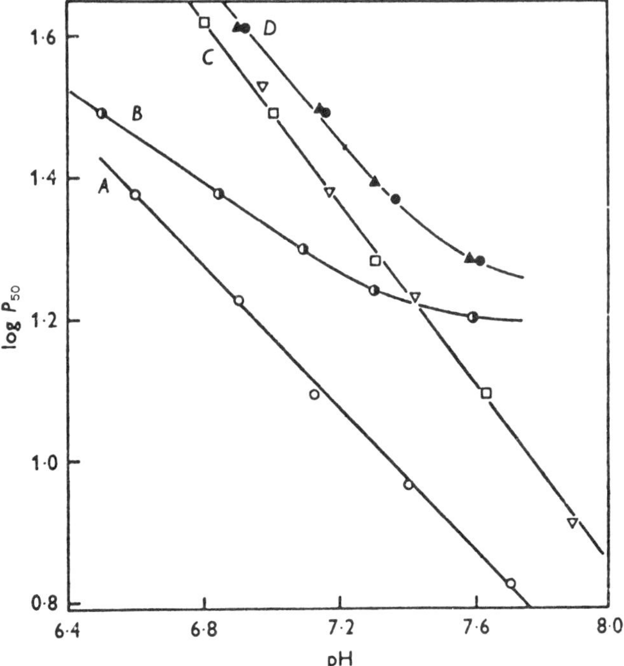

Figure 2–7. The effect of pH, PCO_2, and organic phosphates on the oxygen affinity of human hemoglobin. *A* (○) represents phosphate-free Hb, $PCO_2 = 0$; *B* (◑) represents phosphate-free hemoglobin, $PCO_2 = 40$ mm Hg: *C* represents hemoglobin containing equimolar ATP (□) or 2,3-DPG (▽), $PCO_2 = 0$; *D* represents hemoglobin containing equimolar ATP (●) or 2,3-DPG (▲), $PCO_2 = 40$ mm Hg. (From Kilmartin, J. V., and Rossi-Bernardi, L.: Physiol. Rev. 53:836, 1973.)

CO_2 is released from the β chain than from the α chain (Kilmartin et al., 1973b). Arnone (1974) has completed x-ray diffraction analysis of crystals of human deoxyhemoglobin in the presence and absence of CO_2. He was able to demonstrate the carbamino complex at the N termini of the β chains. No gross perturbation in the tertiary structure of the subunit was observed. Unexpectedly, no carbamate formation at the N termini of the α chains was demonstrated.

It is difficult to determine how significant a role carbamino formation plays in CO_2 transport. Certainly the reciprocal binding of CO_2 and O_2 is physiologically appropriate. That is, as oxygen is given up to respiring tissues, direct CO_2 uptake by hemoglobin is enhanced. As we mentioned in the section on the Bohr effect, CO_2 is transported primarily as bicarbonate ions and protons bound to hemoglobin. Under physiologic conditions only about 10 per cent of CO_2 produced by respiring tissues is transported as a carbamino complex with hemoglobin (Bauer and Schroeder, 1972). An earlier estimate by Roughton was too high because it failed to account for the fact that CO_2 and 2,3-diphosphoglycerate compete for the same binding site on the β chain (see next section and Figure 2–7).

THE INTERACTION OF HEMOGLOBIN WITH ORGANIC PHOSPHATES

Early experiments by Barcroft (1928) established that oxygen affinity of hemoglobin depended in part on the ionic strength of the solution. More recently, Antonini and his associates in Rome investigated in detail the effects of a number of salts on the functional behavior of hemoglobin (Rossi-Fanelli et al., 1961). They established that at a given pH, the oxygen affinity of hemoglobin decreased progressively with increasing concentration of anion. Inorganic phosphate was shown to have a more marked effect than univalent anions. With this background, it is difficult to understand why the effects of the specific anions which exist in the red cell were not explored until 1967. The erythrocyte of the human and most other mammals has a very high concentration of the glycolytic intermediate 2,3-diphosphoglycerate (2,3-DPG). Although it is the most abundant organic phosphate of the red cell, it is present in only trace amounts in other tissues. Its concentration within the red cell is normally about 5 mMoles per liter of packed cells, roughly equivalent to the concentration of hemoglobin tetramer and about fourfold that of ATP. All other organic phosphates are present in much lower concentrations. In 1967 Chanutin and Curnish and Benesch and Benesch independently demonstrated that 2,3-DPG is a potent modifier of hemoglobin function. Hemoglobin which had been carefully "stripped" of all red cell organic phosphates had an unexpectedly high oxygen affinity, although heme-heme interaction (Benesch et al., 1968a) and the Bohr effect (Benesch et al., 1969) remained intact. As shown in Figure 2–8, the addition of a low concentration of 2,3-DPG (0.2 to 2.0 mM) results in a progressive decrease in oxygen affinity. ATP is almost as effective as 2,3-DPG. The relative potency of other organic phosphates in lowering the oxygen affinity of hemoglobin is roughly proportional to their anionic strength.

THE BINDING OF 2,3-DPG TO HEMOGLOBIN

The structure of 2,3-DPG is shown in Figure 2–9. It has 5 titratable acid groups. As the titration curve shows, at physiologic pH, 2,3-DPG has about 3.5 negative charges. Thus, it qualifies as a potent polyanion. On this basis, the Benesches considered it likely that 2,3-DPG interacted electrostatically with positively charged groups on the hemoglobin molecule. They measured the binding of 2,3-DPG to

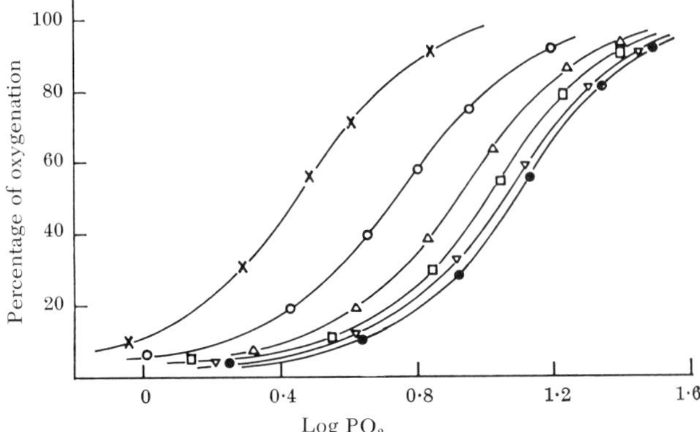

Figure 2–8. The effect of 2,3-DPG on the oxygenation of phosphate-free hemoglobin. X = no 2,3-DPG; ○ = 0.2 mM 2,3-DPG; △ = 0.4 mM 2,3-DPG; □ = 0.6 mM 2,3-DPG; ▽ = 0.8 mM 2,3-DPG; ● = 1.0 mM 2,3-DPG. (From Benesch, R., and Benesch, R. E.: Nature *221*:618, 1969.)

hemoglobin by means of a modified form of equilibrium dialysis (Benesch et al., 1968b). As shown in Figure 2–10, 2,3-DPG bound to deoxyhemoglobin in a 1:1 molar ratio.[5] From this diagram it can be seen that half of the hemoglobin was bound when the concentration of free 2,3-DPG was 2.5×10^{-5} M. Thus, the equilibrium dissociation

[5]One mole of 2,3-DPG per mole of deoxyhemoglobin tetramer.

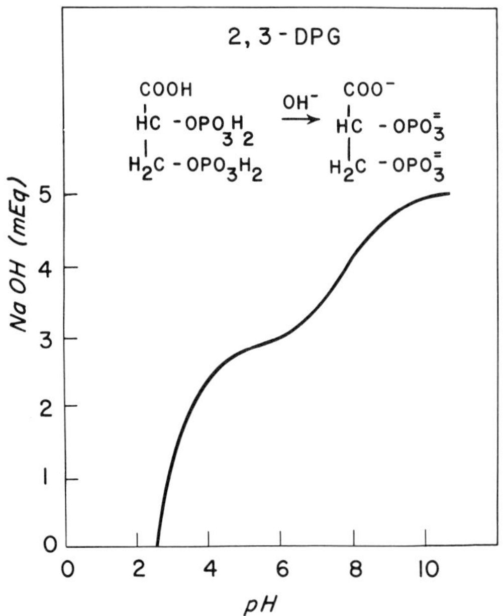

Figure 2–9. Structure of 2,3-DPG and titration curve showing 5 titratable protons.

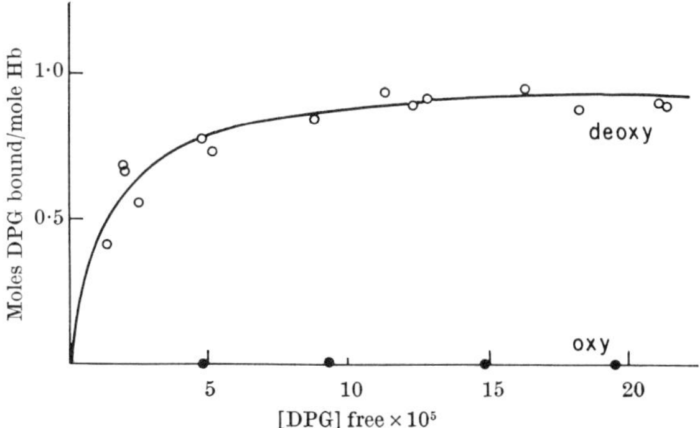

Figure 2–10. The binding of 2,3-DPG to oxy- and deoxyhemoglobin. (From Benesch, R., and Benesch, R. E.: Nature *221*:618, 1969.)

constant K_D for the binding of 2,3-DPG to deoxyhemoglobin can be expressed as follows:

$$\frac{[Hb][DPG]}{[HbDPG]} = K_D = 2.5 \times 10^{-5}M$$

In contrast, under the same experimental conditions, virtually no oxyhemoglobin bound 2,3-DPG (Fig. 2–10). Other liganded forms of hemoglobin such as carboxy- and cyanmet hemoglobins behaved similarly (Benesch et al., 1968b). Subsequently, it was shown that ATP binds to hemoglobin competitively with 2,3-DPG and, like 2,3-DPG, in a 1:1 molar ratio (Lo and Schimmel, 1969). It should be emphasized that these binding studies were done under physiologic conditions of pH and ionic strength. At low pH and low ionic strength, 2,3-DPG and other polyanions bind nonspecifically to both deoxyhemoglobin and oxyhemoglobin (Berman et al., 1971). For this reason, some studies on the binding of 2,3-DPG and hemoglobin are difficult to interpret (Chanutin and Hermann, 1969; Luque et al., 1969). Recently, Garby and deVerdier (1971) and Hedlund and Lovrien (1974) have presented evidence that at very high hemoglobin concentrations, approaching that of the red cell, the binding of 2,3-DPG to deoxyhemoglobin is considerably weaker. These results imply that some type of nonideality such as interaction between hemoglobin tetramers may perturb the equilibrium between organic phosphates and hemoglobin. Recent data of Hamasaki and Rose (1974) fail to confirm weaker binding of 2,3-DPG to hemoglobin at high protein concentrations.

In addition to protons and CO_2, 2,3-DPG is another cofactor which binds to hemoglobin reciprocally with oxygen. Accordingly, linkage equations (Garby et al., 1972) similar to those for the Bohr effect and carbamino formation can be written. The following net reaction pertains:

$$\text{HbDPG} + 4O_2 \rightleftharpoons \text{Hb}(O_2)_4 + \text{DPG}$$

This equilibrium is identical in form to those shown previously for H^+ and CO_2 interaction. The equilibrium constant which the Benesches obtained from direct measurement of the binding of 2,3-DPG to deoxyhemoglobin was in excellent agreement with the constant derived indirectly from the measurement of oxygen affinity in the absence and presence of 2,3-DPG. This is entirely analogous with the two experimental approaches for measuring the Bohr effect (see above).

The 2,3-DPG Binding Site

In view of its potent effect on the oxygen dissociation curve, 2,3-DPG must act as an allosteric modifier of hemoglobin function. It was therefore of prime importance to determine the precise site on the hemoglobin molecule at which 2,3-DPG binds. Since hemoglobin is a large molecule with a twofold axis of symmetry, the 1:1 stoichiometry of 2,3-DPG to hemoglobin tetramer was somewhat unexpected. The Benesches (1968a) found that the deoxy and oxy forms of hemoglobin H (β_4) bound 2,3-DPG in the same 1:1 molar ratio, whereas isolated α chains showed no significant interaction with 2,3-DPG. From these observations, they concluded that 2,3-DPG binds to the β chains of deoxyhemoglobin, probably somewhere in the central cavity.

Considerable evidence indicated that the N-terminal amino groups of the β chain were involved. Human hemoglobins A_{Ic} and F_I, which are blocked at the N terminus of their non-α chains, have markedly impaired reactivity to 2,3-DPG (Bunn and Briehl, 1970). Furthermore, cat hemoglobin B which is acetylated at the β N terminus interacted less readily with 2,3-DPG than cat hemoglobin A (Bunn, 1971; Taketa et al., 1971). Benesch et al. (1972) showed that pyridoxal phosphate, when added to deoxyhemoglobin, acted as an affinity label and became covalently linked to the N terminus of the β chain by means of a Schiff base. This modified hemoglobin showed a considerable reduction in oxygen affinity. Finally, 2,3-DPG and CO_2 were shown to be competitors in their binding to hemoglobin (Bauer, 1969; Rossi-Bernardi et al., 1972; Tomita and Riggs, 1971). The long recognized but unexplained high O_2 affinity of blood of the fetus and neonate is based upon the impaired reactivity of human Hb F (F_{II}) with 2,3-DPG (Bauer et al., 1968; Bunn and Briehl, 1970; Tyuma and Shimizu, 1969). Among the differences in primary sequence between the β and γ chains are the different residues at β143(H21)-histidine in the β chain and uncharged serine in the γ chain. Fitting 2,3-DPG to a high-resolution (2.5 Å) model of deoxyhemoglobin, Perutz (1970b) concluded that the organic polyanion could form salt bonds with the β N-terminal amino groups, the imidazoles of β143-histidine, and the amino groups of β82(EF6)-lysine. By contrast, in oxyhemoglobin the β H helices are too close together and the β N termini are too far apart to permit a satisfactory fit. Recently, Arnone (1972) has analyzed crystals of deoxyhemoglobin bound to 2,3-DPG by x-ray diffraction and established this to be the correct binding site. A diagram of the 2,3-DPG binding site is shown in Chapter 1 (Fig. 1–10).

In summary, 2,3-DPG binds firmly to a specific site on deoxyhemoglobin, whereas the conformational change induced by oxygenation results in much weaker binding to oxyhemoglobin. One can then ask how well does 2,3-DPG bind to partially oxygenated forms of hemoglobin and at what point in oxygenation is the cofactor ejected? In general, it is difficult to design appropriate experiments that provide information on the properties of the partially liganded intermediates. One can prepare hemoglobin derivatives, such as $\alpha_2^{CNMet}\beta_2$ and $\alpha_2\beta_2^{CNMet}$, in which the α or β chains are frozen in the r tertiary structure. These analogs of partially oxygenated hemoglobin bind 2,3-DPG, although more weakly than native deoxyhemoglobin (Bauer et al., 1973; Haber and Koshland, 1971). The two-state allosteric model (see below) predicts that 2,3-DPG binds firmly to partially oxygenated hemoglobins which still possess the T quaternary conformation. When the tetramer flips into the R conformation, 2,3-DPG would be ejected. Thus, interaction with organic phosphates could be considered a probe of quaternary structure. Experimental results utilizing spin-labeled analogs of 2,3-DPG are in accord with this model (Ogata and McConnell, 1971, 1972). There are both kinetic (Salhany et al., 1972) and equilibrium studies (Caldwell et al., 1971) which indicate that 2,3-DPG is released following the binding of the third oxygen to the tetramer. In contrast, ^{31}P-NMR studies on the binding of 2,3-DPG to partially liganded intermediates of human hemoglobin do not support a simple two-state allosteric model (Huestis and Raftery, 1972). These data indicate that 2,3-DPG binds to species such as Hb(CO), $Hb(CO)_2$, and $Hb(CO)_3$ with affinities intermediate between that for deoxyhemoglobin and that for $Hb(CO)_4$.

THE EFFECT OF TEMPERATURE

Early measurements of the oxygenation of hemoglobin both in red cells and in dilute solution established that oxygen affinity varies inversely with temperature. Precise determinations of the oxygen binding curve at different temperatures permit the calculation of the thermodynamic parameters, enthalpy (Δ H) and entropy (Δ S), involved in the binding of ligands to hemoglobins. As mentioned before, the conformational isomerization which is responsible for heme-heme subunit interactions involves primarily a change in entropy. The binding of 2,3-DPG to deoxyhemoglobin results in a significant decrease in entropy, suggesting a higher "ordering" of the molecule (Benesch et al., 1969).

The relationship between temperature and oxygen affinity appears to be physiologically appropriate. Thus, under conditions of relative hypothermia metabolic demands are relatively low. Because of the left shift in the oxygen dissociation curve, less oxygen is released to tissues. Conversely, during pyrexia, the right-shifted curve should result in increased oxygen unloading, helping to meet the higher requirement which fever is known to engender. In homeotherms such as man and other mammals, only a slight variation in body temperature is possible. In order for this phenomenon ($\Delta P_{50}/\Delta T$) to be physiologically significant, it must be pronounced. This is the case for human hemoglobin where a 10° increase in temperature results in nearly a twofold increase in P_{50}. Conversely, it may be advantageous for oxygen binding in poikilotherms to be less dependent on temperature. It is of interest that the P_{50} of frog blood (Barcroft, 1928) increases much less with increased temperature and that the oxygen binding curve of the tuna fish is almost invariant with increased temperature (Rossi-Fanelli and Antonini, 1960). Finally, one may consider the hemoglobins of arcid clams, the P_{50} values of which actually *decrease* with increasing temperature (Collett and O'Gower, 1972). Such "anomalous" behavior may be of considerable advantage to this mollusk. The amount of oxygen which can be physically dissolved in water decreases markedly with increasing temperature. Thus, when submerged in warm water shoals, the increased oxygen affinity of the hemoglobin of the clams may enable them to scavenge more oxygen from the sea water!

FUNCTIONAL PROPERTIES OF ISOLATED CHAINS

As discussed in detail at the beginning of this chapter, the functional properties of hemoglobin are strongly dependent on interactions between the α and β globin subunits. It is no surprise that the functional properties of isolated chains are markedly different from those of the intact tetramer.

Alpha and beta chains can be prepared from human hemoglobin after treating a hemolysate with p-chloromercuribenzoate, which forms a complex with the globin sulfhydryl groups (Bucci and Fronticelli, 1964). Upon chemical removal of the mercury compound, these preparations probably represent native hemoglobin subunits. Naturally occurring free β chains can be found in hemolysates of some individuals with α thalassemia. The functional properties of so-called hemoglobin H have been found to be identical with those of β chains prepared from normal A hemoglobin.

Like myoglobin, isolated α chains are largely monomers (16,100 M.W.) (Ranney et al., 1965). In contrast, β chains aggregate to form a β_4 tetramer (hemoglobin H). Despite this, all three heme proteins have similar oxygen binding properties (Benesch et al., 1968b; Brunori et al., 1966; Tyuma et al., 1966):

1. High oxygen affinity.
2. Absence of heme-heme interaction.
3. Absence of Bohr effect.
4. No effect of 2,3-DPG on oxygenation.

As one might expect, the oxygen binding curve is in the form of a rectangular hyperbola. β_4 has a somewhat higher oxygen affinity than α chains (Ranney et al., 1965). Although, as mentioned above, 2,3-DPG does not bind at all to α chains, it binds equally readily to the oxy and deoxy forms of β_4 (Benesch et al., 1968a). Thus, the interaction of 2,3-DPG with β_4 is not oxygen-linked. This is not surprising, since x-ray studies indicate that hemoglobin H does not change quaternary conformation on oxygenation (Perutz and Mazzarella, 1963).

Even when fully deoxygenated, α chains and β_4 are probably in the r (relaxed) tertiary conformation. The deoxy forms of these hemoglobins have a characteristic absorption spectrum in the 406 to 450 nm range. Very similar spectral properties have been found for various chemically modified and mutant hemoglobins which are unable to assume a T conformation upon deoxygenation.

OTHER PROPERTIES OF HEMOGLOBIN

There is now a large body of information on the various physical and chemical properties of hemoglobin. In general, it is striking how many of these are dependent on the quaternary structure, that is, whether hemoglobin is in the T (deoxy) or R (oxy) conformation. A broad comparison is shown in Table 2–1. Many of the differences in the chemical properties of oxy- and deoxyhemoglobin can be interpreted and even predicted in terms of the three-dimensional atomic models proposed by Perutz and his associates. For example, the decreased reactivity of the sulfhydryl group of β93-cysteine in deoxyhemoglobin is due to the fact that this group is partially hidden and less accessible to attack by sulfhydryl reagents. This residue (βF9), adjacent to the proximal (F8) histidine, is an invariant residue,

TABLE 2–1. *Physical and Chemical Differences Between Oxyhemoglobin and Deoxyhemoglobin*

	OXYHEMOGLOBIN	DEOXYHEMOGLOBIN	REFERENCES
PHYSICAL PROPERTIES			
Visible spectrum: absorbance peak(s)	576,540 nm	555 nm	
Soret spectrum: absorbance peak	415 nm	430 nm	
Magnetic susceptibility	Low (diamagnetic)	High (paramagnetic)	
CHEMICAL PROPERTIES			
Solubility	High	Lower	
Dissociation into $\alpha\beta$ dimers	Fast	Slow	Benesch et al. (1962)
Binding to haptoglobin	Fast	Slow	Nagel et al. (1965)
Digestion by carboxypeptidase	Fast	Slow	Zito et al. (1964)
Reactivity of β93-cysteine SH	Fast	Slow	Morell et al. (1962); Benesch and Benesch (1962)
Reactivity to bromothymol blue	Slow	Fast	Antonini et al. (1963)
Reactivity to cyanate	Slow	Slower	Lee and Manning (1973); Jensen et al. (1973b)
FUNCTIONAL PROPERTIES			
Affinity for heme ligands	High	Low	
Affinity for protons	Low	High	
Relative affinity for CO_2	Low	High	
Affinity for organic phosphates	Low	High	

present in all mammalian hemoglobins of known structure.[6] The functional significance of this group is not understood.

As shown in Table 2–1, deoxyhemoglobin dissociates into dimers much less readily than oxyhemoglobin:

Deoxyhemoglobin	$\alpha_2\beta_2 \overset{\rightharpoonup}{\longleftarrow} 2\alpha\beta$	
Oxyhemoglobin	$\alpha_2\beta_2 \rightleftharpoons 2\alpha\beta$	

This difference is due primarily to the inter-subunit salt bonds, including 2,3-DPG, which stabilize the deoxy structure (see Perutz, 1970a, and Chapter 1). The dissociation of hemoglobin into dimers appears to be necessary for its binding to haptoglobin (Nagel and Gibson, 1971) and for the filtration of hemoglobin through renal glomeruli (Bunn et al., 1969a).

The stereochemical bases for the differential binding of protons and 2,3-DPG to oxy- and deoxyhemoglobins are discussed in earlier sections of this chapter.

HEMOGLOBIN AS AN ALLOSTERIC PROTEIN

Hemoglobin can be considered a prototype of an allosteric protein. In this type of protein, binding of ligand at one site alters the affinity for ligand at another site on the molecule. Generally, allosteric proteins contain multiple interacting subunits. Furthermore, such proteins undergo an alteration in conformation upon successive binding of ligand. A number of enzymes are known to have multiple subunits and, in some, cooperativity between subunits has been demonstrated. Besides hemoglobin, several enzymes qualify as allosteric proteins (Hammes and Wu, 1971). These include aspartate transcarbamylase, phosphorylase, and glutamate dehydrogenase. Allosteric enzymes cannot be analyzed by simple Michaelis-Menten kinetics. Because of subunit cooperativity, the binding of one molecule of substrate enhances the affinity at another site on the enzyme for the same substrate, resulting in a sigmoid binding curve. This is known as *homotropic interaction.* In this way, the reaction rate can be closely regulated by small changes in substrate concentration. In addition, allosteric enzymes may be controlled by the participation of allosteric modulators, either activators or inhibitors, which bind at sites different from the substrate binding site. This is known as *heterotropic interaction.* In the case of hemoglobin, the binding of oxygen increases the affinity of the remaining hemes for oxygen (homotropic interaction) and lowers the affinity of various effectors

[6]One exception is the Barbary sheep which has histidine at βF9.

(modulators) such as protons, 2,3-DPG, and CO_2 at other sites on the hemoglobin molecule (heterotropic interactions).

Two models have been proposed to explain the molecular basis of allosteric control. Monod, Wyman, and Changeux (1965) (MWC) have suggested that such a protein exists in an equilibrium between two conformers (R and T states) which differ in affinity for ligand or substrate. The binding of ligand to the subunits of the protein results in a concerted transition in conformation, so that the affinity of the unreacted subunits for ligand changes abruptly. Thus, the equilibrium between the two conformers is markedly altered by the binding of ligand. Effectors have a different affinity for the R and T states and thus will also affect the conformational equilibrium. The simplest form of the two-state MWC model is shown diagrammatically in the two vertical rectangles in Figure 2–11. In the model proposed by Koshland, Nemethy, and Filmer (KNF) (1966), the binding of ligand

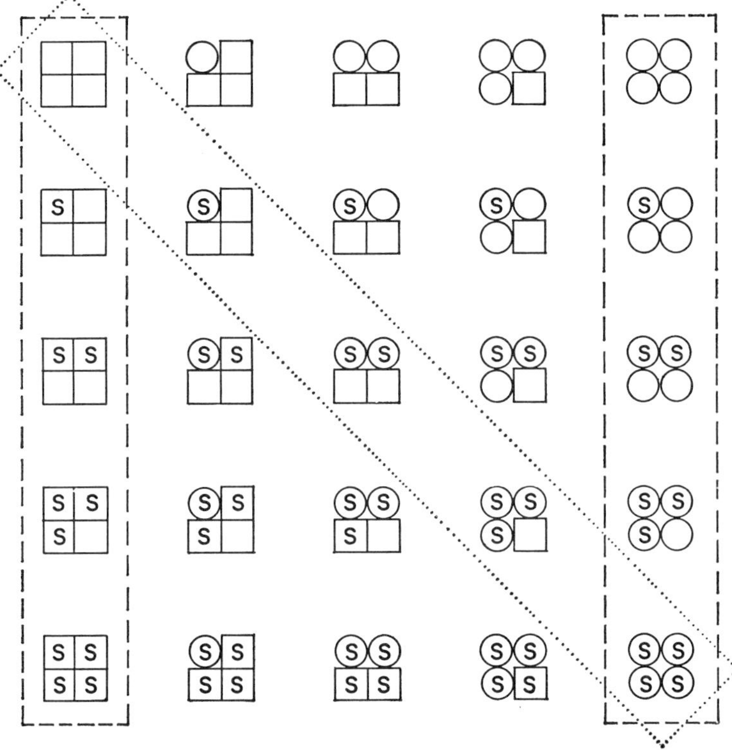

Figure 2–11. A general allosteric model for the binding of substrate (S) to a four-subunit enzyme. In the case of hemoglobin, $S = O_2$. The squares represent the t conformation and the circles the r conformation. The model proposed by Monod et al. is shown by the dashed lines and that proposed by Koshland et al. is shown by the dotted lines. (From Hammes, G. G., and Wu, C.: Science *172*:1205, 1971.)

to each subunit of the molecule results in a change in the tertiary structure of that subunit. This conformational alteration affects the affinity of neighboring subunits for ligands. This "induced fit" results in several intermediate conformational species, depending upon the number of ligand binding sites in the molecule. This is illustrated by the diagonal in Figure 2–11. In contrast, the MWC model postulates the existence of only two conformational species.

From studies on hemoglobin, a great deal of experimental evidence has been marshaled in support of one or both of these two allosteric models. As mentioned in the section above, there are marked differences in the physical and chemical properties of oxy- and deoxyhemoglobin. Many of these properties serve as useful probes of quaternary structure (R vs. T). The cooperative nature of oxygen binding to hemoglobin results in the predominance of fully liganded and fully deoxygenated molecules throughout the saturation curve: the concentration of partially liganded hemoglobin is always low. While a model involving sequential change in structure might predict a linear relationship between fractional ligand concentration and parameters sensitive to hemoglobin structure (e.g., release of Bohr protons, change in EPR spectra), vanishingly small concentrations of partially liganded intermediates would not cause large deviations from linearity. While the two-state model fits most observations within the limits of experimental error, the results of many studies of the kinetics of ligand binding cannot be satisfactorily explained by the two-state model. Thus, there is still considerable uncertainty about the means by which subunit cooperativity or heme-heme interaction takes place. The solution of this problem may permit a better understanding of how other, more complex allosteric proteins work.

Chapter 3

OXYGEN AND CARBON DIOXIDE TRANSPORT IN THE RED CELL IN HEALTH AND DISEASE

In the previous chapter we have discussed in detail the chemistry of hemoglobin with particular emphasis on its interaction with gaseous ligands such as oxygen and carbon monoxide and with various allosteric effectors: hydrogen ion, carbon dioxide, and organic phosphates. Most of this information was developed from experiments done on dilute solutions of hemoglobin under artificially controlled conditions of temperature, pH, and ionic strength. It is no surprise that the properties of hemoglobin are significantly affected by conditions peculiar to the living red cell. In order to approach understanding of hemoglobin's physiologic function, it is necessary to study whole blood under in-vivo conditions. In this chapter we will consider the physiology of oxygen transport and especially the uptake and release of oxygen by the circulating red cell. We will discuss the metabolic control of red cell 2,3-DPG and its perturbation in various pathologic states. From this information, we can draw some conclusions about the importance of red cell oxygen affinity under physiologic conditions and determine whether displacements of the oxygen binding curve can be significant in the adaptation of the organism to hypoxia.

OXYGEN TRANSPORT

At sea level, the air we breathe contains 20.95 per cent oxygen. This ambient oxygen tension (PO_2) is approximately 0.21×760 or

160 mm Hg. As air is drawn into the upper air passage, it becomes fully saturated with water. Within the airways and lungs, the inspired air mixes with both dead space gas and alveolar gas which is continuously altered by uptake of O_2 and evolution of CO_2 from mixed venous blood. Accordingly, the PO_2 in the alveolar air drops to about 95 mm Hg.

The amount of oxygen transported across the alveolar capillary membrane per unit time is a product of the diffusing capacity of the membrane per unit time and the PO_2 difference between alveolar gas and pulmonary capillary blood. This membrane is about 0.2 micron thick, consisting of surfactant, alveolar epithelium, basement membrane, interstitial tissue, basement membrane, and capillary endothelium (Waltemath, 1970). Oxygen is transported passively across the alveolar capillary membrane. In normal lung tissue, the resistance to gas movement across this membrane is negligible. In order for there to be a measurable difference between alveolar and end-capillary oxygen tension, the membrane thickness would have to be many fold greater (Comroe, 1965).

In a normal individual at rest, the red cell spends about 0.75 second in transit through pulmonary capillaries. It has been estimated that equilibration with alveolar gas is nearly complete within 0.35 second (Comroe et al., 1962). One factor which contributes slightly to an alveolar-capillary oxygen gradient is lung tissue, including metabolically active macrophages that take oxygen directly from alveolar gas. Although the red cell membrane delays the transport of oxygen somewhat, the presence of hemoglobin facilitates the diffusion of oxygen inside the red cell. At a concentration of 34 g per 100 ml, the hemoglobin molecules are closely packed inside the erythrocyte. Nevertheless, they have sufficient rotation and translation to serve as a "bucket brigade" and hasten the passage of oxygen into the interior of the red cell (Scholander, 1960). As mentioned in the previous chapter, expulsion of CO_2 in the pulmonary circulation results in an increase in intracellular pH. Because of the Bohr effect, the oxygen affinity of the hemoglobin increases, facilitating transport of oxygen into the red cell.

Blood from pulmonary capillaries becomes mixed with blood from bronchial, pleural, and thebesian veins. Normally, this shunt amounts to about 1 to 2 per cent of the pulmonary circulation and results in a further drop in PO_2 in the pulmonary vein to about 90 mm Hg. This oxygen pressure is maintained until the blood reaches the systemic capillaries.

WHY RED CELLS?

This chapter will focus on the various factors that determine the oxygen binding properties of human blood under physiologic conditions. It is reasonable to ask why hemoglobin of man, and indeed of all other vertebrates, is so neatly packaged in corpuscles. If hemoglobin were circulating free in plasma at a concentration of 15 g per 100 ml, the oncotic pressure would be prohibitively high. One of the primary functions of the red cell membrane is to extrude intracellular cation and water in order to prevent osmotic lysis. For hemoglobin to function in free solution, it would have to be in the form of large polymers such as the hemocyanins of mollusks. It has often been stated that hemoglobin in solution would have a significantly higher viscosity compared to blood having the same oxygen-carrying capacity. This has been shown to be untrue for human hemoglobin (Schmidt-Nielsen and Taylor, 1968). However, the viscosity of a comparable concentration of a high molecular weight polymeric hemoglobin would be prohibitively high. Castle and Jandl (1966) have pointed out that the viscosity of whole blood varies with the hematocrit in such a way that maximal oxygen transport occurs when the packed cell volume is in the normal range.

The design of the red cell appears optimal. Its overall contour allows efficient diffusion of gas throughout the cell interior. The excess of surface area relative to volume enables the cell to distort its shape in such a way that it can readily traverse small-bore capillaries. Such distensibility would be impossible if the erythrocyte were spherical. Thus, the packaging of hemoglobin into pliable, biconcave discs appears to solve a number of problems in the transport of oxygen and carbon dioxide.

DETERMINANTS OF OXYGEN UNLOADING

The unloading of oxygen to tissues is governed by three independent variables which can be expressed quantitatively in the Fick equation:

$$VO_2 = 0.139 \cdot Q \cdot Hb \cdot (S_aO_2 - S_{\bar{v}}O_2)$$

where VO_2 is the amount of oxygen released (l/min), 1.39 is the amount in milliliters of O_2 bound by 1 gram of fully saturated hemoglobin, Q is blood flow (l/min), and S_aO_2 and $S_{\bar{v}}O_2$ are arterial and mixed venous oxygen saturations (%). Here the small amount of O_2 that is physically dissolved in blood is disregarded.

The *hemoglobin concentration* of the blood is the resultant of the balance between erythropoiesis and red cell destruction (or loss). As discussed in detail below, increased red cell mass mediated by erythropoietin represents an important adaptation to hypoxia.

The *blood flow* to a given tissue or organ is controlled by a complex interplay of local, neural, and hormonal factors. Alteration in blood flow to a given organ is generally appropriate to its metabolic demands. For example, during vigorous muscular exercise, increased cardiac output accompanies enhanced blood flow through exercising muscle. Unused capillaries are recruited in order to maximize oxygen delivery and clearance of metabolic wastes. Considerable alterations in the distribution of blood flow often occur without any significant change in the cardiac output. Familiar examples include the increased blood flow to the intestine following meals and the marked effect of ambient temperature upon circulation to the skin. Because of the body's wisdom in tailoring regional circulation to the local and temporal demands, the determinants of blood flow at the tissue level are very complex. Thus, it is very difficult to obtain a good estimate of blood flow through a given capillary bed.

The third factor in the Fick equation ($S_aO_2 - S_{\bar{V}}O_2$) is a quantitative expression of the *fractional unloading of oxygen from hemoglobin* during the flow of blood from artery to vein. This parameter is dependent upon the blood's oxyhemoglobin dissociation curve, which determines the amount of oxygen the blood can release for a given decrement in PO_2. Under physiologic conditions, the dissociation curve is poised so that blood becomes nearly fully saturated with oxygen during the circulation through the lungs. During flow through systemic capillaries a steeper portion of the curve is encompassed, permitting a relatively large amount of oxygen to be unloaded over a relatively small drop in PO_2. This allows oxygen to be released into the plasma at sufficiently high concentration to provide an adequate gradient into the interior of cells. Lawson and Forster (1967) have estimated that in the tissue capillaries the oxygen tension of the red cell is about 1 mm Hg greater than that of the plasma. The PO_2 gradient between the plasma and the interior of cells must be highly variable, depending upon a number of independent factors, including capillary blood flow, capillary density, diffusion barriers, and the metabolic activity of the cell. Each capillary supplies a cylinder of tissue. It is not surprising that estimations of the cylinder radii differ widely for various tissues (Krogh, 1919).

In most tissues the transport of oxygen into the cell is diffusion-limited. The transfer of O_2 through tissue protoplasm may be faster than through an equivalent thickness of water (Longmuir and Bourke, 1960). Skeletal and cardiac muscles have high concentrations of myoglobin within the cell cytoplasm. Because of its high O_2 affinity, this heme protein scavenges and stores oxygen. Myoglobin also facilitates the transport of oxygen into the cell (Wittenberg, 1965) in a manner similar to that described above for hemoglobin within the red cell.

The PO_2 within the muscle cells of the myocardium has been estimated to be 5 mm Hg (Coburn et al., 1973). About 0.5 mm Hg is required for normal respiration of isolated mitochondria (Chance et al., 1962). If O_2 tension falls below 0.1 mm Hg, tissue respiration ceases and cell death occurs. Thus, oxygen is generally present in excess at the mitochondrial level. Under normal circumstances, cellular respiration is thought to be limited by ADP levels rather than by availability of oxygen, substrate, or respiratory chain enzymes.

DETERMINANTS OF WHOLE BLOOD OXYGEN AFFINITY

The oxygen affinity of hemoglobin is generally measured as P_{50}, the partial pressure of O_2 at which hemoglobin is half oxygenated (and half deoxygenated). Measurement of P_{50} takes no account of the shape of the O_2 dissociation curve (heme-heme interaction), but designates the position of the mid-portion of the curve. As O_2 affinity increases, P_{50} of course becomes smaller. Under physiologic conditions (T = 37° C, PCO_2 = 40 mm Hg, pH = 7.4), blood from normal males has a P_{50} of about 26 mm Hg. When measurements are made in the same laboratory, the standard error of the mean is relatively low

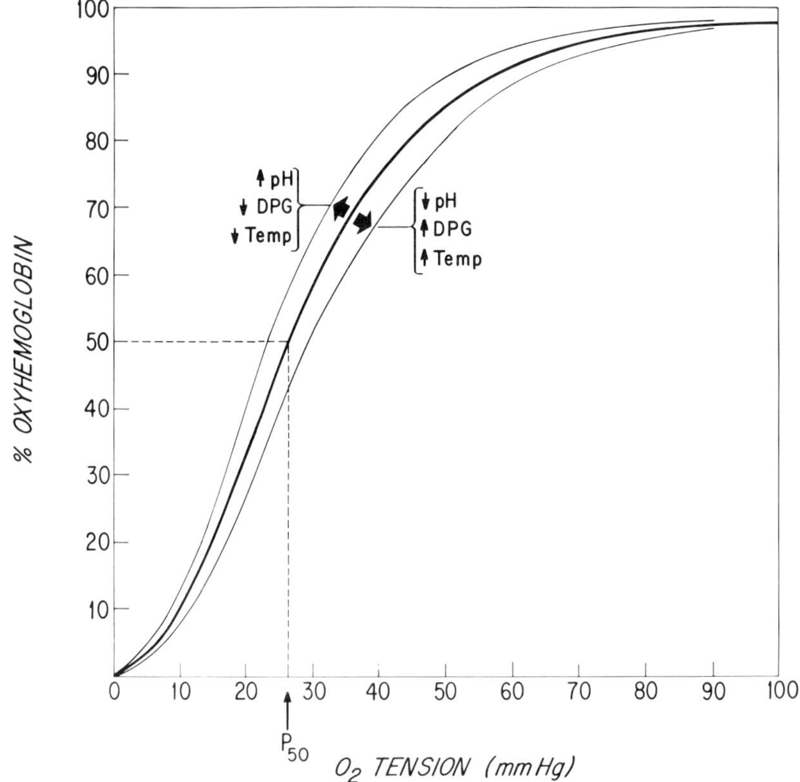

Figure 3–1. The principal factors which influence the position of the oxyhemoglobin dissociation curve.

(~ 0.4), indicating only a small amount of variation of P_{50} values in normals (Bartels et al., 1961). Females tend to have somewhat higher P_{50} levels (mean 28.0 mm Hg ± 0.4 S.E.M. [Humpler and Armor, 1973]). These values depend somewhat on the method used to measure whole blood oxygen affinity. As we will discuss in detail below, P_{50} values vary considerably in a number of clinical disorders. Widely varying oxygen affinities have been noted in the blood of different mammals. Small mammals such as the mouse tend to have higher P_{50} values (45 mm Hg) than large species such as the elephant (21 mm Hg) (Schmidt-Nielsen and Larimer, 1958) (see pp. 99 and 100).

The three primary determinants of oxygen affinity of whole blood are depicted in Figure 3–1:

1. Temperature
2. pH
3. Red cell 2,3-DPG

Effect of Temperature

The effects of temperature on the oxygen affinity of whole blood and of dilute solutions of purified hemoglobin A are very similar. For example, an increase in temperature from 20° C to 30° C increases the P_{50} of normal human blood 88 per cent (Astrup et al., 1965) and that of phosphate-free hemoglobin A (pH 7.2) 93 per cent (Benesch et al., 1969). The physiological relevance of the change in oxygen affinity with temperature is discussed in Chapter 2.

pH and the Bohr Effect

The Bohr effect can be readily demonstrated in whole blood by measurement of P_{50} at various values of pH. For normal human blood at 37° C, PCO_2 = 40 mm Hg, $\Delta \log P_{50}/\Delta pH \cong -0.50$ (Astrup et al., 1965). This value happens to be quite close to that determined for dilute solutions of phosphate-free hemoglobin (Benesch et al., 1969). The stereochemical basis and the physiological significance of the Bohr effect have also been covered in the previous chapter. Because of the direct binding of CO_2 in the formation of carbamino complexes, the PCO_2 of whole blood can alter its oxygen affinity independent of its effect on pH (see below). Changes in red cell 2,3-DPG (Benesch et al., 1969; Riggs, 1971; Wranne et al., 1972; Artierson et al., 1974) and PCO_2 (Riggs, 1971; Wranne et al., 1972; Artierson et al., 1974) can result in significant alteration in the Bohr effect.

Effect of 2,3-DPG

The red cell's concentration of 2,3-DPG is the third important determinant of the oxygen affinity of whole blood. The level of 2,3-

DPG in normal adult red cells is about 15 ± 1.5 μmoles per gram hemoglobin or 5 mmoles per liter packed red cells. There is some variability in red cell 2,3-DPG values depending upon the methods employed. Females may have a slightly higher level than males. Young children (< 5 years) tend to have slightly higher red cell 2,3-DPG concentration than adults, perhaps because of a higher level of plasma inorganic phosphate (Card and Brain, 1973). Conversely, red cell 2,3-DPG declines significantly in elderly individuals, again in parallel with decreased plasma inorganic phosphate (Purcell and Brozovic, 1974).

Since whole blood oxygen binding curves are customarily done under standard physiologic conditions (37° C, pH = 7.4, PCO_2 = 40 mm Hg), variations in P_{50} are due primarily to alterations in red cell 2,3-DPG.[1] This has been documented for blood specimens from patients with a variety of disorders associated with a wide range of values for O_2 affinity (Oski and Gottlieb, 1971). As expected from the measurements of oxygen equilibria of dilute hemoglobin solutions, the P_{50} of whole blood increases directly with 2,3-DPG. However, as shown in Figure 3–2, this increase is significantly modified by the conditions that pertain in the intact red cell. Garby and deVerdier (1971) and Hedlund and Lovrien (1974) showed that the binding affinity of 2,3-DPG to deoxyhemoglobin decreases significantly at hemoglobin concentrations approaching those of the red cell. Furthermore, the studies of Berger et al. (1973) indicate that there may be

[1]Unless otherwise stated, P_{50} values in this chapter have been corrected to standard conditions.

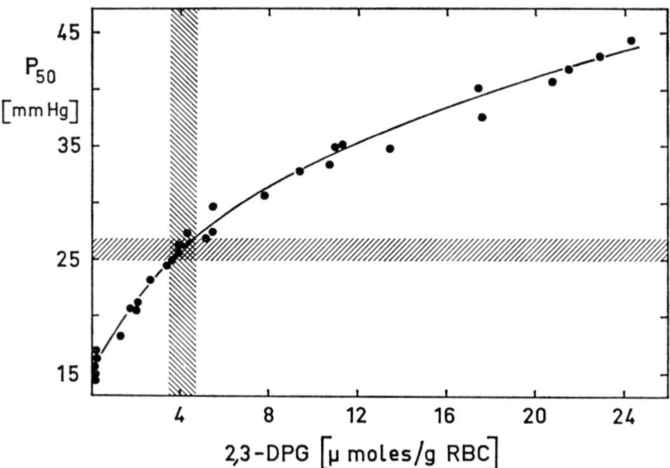

Figure 3–2. The relationship between red cell 2,3-DPG and oxygen affinity. Shaded area indicates normal range. (From Duhm, J.: Pflügers Arch. *326*:341, 1971.)

significant binding of 2,3-DPG to oxyhemoglobin under these circumstances.

Two,3-DPG has an important effect on intracellular oxygen affinity that is independent of its preferential binding to deoxyhemoglobin. As Guest and Rapoport (1939) and Battaglia et al. (1970) have pointed out, the fact that 2,3-DPG is a highly charged impermeant anion makes it strongly affect the difference in pH between the inside and outside of the cell. Indeed, 2,3-DPG and hemoglobin itself are the two principal impermeant anions of the erythrocyte. The distribution of permeant ions between these two compartments obeys the Gibbs-Donnan law as expressed in the following equation:

$$\frac{H_e^+}{H_i^+} = \frac{OH_i^-}{OH_e^-} = 0.92\,\frac{Cl_i^-}{Cl_e^-} = 0.93\,\frac{HCO_3^-)_i}{(HCO_3^-)_e}$$

where e = extracellular concentration and i = intracellular concentration. This relationship follows from a consideration of the chemical activities of the permeant ions at equilibrium and the requirement for electrical neutrality inside and outside the cell. The factors 0.92 and 0.93 are due to small differences between the activities and concentrations of the anions. Because of the presence of hemoglobin and 2,3-DPG inside the red cell, the ratio of intracellular to extracellular chloride ion is approximately 0.7. From the above equation one can calculate that the pH_i should be about 0.15 unit lower than pH_e. This is in good agreement with direct measurements showing that at a plasma pH of 7.4 (37° C) the intracellular pH is about 7.20 to 7.25 (Waddell and Bates, 1969).

Because of the Bohr effect, the oxygen affinity of whole blood is dependent not only on the plasma pH but also upon the difference between intracellular and extracellular pH. This ΔpH increases in direct proportion to red cell 2,3-DPG (Duhm, 1971; Salhany et al., 1971). Red cells having a sixfold increase in 2,3-DPG have an intracellular pH of 6.85 when extracellular pH is 7.40. Thus, 2,3-DPG has a dual effect in lowering oxygen affinity: it interacts directly with hemoglobin and it lowers intracellular pH relative to extracellular pH. As Figure 3–2 shows, at levels greater than 5 mmoles per liter packed red cells, 2,3-DPG has a smaller effect on oxygen affinity which is due almost entirely to a progressive lowering of intracellular pH. These considerations explain why the relationship between red cell 2,3-DPG and P_{50} shown in Figure 3–2 is biphasic.

Other Determinants of Red Cell Oxygen Affinity

In comparison to temperature, pH, and red cell 2,3-DPG, other factors are much less important determinants of red cell oxygen affinity.

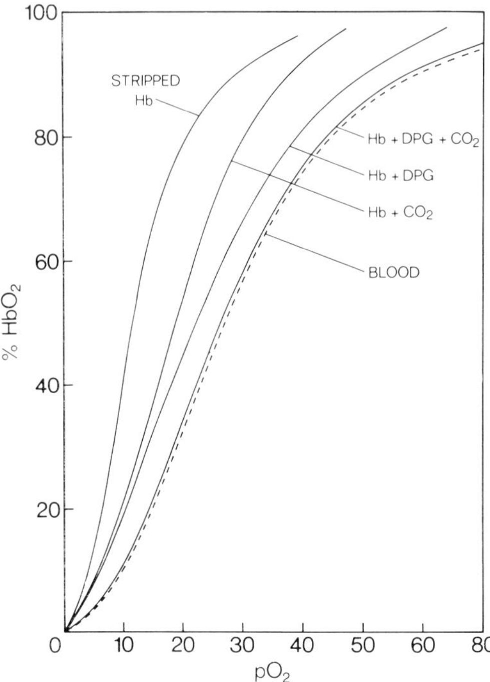

Figure 3–3. The effect of 2,3-DPG and CO_2 on the oxygen binding of phosphate-free human hemoglobin (37° C, pH 7.2). At physiologic concentrations of 2,3-DPG and PCO_2, the oxygen affinity of the hemoglobin solution is very close to that of the intact red cell. (From Kilmartin, J. V., and Rossi-Bernardi, L.: Physiol. Rev. *53*:836, 1973.)

(a) *Carbon dioxide* affects red cell oxygen affinity independent of its contribution to intracellular pH. The nature of the interaction between CO_2 and hemoglobin is discussed in Chapter 2. Under physiologic conditions, the PCO_2 of 40 mm Hg contributes significantly to the P_{50} of normal blood. As shown in Figure 3–3, the P_{50} of a concentrated solution of stripped (phosphate-free) hemoglobin, at pH 7.2, increases from 10 mm Hg to 20 mm Hg with the addition of 2,3-DPG (1.2 moles per hemoglobin tetramer) (Kilmartin and Rossi-Bernardi, 1973). If the PCO_2 of this solution is then increased from 0 to 40 mm Hg, and the pH is kept at 7.2, the P_{50} of the solution rises to 25 mm Hg. This is very close to the value obtained for normal human blood (26 mm Hg). From these results, it is apparent that wide deviations of PCO_2 from normal would be required to affect significantly the oxygen affinity of red cells directly through the formation of carbamino complexes. The range of PCO_2 values encountered in various clinical states would have little direct influence on whole blood oxygen affinity. The indirect effect of PCO_2 on pH is much more significant.

(b) *ATP* is the second most abundant organic phosphate in human red cells. Normally, its concentration is about one-fourth that of 2,3-DPG. ATP per se is almost as strong a modifier of hemoglobin as 2,3-DPG (Benesch and Benesch, 1967; Chanutin and Curnish, 1967; Bunn et al., 1971). However, because ATP has a much higher affinity for divalent cations than has 2,3-DPG, the bulk of red cell ATP is bound to magnesium ion (Rose, 1968; Bunn et al., 1971; Berger et al., 1973). The MgATP complex has no significant effect on the oxygenation of hemoglobin (Bunn et al., 1971). Thus, red cell ATP probably has no effect on the oxygen affinity of whole blood. In contrast to human red cells, ATP is the prime mediator of oxygen affinity of fishes and most amphibians.

(c) *MCHC* (the mean corpuscular hemoglobin concentration) probably has a small effect on the oxygen affinity of red cells. The oxygen affinity of phosphate-free hemoglobin decreases slightly with increasing hemoglobin concentration (Benesch et al., 1969). Although a significant positive correlation between MCHC and P_{50} has been reported (Bellingham et al., 1971), its functional significance is uncertain. May and Huehns (1972) and Murphy et al. (1974) measured the oxygen affinity of normal red cells that had been artificially swollen and contracted by suspension in hypo- and hypertonic media. No significant change in P_{50} was observed when corrections for changes in intracellular pH were applied. These results indicate that the oxygen affinity of red cells is not significantly affected by changes in the intracellular concentration of hemoglobin.

From these considerations, one would conclude that the P_{50} of normal human red cells is determined within rather narrow limits by temperature, plasma pH, PCO_2, and red cell 2,3-DPG. Since all but the latter are fixed experimentally or corrected for in the measurement of oxygen binding to whole blood, it follows that P_{50} is dependent primarily on red cell 2,3-DPG. In general this appears to be true in a wide variety of clinical settings. Nevertheless, some interesting exceptions have been noted. Red cells from the fetus and the newborn have increased oxygen affinity because of impaired interaction between 2,3-DPG and hemoglobin F (see p. 93). The red cells of patients with diabetes mellitus have a lower P_{50} than one would predict from red cell 2,3-DPG levels (Arturson et al., 1975), probably related to the presence of increased concentration of hemoglobin A_{Ic} in diabetics (Rahbar, 1968; Trivelli et al., 1971). Hemoglobin A_{Ic} also fails to interact normally with 2,3-DPG (Bunn and Briehl, 1970). Erythrocytes of patients with hereditary spherocytosis (HS) have somewhat higher P_{50} values than one would expect from red cell 2,3-DPG levels (Fernandez and Erslev, 1973); this has been attributed to the significant increase in MCHC in HS cells. If the human red cell contains structurally abnormal hemoglobin, its oxygen binding properties may be significantly altered. This includes many of the hemoglobin variants (see Chapters 8 and 9) as well as acquired abnormalities in hemoglobin structure. Some conditions in which altered oxygen affinity of whole blood remains unexplained are (1) blood from the coronary sinus of some patients with coronary artery disease who are undergoing atrial pacing (Shappell et al., 1970), and (2) blood from patients with decompensated hepatic cirrhosis (Zimmon, 1972).

Red cell oxygen affinity also may be altered in the presence of certain *exogenous agents.* Several of these influence the oxygenation of the red cell by affecting intracellular pH. The P_{50} of red cells is promptly and significantly increased by the addition of small amounts of propranolol (1 to 5×10^{-4}M) (Oski et al., 1972; Pendleton et al., 1972), which has no effect on the oxygen affinity of hemoglobin solutions. Propranolol appears to lower red cell oxygen affinity by causing a massive leakage of potassium ions, thus lowering the pH inside the cell because of an alteration in the Donnan equilibrium (Agostoni et al., 1973). The decrease in oxygen affinity observed after the addition of hypertonic solutions of neutral salts (Valtis and Kennedy, 1954; Dawson, 1972) can also be explained by a relative decrease in intracellular pH (Murphy et al., 1974). High concentrations of iodinated dyes, used as contrast media in radiology, *increase* blood oxygen affinity (Rosenthal et al., 1973). These agents are relatively impermeant anions which decrease the pH gradient between the inside and outside of the red cell, an effect opposite to that of propranolol (Lichtman et al., 1975; Rosenthal and Mesrobian, 1975).

A number of exogenous agents are known to increase the oxygen affinity of intact red cells. Cyanate increases oxygen affinity by carbamylating the N-terminal amino groups of α and β chains, sites that are crucial to the molecule's function (Kilmartin and Rossi-Bernardi, 1969; DeFuria et al., 1972). Small concentrations (1.5 mM) of zinc chloride increase the oxygen affinity of both intact red cells and hemoglobin solutions (Oelshlegel et al., 1973). Red cell oxygen affinity is also increased in a hyperbaric environment (50 Atm) (Kiesow et al., 1973). The mechanisms for these latter two observations have not yet been worked out.

METABOLIC CONTROL OF RED CELL 2,3-DPG

Since the level of 2,3-DPG within the red cell is a prime determinant of whole blood oxygen affinity, it seems appropriate to examine the factors involved in the regulation of this glycolytic intermediate. This information is necessary for an understanding of how the concentration of red cell 2,3-DPG changes in response to environmental perturbations.

RED CELL METABOLISM

The red cell's sole *raison d'être* is the efficient transport of oxygen from lung tissues and CO_2 in the reverse direction. As emphasized in the preceding section, the red cell is especially well engineered for this purpose. It has differentiated to the extent that only essential metabolic pathways are in operation. Thus, the adult erythrocyte has a relatively simple organization: a metabolically active membrane enclosing a homogeneous cytoplasm that contains by weight 34 per cent hemoglobin and about 2 per cent nonheme proteins, primarily carbonic anhydrase and glycolytic enzymes. The red cell has very limited metabolic obligations: (a) maintenance of the sodium-potassium pump in order to prevent colloid osmotic lysis (see above); (b) maintenance of hemoglobin in the reduced (ferrous) state, since the oxidized form, methemoglobin (ferrihemoglobin), is unable to bind oxygen; (c) repair of the membrane by acylation of phospholipids (Shohet et al., 1968); and (d) protection of the cell membrane and interior against oxidant stress. These functions can be accomplished with a relatively low expenditure of ATP (the metabolic currency of the cell) and reducing equivalents, NADH and NADPH.

During its maturation in the bone marrow, the red cell loses its organelles and, with them, the capability for mitochondrial respiration and fatty acid and protein synthesis. Only two metabolic pathways remain intact in the mature erythrocyte: anaerobic glycolysis (the Embden-Meyerhof pathway) and the pentose phosphate pathway (hexose monophosphate shunt). These metabolic processes are diagrammed in Figure 3–4. Under physiologic conditions, glucose is the only important substrate for red cell metabolism. It enters the cell by facilitated diffusion. Once phosphorylated, the glycolytic intermediates are locked within the cell until they are metabolized to pyruvate and lactate. These two nonphosphorylated products are free

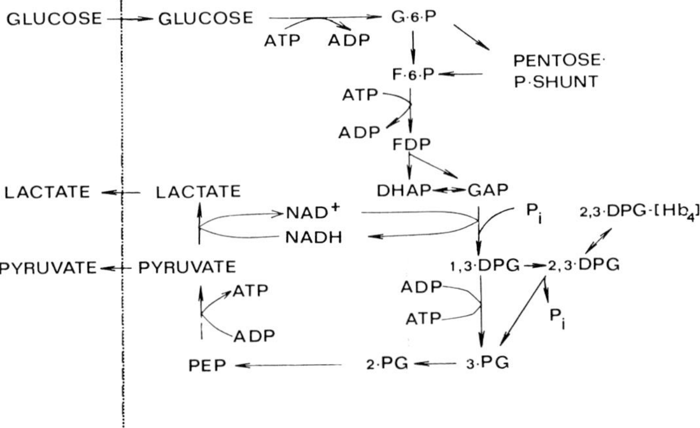

Figure 3–4. Glycolytic pathway within red cells. Glucose enters red cell and is metabolized to lactate and pyruvate, which escape from the cell. (From Rörth, M.: Series Haemat. 5:1, 1972.)

to diffuse out of the red cell and constitute the prime source of plasma pyruvate and lactate under resting conditions.

In the red cell, 2,3-DPG is by far the most abundant organic phosphate. In this respect, the red cell differs dramatically from other tissues in which 2,3-DPG is present only in the minute concentration which is required for it to serve as a cofactor in the monophosphoglycerate mutase reaction (see Figure 3–5).

Regulation of Red Cell 2,3-DPG

During red cell glycolysis, the intermediate 1,3-diphosphoglycerate is at a crossroad. As depicted in Figure 3–4, it can be converted to 3-phosphoglycerate with the concomitant conversion of ADP to ATP, or it can be isomerized to 2,3-DPG. The latter reaction is energetically wasteful, involving the loss of a high-energy phosphate bond. By hydrolysis 2,3-DPG is catabolized to 3-phosphoglycerate and inorganic phosphate. These two reactions constitute the Rapoport-Luebering shunt (Rapoport and Luebering, 1951) (Fig. 3–5).

In essence, the level of red cell 2,3-DPG is determined by three factors: (a) the rate of formation of substrate 1,3-DPG; (b) the relative amount of 1,3-DPG going into the Rapoport-Luebering shunt versus that undergoing conventional glycolysis; and (c) the rate at which 2,3-DPG is hydrolysed. It is apparent that the concentration of 2,3-

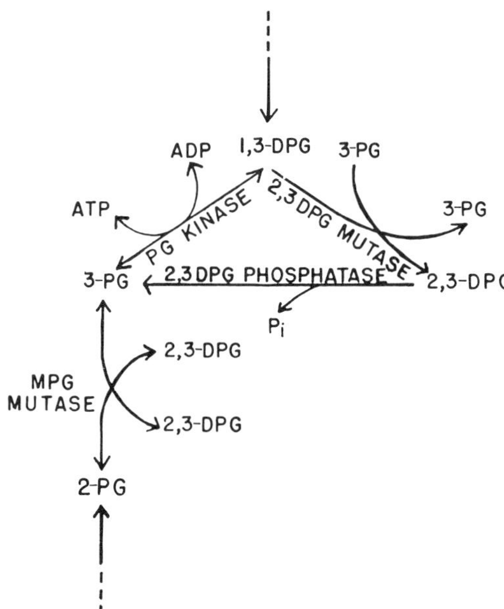

Figure 3–5. The Rapoport-Luebering cycle. 1,3-diphosphoglycerate (1,3-DPG) can be isomerized to 2,3-DPG or, alternatively, can be converted directly to 3-phosphoglycerate (3-PG) with the formation of one equivalent of ATP. (From Keitt, A. S.: Amer. J. Med. *41*: 762, 1966.)

DPG is the resultant of a complex array of independent and interdependent factors, a number of which are altered by environmental stimuli. We shall consider these in order.

Glycolysis

The synthesis of 2,3-DPG in the red cell is directly dependent upon the rate of glycolysis—i.e., the rate at which glucose is converted to lactate. From measurements of various glycolytic intermediates before and after a given change in incubation conditions, one can demonstrate which enzymatic steps of the glycolytic sequence remain in equilibrium and which are perturbed by the change. The latter, called crossover points, indicate those enzymes which are subject to metabolic control (Williamson, 1970). In the red cell, phosphofructokinase (PFK) is a particularly sensitive step. The positive and negative effectors which help control the activity of this enzyme are shown by the following reaction:

$$\text{Fructose-6-PO}_4 + \text{MgATP} \xrightarrow[-:\text{ATP, H}^+]{+:\text{ADP, P}_i} \text{Fructose-1,6-diphosphate} + \text{MgADP}$$

This reaction is unusual in that it is activated by product (ADP) and inhibited by substrate (ATP). In addition, PFK is activated by inorganic phosphate and inhibited by hydrogen ion. Thus, the rate of red cell glycolysis varies directly with pH and with inorganic phosphate. Both in vivo (in appropriate clinical states discussed below) and in vitro, corresponding changes in red cell 2,3-DPG have been observed (Minikami, 1969; Keitt, 1966).

The Ratio of NAD to NADH

The ratio of NAD to NADH is an important determinant of the rate of synthesis of 1,3-DPG (see Figure 3–4). Thus, the incubation of red cells with appropriate oxidants such as pyruvate (Duhm, 1971; Oski et al., 1971) or methylene blue (Dawson and Kocholaty, 1972) will increase this ratio and, by enhancing levels of 1,3-DPG, will promote synthesis of red cell 2,3-DPG. This observation has been exploited in the design of a suitable medium for preservation of red cells (see p. 95).

The Ratio of ADP to ATP

Which of the two reaction pathways 1,3-DPG takes is determined in part by the ratio of ADP to ATP. A relative increase in ADP will favor the conversion of 1,3-DPG to 3-phosphoglycerate. Conversely, if ADP is relatively decreased, the synthesis of 2,3-DPG will be favored. This probably explains why levels of red cell 2,3-DPG and ATP are often reciprocal. The determination of the ADP/ATP ratio involves a complex interaction between the glycolytic rate and the metabolic demands of the cell.

Activity of Diphosphoglycerate Mutase

The other important factor determining the metabolic fate of 1,3-DPG is the activity of the diphosphoglycerate mutase:

$$\text{1,3-DPG} \xrightarrow{\text{DPG mutase}} \text{2,3-DPG}$$

This enzyme has been purified from human red cells and studied extensively by Zelda Rose (1968), who has shown that this enzyme is markedly inhibited by its product, 2,3-DPG. With a K_i of 0.8 μM, the reaction in the normal human red cell containing about 3.2 mM of free 2,3-DPG would be proceeding at only 1/500th of its maximal velocity. If this is so, only a very small fraction of 1,3-DPG would enter the Rapoport-Luebering cycle. In contrast, it has been estimated from pulse-labeling experiments with intact red cells that as much as 50 per cent of glycolysis proceeds through the cycle (Keitt, 1966).

In general, one must be cautious about using kinetic constants derived from purified enzymes to estimate the reaction rate in vivo. The isolation of the enzyme per se could alter its kinetic properties, and there may be additional and as yet unknown factors present in the intact cell which could significantly affect the enzyme's function. There is good reason to believe that in human red cells 2,3-DPG exerts much less of an inhibitory effect than predicted from studies on the isolated enzyme. Red cells incubated with appropriate substrates (inosine, pyruvate, phosphate) rapidly increase 2,3-DPG up to four fold, despite this product inhibition. The activity of the mutase increases directly with pH up to pH 9.75 (Rose, 1968, 1973). The increase in red cell 2,3-DPG induced by alkalosis is probably due in part to this pH effect on the mutase as well as the stimulation to glycolysis discussed above. The activity of diphosphoglycerate mutase is markedly diminished in red cells of mammals such as the cat and the ruminants, which contain very low levels of red cell 2,3-DPG ($<$0.5 mmoles/liter RBC) (Harkness et al., 1969). Thus, the activity of this enzyme in vivo is probably an important determinant of the concentration of 2,3-DPG within the red cell.

In addition to the formation of 2,3-DPG by diphosphoglycerate mutase, there may also be net synthesis of 2,3-DPG by *mono*phosphoglycerate mutase (Laforet et al., 1974). This interesting possibility adds even greater complexity to the metabolic control of red cell 2,3-DPG.

Activity of Diphosphoglycerate Phosphatase

Diphosphoglycerate phosphatase hydrolyzes 2,3-DPG to 3-phosphoglycerate:

$$\text{2,3-DPG} + H_2O \xrightarrow{\text{DPG phosphatase}} \text{3-PG} + P_i$$

This enzyme has been purified and studied by Harkness and Roth (1969) and by Rose and Liebowitz (1970a). It must be distinguished from monophosphoglycerate mutase, which has some DPG phosphatase activity, particularly in the presence of activators such as 2-phosphoglycolate (Rose and Liebowitz, 1970b) or pyrophosphate (Keitt, 1971). Diphosphoglycerate phosphatase is activated by a number of anions, including chloride and inorganic phosphate (Harkness et al., 1969), whereas monophosphoglycerates (2-PG and 3-PG) are competitive inhibitors (Harkness et al., 1969). Certain sulfur anions such as bisulfite and dithionite (Harkness et al., 1969) as well as 2-phosphoglycolate are potent activators of this enzyme. The 2,3-DPG content of normal human red cells can be rapidly lowered in vitro by incubation with bisulfite (Parker, 1969). Diphosphoglycerate phosphatase has a pH optimum at about 6.2 (Rose and Liebowitz, 1970a). This is a third factor (along with the above mentioned effects of pH on DPG mutase and on glycolysis) which explains the direct relationship between red cell 2,3-DPG and pH. Under physiologic conditions, the activity of diphosphoglycerate phosphatase is probably controlled by the levels of inorganic phosphate, the monophosphoglycerates, as well as by the intracellular pH. Rose and Liebowitz (1970a) have calculated the velocity of the enzyme under apparent in-vivo conditions at 0.08 μmole per hour, which is 10 per cent of the V_{max} of the enzyme.

Identity of the Two Enzymes

Diphosphoglycerate mutase and diphosphoglycerate phosphatase have identical electrophoretic (Rosa et al., 1973, 1975) and chromatographic properties and may indeed be the same protein. Sasaki et al. (1975) and Kappel and Hass (1975) purified this protein from human erythrocytes to homogeneity and demonstrated enzymatic activity for both reactions.

METABOLIC "FUNCTIONS" OF 2,3-DPG

It is apparent that 2,3-DPG fulfills a number of physiological and metabolic functions in the erythrocyte. By far the most important, of course, is the mediation of oxygen affinity by direct binding to a specific site on hemoglobin. Secondly, because it is a highly charged impermeant anion, 2,3-DPG effectively lowers intracellular pH. These two phenomena are discussed in detail above. Thirdly, because 2,3-DPG is present in such high concentrations in the red cell, it may serve as an energy source under certain circumstances such as during storage of bank blood (see below). Finally, 2,3-DPG affects the activity of a number of other red cell enzymes. Among the glycolytic enzymes, it inhibits hexokinase (Dische, 1964; Brewer, 1969; Beutler, 1971; Harkness et al., 1971; cf. deVerdier and Garby, 1965), phosphofructokinase (Beutler, 1971; Harkness et al., 1971; cf. Staal and Koster, 1972), aldolase (Beutler, 1971), glyceraldehyde-3-phosphatase (Beutler, 1971; Harkness et al., 1971), and phosphoglucomutase (Beutler, 1971; Harkness et al., 1971). The first four of these are proximal to 2,3-DPG synthesis. Thus, the inhibition of these enzymes by 2,3-DPG may serve as a form of negative feedback, controlling 2,3-DPG formation (Beutler, 1971). In addition, other red cell enzymes are inhibited by 2,3-DPG, including AMP deaminase (Askari and Roa, 1968; Lian and Harkness, 1974), phosphoribosyl pyrophosphate synthetase (Hershko et al, 1969; Yip and Balis, 1975), and IMP:pyrophosphate phosphoribosyl transferase and AMP:pyrophosphate phosphoribosyl transferase (Yip and Balis, 1975). By inhibiting the catabolism of AMP, 2,3-DPG helps to preserve the red cell pool of adenine nucleotides.

Because 2,3-DPG can chelate with divalent cations, it may play a role in determining the concentration of free and bound magnesium ion within the red cell. One can consider hemoglobin and Mg^{++} as competitors for binding to the two main organic phosphates, 2,3-DPG and ATP. From a knowledge of the stability constants for the various complexes under physiologic conditions, one can estimate

TABLE 3–1. *Distribution of ATP, 2,3-DPG, Mg^{++}, and Mg-Phosphate Complexes in Human Erythrocytes**

Species	Oxygenated (mmol/l [% total])	Deoxygenated (mmol/l [% total])
Free ATP	0.18 (9.0)	0.11 (5.6)
MgATP	1.44 (70.0)	1.43 (71.5)
HbATP	0.23 (11.5)	0.26 (13.0)
HbATP·Mg	0.19 (9.5)	0.20 (10.0)
Free DPG	3.19 (44.3)	1.19 (16.5)
MgDPG	1.24 (17.2)	0.76 (10.6)
HbDPG	2.77 (38.4)	5.25 (72.9)
Free Mg^{++}	0.67 (19.1)	1.12 (32.0)
MgATP	1.44 (40.0)	1.43 (40.9)
MgDPG	1.24 (35.4)	0.76 (21.7)
HbATP·Mg	0.19 (5.4)	0.20 (5.7)

*From Gerber et al., 1973.

the distribution of the various species in the oxygenated and deoxygenated red cell (Bunn et al., 1971; Gerber et al., 1973) (Table 3–1). It appears that the inhibition by 2,3-DPG of phosphofructokinase may be due to its ability to chelate magnesium and thus reduce the concentration of the substrate MgATP. The change in free magnesium with deoxygenation may affect the activity of reactions involving MgADP, such as phosphoglycerate kinase and pyruvate kinase.

2,3-DPG and Hypoxia

One of the most intriguing features of the metabolic control of red cell 2,3-DPG is the fact that this organic phosphate becomes elevated in various pathologic and experimental states of hypoxia. Moreover, this change is physiologically appropriate, since the resultant shift to the right in the oxygen dissociation curve permits increased unloading of oxygen to tissues. Two mechanisms have been proposed for this adaptation (Fig. 3–6). Hypoxia is generally accompanied by a respiratory alkalosis. In addition, enhanced extraction of oxygen during capillary circulation results in a further increase in red cell pH because of proton binding by deoxyhemo-

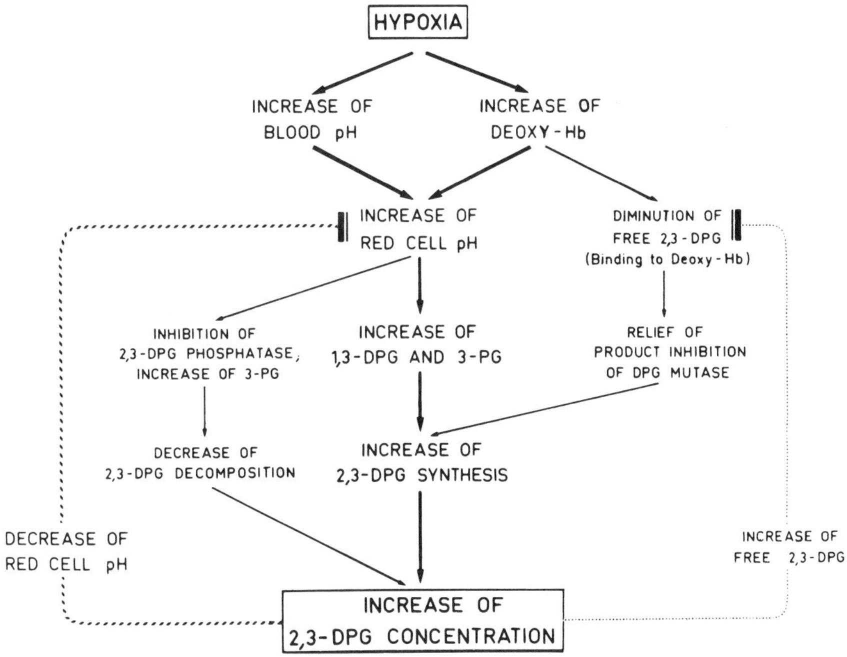

Figure 3–6. Probable mechanisms for increased red cell 2,3-DPG induced by hypoxia. (Courtesy of Dr. J. Dühm.)

globin. As discussed above, red cell 2,3-DPG increases not only because alkalosis stimulates glycolysis but also because of direct effects of pH on the two 2,3-DPG enzymes. It has been shown both in man (Lenfant et al., 1971) and in experimental animals (Duhm and Gerlach, 1971) that acute hypoxia will not induce an increase in red cell 2,3-DPG if alkalosis is prevented.

In addition, the increase in deoxyhemoglobin in hypoxic states decreases the level of free 2,3-DPG in the red cell (Fig. 3–6). This affords partial relief of the strong inhibition which 2,3-DPG exerts on its own synthesis. Applying the Michaelis-Menten equation for competitive inhibition to the diphosphoglycerate mutase reaction,[2]

$$v = \frac{V_{max}}{1 + \frac{K_m}{(1,3\text{-DPG})}\left(1 + \frac{2,3\text{-DPG}}{K_i}\right)},$$

it can be calculated that the velocity of the enzyme would be enhanced about 50 per cent going from the oxygenated to the completely deoxygenated state. Even in severe hypoxemia, oxygen extraction is seldom greater than 50 per cent (except in the coronary circulation). Thus, the increase in 2,3-DPG synthesis induced by deoxygenation in vivo would be correspondingly less. Oski et al. (1970) have shown that under conditions in which pH has been carefully controlled, deoxygenation of hemoglobin A favors the synthesis of 2,3-DPG. In a parallel experiment, this augmentation was not observed with hemoglobin F, presumably because it fails to bind strongly to 2,3-DPG.

It is likely that the former mechanism (pH increase) is the more important means by which hypoxia increases red cell 2,3-DPG. Duhm and Gerlach (1971) showed that in red cells containing low levels of 2,3-DPG but high levels of the triose phosphate precursors, deoxygenation made no difference in the rate of 2,3-DPG formation during incubation in pyruvate. Another approach to this question is to examine 2,3-DPG levels in individuals who are hypoxic and yet do not have increased oxygen extraction. For example, there are families in which polycythemia accompanies the presence of a hemoglobin variant with increased oxygen affinity (see Chapter 9). Red cell 2,3-DPG levels have been measured in about six of these and have been consistently normal (Lokich et al., 1973). In like manner, carbon monoxide can cause a significant shift to the left in the oxygen dissociation curve. Animals chronically exposed to carbon monoxide were found to have increased red cell 2,3-DPG (Dinman et al., 1970). A patient with congenital methemoglobinemia due to diaphorase I

---

[2] K_m (1,3-DPG) = 3.1 μM; K_i (2,3-DPG) = 20 μM (Rose, 1973); 1,3-DPG = 500 μM (Rose and Warms, 1970); and 2,3-DPG = 3,190 μM in oxygenated red cells and 1,190 μM in deoxygenated red cells (Berger et al., 1973).

deficiency had a 70 per cent increase in 2,3-DPG which approached normal on treatment with methylene blue (Versmold et al., 1973). These observations are interesting but do not provide firm evidence concerning the mechanism by which hypoxia induces increased red cell 2,3-DPG. Red cells having increased O_2 affinity lack both the pH increment contributed by the Bohr effect and the enhanced binding of 2,3-DPG by deoxyhemoglobin.

Even though chronic hypoxemia results in marked changes in red cell 2,3-DPG, it is unlikely that the transient oxygenation and deoxygenation of blood circulating through the lungs and tissues has any significant bearing on red cell metabolism. The turnover of most red cell enzymes is too slow to be influenced by any such oscillations in pH, free 2,3-DPG, etc. The report showing significant differences between arterial and venous 2,3-DPG (Hamasaki et al., 1971) has not been corroborated in other laboratories (Ravin et al., 1973).

In-Vivo Red Cell Aging

During the red cell's 120-day life span, oxygen affinity increases considerably (Edwards et al., 1961). Red cells become more dense as they age in vivo. Accordingly, "young" and "old" red cells can be separated by centrifugation. Young (top layer) red cells have a P_{50} of 33.5 mm Hg compared to a P_{50} of 27 mm Hg for old (bottom layer) cells (Edwards et al., 1961). By developing a special microspectrophotometric technique for measuring the oxygen affinity of individual red cells, Waldeck (1967) has obtained P_{50} values which approximate this range. After hemolysates of young and old cells are dialysed against a salt solution, there is no longer any difference in oxygen affinity (Edwards and Rigas, 1967). The dialysable substance that accounts for the difference in P_{50} is 2,3-DPG (Murphy et al., 1974). Several studies have shown significantly higher levels of 2,3-DPG in young cells compared to old red cells (Bernstein, 1959; Bunn et al., 1969b; Haidas et al., 1971; cf. Hjelm, 1969). These differences adequately explain the observed change in P_{50} with red cell aging. The fact that 2,3-DPG of normal whole blood specimens does not correlate with an age-related enzyme (erythrocyte glutamic-oxalacetic transaminase) (Edwards et al., 1971) cannot be considered as evidence to the contrary.

ALTERATIONS OF OXYGEN AFFINITY IN VARIOUS CLINICAL STATES

Over the past few decades, whole blood oxygen affinity has been measured in a wide variety of clinical disorders. One conclusion

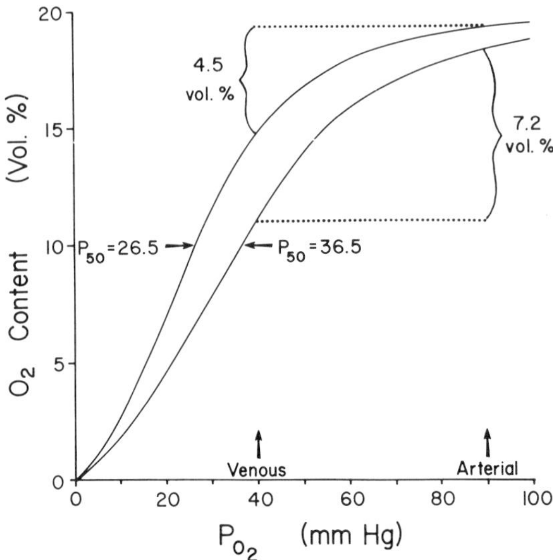

Figure 3–7. Enhancement of oxygen unloading due to a decrease in red cell oxygen affinity. Normal oxygen binding curve: $P_{50} = 26.5$ mm Hg; Right-shifted curve: $P_{50} = 36.5$ mm Hg. (From Klocke, R. A.: Chest 62:795, 1972.)

which emerges from all these data is that oxygen affinity is decreased in patients with various types of hypoxia. In all instances, the "shift to the right" has been found to be due to increased red cell 2,3-DPG. As discussed in the previous section, the mechanism by which this phenomenon occurs is not fully understood. Yet, as Figure 3–7 shows, it may serve as an adaptation to hypoxia. In certain clinical situations described below, the decreased oxygen affinity of the blood enables an increased amount of oxygen to be unloaded to tissues. In this section we will consider a number of adaptational and clinical conditions in which displacement of the oxygen dissociation curve has been reported.

ANEMIA

From the relationship $VO_2 = 0.139 \cdot Q \cdot Hb \cdot (S_aO_2 - S_{\bar{v}}O_2)$ it is apparent that if there is a primary deficit in red cell mass (Hb), oxygen delivery to an organ or tissue (VO_2) can be maintained by an increase in blood flow or in O_2. Patients with mild or moderate anemia maintain a normal cardiac output. If the packed cell volume falls below 25 per cent, cardiac output increases in proportion to the severity of the anemia. However, even with lesser degrees of anemia, alterations in the distribution of blood flow occur so that circulation to vital organs is enhanced. The second mode of compensation, in-

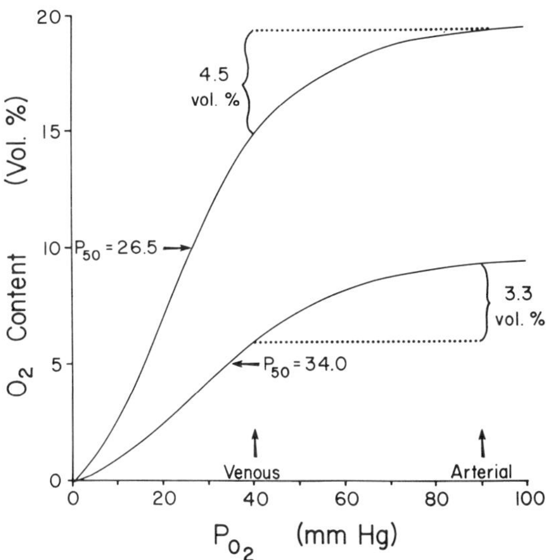

Figure 3–8. Enhancement of oxygen unloading by decreased red cell oxygen affinity in a patient with anemia. Anemic patient with a 50 per cent reduction in hemoglobin concentration has only a 27 per cent reduction in oxygen unloading. (From Klocke, R. A.: Chest *69*:795, 1972.)

creased oxygen extraction, is made possible by a decrease in whole blood oxygen affinity. Unlike individuals at altitude and those with chronic lung disease or cyanotic heart defects (discussed below), anemic patients have normal arterial oxygen saturation. Therefore, a "shift to the right" permits a steeper portion of the oxygen dissociation curve to be encompassed. It is apparent from the oxygen dissociation curves shown in Figure 3–8 that in the anemic patient the "shift to the right" compensates in part for the decrease in red cell mass. The patient shown in this figure has a hemoglobin level that is half normal. However, because of this compensation, the amount of oxygen unloaded at a given venous PO_2 is 73 per cent normal.

In patients with anemias of different etiology and severity, red cell 2,3-DPG varies inversely with hemoglobin concentration (Hjelm, 1969; Valeri et al., 1969; Torrance et al., 1970; Koch and Schroeter, 1973). Indeed, this correlation has even been established in normal subjects (Eaton and Brewer, 1968; Koch and Schroeter, 1973). Thus, the product of hemoglobin concentration and oxygen extraction is fixed within rather narrow limits. Card and Brain (1973) have postulated that the hemoglobin and red cell mass in children are set at a slightly reduced level because decreased oxygen affinity enhances oxygen unloading.

Red cell age probably has a bearing on the level of 2,3-DPG in anemic patients. Since 2,3-DPG decreases as cells age (see above), patients with hemolysis should have higher levels than those with anemia of similar severity due to failure of red cell production. Data of Opalinski and Beutler (1971) and Humpeler et al. (1974) indicate that this is true (Table 3–2). Nevertheless, patients with aplastic anemia and presumably a near-normal mean red cell age have elevated 2,3-DPG. This is observed even in patients who are dependent upon transfusions of 2,3-DPG–depleted red cells (Dickerman et al., 1973b).

Lichtman et al. (1974c) have shown that anemic patients have a respiratory alkalosis which offsets the effect of elevated 2,3-DPG on red cell oxygen affinity. Thus, these individuals generally have a normal in-vivo oxygen dissociation curve. However, it does not follow that 2,3-DPG is not an important compensation in anemic patients. After all, if red cell 2,3-DPG remained fixed, these patients would have left-shifted curves and, consequently, impaired oxygen release.

In most types of anemia, red cell 2,3-DPG is predicated on the deficit in red cell mass (Valeri and Fortier, 1969) and perhaps on red cell age. However, there are interesting exceptions. In congenital nonspherocytic hemolytic anemia due to a deficiency in one of the glycolytic enzymes, red cell 2,3-DPG may be determined by the primary metabolic abnormality. Patients with pyruvate kinase deficiency have unusually high red cell 2,3-DPG (Keitt, 1966), while those with hexokinase deficiency have subnormal 2,3-DPG (Keitt, 1969). In hereditary spherocytosis the 2,3-DPG is unexpectedly low, perhaps because red cells are sequestered in the unfriendly environment of the spleen (Palek et al., 1969). Following splenectomy, red cell 2,3-DPG rises to normal (Astrup, 1969; Fernandez and Erslev, 1972).

Polycythemia

There are widely conflicting reports on red cell 2,3-DPG in patients with polycythemia vera ranging from 55 per cent (Hakim et al., 1972) to 145 per cent of normal (Hjelm and Wadman, 1972; Koch and Schröter, 1973). There is no apparent explanation for this discrepancy. As mentioned above, patients with polycythemia related to pulmonary disease or cardiac right-to-left shunt have increased 2,3-DPG, while those with functionally abnormal hemoglobin variants have normal levels.

High Altitude Adaptation

Individuals exposed to low ambient oxygen tension adapt to this environmental stress in several ways. Pulmonary ventilation increases and polycythemia develops. The overall cardiac output is unchanged, although there may be redistribution of blood flow to

TABLE 3–2. *Levels of Red Cell 2,3-DPG in Various Types of Anemia**

Group	Diagnosis	Number of Patients	Hb (g/100 ml)	Arterial pH	2,3-DPG	
					μmol/g Hb	*mmol/l RBC*
1	Iron Deficiency	9	8.2	7.39	27.9	7.15
2	Hepatic Cirrhosis	8	8.7	7.43	22.4	6.15
3	Hemolytic Anemia	7	7.5	7.38	24.0	7.66
4	Leukemia	22	8.3	7.42	18.5	5.68
5	Aplastic Anemia	11	8.0	7.41	19.9	6.11
6	Uremia	16	6.9	7.32	15.6	4.95
NORMALS		50	15.8	7.38	13.2	4.10

*From Humpeler et al., 1974.

vital organs. The acclimatized individual is able to maintain normal oxygen consumption and exercise tolerance even at an altitude of 5000 meters (arterial PO_2 = 40 mm Hg). This subject has been reviewed recently by Lenfant and Sullivan (1971).

It has long been known that individuals living at high altitudes have decreased whole blood oxygen affinity. The mechanism for this "shift to the right" has been nicely worked out by Lenfant and his associates (1968). A group of normal volunteers were taken from sea level to an altitude of 4530 meters. As Figure 3–9 shows, the whole blood P_{50} increased rapidly, reaching a maximum of about 31 mm Hg* by 36 hours. This change in oxygen affinity was accompanied by a parallel rise in red cell 2,3-DPG. The P_{50} and 2,3-DPG of these volunteers and natives living at this altitude fell to normal levels within 48 to 72 hours after descent to sea level. This study was the first to demonstrate that 2,3-DPG mediated a decrease in oxygen affinity following a hypoxic stimulus. In a later study this group showed that this response was abolished if volunteers were given acetazolamide, which presumably prevented the development of respiratory alkalosis (Lenfant et al., 1971) (see above, 2,3-DPG and Hypoxia). Eaton, Brewer, and Grover (1969) measured red cell 2,3-DPG in a large number of individuals living at sea level and at 3300 meters (Leadville, Colorado). They found that 2,3-DPG was somewhat elevated in the individuals living at altitude. Those that had exces-

*Corrected to pH 7.4.

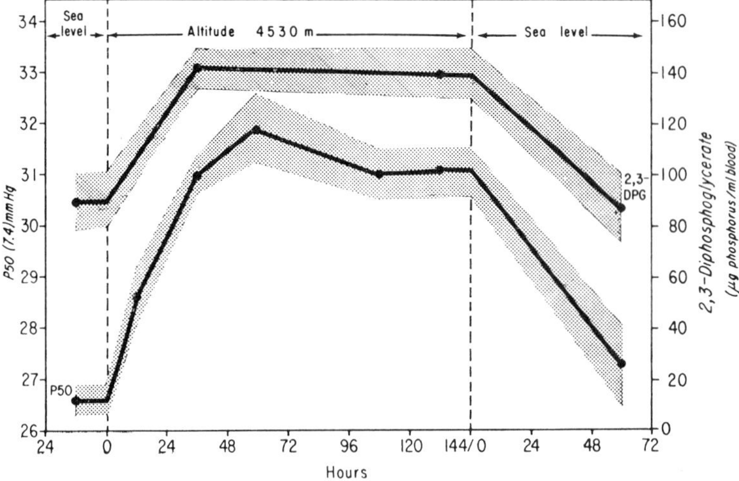

Figure 3–9. The effect of exposure to altitude on red cell 2,3-DPG and red cell oxygen affinity. (From Lenfant, C., et al.: J. Clin. Invest. *47*:2652, 1968.)

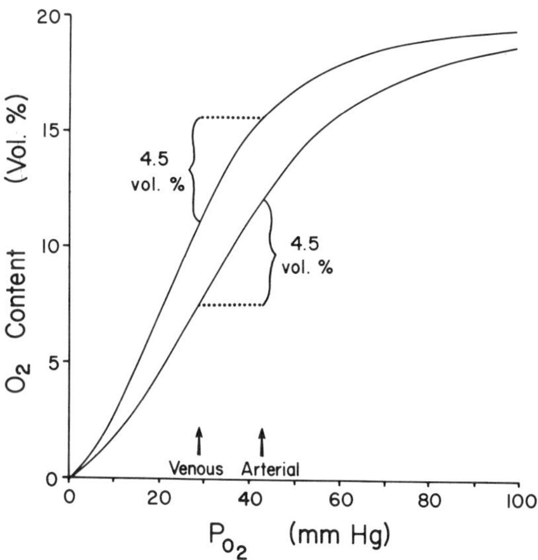

Figure 3–10. Failure of right-shifted oxygen binding curve to enhance oxygen unloading in patients with arterial hypoxemia. (From Klocke, R. A.: Chest 62:795, 1972.)

sive polycythemia had a more impressive increase in red cell 2,3-DPG. Exposure to high altitude does not affect the concentration of other organic phosphates in the red cell (Torrance and Bartlett, 1970).

After a thorough analysis of the various factors determining oxygen delivery to individuals acclimatized at high altitudes, Lenfant and Sullivan (1971) concluded that the "shift to the right" of the oxygen dissociation curve is of very little adaptive value. As Figure 3–10 shows, the portion of the oxygen dissociation curve which is encompassed between a low arterial PO_2 (43 mm Hg) and a mixed venous PO_2 of 30 mm Hg are equally steep at whole blood P_{50}'s of 26 and 36 mm Hg. At low alveolar oxygen tension, the arterial saturation is significantly reduced by red cells having an increased P_{50}. This decrease in oxygen-carrying capacity offsets whatever enhancement there is in oxygen desaturation in the capillaries. Thus, the A-V oxygen content may be minimally affected by the increase in P_{50}. The extent to which this is true varies from one organ to another (Klocke, 1972). Polycythemia is a much more significant adaptation to altitude, since it enhances oxygen-carrying capacity. It is interesting that those Leadville citizens who had the most severe polycythemia had the highest levels of 2,3-DPG. As Eaton et al. (1974) have pointed out, the resultant "right shift" is probably inappropriate and may even aggravate the degree of hypoxia. Animals adapted to high altitude such as certain Camelidae (llama, vicuna) (Chiodi, 1971) and mouflon sheep (Huisman et al., 1958b) have left-shifted oxygen dissociation curves. These animals, then, have a maximum oxygen-carrying capacity without the necessity to develop polycythemia. They probably have become adapted to utilizing oxygen at reduced tension. Recently, Eaton et al. (1974) showed that rats survived better at simulated high altitudes (9200 meters) if their whole blood oxygen affinity was *increased* by chemically modifying the hemoglobin with oral administration of sodium cyanate.

PULMONARY DISEASE

In one of the first surveys of red cell 2,3-DPG in various clinical disorders, Oski and his associates (1969) showed that patients with chronic obstructive pulmonary disease had significantly elevated levels (5.2 mmoles/l RBC versus normal of 4.1 mmoles/l RBC). This undoubtedly accounts for the shift to the right that has been observed in some of these patients. Edwards and his associates (1968) have presented carefully measured oxygen binding curves showing that the decreased oxygen affinity in these patients enhances oxygen unloading. In general, this advantage cannot be great in patients with arterial hypoxemia for reasons cited in the section above. (See also Flenley et al., 1975.) There is a wide variation of P_{50} and 2,3-DPG values in patients with chronic pulmonary disease (Keitt et al., 1974; Flenley et al., 1975). Those patients with secondary polycythemia tended to have increased P_{50} values while those with normal hematocrits had decreased P_{50} values. This is a complex group of patients to analyze, since they vary greatly in acid-base status and 2,3-DPG is very sensitive to alterations in plasma and red cell pH. For these reasons, it is not surprising that in these groups of patients, red cell 2,3-DPG does not closely parallel the degree of hypoxia. Keitt et al. (1974) found that red cell 2,3-DPG had a marginally significant correlation with arterial PO_2 in patients with chronic obstructive pulmonary disease. However, acute changes in red cell 2,3-DPG which were observed after the administration or withdrawal of oxygen therapy correlate closely with changes in arterial pH. In contrast to patients with chronic lung disease, acute asthmatics have normal red cell 2,3-DPG but slightly increased hemoglobin levels (Gallagher, 1971).

CARDIAC DISORDERS

Cardiac function is obviously of critical importance in maintaining oxygen homeostasis. Hypoxia can be seen in a variety of cardiac disorders. Patients with *cyanotic congenital heart disease* shunt blood from the right heart to the left, bypassing the pulmonary circulation. Accordingly, arterial oxygen tension is reduced. Five such patients having a mean arterial oxygen saturation of 72 per cent had a 74 per cent increase in red cell 2,3-DPG (Oski et al., 1969). Similar elevations in 2,3-DPG have also been reported in another series (Ravin et al., 1973). It is doubtful whether the resultant decrease in oxygen affinity is of significant advantage to these patients, for reasons analogous to those discussed in the previous sections concerning hypoxemia secondary to high altitude or pulmonary disease. Following surgical correction of cyanotic heart defects, red cell 2,3-DPG falls promptly to normal (Ravin et al., 1973). This may be due in part to reversal of the hypoxia but also to the transfusion of stored blood (see below) and perhaps alterations in red cell metabolism following surgery (Young et al., 1973).

The development of congestive failure is accompanied by decreasing cardiac output and impaired perfusion of tissues. Woodson and his associates (1970) have measured cardiac and hemoglobin function in 39 cardiac patients and found that P_{50} was significantly increased in those whose cardiac index fell below 2.3 liters/min/m^2. When patients' hemoglobin levels were considered, an inverse linear relationship between "hemoglobin flow" (Hb × cardiac output) and P_{50} was found. Cardiac patients with a functional classification of III or IV had significant elevations in red cell 2,3-DPG and P_{50}. As previously discussed, oxygenation is related to a product of blood flow × hemoglobin × (S_aO_2–$S_{\bar{v}}O_2$). For patients with cardiac failure in whom blood flow is compromised, enhanced oxygen extraction serves as a compensation.

Decreased oxygen affinity (as measured by P_{50} under standard conditions) has also been noted in patients who have sustained an *acute myocardial infarction.* The degree of the increase in P_{50} correlated with the size of the infarct (Kostuk et al., 1973). However, the "shift to the right" in these patients could not be explained by increased red cell 2,3-DPG. Lichtman et al. (1974a) performed thorough hemodynamic studies on 23 patients following acute myocardial infarction. Increased extraction of oxygen was found to be inversely proportional to "hemoglobin flow" (Hb × cardiac output). About a third of the enhanced oxygen extraction could be explained by a slight decrease in whole blood oxygen affinity.

In contrast to patients with congestive heart failure, those with circulatory collapse due to *cardiogenic and septic shock* may have decreased red cell 2,3-DPG (Miller et al., 1970; Chillar et al., 1971) and, consequently, decreased P_{50} values (Miller et al., 1970). These abnormalities appeared to be related to the presence of acidosis (Chillar et al., 1971). Those patients with low red cell 2,3-DPG had a more severe clinical status and prognosis (Miller et al., 1970; Chillar et al., 1971). Miller et al. (1970) have attributed the impairment of oxygen extraction in septic shock to increased oxygen affinity rather than to peripheral arteriovenous shunting. However, the in-vivo P_{50} of these patients is often close to normal, since the direct effect of acidosis on P_{50} counterbalances the increased O_2 affinity (Agostoni et al., 1975).

It is worth examining the relationship between altered oxygen affinity and the coronary circulation, since the myocardium normally extracts more oxygen than any other tissue. A primary "shift to the left" does not appear to be deleterious to cardiac function. Those individuals having familial polycythemia due to high-affinity hemoglobin variants (see Chapter 9) have no apparent increase in the frequency of episodes of angina pectoris or other cardiac manifestations. However, increased oxygen affinity may be deleterious to patients with pre-existing coronary artery disease. A group of dogs with experimental coronary artery obstruction developed electrocardiographic evidence of ischemia when given blood depleted of 2,3-DPG (Holsinger et al., 1973). Eliot and his associates (Eliot and Bratt, 1969; Eliot et al., 1970) have studied a group of patients with angina pectoris but normal coronary arteries and found that their dialysed hemolysates had significantly *decreased* oxygen affinity. However, more recently whole blood P_{50}'s on similar groups of patients were found to be within normal limits (Vokonas et al., 1974; deVerdier et al., 1975). Shappell et al. (1970) measured the oxygen affinity of blood from the coronary sinus of patients with angina pectoris. During atrial pacing, the P_{50} rose (range 0.6 to 2.9 mm Hg) while 2,3-DPG levels did not change. The mechanism underlying these observations is unknown. More recently, Colvard and Longmuir (1973) noted a significant increase in P_{50} during atrial pacing in about one-third of patients with angina. It would be of considerable interest if oxygen affinity were regulated at a local level by some type of feedback control.

Whole blood oxygen affinity may be affected by agents used in the treatment of angina pectoris. The effect of propranolol on red cell oxygenation has been discussed in an earlier section of this chapter (Determinants of Whole Blood Oxygen Affinity). Nitroglycerin may affect oxygen affinity in the coronary circulation. Following the intracoronary perfusion of the drug in dogs, Gross and Hardman (1975) observed a significant increase in the P_{50} of blood from the coronary sinus. The mechanism of this effect is unclear.

DISORDERS OF ACID-BASE BALANCE

In their survey of red cell metabolites in various clinical conditions, Guest and Rapoport (1939) showed that 2,3-DPG was increased in patients with alkalosis and decreased in those with acidosis. Forty years later their observation has been amply con-

TABLE 3–3. Effect of Blood pH on Oxygen Affinity

CLINICAL STATE	RED CELL 2,3-DPG	DPG EFFECT ON P_{50}	DIRECT pH EFFECT ON P_{50}	"IN-VIVO" P_{50}
Acidosis	↓	↓	↑	Normal
Alkalosis	↑	↑	↓	Normal

firmed (Bellingham et al., 1970; Bellingham et al., 1971; Alberti et al., 1972). The importance of pH in the regulation of 2,3-DPG has been stressed in a previous section. Astrup and his associates (Astrup, 1969, 1970; Astrup et al., 1970) have presented a convincing argument that it is the prime determinant of red cell 2,3-DPG in various clinical disorders. It is apparent that the pH-induced changes in red cell 2,3-DPG influence oxygen affinity in a direction opposite to the direct influence of pH (Bohr effect) (Table 3–3). The net result is that in most chronic acid-base disorders, in-vivo P_{50} is normal. Thus, 2,3-DPG serves as a buffer to maintain uniform oxygen release irrespective of the patient's plasma pH. However, as Bellingham et al. have pointed out, when this delicate balance is upset by acute changes in a patient's acid-base status, significant and perhaps deleterious changes in in-vivo oxygen affinity can occur. For example, if metabolic acidosis is rapidly corrected by the infusion of bicarbonate or lactate, the prompt rise in plasma pH is reflected in a corresponding increase in oxygen affinity as dictated by the Bohr effect (Bellingham et al., 1970; Bellingham et al., 1971). There is a lag of several hours before the increase in pH results in higher levels of red cell 2,3-DPG. Meanwhile, the in-vivo P_{50} is decreased and may compromise oxygen release, particularly in patients who lack other compensatory mechanisms for insuring optimal tissue oxygenation.

The regulation of erythropoiesis may depend in part on the acid-base status of the organism. It has been a puzzle why levels of erythropoietin rise sharply immediately following exposure to a hypoxic environment but then fall within 12 to 18 hours toward baseline. Miller et al. (1970) have shown that humans exposed to a simulated altitude of 4500 meters developed alkalosis, accompanied by a temporary drop in P_{50} of about 2 mm Hg until 2,3-DPG increased and normalized the in-vivo oxygen affinity. The acute rise in serum erythropoietin was blunted when alkalosis was prevented by the administration of acetazolamide. These results suggest the interesting possibility that the initial high levels of erythropoietin could be due in part to the transient "shift to the left." However, it is difficult to understand how this modest increase in oxygen affinity could contribute significantly to the individual's degree of hypoxia in view of the discussion in an earlier section on oxygen affinity in hypoxemic states (see Figure 3–10). The above experiments do not rule out the possibility that pH or acetazolamide itself has a direct effect on erythropoietin production.

Hyperphosphatemia and Hypophosphatemia

Inorganic phosphate (P_i) plays an important but complex role in red cell metabolism. P_i stimulates glycolysis by activating the important regulatory enzyme phosphofructokinase. In addition, phosphate is a substrate in the synthesis of 1,3-diphosphoglycerate. For these reasons, red cell 2,3-DPG synthesis is enhanced by inorganic phosphate. Red cells incubated in the presence of glucose and inorganic phosphate maintain higher 2,3-DPG levels than those incubated with glucose alone (Keitt, 1966). In 1939, Guest and Rapoport found that patients with hypophosphatemia had low levels of red cell 2,3-DPG and ATP. More recently, decreased 2,3-DPG and a concomitant increase in oxygen affinity have been seen in patients with hypophosphatemia secondary to diarrhea (Jacob and Amsden, 1971; Lichtman et al., 1971), hyperparathyroidism (Sheldon et al., 1971), and inadequate phosphate supplements during hyperalimentation (Sheldon et al., 1971; Travis, 1971). In addition, hemolysis may be encountered in association with rigid, ATP-depleted red cells (Jacob and Amsden, 1971).

Elevations in red cell ATP and 2,3-DPG have been observed in patients with hyperphosphatemia. Those in whom increased serum phosphate is due to chronic renal failure may fail to show these changes because of co-existent acidosis (see below). Children up to the age of 12 have plasma phosphate levels which are 50 per cent higher than those of adults. The resulting increase in red cell ATP and more modest elevation in 2,3-DPG account for the slight (1.6 mm Hg) right shift in their oxygen dissociation curve (Card and Brain, 1973). Card and Brain attribute the physiologic "anemia" of childhood to enhanced oxygen unloading secondary to this decrease in oxygen affinity.

Renal Failure

Patients with uremia have a complex array of physiological and metabolic abnormalities. They have varying degrees of anemia, metabolic acidosis, and hyperphosphatemia. All these factors affect the concentration of red cell 2,3-DPG. As a group, uremic patients have decreased oxygen affinity (Palek et al., 1969; Torrance et al., 1970; Mitchell and Pegrum, 1971) which is due to increased levels of 2,3-DPG (Hunt and Chanutin, 1964; Torrance et al., 1970; Lichtman et al., 1971). Uremic patients have about the same (Torrance et al., 1970) or somewhat lower (Lichtman et al., 1971; Humpeler et al., 1974; Lichtman et al., 1974b, 1974c) elevations of red cell 2,3-DPG compared to patients with other types of anemia of similar severity. As one might expect, those uremic patients with acidosis tend to have relatively low values while they are relatively high in those with hyperphosphatemia (Astrup et al., 1970; Lichtman et al., 1971). Lichtman et al. (1971) have shown that patients with renal failure have about a twofold elevation in red cell ATP. Furthermore, following incubation of uremic plasma with normal red cells, ATP increased about 50 per cent. This was shown to be due to increased P_i in uremic plasma. As we have stated in the introduction to this chapter, ATP probably has no influence on the P_{50} of normal red cells. Moreover, the elevated levels of ATP in uremic patients do not appear to influence oxygen affinity (Lichtman et al., 1974b).

Hemodialysis of uremic patients can result in a significant reduction in serum phosphate and in red cell 2,3-DPG (Raich et al., 1973). This occurred despite a concomitant increase in plasma pH. This observation was not confirmed in a subsequent study (Lichtman et al., 1974b). Reduced 2,3-DPG has also been found in patients whose hyperphosphatemia has been corrected by aluminum hydroxide gels.

Hepatic Cirrhosis

Patients with advanced cirrhosis of the liver have decreased whole blood oxygen affinity (Keys and Snell, 1938; Caldwell et al., 1965; Mulhausen et al., 1967) in association with increased red cell 2,3-DPG (Hurt and Chanutin, 1965). Astrup and Rörth (1973) showed that the increase in 2,3-DPG in these patients was proportional to the degree of anemia. However, at a given hemoglobin level, 2,3-DPG was significantly higher in cirrhotic patients than in those without liver disease. The reason for this is not clear. Varying concentrations of ammonium ion did not affect levels of red cell 2,3-DPG in vitro (Astrup and Rörth, 1973). Patients with advanced hepatic decompensation have decreased arterial oxygen saturation that cannot be explained by moderately decreased oxygen affinity. Perhaps venous-arterial shunting contributes to the elevated 2,3-DPG in these patients. In contrast to the above study, Zimmon (1972) has concluded that the shift to the right in patients with hepatic encephalopathy cannot be attributed to elevated red cell 2,3-DPG and that some other factor in cirrhotic plasma can effectively lower oxygen affinity. Cross incubation experiments implicated a plasma factor as responsible for the elevated P_{50} of patients with hepatic encephalopathy.

ENDOCRINE DISORDERS

Patients with thyrotoxicosis have an increased rate of metabolism and therefore may have hypoxia at the subcellular level. Accordingly, decreased oxygen affinity would serve as an appropriate compensation. Moderate increases in P_{50} (2 to 3 mm Hg) have been observed in patients with Graves' disease (Miller et al., 1970) as well as in euthyroid human volunteers (Miller et al., 1970; Gahlenbeck and Bartels, 1968) and rats who were given triiodothyronine (T_3) (Gahlenbeck and Bartels, 1968; Gahlenbeck et al., 1968). Furthermore, following the incubation of rat blood with supraphysiologic amounts of T_3, a significant increase in P_{50} was observed (Gahlenbeck et al., 1968). Mills et al. (1966) found that in volunteers given T_3, red cell 2,3-DPG increased 15 per cent. Increased red cell 2,3-DPG has also been observed in patients with hyperthyroidism (Miller et al., 1970; Snyder and Reddy, 1970a). However, rats given T_3 in doses known to increase P_{50} (Gahlenbeck et al., 1968) showed no significant change in red cell 2,3-DPG (Duhm et al., 1969; cf. Brewer et al., 1972).

Snyder and Reddy (1970b) showed that in a cell-free system containing a partially purified enzyme preparation the conversion of 1,3-DPG to 2,3-DPG was enhanced by the addition of thyroxine (10^{-12} M) or T_3 (10^{-14} M). These results indicate that thyroid hormone stimulates diphosphoglycerate mutase activity. However, Rose (1973), Czernik et al. (1974), and Torrance (1974) were not able to reproduce these results.

Thyroid hormone may affect red cell 2,3-DPG levels in the neonatal period. During the first four days of life, red cell 2,3-DPG increases 25 per cent while total thyroxine and free thyroxine increase 70 per cent and 100 per cent, respectively (Riegel et al., 1973; Versmold et al., 1973). However, this association may well be fortuitous.

The importance of thyroid hormone in regulating red cell 2,3-DPG remains unsettled. Not all patients with thyrotoxicosis have elevated levels. If patients with borderline low hemoglobin values are excluded, Monti (1974) found no significant difference between 17 hyperthyroid females and 10 normal females. We have found that among six patients with thyrotoxicosis, five had normal values for red cell 2,3-DPG. Furthermore, four patients with myxedema also had normal concentrations.

Patients with panhypopituitarism have anemia accompanied by inappropriately low levels of red cell 2,3-DPG (Rodriguez and Shahidi, 1971). This has also been observed in a patient with isolated growth hormone deficiency (Rodriguez and Shahidi, 1971). Administration of thyroxine and human growth hormone acted synergistically to increase red cell 2,3-DPG to normal levels. The same laboratory has reported a marked rise in 2,3-DPG of uremic patients given testosterone (Parker et al., 1972). This increase was far in excess of that attributable to an influx of young red cells. Gorshein et al. (1974) and Smolens et al. (1975) have shown that androgens will induce an increase in red cell 2,3-DPG in animals, independent of erythropoietin (Smolens et al., 1975). Molinari et al. (1973) observed a significant rise in red cell 2,3-DPG after incubation with various androgens in vitro.

There is not much information on the effect of adrenal hormones on intracellular hemoglobin function. Rabbits treated with aldosterone had a 2.7 mm Hg increase in P_{50} (Bauer and Rathschlag-Schaefer, 1968). A somewhat smaller shift to the right was observed following administration of cortisol. No change in the concentrations of red cell cation was observed. In this study 2,3-DPG was not measured. Red cell P_{50} was not affected by incubation with these hormones. High doses of prednisone have resulted in significant increases in 2,3-DPG in patients with leukemia and the nephrotic syndrome (Silken, 1975).

Brewer et al. (1972) have reported that adrenalin increases the level of red cell 2,3-DPG in rats. They also observed an increase following administration of thyroid hormone, in contrast to the study of Duhm et al. (1969).

During pregnancy, maternal red cell 2,3-DPG rises 25 per cent (Rörth, 1972). It is uncertain whether this increase is mediated by either ovarian or placental hormones. As Rörth (1972) has pointed out, this coincides with the development of respiratory alkalosis secondary to hyperventilation. The low maternal PCO_2 may facilitate the efflux of CO_2 from the fetus. It is likely that the increase in maternal red cell 2,3-DPG and mild alkalosis result in a normal oxygen affinity in vivo.

Oxygen Affinity in the Fetus and Newborn

The oxygen dissociation curve of blood from the human fetus and newborn is shifted to the left of that of maternal blood. This difference in oxygen affinity has also been observed in a variety of other mammals. The only exception reported to date is the cat (Novy and Parer, 1969). The higher oxygen affinity of fetal blood has been considered to be physiologically advantageous in facilitating oxygen transport across the placenta. However, this phenomenon may be of limited significance in man. There are now several instances in which mothers having a markedly left-shifted oxygen binding curve due to the presence of a hemoglobin variant have borne entirely normal offspring who didn't inherit the variant. Here, the maternal blood presumably had a higher oxygen affinity than the fetal blood.

The mechanism underlying the increased oxygen affinity of fetal red cells is interesting. The red cells of the newborn contain about 80 per cent hemoglobin F ($\alpha_2\gamma_2$). This hemoglobin, when purified and studied in a phosphate-free buffer, has a slightly *lower* oxygen affinity than hemoglobin A. However, 2,3-DPG binds less strongly to deoxyhemoglobin F (deVerdier and Garby, 1969). Consequently, a given concentration of 2,3-DPG is less effective in lowering oxygen affinity (Bauer et al., 1968; Tyuma and Shimizu, 1969). The diminished interaction between 2,3-DPG and hemoglobin F is probably due to the fact that at position βH21, an important binding site, the γ chain has nonpolar serine rather than a positively charged histidine residue. Neonatal red cells have normal to slightly increased levels of 2,3-DPG. However, this cofactor is not doing its job in newborn erythrocytes, and as a consequence oxygen affinity is significantly higher than "normal."

Following birth, the oxygen affinity of the baby's blood decreases rapidly (Delivoria-Papadopoulos et al., 1971b) (Table 3–4). During the first week of life, red cell 2,3-DPG increases 25 per cent (Riegel et al., 1973; Delivoria-Papadopoulos et al., 1971a). Although this increment in 2,3-DPG would not have much direct interaction with the fetal hemoglobin, it should lower intracellular pH and thereby decrease oxygen affinity. This rapid change in P_{50} seems appropriate for the increased metabolic demands following birth. A rapid rise in red cell 2,3-DPG during the neonatal period has been observed in several other species, including the goat (Battaglia et al., 1970), the pig (Delivoria-Papadopoulos et al., 1972), the horse (Bunn and Kitchen, 1973), and the dog (Dhindsa et al., 1972). The mechanism for this phenomenon is not clear. During the first six months of life, hemoglobin F decreases from 77 per cent to about 5 per cent of the total. This results in a further increase in P_{50} (see Table 3–4).

Under certain circumstances, the increased oxygen affinity of

TABLE 3–4. *Postnatal Changes in P_{50}, Red Blood Cell 2,3-DPG, and Fetal Hemoglobin in Term Infants**

Age of Infant	P_{50} (mm Hg)	2,3-DPG (μmol/ml RBC)	Fetal Hb (%)
1 day	19.4 ± 1.8	5.4 ± 1.00	77.0 ± 7.3
5 days	20.6 ± 1.7	6.6 ± 0.99	76.8 ± 5.8
3 weeks	22.7 ± 1.0	5.4 ± 0.73	70.0 ± 7.3
6 to 9 weeks	24.4 ± 1.4	5.6 ± 0.75	52.1 ± 11.0
3 to 4 months	26.5 ± 2.0	5.8 ± 1.20	23.2 ± 16.0
6 months	27.8 ± 1.0	5.1 ± 1.60	4.7 ± 2.2
8 to 11 months	30.3 ± 0.7	7.4 ± 0.49	1.6 ± 1.0
Normal adult	27.0 ± 1.1	5.1 ± 0.42	<2.0 %

*From Oski and Gottlieb, 1961.

newborn's blood may be a handicap. Oski and his associates (Delivoria-Papadopoulos et al., 1971a) have found that the mortality of premature newborns (weighing between 750 and 1250 grams at birth) is reduced if these infants are given an exchange transfusion of fresh adult blood having near-normal oxygen affinity. These investigators are also studying this therapy in newborns with respiratory distress syndrome. Infants with this disorder have even more left-shifted curves and lower red cell 2,3-DPG than have normal infants of comparable age and weight.

Transfusion of Stored Blood

During the first week of storage of blood in acid-citrate-dextrose (ACD), red cells become depleted of 2,3-DPG and, as a result, have increased oxygen affinity (Valtis and Kennedy, 1954; Gullbring and Strom, 1956; Akerblom et al., 1968; Bunn et al., 1969b). Thus, patients who are transfused with large amounts of such blood will have a "left-shifted" oxygen hemoglobin dissociation curve (Valtis and Kennedy, 1954). The clinical significance of this phenomenon has not been established. At the least, it is safe to say that the recipient does not derive the full physiologic benefit from blood depleted in 2,3-DPG. Following infusion of such donor cells into normal volunteers, their content of 2,3-DPG returns to normal within 6 to 24 hours (Beutler and Wood, 1969; Valeri and Hirsch, 1969). Considerable attention is now being focused on ways of modifying storage media in order to preserve red cell 2,3-DPG and normal hemoglobin function. It has been shown that 2,3-DPG and P_{50} are better maintained in citrate-phosphate-dextrose (CPD) (Huisman et al., 1969) because of the higher pH of this medium (Dawson et al., 1970). In 1971, 10 per cent of the blood banks in the United States used CPD as a preservative while 90 per cent continued to use ACD. By 1975, the reverse was true; CPD is now employed by 90 per cent of American blood banks. Although the shelf life is the same for the two preservatives (21 days), CPD enables red cells to function more physiologically during the first week of storage and therefore is a superior preservative.

Recently, several laboratories have been investigating the inclusion of various substrates to blood storage media that will allow the maintenance of physiologic levels of 2,3-DPG and ATP for longer periods. The addition of inosine to the storage medium provides ribose-1-phosphate, a substrate which feeds directly into the glycolytic pathway (Fig. 3–11). The resulting increase in 2,3-DPG is potentiated by the addition of pyruvate (Duhm, 1971; Oski et al., 1971b), methylene blue (Dawson and Kocholaty, 1972), or fructose (Torrance, 1973), all of which undergo reduction, coupled with oxidation of NADH to NAD, thereby providing cofactor for the glyceralde-

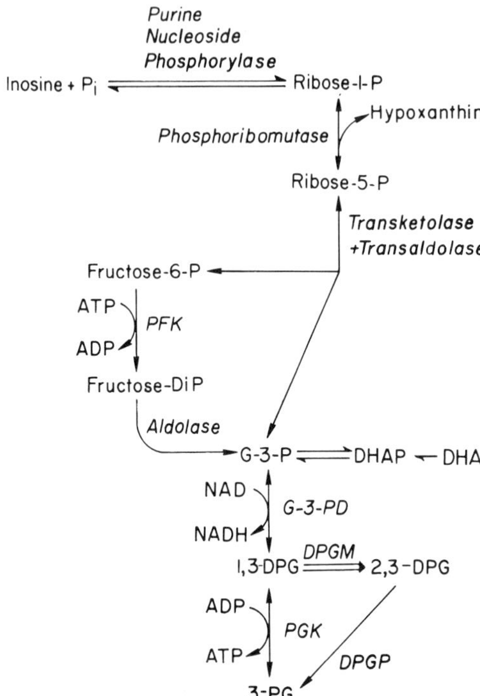

Figure 3–11. The pathway of red cell inosine metabolism to 2,3-DPG. Also shown in this figure is the Rapoport-Luebering cycle, wherein 1,3-DPG can be converted to 3-PG either directly or via 2,3-DPG. The conversion of dihydroxyacetone (DHA) to dihydroxyacetone phosphate (DHAP) is also shown. PFK, phosphofructokinase; G-3-PD, glyceraldehyde-3-phosphate dehydrogenase; PGK, phosphoglycerate kinase; DPGM, diphosphoglycerate mutase; DPGP, diphosphoglycerate phosphatase; P_i, inorganic phosphate; G-3-P, glyceraldehyde-3-phosphate; 3-PG, 3-phosphoglycerate. (Modified from Oski, F. A., Travis, S. E., et al.: Blood 37: 52–58, 1971b, by permission of Grune & Stratton.)

hyde-3-phosphate dehydrogenase reaction. The transfusion of large amounts of blood stored in inosine may be limited by hyperuricemia resulting from the catabolism of this purine. More recently, dihydroxyacetone has been proposed as an additive (Wood and Beutler, 1974). The red cells contain a kinase which permits this compound to be phosphorylated to dihydroxyacetone phosphate (DHAP). As shown in Figure 3–4, DHAP is a normal intermediate in glycolysis and serves as an effective substrate for the synthesis of 2,3-DPG. Beutler (Wood and Beutler, 1974) has shown that dihydroxyacetone is useful in preserving 2,3-DPG in stored red cells. One great advantage of this preservative is that it would not engender hyperuricemia.

The efficiency of conventional blood banking is severely limited by the finite shelf life of the stored units. Discarding of ACD and CPD blood after 21 days' storage is a major waste of a precious resource. The levels of 2,3-DPG and ATP in outdated blood can be restored to normal by incubation with appropriate substrates such as inosine, dihydroxyacetone, pyruvate, or methylene blue. If such rejuvenated blood is frozen in glycerol, the levels of 2,3-DPG and ATP are well maintained. Upon thawing, the added substrates and waste products are removed along with the glycerol. This "recycling" extends the effective shelf life of stored red cells indefinitely without sacrifice of either erythrocyte survival or function.

OVERALL SIGNIFICANCE OF ERYTHROCYTE OXYGEN AFFINITY

This chapter has been concerned with shifts in oxygen affinity which can occur in various physiologic and pathologic states. Before deciding whether these alterations have adaptive significance, we must take a critical view of the overall importance of whole blood oxygen affinity as a determinant of tissue oxygenation. This question defies an easy answer. It is very difficult to measure the oxygen supply and demand for a given organ or tissue under conditions in which oxygen affinity, hemoglobin concentration, and blood flow can be adequately controlled. In this section we will review some experimental and clinical studies which address themselves to this problem.

As we mentioned earlier, mitochondrial respiration is normally not limited by availability of oxygen. It is estimated that the PO_2 within canine myocardial cells is about 5 mm Hg (Coburn et al., 1973). Intracellular PO_2 has to drop to the range of 0.5 mm Hg before cellular respiration is affected (Chance et al., 1962). It is apparent that there is a large gradient in oxygen tension between the capillary where oxygen is released from red cells and the intracellular organelles which utilize oxygen. Assuming that blood flow and oxygen utilization remain unchanged, an increase in oxygen affinity should result in a predictable decrease in capillary PO_2. Would a drop in capillary PO_2 from, say, 40 mm Hg to 30 mm Hg result in a significant alteration in intracellular PO_2? A consideration of electrical power provides a crude analogy. If the voltage of the high-tension wires from a hydroelectric plant is decreased from 400,000 V to 300,000 V, this drop in power would be reflected proportionately by a decrease in house voltage from 120 V to 90 V. Thus, a significant drop in capillary PO_2 would necessarily reduce the pressure gradient and, consequently, the flux of oxygen into cells. Whether such a reduction is metabolically significant must depend on the oxygen requirement of the tissue and on whether compensatory adjustments in blood flow (which would decrease the radius of the tissue cylinder) can maintain intracellular oxygenation. In general, the experimental and clinical studies to date indicate that displacements in oxygen affinity become important only if other modes of compensation are significantly compromised.

From the information which is now on hand, it appears as if rather marked increases in oxygen affinity have little or no effect on the overall circulation and metabolism of individuals or experimental animals that are otherwise normal. Riggs et al. (1973) performed exchange transfusions on monkeys with blood that had been depleted of 2,3-DPG. As a result, mean P_{50} dropped from 33.9 ± 1.1 (S.D.) mm Hg to 27.2 ± 5.9 mm Hg. However, there was no change in red cell mass, cardiac output, oxygen consumption, or base deficit. Therefore, despite the lowering of venous oxygen tension, the shift to the left didn't seem to affect overall oxygen or acid-base homeostasis. Rand et al. (1973) compared rabbits with both normal and increased red cell oxygen affinity subjected to graded atmospheric hypoxia at fixed ventilation. The group having low-DPG red cells showed higher cardiac output than did the control group. However, there were no significant differences in the measured PO_2 of various tissues, including the brain, kidney, and muscles. In contrast, Guy et al. (1974) found that the oxygen tension in skin bubbles produced in rats fell significantly following exchange transfusion with blood having increased oxygen affinity. However, oxygen tension to more vital tissues may well have been preserved. Cassel et al. (1973) measured metabolites in brain tissue of control rabbits and of those having marked increases in oxygen affinity induced by the administration of cyanate. No significant differences were observed. These studies indicate that animals with increased oxygen affinity have sufficient compensatory mechanisms to maintain oxygenation to vital organs. Indeed, as mentioned above, there is doubt as to whether increased oxygen affinity poses any handicap at all in animals or humans with arterial hypoxemia. In fact, Eaton et al. (1974) observed that rats whose P_{50} was lowered 43 per cent by the administration of oral sodium cyanate had significantly improved survival when subjected to low ambient oxygen tension. In contrast to the results of Rand et al. (1973), the group with high oxygen affinity had lower heart rates than the control rats subjected to an identical hypoxic stress.

Woodson and his associates (1973) have examined the effect of whole blood oxygen affinity on the work performance of rats. They devised a treadmill which gave an accurate and reproducible end point of muscle exhaustion. All measurements were made on animals breathing room air. The duration of maximal exercise was shown to be linearly related to an animal's red cell mass. Rats with significantly increased oxygen affinity showed a lower exercise tolerance. The authors concluded that a 12 mm Hg (34 per cent) decrease in P_{50} was equivalent to a 10 per cent decrease in red cell mass. Thus, severe impairment of tissue oxygenation was seen in animals having a combination of increased oxygen affinity and reduced red cell mass. The obvious clinical inference that one might draw is that a significant "shift to the left" is deleterious to those patients who cannot compensate by developing circulatory adjustments and/or secondary erythrocytosis.

As we have mentioned, patients with increased oxygen affinity due to a hemoglobin variant have no apparent clinical manifestations other than secondary erythrocytosis. They maintain normal oxygen consumption and a normal (Novy et al., 1967) or slightly increased (White et al., 1973; Oski, unpublished data) resting cardiac output (see Chapter 9). However, if robbed of their primary mode of compensation by phlebotomy to a normal red cell mass, these individuals have impaired exercise tolerance and a more pronounced increase in cardiac output (Oski, unpublished data).

Recently, Oski and his associates (1971a) had the unique opportunity of comparing two adolescents with differing types of congenital nonspherocytic hemolytic anemia associated with marked differences in red cell 2,3-DPG. The patient with red cell pyruvate kinase (PK) deficiency had a markedly "right-shifted" oxygen binding curve (P_{50} = 38 mm Hg) due to the greatly increased red cell 2,3-DPG which almost always accompanies this disorder. In contrast, the patient with hexokinase (HK) deficiency had a left-shifted curve (P_{50} = 19 mm Hg) due to a decrease in red cell 2,3-DPG. Otherwise, the two patients were reasonably well matched for age and severity of anemia (9.8 to 10 g/100 ml hemoglobin). These two enzymopathies appear to be localized to the red cell. During graded exercise the patient with HK deficiency developed much lower mixed venous oxygen tension and higher cardiac output (Fig. 3–12) than the patient with PK deficiency. These hemodynamic differences are reflected in the clinical status of the two patients. The one with HK deficiency is a semi-invalid, whereas the PK-deficient individual plays on his junior high school soccer team.

In considering the overall importance of oxygen affinity on oxygen homeostasis, it is worth surveying other mammals to see how they solve this problem. Whole blood oxygen affinity has been

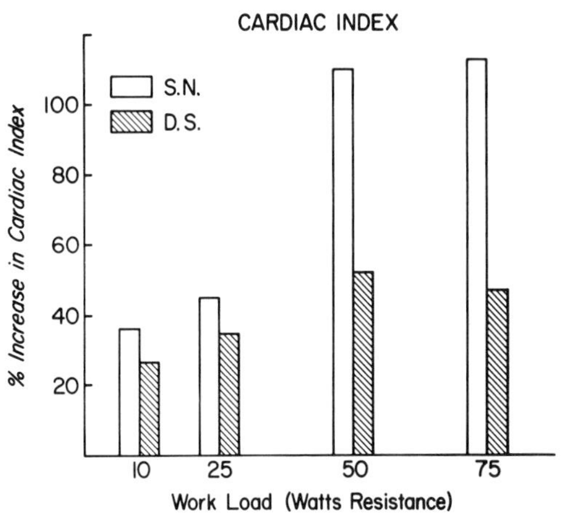

Figure 3–12. The effect of graded exercise on cardiac output in two patients: S.N., with hexokinase deficiency and increased red cell oxygen affinity, and D.S., with pyruvate kinase deficiency and decreased red cell oxygen affinity. (From Oski, F. A.: Unpublished figure.)

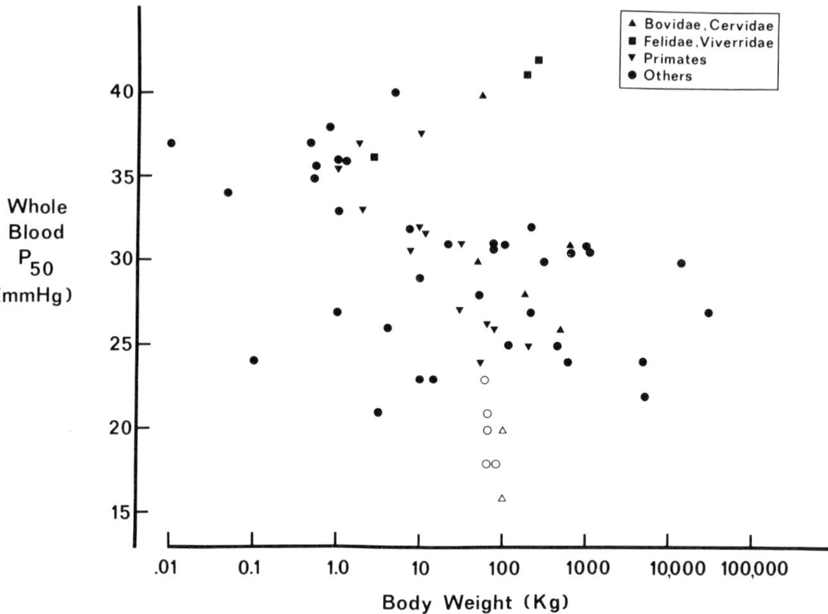

Figure 3–13. Variability in red cell oxygen affinity among mammals of different size. Open symbols are animals adapted to high altitude. (From Bunn, H. F., et al.: Ann. N.Y. Acad. Sci. *241*:498, 1974a.)

measured on at least 70 different mammalian species. Although, as Figure 3–13 shows, there is a considerable amount of scatter, P_{50} appears to vary inversely with body weight. This relationship seems appropriate, since smaller mammals having higher metabolic rates would benefit from enhanced oxygen unloading. Red cell hemoglobin function is mediated by high concentrations of 2,3-DPG in all mammals with the exception of two suborders: the ruminants (Bovidae and Cervidae) and the Feloidea (cats, hyenas and civets) (Bunn et al., 1974a). They have only a trace amount of 2,3-DPG in their red cells. Physiologic oxygen binding in these mammals is dependent upon the presence of hemoglobin(s) of intrinsically low oxygen affinity. Interestingly, animals adapted to high altitude, such as mountain sheep and certain Camelidae, have increased oxygen affinity (Fig. 3–13).

Chapter 4

HEMOGLOBIN BIOSYNTHESIS

GENETICS OF HUMAN HEMOGLOBIN SYNTHESIS

NORMAL HUMAN HEMOGLOBINS AND THEIR GENES

The protein portion of the various normal human hemoglobin molecules (Table 1–1) is made up of two α (or α-like) and two non-α polypeptide chains which are the products of separate and distinct genes or genetic loci.

Two embryonic hemoglobins, Gower-1 (? ϵ_4 or $\zeta_2\epsilon_2$) and Gower-2 ($\alpha_2\epsilon_2$), contain epsilon chains and are found only during the first 10 to 12 weeks of fetal development (Huehns et al., 1961, 1964; Hecht et al., 1966; Lorkin, 1973). They are presumably synthesized by erythroid cells derived from the yolk sac (Yoffey, 1971; Weatherall et al., 1974). Oxygen dissociation studies (Huehns and Farooqui, 1975) suggest that Hb Gower-1 may consist of two zeta chains and two epsilon chains rather than four epsilon chains, as initially proposed. In embryo and in normal cord blood (in trace amounts) one can detect another embryonic hemoglobin, Hb Portland-1 (Capp et al., 1967, 1970; Hecht et al., 1967), which is composed of two α-like chains (zeta chains) and two γ chains ($\zeta_2\gamma_2$). Increased levels of Hb Portland-1 are found in cord blood of infants with α thalassemia:Hb Barts-hydrops syndrome (Weatherall et al., 1970; Todd et al., 1970). The structure of zeta chains has been studied in a number of animal species: it is similar in structure in different species and shares a great deal of homology with the sequence of α globin chains (Melderis et al., 1974). The similarity in structure of human α and ζ chains has led to the conclusion that ζ chains probably constitute an α-like embryonic chain (Kamuzora et al., 1974; Kamuzora and Lehmann, 1975).

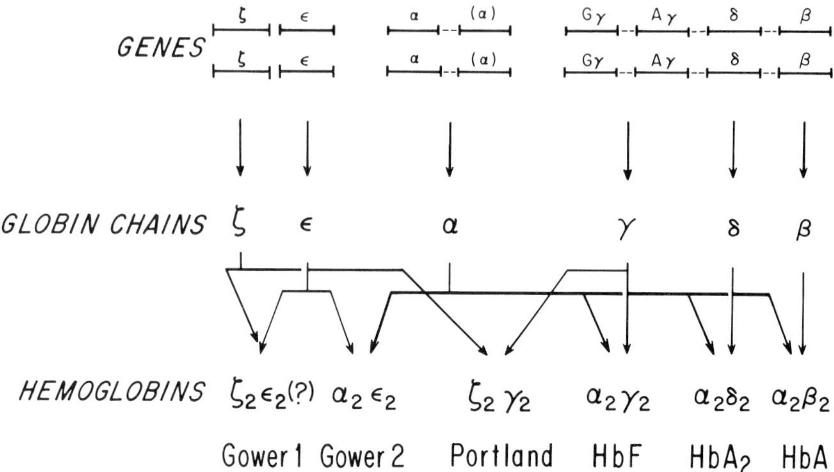

Figure 4–1. Schematic representation of the genes for the different human globin chains and their gene products.

Fetal hemoglobin, Hb F, consists of two α and two γ chains, and its appearance coincides with the shift in the site of erythropoiesis from the yolk sac to the liver and spleen. The adult hemoglobins, Hb A ($\alpha_2\beta_2$) and Hb A_2 ($\alpha_2\delta_2$), are normally the predominant hemoglobins present after the first year of life and are synthesized by erythroid precursor cells in the bone marrow. The synthesis of Hb A or Hb F is, however, not strictly limited to cells of marrow vs. liver or spleen origin. There exists at least one pair of allelic genes for each of these globin chains, as illustrated in Figure 4–1, and in the case of the α and γ globin chains there is evidence of gene duplication.

Alpha-chain Genes

Duplication of the α-chain locus has been demonstrated in many animal species, but there is still some controversy over the existence (or the incidence) of duplication of the human α-chain structural gene (Wasi, 1973). The most convincing evidence in favor of α-chain gene duplication consists of reports of families in which individuals have two different α-chain variants in addition to Hb A: (1) in a Hungarian family, three siblings were found to be heterozygous for two different α-chain variants (Hb J-Buda and Hb G-Pest) and still had approximately 50 per cent Hb A (Hollan et al., 1972); (2) in a number of individuals from a tribe in India two different α-chain variants (Hb Rampa and Hb Koya Dora) were found in addition to normal Hb A (DeJong et al., 1975); (3) red cells of an individual of black ancestry who was doubly heterozygous for the α-chain variants Hb G-Philadelphia and Hb-Seal Rock also contained Hb A (Bradley et al., 1975); (4) a presumed homozygote for the α-chain variant Hb Constant Spring also had substantial amounts of Hb A (Lie-Injo, 1974). The finding of two abnormal α chains in addition to normal α chains in heterozygotes for the α-chain variant Hopkins-2 has been used as further evidence of duplication of the human α gene (Ostertag et al., 1972b). The genetics of the α-thalassemia syndromes, especially Hb H disease (Lehmann and Carrell, 1968; Kattamis and Lehmann, 1970; Lehmann, 1970) in association with Hb Constant Spring (Wasi, 1973), also strongly support the concept of α-chain duplication without providing conclusive evidence for it. Finally, α-chain duplication is suggested by the fact that heterozygotes for most (but not all) α-chain variants have a lower percentage of the abnormal hemoglobin than do heterozygotes for β-chain structural variants (Lehmann and Carrell, 1968, 1969; White, 1972) (see Figure 6–4).

The evidence against α-chain gene duplication is the finding, in a Melanesian family, of the absence of Hb A in two homozygotes for the α-chain variant Hb J-Tongariki (Abramson et al., 1970). Three other individuals homozygous for Hb J-Tongariki have been found in New Guinea and they all lack Hb A (Beaven et al., 1972). Absence of Hb A in a patient homozygous for Hb G-Philadelphia, in Hb Q/α thalassemia (reviewed by Wasi, 1973) and in one case of Hb G/α thalassemia (Rieder et al., 1976) also favors the theory of a single α-chain locus, unless one postulates the existence of an α-thalassemia gene in cis with the α-chain variant (Wasi, 1973).

On the basis of all this evidence, one must conclude that α-chain gene duplication almost certainly occurs in some, but not necessarily all, human populations. Variations in the levels of the variant Hb present in black patients heterozygous for Hb G-Philadelphia (Baine et al., 1976) and in Algerian patients with Hb J-Mexico (Trabuchet et al., 1976) suggest, in fact, that even in individuals of the same race, there may be heterogeneity in the number of α-chain loci (see Chapter 5).

Gamma-chain Genes

The presence of at least two structural genes for the gamma chain has been established by the finding, in individuals of a number of different populations, of two types of γ chains which have either glycine or alanine in position 136 of their amino acid sequence (Schroeder et al., 1968, 1972); these two different γ chains are referred to as the $^{G}\gamma$ and $^{A}\gamma$ chains, respectively. The $^{G}\gamma$ and $^{A}\gamma$ chains are the products of different genes and not due to a post-transcriptional process, because γ-chain variants are of either the $^{G}\gamma$ or the $^{A}\gamma$ type, but not both. The ratio of $^{G}\gamma$ to $^{A}\gamma$ chains in the Hb F of cord blood of neonates is 3:1, whereas in the Hb F of adult blood it is 2:3. When increased fetal hemoglobin is present in the course of various hematological conditions in the adult, either the 3:1 or the 2:3 ratio may be found. The reason for this variable ratio is not known; it may be related to the presence of more than one copy of either or both of the γ genes or may be due to other unknown regulatory mechanisms.

Huisman, Schroeder, and their colleagues (1972a) have proposed an interesting model for the number of γ-chain genes, based on the study of the type ($^{A}\gamma$ vs. $^{G}\gamma$) and the relative proportions (% of total Hb F) of the various fetal hemoglobin structural variants (Huisman et al., 1972a; Schroeder et al., 1973). According to this model there would be four nonallelic structural genes for the γ chain: two $^{A}\gamma$ and two $^{G}\gamma$ genes, each with a different quantitative output of a gene product. These genes have been labeled $^{G}{}_{m}\gamma$, $^{G}{}_{l}\gamma$, $^{A}{}_{m}\gamma$, $^{A}{}_{l}\gamma$ (where m and l indicate *m*ore and *l*ess) or $^{G}\gamma$, $^{g}\gamma$, $^{A}\gamma$, $^{a}\gamma$ (where the capital and lower case letters indicate genes with a relatively high or low output of gene product, respectively). These genes would be arranged in the following order on the chromosome (going from N-terminal to C-terminal coding sequences of the genes, or from left to right as in Figure 4–1): $^{G}\gamma$, $^{g}\gamma$, $^{A}\gamma$, $^{a}\gamma$. If the production rate by $^{a}\gamma$ (the lowest output of the four genes) is arbitrarily given a value of one, the proportion of $^{G}\gamma$ and $^{A}\gamma$ in fetal and adult red cells may be explained by the following scheme:

		GENE			
		$^{G}{}_{m}\gamma$	$^{G}{}_{l}\gamma$	$^{A}{}_{m}\gamma$	$^{A}{}_{l}\gamma$
	or	$^{G}\gamma$	$^{g}\gamma$	$^{A}\gamma$	$^{a}\gamma$
Production in fetal cells		4	2	2	1
Production in adult cells		0	2	2	1

This model is totally arbitrary and is based on the probably erroneous assumption that the cellular content of an abnormal gene product is directly proportional to the number of genes coding for that protein. The model does, however, provide a plausible explanation for the fact that fetal red cells have a $^{G}\gamma$:$^{A}\gamma$ ratio of approximately 3:1 (70:30), whereas adult red cells have a ratio of 2:3. If it is correct, the model may prove quite useful in furthering our understanding of the fetal to adult hemoglobin "switch" and the distribution of fetal hemoglobin subtypes in hereditary persistence of fetal hemoglobin (HPFH) and thalassemia.

Chromosomal Arrangement of Human Globin Genes

The precise location of the globin-chain genes on human chromosomes is not known. There is a report of presumptive identification of the chromosomes bearing the human globin genes by means of in-situ hybridization of radioactive rabbit globin mRNA to metaphase chromosomes of human lymphocytes (Price et al., 1972). However, there are serious criticisms of the work (Bishop and Jones, 1972; Prensky and Holmquist, 1973). There is slight evidence favoring linkage of the beta (and delta) locus with the Duffy blood group locus (Nance et al., 1970), and it is known that the Duffy locus is located on chromosome No. 1 (Donahue et al., 1968). Although there is increased fetal hemoglobin associated with the D1 trisomy (trisomy 13), this is thought to result from a defect in normal fetal maturation rather than being an indication of localization of the gamma genes on chromosome 13 (Wilson et al., 1967; Bard, 1972).

Linkage studies show clearly that the α and β genes are not closely linked to each other and may even be on different chromosomes (Smith and Torbert, 1958; Wong and Huisman, 1972). Localization of α and β genes on different chromosomes has recently been confirmed by analysis of somatic cell hybrids (Deisseroth et al., 1976). However, the beta and delta genes are closely linked to one another as evidenced by the study of a number of families in which both a delta- and a beta-chain variant occur: there was no recombination, in 41 opportunities, between the two loci (Boyer et al., 1963). The occurrence of a delta-beta hybrid globin chain in Hb Lepore (Gerald and Diamond, 1958), presumably the result of a nonhomologous crossover between δ- and β-structural genes (Baglioni, 1962), also supports the close proximity of these two genes. The Lepore globin chain has the N-terminal sequence of the δ chain and the C-terminal sequence of the β chain, and in homozygotes for Hb Lepore, there is total absence of normal Hb A and Hb A_2. These findings definitively situate the δ-chain gene to the N-terminal coding side of the β-chain gene. The origin of the Lepore $\delta\beta$ chain is illustrated diagrammatically in Figure 5–3A and is discussed in detail in Chapter 6; the clinical and biochemical features of this condition are discussed in Chapter 5.

The precise location of the γ genes is not certain but there is evidence to indicate close proximity of the γ genes to the β and δ genes:

(1) In families where a β-chain structural variant (or β thalassemia) occurs in association with hereditary persistence of fetal hemoglobin (HPFH), β-chain and HPFH genes behave as alleles, indicating close linkage between the two loci (Weatherall and Clegg, 1972).

(2) In individuals homozygous for HPFH or doubly heterozygous for HPFH and a β- or δ-chain structural variant, there is no synthesis of normal β or δ chain associated with the HPFH gene (Weatherall and Clegg, 1972). This is the so-called "cis-effect," i.e., the β- and δ-chain genes in the cis position of the HPFH gene are usually totally inactive.

(3) Finally, there exists Hb Kenya, a fused $\gamma\beta$ globin chain (Huisman et al., 1972b) which has the N-terminal sequence of the γ chain and the C-terminal sequence of the β chain. The Kenya $\gamma\beta$ chain presumably resulted from nonhomologous crossing over of the γ- and β-structural genes in a manner analogous to the $\delta\beta$ crossover of Hb Lepore (see Figure 5–10 and Chapter 6). Individuals heterozygous for Hb Kenya (or doubly heterozygous for Hb Kenya and Hb S) synthesize Hb F only of the $^G\gamma$ type, presumably from the remaining intact γ-chain genes in cis to the fused Kenya $\gamma\beta$-chain gene. These findings indicate that the $^A\gamma$ gene(s) is involved (or deleted) in the crossover event and is therefore localized (perhaps, but not necessarily, with the $^G\gamma$ gene[s] as well) to the N-terminal coding side of the δ- and β-chain genes (Fig. 4–1). The clinical features of the Hb Kenya syndromes are discussed in Chapter 5.

The close proximity of the γ-, δ-, and β-chain genes on the same chromosome and the similarities in the amino acid sequences of these globin chains (10 amino acids different out of 146 between δ and β chains and 39 differences between γ and β) support the theory that the δ- and γ-chain genes may have evolved as a result of reduplication of the β-chain gene.

The location and relationship of the epsilon- and zeta-chain genes to one another and to other globin-chain genes are not known.

ONTOGENY OF HEMOGLOBIN SYNTHESIS

Changes in Hemoglobin During Development

The time of appearance and relative proportions of the various globin chains present during fetal and neonatal development are schematically represented in Figure 4–2. Alpha chains appear early and persist throughout development. Epsilon chains can be detected in the fetus from an early age but they disappear by the 10th to 12th week of gestation (Huehns et al., 1964; Lorkin, 1973) when γ chains begin to appear in large quantity. The time of onset and pattern of zeta-chain synthesis has not yet been determined in humans; its synthesis probably parallels that of ϵ chains, but it must persist at a low level in the later stages of fetal development because of the finding of trace amounts of Hb Portland-1 in normal cord blood. Alpha- and γ-chain synthesis predominates after the first 10 to 12 weeks of fetal development. A small amount of β-chain synthesis can be detected in fetuses as early as 6 to 8 weeks of gestation (Hollenberg et al., 1971; Basch, 1972; Kan et al., 1972a; Pataryas and Stamatoyannopoulos, 1972; Kazazian and Woodhead, 1973; Wood and Weatherall, 1973; Cividalli et al., 1974a). However, β chains appear in substantial amounts only near term. Studies of globin synthesis in cord blood

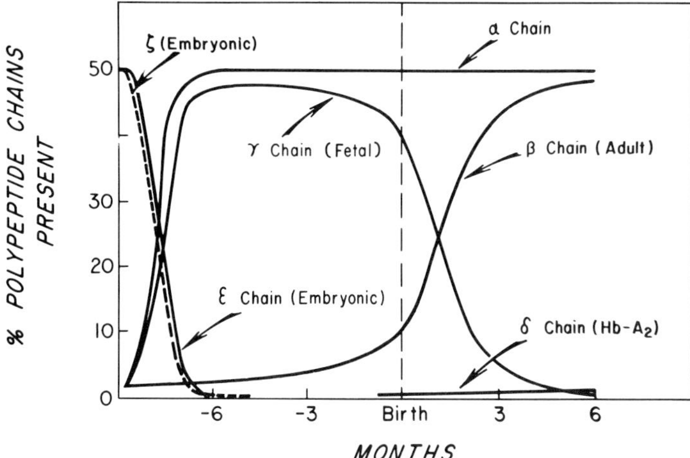

Figure 4-2. Diagrammatic representation of the changes in human globin synthesis during prenatal and neonatal development. (Modified from Beck, W. S. (ed.): Hematology. 2nd ed. Boston, MIT Press, 1976.)

(Bard et al., 1970; Kan et al., 1972b; Bard, 1975) show that there is approximately one-third to one-half as much β- as γ-chain synthesis at term. During the first 3 months of life, β-chain synthesis rapidly increases as γ-chain synthesis ceases. By 6 months of age β-chain synthesis has usually achieved its maximal adult rate, and γ-chain synthesis is normally reduced to 1 per cent or less of the total hemoglobin. This phenomenon is variable, however (Colombo et al., 1976), and in some normal children higher levels of Hb F (2 to 5 per cent) persist for 12 to 24 months (Chernoff and Singer, 1952). Delta-chain synthesis probably starts only late in the third trimester of intrauterine life, and cord blood contains only trace amounts of Hb A_2. Its synthesis increases gradually during the first 6 to 12 months of life until it reaches the normal adult level (approximately 2.5 per cent of the total hemoglobin). The reason for this low level of δ-gene expression is unknown. As will be discussed later in relation to Hb Lepore (Chapter 5), the synthesis of δ chains is active only in nucleated erythroid precursor cells and is virtually absent in reticulocytes; the cause of this phenomenon is also unexplained.

The sequence of appearance of the various globin chains is important for the understanding of the development of clinical manifestations in the thalassemia syndromes and other hemoglobinopathies. A deficiency in α-chain or γ-chain synthesis should be obvious at birth, whereas β-chain deficiency will not become clinically manifest until several months of age. Similarly, β-chain structural variants such as Hb S will not accumulate in sufficient quantities to cause clinical symptoms until the latter half of the first year of life. On the other hand, the low but measurable levels of β-chain synthesis in normal fetuses make possible the prenatal diagnosis of β-chain hemoglobinopathies before the 20th week of gestation (see Chapter 5).

There is definite physiological advantage for the developing fetus to have Hb F rather than Hb A. Hemoglobin F, because of its structure and its decreased ability to bind 2,3-DPG, has a relatively high oxygen affinity. Therefore, in the low oxygen tension environment of the placenta, Hb F can effectively compete with Hb A for its oxygen (see Chapter 3). The possible biological or physiological significance of Hb A_2 and the embryonic hemoglobins is unknown.

THE SWITCHOVER FROM FETAL TO ADULT HEMOGLOBIN SYNTHESIS

The mechanism of the "switch" from γ- to β-chain synthesis is unknown. The switch seems to be regulated more by gestational age than by the extrauterine environment, since prematurity seems to have little effect on the process (Bard, 1971, 1973). However, various forms of anoxia (Cooper and Hoagland, 1972), intrauterine growth retardation (Bard, 1970), maternal anoxia (Bromberg et al., 1956), and the D1 trisomy syndrome (Wilson et al., 1967; Bard, 1972) seem to delay the switch. The cord blood of infants with erythroblastosis fetalis contains increased amounts of Hb A compared to normal cord blood (Cooper and Hoagland, 1972; Fraser, 1972). However, this finding is not universal (Bhoyroo and Storrs, 1971), and it is not related to the actual levels of synthesis of γ and β chains by the reticulocytes of the infants: the relative amounts of Hb A and Hb F synthesized are not different from those of normal neonates of the same gestational age (Bard et al., 1971; Kan et al., 1972b). The preponderance of Hb A probably results from the destruction of the older Hb F-containing cells. Previous intrauterine transfusion (Bard et al., 1970) or exchange transfusion at birth (Fraser, 1972) does not seem to affect the relative synthesis of Hb A and Hb F at birth or during neonatal development. In normal cord blood, small amounts of Hb Bart's (γ_4) can be detected; this finding suggests that in the γ to β switching process there is some imbalance between α and $\beta + \gamma$ synthesis, with a small relative excess of γ chains produced (Weatherall, 1963). An even greater excess of γ- to α-chain synthesis has been observed during the course of fetal development in sheep (Kazazian et al., 1976).

Once the switch has occurred it is not usually reversible, although in certain medical conditions (Cooper and Hoagland, 1972; Lorkin, 1973) usually associated with some hematological stress, an increase in fetal hemoglobin is observed (see Chapter 1). In such instances the Hb F is heterogeneously distributed among the red cells and usually only a small proportion of the red cells contains significant amounts of Hb F. In the neonatal "switch" there is true reciprocal relationship between Hb A and Hb F production. However, in cases of persistence or reactivation of Hb F synthesis associated with other medical conditions, the synthesis of Hb A does not decrease proportionally, and the Hb F is accumulated as an "extra package" which increases the Hb content of the cell (Weatherall et al., 1974). In certain conditions, however, such as juvenile chronic myeloid leukemia and rare cases of erythroleukemia (Weatherall et al., 1968; Maurer et al., 1972; Weatherall et al., 1975b), there is near total reversion to a state of fetal red cell protein synthesis, with a decrease in Hb A and Hb A_2, a decrease in carbonic anhydrase and I-antigen titer, and an increase in i-antigen titer.

Changes in the types of hemoglobin synthesized during fetal development are associated with changes in the site of erythropoiesis. Embryonic hemoglobins are presumably synthesized in cells of yolk sac origin; fetal hemoglobin is synthesized when erythropoiesis is maximal in liver and spleen but adult hemoglobin synthesis increases when erythropoiesis shifts from liver and spleen to bone marrow. However, there is no evidence that the type of hemoglobin synthesized by an erythroid cell is strictly determined by the site or organ of its origin. In fact, fetal and adult hemoglobins are both present in many neonatal red cells (Shepard et al., 1962; Tomada, 1964). Furthermore, the ratio of Hb F to Hb A synthesis is the same in fetal erythroid cells derived from marrow, liver, and spleen at all stages of development (Wood and Weatherall, 1973). When extramedullary hematopoiesis develops in the adult there is rarely a significant amount of fetal hemoglobin synthesis. Furthermore, when increased fetal hemoglobin synthesis occurs in the course of various hematological disorders, there is rarely any associated extramedullary hematopoiesis. Another striking example of the lack of site specificity of fetal hemoglobin synthesis is the finding that in leukemic patients recovering from chemotherapy and in patients receiving homologous adult bone marrow transplants, there is an initial burst of fetal hemoglobin synthesis by the regenerating or engrafted marrow cells which then switches to Hb A synthesis (Alter et al., 1975; Weatherall et al., 1975b).

The finding of increased maternal synthesis of fetal hemoglobin during pregnancy (Pembrey et al., 1973) suggests the possible role of a humoral factor in the control and maintenance of fetal hemoglobin synthesis. There is, however, no definitive information on the possible nature of this putative humoral factor or its origin from either fetus, mother, or placenta. The maternal synthesis of Hb F occurs as a short burst for a few weeks in the first trimester and accounts for approximately 5 per cent of total Hb synthesis during that time; it coincides with the time of peak excretion of human chorionic gonadotropin (Pembrey et al., 1973).

The role of erythropoietin in the control of fetal erythropoiesis and the Hb A→Hb F switch remains controversial. No definite role has been demonstrated for erythropoietin in the activation of neonatal Hb A synthesis. It is generally agreed that yolk sac erythroid cells are insensitive to erythropoietin. However, fetal liver erythroid cells are responsive to the hormone. In humans, fetal liver erythroid cells do show sensitivity to erythropoietin in short-term culture systems (Basch, 1972; Shchory and Weatherall, 1975). The degree of responsiveness varies with the fetal age, but no change in the ratio of Hb A to Hb F synthesis in vitro was observed as a result of the erythropoietin stimulation (Basch, 1972). Nevertheless, erythropoietin can be detected in vivo in blood, urine, and amniotic fluid of human fetuses in the third trimester, and these levels are increased in hypoxic and hemolytic states (Finne and Halvorsen, 1972). These findings suggest that erythropoietin may play a role in the regulation of erythropoiesis in the third trimester of intrauterine life, although its role in the Hb F to Hb A switch remains to be demonstrated.

In sheep and goats, the induction of fetal anemia will result in an increase in erythropoietin levels in the fetuses, probably from an extrarenal source (Zanjani et al., 1974a). Furthermore, the administration of antierythropoietin serum results in suppression of erythropoiesis in fetal sheep (Zanjani et al., 1974b). Bleeding of fetal sheep can actually cause premature activation of the fetal to adult switch (Kazazian et al., 1976) but it is not known if this effect is directly mediated by erythropoietin.

A different type of hemoglobin switching phenomenon in goats and sheep is, however, directly mediated by erythropoietin: the Hb A to Hb C switch which occurs in certain types of sheep and goats when they are made anemic (Blunt and Evans, 1963; Van Vliet and Huisman, 1964). The change of Hb type under the stress of anemia is associated with suppression of the synthesis of β^A chains of Hb A and activation of synthesis of another globin chain, the β^C chain of Hb C, which is different from the non-α chain of ovine fetal Hb (Boyer et al., 1967; Wilson et al., 1966). This phenomenon has been conclusively shown to be mediated by erythropoietin (Thurmon et al., 1970; Adamson and Stamatoyannopoulos, 1973). The switch operates at the level of individual cells and not at a clonal level, since both Hb A and Hb C can be detected in the same red cells (Garrick et al., 1973; Nienhuis and Bunn, 1974). This phenomenon does not represent a true fetal to adult (or adult to fetal) switch but it does provide an experimental system for the study of molecular mechanisms involved in the process of differential globin gene expression.

Another consideration in the control of switching from γ- to β-chain synthesis is whether the γ- and β-chain genes on the same chromosome are active at the same time. Even though neonatal cells individually contain both Hb F and Hb A, it is not known with certainty if all the cells' γ- and β-chain genes are active simultaneously or whether γ-chain synthesis and β-chain synthesis are each specified by a different chromosome. This problem was studied by Kabat (1974) in red cells from neonates heterozygous for Hb S ($\alpha_2\beta_2{}^S$). He found that individual red cells of these infants probably contain either Hb A + Hb S, Hb A + Hb F, or Hb S + Hb F, but not all three hemoglobins simultaneously. He concluded that it is unlikely that γ- and β-chain genes on the same chromosome are simultaneously active in the neonatal period. One can, however, question the sensitivity of the cytological methods used to detect the various hemoglobins. It is possible that very small quantities of a given type of hemoglobin could be present in a given cell but go undetected by purely cytological techniques. Even if this were the case, however, the results still indicate that the majority of the red cells in AS neonates do not contain substantial amounts of all three possible hemoglobins (A, S, and F).

Yet another issue in the fetal to adult hemoglobin switch is the nature of the low level (1 per cent) of Hb F synthesis observed in normal adults. Do most red cells synthesize very low levels of Hb F, or do small numbers of red cells synthesize the bulk of Hb F? Boyer et al. (1975) and Wood et al. (1975) have studied this phenomenon using sensitive immunochemical techniques. The results indicate that normal adults contain small numbers of cells which show substantial immunofluorescence using anti-Hb F antibodies, whereas most cells show no fluorescence. These findings suggest that adult synthesis of Hb F is limited to a small clone of cells. Such fetal clones could expand in response to various hematological stresses.

In hereditary persistence of fetal hemoglobin (HPFH) the fetal to adult hemoglobin switchover does not occur. The red cells of adult black patients homozygous for this disorder contain 100 per cent Hb F. The complete absence of Hb A (and Hb A_2) in such homozygotes indicates that the defect is not simply a failure of switching over from the low levels (10 per cent) of Hb A synthesis in utero to the adult levels; there is a total lack of expression of the affected β (and δ) globin gene. In fact, this condition has been shown, in black homozygotes, to be associated with a β-globin gene deletion (Kan et al., 1975d; Forget et al., 1976b). HPFH is, however, genetically and biochemically heterogeneous: in some cases, β-chain synthesis in cis to the HPFH gene has been observed (see Chapter 5). Although most cases of HPFH synthesize both ${}^A\gamma$ and ${}^G\gamma$ chains in the usual *adult* ratio, cases have been described in which only ${}^G\gamma$ or ${}^A\gamma$ chains are synthesized. The genetic, clinical, and biochemical findings observed in HPFH will be discussed in more detail in Chapter 5.

In conclusion, we know very little about the precise molecular mechanisms which are involved in the fetal to adult hemoglobin switch in humans. Better knowledge of these mechanisms is of great practical as well as theoretical interest, because the ability to manipulate and preserve γ-chain synthesis into adult life might provide an effective future means of treatment of β thalassemia and other β-chain hemoglobinopathies such as sickle cell anemia.

GLOBIN-CHAIN BIOSYNTHESIS

Mechanism of Polypeptide-Chain Synthesis

The major steps involved in protein synthesis are illustrated schematically in Figure 4–3 and pertain to the synthesis of globin as well as of any other polypeptide chain. The genetic information for the structure of a given protein is encoded in the nucleotide sequence of the DNA, which makes up a gene located on a chromosome within the cell nucleus. Each amino acid is specified by a

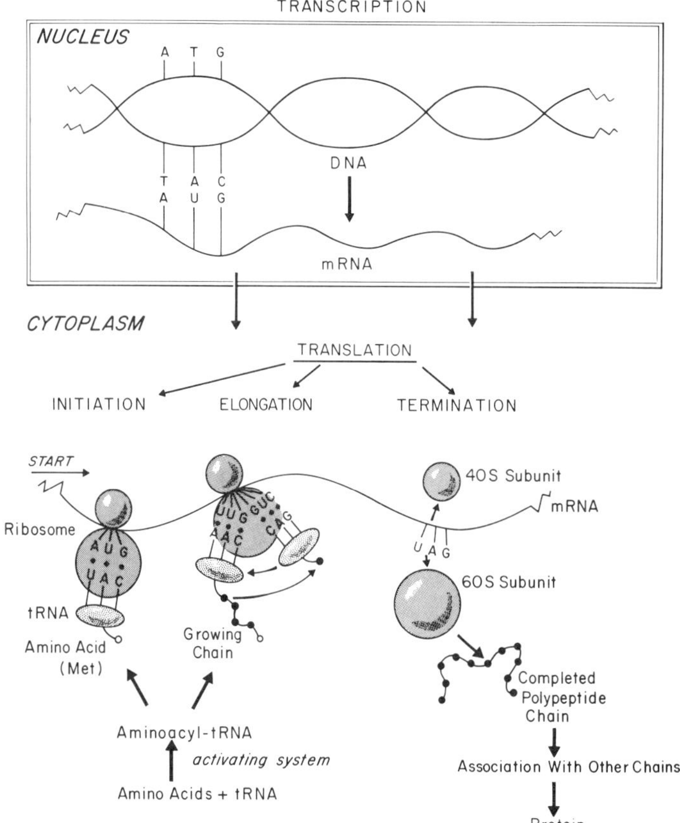

Figure 4–3. Schematic representation of the mechanism of polypeptide-chain biosynthesis.

TABLE 4–1. *The Messenger RNA Codons for the Various Amino Acids**

Alanine	*Arginine*	*Asparagine*	*Aspartic acid*	*Cysteine*
GCU	CGU	AAU	GAU	UGU
GCC	CGC	AAC	GAC	UGC
GCA	CGA			
GCG	CGG			
	AGA			
	AGG			
Glutamic acid	*Glutamine*	*Glycine*	*Histidine*	*Isoleucine*
GAA	CAA	GGU	CAU	AUU
GAG	CAG	GGC	CAC	AUC
		GGA		AUA
		GGG		
Leucine	*Lysine*	*Methionine*	*Phenylalanine*	*Proline*
UUA	AAA	AUG	UUU	CCU
UUG	AAG		UUC	CCC
CUU				CCA
CUC				CCG
CUA				
CUG				
Serine	*Threonine*	*Tryptophan*	*Tyrosine*	*Valine*
UCU	ACU	UGG	UAU	GUU
UCC	ACC		UAC	GUC
UCA	ACA			GUA
UCG	ACG			GUG
AGU				
AGC				

SPECIAL CODONS

Chain initiation	*Chain termination (nonsense codons)*
AUG	UAA
	UAG
	UGA

*Adapted from Watson, 1970. The first letter shown for each triplet codon represents the 5′ extremity of the mRNA codon. Note that AUG serves both as chain initiation codon and as methionine codon.

sequence of three nucleotide bases, called a codon (Table 4–1). A given amino acid can be specified by many different codons, but each codon is specific for only one amino acid and for a different specific transfer RNA (tRNA) molecule necessary for transporting that amino acid. The genetic information is relayed to the cytoplasm of the cell, where protein synthesis must occur, by the synthesis of a strand of RNA called messenger RNA, or mRNA. The mRNA is complementary to, or the mirror image of, the DNA according to Watson-Crick base pairing (C gives G, A gives U, G gives C, and T gives A). The synthesis of mRNA from DNA by the enzyme RNA polymerase is called the process of transcription.

The mRNA is then transported from the nucleus to the cytoplasm where it binds to ribosomes, which are the subcellular organelles on which protein synthesis occurs. The following process by which the mRNA directs the synthesis of a specific polypeptide chain is called translation, and it involves a number of different steps. The initial step of mRNA binding to ribosomes is called initiation: it is a complex enzymatic reaction which brings together the mRNA; the smaller (40S) ribosomal subunit; a special initiator tRNA, which carries the amino acid methionine; and the larger (60S) ribosomal subunit. The reaction requires a number of separate protein factors (initiation factors), GTP, and ATP. In mammalian systems, just as in bacterial systems, the first amino acid incorporated into a protein chain is methionine, but contrary to the bacterial systems this initial amino acid does not have a blocked (formylated) amino group and it is later cleaved from the nascent polypeptide chain during its elongation. The completed mammalian polypeptide chain, therefore, does not necessarily have an N-terminal methionine.

Once initiated, the synthesis of a protein chain continues by the process of elongation, which involves the sequential addition of amino acids to the initial amino acid by peptide bond formation, resulting in gradual lengthening of the polypeptide chain. Protein synthesis begins at the N-terminal amino acid residue and proceeds toward the C-terminal residue of the polypeptide chain. Each amino acid is brought to its specific position by a specific tRNA to which it is attached (the complex is called aminoacyl-tRNA). The aminoacyl-tRNA binds to the ribosome and the specific codon sequence of the mRNA by a complementary nucleotide sequence of its own, called the anticodon, which is located in a specific site of the tRNA. The nascent peptide chain which is attached to the previous tRNA is transferred to the new tRNA, and a peptide bond is formed with the new amino acid. This new peptidyl-tRNA complex then moves to the position of the previous tRNA, which is released as the ribosome moves along to the next codon. A new aminoacyl-tRNA binds to this new codon, and the process is repeated. This process involves a complex set of reactions which involve many enzyme factors and GTP. Chain elongation continues until the ribosome, traveling down the messenger RNA in "ticker-tape" fashion, reaches a specific nucleotide codon which signifies chain termination, at which time the polypeptide chain is released from the ribosome which dissociates into two subunits and separates from the mRNA. The polypeptide chain then assumes its secondary and tertiary structure and may bind to other polypeptide subunits and other cellular components to form a mature protein. The details of this complicated process of eukaryotic protein synthesis have recently been reviewed (Benz and Forget, 1974).

The synthesis of globin is accomplished by this same basic

mechanism. In fact, much of the process of eukaryotic protein synthesis was elucidated by the study of globin-synthesizing cells and cell-free systems. Once synthesized, the globin chains bind heme and combine with one another to form appropriate tetramers of complete hemoglobin molecules. In the following sections we will discuss the details in the process of protein synthesis which specifically apply to the mechanism and control of globin-chain synthesis itself.

Control of Globin Gene Transcription and Globin mRNA Synthesis

With very few exceptions to be discussed later, the types and amounts of globin chains synthesized by erythroid cells are determined by the nature and amount of globin-chain mRNA present in that cell. The cell therefore controls globin-chain synthesis primarily by regulating the transcription of globin gene DNA into its specific complementary mRNA.

The specific factors responsible for the activation and suppression of globin gene transcription are not known. However, some of the details of globin mRNA biogenesis are known and do shed some light on the nature of the process of transcription. Transcription of chromatin isolated from nuclei of various tissues has been studied in cell-free systems by a number of laboratories. Nuclear chromatin consists of DNA (and some RNA) associated with various histone and nonhistone chromosomal proteins. The products of cell-free chromatin transcription appear to be tissue specific: globin mRNA sequences can be detected by RNA-DNA hybridization assays in transcription products of erythroid cell chromatin but not in those of nonerythroid (liver) cell chromatin (Axel et al., 1973; Gilmour and Paul, 1973; Anderson et al., 1974; Barrett et al., 1974; Steggles et al., 1974). These results indicate that the globin gene DNA is somehow exposed and available for transcription by RNA polymerase in erythroid cell chromatin but not in liver cell chromatin.

The factors responsible for specificity of chromatin transcription have been analyzed by fractionation and reconstitution experiments mixing the various constituents of chromatin from different tissues. These experiments have indicated that the acidic nonhistone protein components of chromatin are responsible for the specificity of sequences transcribed: DNA and histones from liver or brain cell chromatin reconstituted with nonhistone acidic proteins from erythroid cell chromatin will yield globin mRNA transcripts in the cell-free system (Paul et al., 1973; Barrett et al., 1974; Chiu et al., 1975). The details of how these proteins might exert their control on DNA transcription are not known. The relevance and specificity of these observations with respect to the transcription process in intact cells are also uncertain, because the in-vitro chromatin transcription products are much smaller in size (length) than the physiologic DNA transcripts (heterogeneous nuclear RNA) of intact cells. In fact, the in-vitro chromatin transcripts are even shorter than the mature cytoplasmic mRNA. There is, however, evidence that chromatin-bound proteins do play a role in regulating transcription in intact cells: in transcriptionally active chromatin of erythroid cells, a defined portion (20 per cent) of the globin gene is specifically covered by protein, whereas in inactive chromatin, the globin gene DNA is randomly covered by protein (Axel et al., 1975).

Like other eukaryotic mRNA's, globin mRNA does not appear to be initially synthesized from globin gene DNA in its final form or size. Most eukaryotic mRNA's are initially synthesized in the form of a very high molecular weight RNA (5,500 to 50,000 nucleotides long), called heterogeneous nuclear RNA (HnRNA) (Darnell et al., 1973). Only a small portion of the HnRNA molecule contains mRNA specific sequences. Mature cytoplasmic mRNA is much smaller (up to 10 times smaller) than the HnRNA, and the bulk of the HnRNA is rapidly turned over or degraded in the cell nucleus (Darnell et al., 1973). There is some evidence that globin mRNA might arise from HnRNA. A number of laboratories have reported studies showing that HnRNA isolated from nucleated avian or murine erythroid cells can be translated into globin in various protein synthesizing systems (Ruiz-Carillo et al., 1973; Williamson et al., 1973; Knöchel and Tiedemann, 1975), and that erythroid cell HnRNA contains globin mRNA sequences detectable by hybridization of the HnRNA to globin-specific synthetic radioactive RNA ("antimessenger" RNA) (Melli and Pemberton, 1972) or DNA (cDNA) (Imaizumi et al., 1973; Scherrer, 1973). The radioactive complementary DNA is cDNA, which is synthesized from purified globin mRNA by the RNA-dependent DNA polymerase, or reverse transcriptase, of avian myeloblastosis virus (Kacian et al., 1972; Ross et al., 1972a; Verma et al., 1972). The critics of this work, however, point out that the results could be explained by the presence of small amounts of aggregated mature globin mRNA which co-migrates with (or is noncovalently bound to) heavy molecular weight HnRNA (Lane et al., 1973; Macnaughton et al., 1974). The proponents of globin HnRNA, on the other hand, claim that their RNA is prepared in conditions of total RNA denaturation which prevent RNA aggregation (Imaizumi et al., 1973; Ruiz-Carrillo et al., 1973). The matter remains the subject of debate and a definitive conclusion cannot yet be drawn.

In the case of human erythroid cells, globin mRNA sequences have been detected by RNA-cDNA hybridization assays in HnRNA isolated from human fetal liver and adult marrow erythroid cells

(Lanyon et al., 1975). The average length of these HnRNA molecules was 6000 nucleotides, or roughly 10 times the length of mature cytoplasmic globin mRNA. The HnRNA from adult marrow cells lacked significant amounts of γ-mRNA sequences while containing the expected amounts of β-chain sequences. If these results are not due to aggregates of mature mRNA (see above), then they indicate that, although the γ- and β-chain genes are situated close to one another on the same chromosome, the precursor to β mRNA is not a polycistronic mRNA initially containing γ-mRNA sequences which are subsequently cleaved and turned over by some post-transcriptional process. The evidence would support the concept of independent control mechanisms for the transcription of the γ-, δ-, and β-chain genes. These experiments also provide some insight into the possible intergene distance between the γ and β loci: it might be at least 5000 to 5500 nucleotides, a distance at least 8 to 10 times greater than the length of the individual γ- and β-chain structural loci themselves.

Little is known of the process by which the putative globin HnRNA becomes mature globin mRNA. In the case of other eukaryotic mRNA's, an important step in the processing of the HnRNA is the addition of poly(A) sequences to the 3′ terminus of the HnRNA (Darnell et al., 1973). If this addition of poly(A) is blocked by the inhibitor cordycepin (3′-deoxyadenosine), newly synthesized mRNA will not appear in the cytoplasmic polyribosomes, even though HnRNA synthesis is not inhibited. When the mRNA-poly(A) sequence is cleaved from the bulk of the HnRNA, it becomes associated with proteins and is transported from nucleus to cytoplasm. These processes are illustrated schematically in Figure 4–4.

In the case of globin mRNA specifically, the details of intranuclear processing of HnRNA are not known. However, globin mRNA does contain a poly(A) sequence at its 3′ terminus (see Cytoplasmic Globin Messenger RNA).

In the case of avian globin mRNA, there is evidence that the mature globin mRNA is not initially cleaved from the HnRNA in its final form or size. A number of intermediate-sized presumptive globin mRNA precursors have been identified in avian erythroid cells (Maroun et al., 1971; Scherrer, 1973; Macnaughton et al., 1974; Spohr et al., 1974). These globin mRNA precursors exist largely in the form of complexes of mRNA and protein (mRNP particles) which may represent intermediate stages in the transport process (Scherrer, 1973).

Disorders or abnormalities in any of these processes—poly(A) adenylation of HnRNA, cleavage or processing of HnRNA, association of mRNA precursors to proteins, processing and transport of precursor mRNP particles, etc.—could conceivably result in distur-

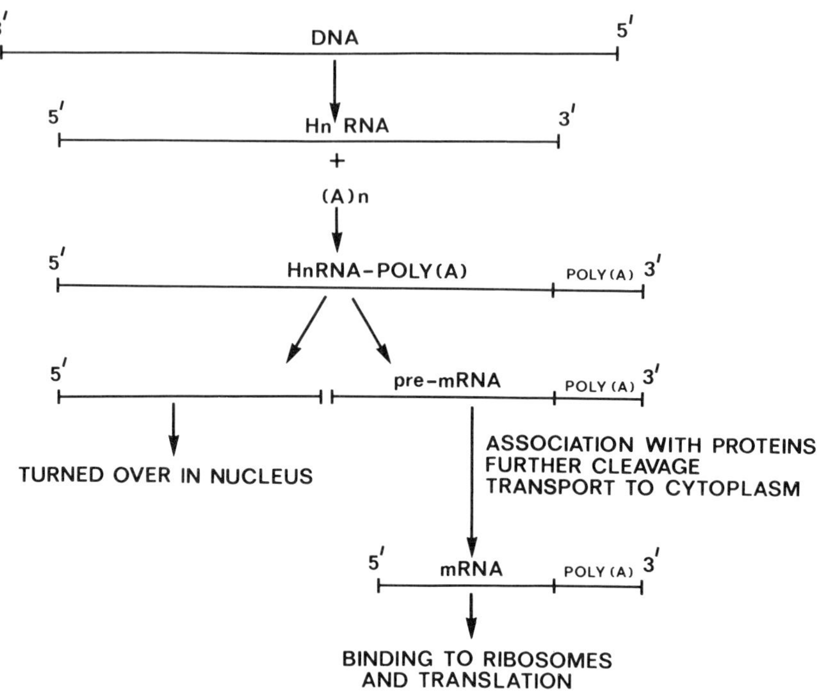

Figure 4–4. Schematic representation of the biosynthesis of globin messenger RNA. (From Benz, E. J., and Forget, B. G.: Sem. Hematol. *11*:463, 1974.)

bances in the delicate control of globin mRNA biogenesis and availability.

Finally, one hypothetical mechanism for the control of globin gene expression in erythroid cells could be gene reiteration or "amplification," with a resulting increase in mRNA output because of increased "gene dosage." Studies of gene quantitation using RNA-DNA hybridization techniques, however, have revealed no evidence of gene reiteration or increase in number of globin genes in erythroid cell DNA compared to nonerythroid cell DNA (Bishop et al., 1972, 1973; Harrison et al., 1972; Packman et al., 1972). Quantitation of human globin genes in DNA isolated from liver and spleen also reveals a limited number of globin genes (Gambino et al., 1974; Ottolenghi et al., 1974, 1975; Taylor et al., 1974; Ramirez et al., 1975b). The remarkable production of globin mRNA by erythroid cells is therefore not the result of gene amplification.

Cytoplasmic Globin Messenger RNA

Like other eukaryotic messenger RNA's, mature cytoplasmic globin mRNA is larger than one would predict if the mRNA contained only the minimal information required to code for the amino acid sequences of the globin chains. Globin mRNA has been isolated from reticulocytes of a number of animal species including man (Benz and Forget, 1971; Nienhuis and Anderson, 1971; Metafora et al., 1972). Its size is rather uniform, corresponding to a sedimentation coefficient of 9 to 10S and a molecular weight of 200,000 to 220,000 (Gould and Hamlyn, 1973; Berns et al., 1974; Kazazian et al., 1974; Morrison et al., 1974; Shearman et al., 1974; Forget et al., 1975a; Hamlyn and Gould, 1975; Kazazian et al., 1975). An mRNA molecule of this size must contain about 650 to 670 nucleotides, roughly 30 per cent more than the 429 and 444 residues (including initiation and termination codons) necessary to code for the globin chains, which contain 141 amino acids (α chains) or 146 amino acids (most non-α chains). The mRNA, therefore, contains untranslated nucleotide sequences (see Figure 6–3), the functions of which remain obscure. Possibly, these untranslated sequences are required for the establishment of the proper coding phase or frame of the mRNA; the maintenance of the conformation (secondary structure) of the mRNA; or the control of other processes such as the transport of mRNA from nucleus to cytoplasm, the binding of the mRNA to various proteins to form ribonucleoprotein particles (mRNP), the binding of the mRNA to ribosomes, etc. It is possible by polyacrylamide-gel electrophoresis in the presence of the denaturing agent formamide to separate α from β mRNA in human as well as mouse and rabbit mRNA (Gould and Hamlyn, 1973; Berns et al., 1974; Kazazian et al., 1974; Morrison et al., 1974; Shearman et al., 1974; Forget et al., 1975a; Hamlyn and Gould, 1975; Kazazian et al., 1975). The α mRNA migrates more rapidly and is therefore smaller than the β mRNA. By this technique one can accurately estimate the molecular weights of the individual mRNA's: the values obtained for rabbit globin mRNA's are 200,000 for α mRNA and 220,000 for β mRNA (Hamlyn and Gould, 1975). Forget et al. (1975a) and Kazazian et al. (1975) have observed a similar difference in the size of human α and β globin mRNA. This difference (approximately 50 base residues) is greater than can be attributed solely to the five additional codons which the β mRNA must contain to give a β chain of 146 amino acids (vs. the 141 amino acids coded for by α mRNA). The β-chain mRNA, by virtue of its size, must therefore contain more untranslated nucleotide sequences than the α-chain mRNA. The human γ-chain mRNA migrates more rapidly than the β mRNA in formamide-acrylamide gels and is therefore presumably shorter than β mRNA, even though it codes for the same number of amino acids (146) (Forget et al., 1975a; Kazazian et al., 1975).

A portion, but not all, of the untranslated sequences of globin mRNA can be accounted for by a poly(A) sequence which is situated at the 3′ terminus of the mRNA (Lim and Canellakis, 1970; Burr and Lingrel, 1971). Poly(A) sequences are virtually a universal finding in eukaryotic mRNA's. Most nonglobin mRNA's contain poly(A) sequences of roughly 200 base residues situated at their extreme 3′ terminus (for a general review, see Darnell et al., 1973). However, in cytoplasmic globin mRNA's the poly(A) sequence is not nearly so long. Globin mRNA from mouse reticulocytes contains a poly(A) sequence of only 50 to 70 base residues (Morrison et al., 1973; Gorski et al., 1974; Mansbridge et al., 1974). Although the size of the poly(A) in globin mRNA appears to be heterogeneous, there is no evidence that the α or β mRNA's differ significantly in the size of their poly(A), either in human globin mRNA (Cann et al., 1974) or in mouse globin mRNA (Gorski et al., 1974; Mansbridge et al., 1974).

In nucleated duck reticulocytes, the poly(A) segment of newly synthesized globin mRNA is approximately 150 nucleotides long (Pemberton and Baglioni, 1972). This newly synthesized mRNA, however, is longer (280,000 M.W. or 866 nucleotides) than the stable polysomal duck globin mRNA (210,000 M.W. or 650 nucleotides), and it has been suggested that the poly(A) segment in duck globin mRNA may become shorter with age (Pemberton and Baglioni, 1973), just as it does in other nonglobin mRNA's (Braverman, 1973; Sheiness and Darnell, 1973). Newly synthesized mouse globin mRNA also has a longer poly(A) segment than the steady-state mRNA, and this poly(A) presumably becomes shorter with age (Gorski et al., 1975; Merkel et al., 1975).

As previously noted, the poly(A) sequence found in mature mRNA's is not transcribed directly from the cell's DNA. It is initially added to the HnRNA as a post-transcriptional event, presumably one base residue at a time (Darnell et al., 1973). The precise function of poly(A) is not known. As we discussed previously, there is considerable evidence that poly(A) may be required for the processing of HnRNA to mRNA, and/or transport of mRNP from nucleus to cytoplasm (Darnell et al., 1973). In the case of globin mRNA, the poly(A) does not appear to be essential for the translation of the mRNA: removal of the poly(A) from globin mRNA by enzymatic digestion does not eliminate its capacity to direct protein synthesis in a cell-free system (Humphries et al., 1974; Sippel et al., 1974; Soreq et al., 1974; Williamson et al., 1974). It is possible, however, that the poly(A) may have a function in maintaining the stability of the mRNA: the activity of globin mRNA from which the poly(A) has been removed appears to decay more rapidly than that of normal globin mRNA, when preincubated in a cell-free lysate (Sippel et al., 1974) or when injected into frog oocytes which normally translate added globin mRNA for very long periods of time (Huez et al., 1974; Marbaix et al., 1975).

The poly(A) segment cannot account for the entire untranslated portion of the 650- to 670-nucleotide–long globin mRNA. When the 50 to 70 bases of the poly(A) region are added to the 430 to 440 residues required to code for the amino acids of the globin chains, there are still 150 to 170 bases unaccounted for. At least 93 of these normally untranslated nucleotides in human α-chain mRNA must be situated near the 3′ extremity of the mRNA in order to account for the mutant α chain of Hb Constant Spring (Clegg et al., 1971b; Milner et al., 1971). This α chain contains 31 extra amino acids at its C-terminal end. As previously stated, the C-terminal portion of a polypeptide is encoded by the region of mRNA near the 3′ terminus of the molecule. The α chain of Hb Constant Spring probably arose from a mutation of a termination codon (UAA or UAG) to a codon (CAA or CAG) specifying the amino acid glutamine (see Chapter 6). Such a phenomenon would permit the translation of normally untranslated sequences of the mRNA until a new termination codon were encountered. In addition, a number of other α- and β-chain variants with elongated C-terminal extremities have presumably arisen by various mutations which allow the translation of normally untranslated 3′ terminal globin mRNA sequences (see Chapter 6).

Direct nucleotide sequence analysis of human globin mRNA (Forget et al., 1974b; Marotta et al., 1974) has revealed a number of untranslated nucleotide sequences of the mRNA, but it is not yet known precisely how many nucleotides are present on the 5′ side or on the 3′ side of the structural region of the mRNA. Proudfoot and Brownlee (1974) have studied the 3′ untranslated sequences of rabbit globin mRNA immediately adjacent to the poly(A). They have identified similar 3′ terminal sequences both in rabbit α and β globin mRNA's and in mouse immunoglobin L-chain mRNA. A particular sequence or secondary structure (or loop) in this region of the mRNA may be a common feature for many mRNA's: perhaps a recognition site for the enzyme which adds poly(A) to the HnRNA, or a signal for the cessation of transcription (Proudfoot and Brownlee, 1974; Proudfoot and Brownlee, 1976a). In the case of rabbit α mRNA (Proudfoot and Brownlee, 1976b), there are 16 nucleotides between the poly(A) and a sequence which is homologous with the amino acid sequence of the C-terminal end of the human α-Constant Spring chain. Similar observations have been made in the case of human α mRNA (Proudfoot and Brownlee, 1976a); these findings indicate that, at least in the case of α-chain mRNA, the bulk of the untranslated sequences (112 nucleotides, including termination codon) are situated to the 3′ terminal side of the structural gene information. There would be only 30 to 50 nucleotides, at most, on the 5′ terminal side of the initiation codon of the α mRNA.

Most of the cytoplasmic globin mRNA in erythroid cells is found attached to polyribosomes which are actively synthesizing globin. However, mRNA has been isolated from ribosome-free supernatant fractions prepared by ultracentrifugation. Ribosome-free cytoplasmic mRNA does not exist in erythroid cells as a naked strand of RNA. Virtually all the globin mRNA which is not bound to polyribosomes is complexed to specific proteins to form mRNA-protein complexes known as messenger ribonucleoprotein particles (mRNP) (Williamson, 1973). Globin mRNP isolated directly from postribosomal supernatant has a sedimentation coefficient of approximately 15S in mammalian anucleate reticulocytes (Bonanou-Tzedaki et al., 1972; Gianni et al., 1972; Jacobs-Lorena and Baglioni, 1972, 1973; Olsen et al., 1972) or 20S in nucleated avian reticulocytes (Gander et al., 1973; Scherrer, 1973). The mammalian globin mRNP's contain almost pure α-chain-specific mRNA; non-α chain globin mRNA constitutes 10 per cent or less of the mRNA in these mRNP's (Bonanou-Tzedaki et al., 1972; Gianni et al., 1972; Jacobs-Lorena and Baglioni, 1972, 1973).

Unlike mammalian globin mRNP's, the RNA of the avian mRNP programs the synthesis of all the duck globin chains rather than only α chains (Spohr et al., 1972; Gander et al., 1973). The avian 20S mRNP contains five to seven discrete proteins attached to a molecule of 9 to 10S globin mRNA, and some of the proteins are phosphorylated (Gander et al., 1973). The intact avian 20S mRNP is inactive in terms of its ability to serve as a template for protein synthesis (Scherrer, 1973) but the mRNA moiety of the mRNP is quite active if it is first released from the protein component (Spohr et al., 1972; Gander et al., 1973). Scherrer (1973) has suggested that the avian 20S mRNP represents a "masked message," that is, messenger RNA which is reversibly inactivated due to the specific proteins which are bound to it. The extent and location of the phosphorylated groups on the mRNP proteins may play a role in the masking-unmasking reactions.

When polyribosomes are treated with EDTA or pyrophosphate, a second type of mRNP particle is released from the polyribosomes. These 14 to 15S "polysomal mRNP" particles contain polysomal 10S globin mRNA bound to two major specific proteins of different molecular weight (Lebleu et al., 1971; Morel et al., 1971; Blobel, 1972), although other minor protein components can also be detected (Morel et al., 1973). These polysomal mRNP proteins appear to be different from the proteins contained in free cytoplasmic mRNP (Gander et al., 1973; Scherrer, 1973) and in nuclear RNP (Lukanidin et al., 1971; Morel et al., 1971). This finding has prompted the suggestion that the mRNA must exchange proteins before or during the process by which free cytoplasmic mRNP transfers mRNA to the ribosome (Scherrer, 1973). The 14 to 15S polysomal mRNP appears to be indistinguishable from deproteinized polysomal globin mRNA in terms of its ability to bind ribosomes (Pragnell and Arnstein, 1970; Lebleu et al., 1971; Nudel et al., 1973) or to promote globin synthesis in cell-free systems (Lingrel et al., 1971; Sampson et al., 1972; Nudel et al., 1973; Ernst and Arnstein, 1975).

The functions of the various proteins bound to globin mRNA are not understood. None of the soluble protein initiation factors required for mRNA translation appear to be included in the protein components of the mRNP (Nudel et al., 1973). One of the mRNP proteins seems to be specifically bound to the poly(A) segment of certain nonglobin mRNA's (Kwan and Braverman, 1972; Blobel, 1973). This protein may play a role in protecting the poly(A) and the mRNA from degradation by maintaining a particular type of secondary structure of the mRNA. At least in the case of avian polyribosome-derived mRNP's, the poly(A) segment of the globin mRNA appears to be bound to mRNP proteins (Favre et al., 1975). However, examination of globin mRNP's by electron microscopy also reveals concentrations of protein at other specific points along the RNA molecule (Dubochet et al., 1973; Morel et al., 1973). The possibility that mRNP's represent mere nonspecific interactions between RNA and proteins is quite unlikely. These mRNP particles probably represent true physiologic elements involved in the handling of cytoplasmic mRNA, the selection of specific classes of mRNA for translation, or the protection of mRNA's from degradation by ribonucleases.

Translation of Globin mRNA and its Control

In general the amounts of α and β globin chains synthesized depend on the amounts of α and β globin mRNA present in the cell. There is little evidence for control of the bulk of cellular α or β globin chain synthesis by "translational control" of the mRNA, i.e., differential control of α or β mRNA translation by various cellular factors or processes. The general mechanism of polypeptide-chain synthesis has been previously outlined (see Ontogeny of Hemoglobin Synthesis and Figure 4–3). The details of this complicated process have been recently reviewed in detail (Benz and Forget, 1974). The process is the same for globin as for other proteins. We will discuss here only those features which are specific for globin synthesis and which may be important for its control.

As previously noted, the synthesis of globin chains, like that of other polypeptide chains, is initiated by the insertion of methionine at the N terminus of the nascent peptide chain (Housman et al., 1970; Jackson and Hunter, 1970; Shafritz and Anderson, 1970; Wilson and Dintzis, 1970; Yoshida et al., 1970). The methionine is coded for by the universal initiation codon of mRNA's AUG, and it is brought to the initiation complex by a specific initiator, transfer RNA ($tRNA_F^{Met}$). The N-terminal methionine is not present, however, in completed globin chains, and it has been demonstrated that it is cleaved from the growing peptide chain when it is 15 to 30 amino acids long (Yoshida et al., 1970; Yoshida and Lin, 1972). Specific enzymes capable of cleaving methionine from nascent globin chains have been identified (Yoshida and Lin, 1972). In the case of human reticulocytes, there is a higher proportion of N-terminal methionine in nascent α and β chains than in rabbit reticulocytes (Suzuki and Itano, 1973a, 1973b). This finding suggests a species difference in this enzymatic processing step or differences in uniformity of elongation or folding of nascent globin chains. The same phenomenon is observed whether the human reticulocytes contain Hb A or Hb S (Suzuki and Itano, 1973b). Thus, an amino acid substitution near the N terminus of the β chain does not affect the removal of the N-terminal methionine.

The process of initial dipeptide and tripeptide synthesis has been extensively studied in rabbit and human reticulocytes (Crystal et al., 1971, 1972, 1973). The amino acids which immediately follow the N-terminal methionine of the nascent globin chains are the amino acids which constitute the N terminus of the completed globin chains. Thus, there is no evidence in the case of hemoglobin for the synthesis of a precursor molecule that contains additional amino acids (other than the N-terminal methionine) which are not found in the mature protein.

One of the more interesting features of globin synthesis is that the translation of α-chain mRNA appears to be less efficiently initiated than that of β-chain mRNA. This fact stems from the observation that nascent α chains are found on polyribosomes of a different size distribution than nascent β chains: polyribosomes bearing nascent α chains have (on the average) 3 ribosomes, whereas those bearing nascent β chains have (on the average) 5 ribosomes (Hunt et al., 1968a, 1968b, 1969; Lodish, 1971, 1974; Lodish and Jacobsen, 1972; Boyer et al., 1974). This phenomenon, initially observed in rabbit reticulocytes, has also been shown to occur in human reticulocytes and bone marrow cells (Clegg et al., 1971a; Nathan et al., 1971; Cividalli et al., 1974b).

The phenomenon can only be explained if β-chain mRNA initiation is more rapid than that of α mRNA, or if α-chain assembly and release is more rapid than that of β chains: the net result in either case would be an increase in the number of ribosomes on a strand of β mRNA at a given time. In fact, the rates of rabbit and human α and β chain elongation (chain assembly) and release (chain termination) have been measured directly and were found to be the same for both chains (Clegg et al., 1968; Rieder, 1971; Lodish and Jacobsen, 1972; Hunt, 1974). The α-chain mRNA must therefore be initiated more slowly and less efficiently than the β mRNA. There is also more direct experimental evidence for the proposed lower initiation potential of α mRNA: the addition of various inhibitors of polypeptide chain initiation to reticulocyte lysates leads to preferential inhibition of α-chain synthesis, as would be predicted if α mRNA initiates less well than β mRNA (Lodish, 1971, 1974). A corollary of this finding is that balanced or equal synthesis of α and β globin chains can only be achieved if the erythroid cell contains an excess of α-chain mRNA relative to β mRNA; this phenomenon would compensate for the less efficient initiation of α mRNA and result in balanced α- and β-chain synthesis (Lodish, 1971; Lodish and Jacobsen, 1972).

This α mRNA excess has been theoretically calculated to be in the range of approximately 1.7:1.0, if α mRNA initiates protein synthesis only 60 per cent as often as β mRNA, as predicted by the model (Lodish and Jacobsen, 1972; Boyer, et al., 1974; Lodish, 1974). The relative amounts of α and β mRNA isolated from normal reticulocytes have been directly assayed by formamide-polyacrylamide–gel electrophoresis, which separates α from β mRNA, and the results indicate that there is a 1.2 to 1.5 excess of α mRNA over β mRNA (Kazazian et al., 1974; Forget et al., 1975a). Molecular hybridization experiments also demonstrate a 20 to 30 per cent excess of α mRNA over β mRNA in normal globin mRNA (Forget et al., unpublished results). The experiments of McKeehan et al. (1974) also indicate the presence of more α mRNA than β mRNA bound to polysomes: the addition of progressively more 40S ribosomal subunits (which have bound mRNA) to a reticulocyte cell-free protein synthesizing system leads to increased synthesis of α chains relative to β chains. The phenomenon of excess α-chain mRNA which is initiated less efficiently than β mRNA also explains the previously mentioned finding of an excess of ribosome-free α-chain mRNA in reticulocytes: if α-chain mRNA is less frequently initiated than β mRNA, then, at any given time, there should be substantially more free cytoplasmic α mRNA waiting to enter into polyribosomes (Lodish, 1974).

It should be noted that differences between α- and β-chain synthesis observed in various experimental systems can, for the most part, be explained by the different properties of α and β mRNA which we have just described, without the need to postulate the existence of chain-specific initiation factors or other translational control mechanisms. Although some workers have presented results suggesting that chain-specific and globin-specific initiation factors may in fact exist (see Benz and Forget, 1974, for review), there is little evidence to suggest that such factors play any role in the regulation of normal globin-chain synthesis (Temple and Lodish, 1975).

More recently a low molecular weight RNA species has been identified which may be involved in the translational control of globin synthesis (Bogdanovsky et al., 1973; Heywood et al., 1974; Kennedy et al., 1974; Bester et al., 1975; Fuhr and Overton, 1975; Salden et al., 1975). However, other evidence suggests that this RNA species most probably has only nonspecific effects on globin and protein synthesis (Berns et al., 1975), and in fact may not be RNA at all (Salden and Bloemendal, 1976). The role of transfer RNA (tRNA) in translational control of globin has also been investigated. Different α/β synthetic ratios can be obtained in a cell-free protein synthesizing system with the use of various fractions of tRNA containing different proportions of the different amino acid acceptor species (Anderson and Gilbert, 1969). There is also a significant difference in the various amounts of the different tRNA species in reticulocyte tRNA as compared to that in tRNA of a less specialized tissue such as the liver (Smith and McNamara, 1971; Smith, 1975). However, these findings do not provide evidence that tRNA normally exerts any translational control of globin synthesis in intact cells.

The possible roles of heme and of the globin chains themselves in the control of globin mRNA translation will be considered in the following sections.

The translation of the δ-chain mRNA of Hb A_2 ($\alpha_2\delta_2$) appears to be subject to an unusual type of control. The synthesis of δ chains appears to be limited to erythroid precursor cells in the bone marrow: there is no detectable synthesis in peripheral blood reticulocytes (Rieder and Weatherall, 1965; Roberts et al., 1972). A similar phenomenon has been observed with respect to the synthesis of the $\delta\beta$-hybrid chain of Hb Lepore (see Chapter 5). It has been postulated that the premature cessation of δ-chain synthesis may be related to instability and premature degradation of its mRNA because of the nature of its 3′- and 5′-terminal untranslated sequences (Roberts et al., 1973). However, in the case of Hb Lepore, although synthesis is absent in peripheral blood, substantial amounts of $\delta\beta$ mRNA can still be detected by molecular hybridization assays (Benz et al., 1975a). These findings indicate that the cessation of Lepore (and perhaps δ) globin chain synthesis may not be necessarily associated with total absence or total degradation of its mRNA.

COORDINATION OF α- AND β-CHAIN SYNTHESIS AND ASSEMBLY OF HEMOGLOBIN TETRAMERS

The synthesis of α and non-α (β+δ+γ) chains must be strictly regulated so that nearly equal amounts of each are produced. Pools of free globin chains in erythroid cells, though present, are very small (Baglioni and Campana, 1967; Zucker and Schulman, 1967; Winterhalter et al., 1969; Gill and Schwartz, 1973), and normal mammalian reticulocytes and bone marrow cells invariably synthesize α and non-α chains in nearly equal amounts (Weatherall and Clegg, 1972).

The balance between α- and non-α–chain synthesis depends on complex and poorly understood mechanisms which counterbalance the relative amounts and translational efficiencies of α chain and non-α chain specific globin mRNA. As we have discussed in the previous section, α mRNA is only 60 per cent as efficient in initiating protein synthesis as β mRNA, and the reticulocyte must therefore contain approximately 1.7 times more α mRNA than β mRNA in order to maintain equal synthesis of α and β chains. However, there is no information on what factors are primarily involved in controlling the amounts of the two different mRNA's present in the cell. It is difficult to imagine precisely how a negative feedback control mechanism could operate in vivo to regulate this process.

Small pools of free α chains and $\alpha\beta$ dimers are present during the post-translational assembly of hemoglobin. The free α-chain pool may play a role in the coordination of α- and non-α–chain synthesis. In cell-free systems derived from rabbit reticulocytes, the addition of free α chains inhibits α-chain synthesis but not β-chain synthesis; conversely, added β chains inhibit β- but not α-chain synthesis (Blum et al., 1967, 1969, 1970, 1972; Shaeffer et al., 1967, 1969). When the endogenous free α-chain pool is first removed from the cell-free system, exogenous α chains both inhibit α-chain synthesis and stimulate β-chain synthesis (Blum et al., 1969, 1970). Human β chains also inhibit rabbit β-chain synthesis; in this case it is possible to show that the inhibition of rabbit β-chain synthesis is simultaneously accompanied by the formation of α(rabbit)-β(human)–hybrid hemoglobins, depletion of the free α-chain pool, decreased release of complete newly synthesized β chains from polyribosomes, and the de-novo appearance of a small pool of free radioactive β chains (Shaeffer et al., 1967, 1969).

These studies suggest that α-chain synthesis is regulated partially through feedback inhibition by free α chains; β-chain synthesis is also subject to feedback inhibition but the inhibition is mediated indirectly by depletion of the free α-chain pool. The free α-chain pool appears to be required for maximal rates of β-chain release from polyribosomes; the α chains may cause the release of β chains from polyribosomes by binding to the completed β chains and forming $\alpha\beta$ dimers (Baglioni and Campana, 1967). Alpha-chain synthesis thus seems to influence β-chain synthesis but β-chain synthesis has little effect on α-chain synthesis. Finally, the requirement of the free α-chain pool for β-chain release is not absolute, since a few free β chains do accumulate despite the removal of the free α-chain pool. This model provides the kind of cross-coordination of α and non-α synthesis which may be required to insure that these chains are produced at nearly equal rates.

Some, but not all, features of the regulatory model derived from the studies of cell-free systems seem to apply in intact cells. O-methyl-threonine (OMT) is an isoleucine analogue which specifically blocks the incorporation of isoleucine into polypeptides and stops polypeptide-chain elongation at each isoleucine codon (Honig, 1967; Kazazian and Freedman, 1968; Rabinovitz et al., 1969). In intact human fetal reticulocytes treated with OMT, γ-chain synthesis is preferentially inhibited because γ chains contain isoleucine, whereas human α and β chains are devoid of isoleucine; α-chain synthesis, however, continues unabated in these cells even though a sizable pool of free α chains accumulates (Honig, 1967; Honig et al., 1969). These findings argue against the existence of efficient feedback mechanisms by which excess α chains in the free α pool limit α-chain synthesis but do support the earlier contention that α-chain synthesis proceeds relatively independently of non-α–chain synthesis (Felicetti et al., 1966; Baglioni and Campana, 1967). Erythroid cells from rabbits with a variant hemoglobin containing normal α chains with isoleucine and mutant β chains with no isoleucine (β^{ileu}-negative) were treated with OMT in a reciprocal experiment (Wolf et al., 1973). In the absence of OMT, the α/β synthetic ratio was 1.0 in both reticulocytes and bone marrow. In reticulocytes, which have a sizable free α-chain pool, OMT inhibited α-chain synthesis but not β-chain synthesis, as expected. However, in bone marrow cells having a much smaller free α-chain pool, the inhibition of α-chain synthesis was followed by a delayed but appreciable reduction in β-chain synthesis. In these intact cells, therefore, optimal β-chain synthesis seemed to require the presence of a free α-chain pool in much the same manner that it did in the experiments with cell-free systems. In a subsequent study using these same mutant rabbits, Garrick et al. (1975) actually showed stimulation of β-chain synthesis in reticulocytes when α-chain synthesis was inhibited by OMT. This phenomenon was interpreted as resulting from relief of competition between α and β mRNA's for limiting components (? initiation factors) required for protein synthesis (Garrick et al., 1975).

In summary, normal non-α–chain synthesis may not proceed independently of α-chain synthesis; rather, it appears to be regulated in part by a free α-chain pool which may be required for optimal rates of release of non-α chains from polysomes. The regulation of α-chain synthesis is still an area of confusion; the straightforward mechanism of feedback inhibition proposed on the basis of data from cell-free systems exposed to exogenous α chains may not strictly apply to intact cells, since human fetal cells continued to accumulate free α chains when treated with OMT. Furthermore, if feedback inhibition does occur in vivo it must be a rather coarse and imperfect control mechanism, since abundant pools of free α chains accumulate in cells from patients with β thalassemia (Weatherall and Clegg, 1972; see Chapter 5). Conversely, the effect of the free α-chain pool on non-α-chain synthesis must be incomplete because free β and γ chains accumulate in α thalassemia (Weatherall and Clegg, 1972; see Chapter 5). Furthermore, as previously noted, inhibition of α-chain synthesis in β^{ileu}-negative rabbits can actually result in a stimulation of β-chain synthesis even after the free α-chain pool has been exhausted (Garrick et al., 1975). On the other hand, biosynthetic studies using thalassemic erythroid cells suggest that there may occur some compensatory inhibition of the synthesis of the nonthalassemic globin chains which accumulate in excess (Cividalli et al., 1974b). These results are compatible with the notion that feedback inhibition mechanisms similar to those just described may indeed exist in normal cells but that these mechanisms are rather easily overwhelmed by lesions which severely disrupt the normal amounts or functions of either globin mRNA or the translational apparatus.

ASSEMBLY OF HEMOGLOBIN TETRAMERS AND POST-TRANSLATIONAL MODIFICATION OF HEMOGLOBIN

Newly synthesized free globin chains are rapidly incorporated into complete hemoglobin tetramers (Rossi-Fanelli et al., 1958; Winterhalter et al., 1969). The process is spontaneous and virtually instantaneous, requiring no enzymes or cofactors other than heme (Rossi-Fanelli et al., 1958a). The exact intermediate steps in the assembly of the tetramer are not understood. However, reticulocyte hemolysates are known to contain a variety of minor globin and hemoglobin components, some of which may represent intermediates in the assembly of hemoglobin from free globin and free heme. This area has been the subject of a detailed review (Winterhalter, 1966).

The exact timing of the combination of globin chains with heme is unknown as is the question of whether heme combines with globin in its physiologically active, divalent form or whether heme first binds to globin in the oxidized (trivalent) state, forming methemoglobin, which is then enzymatically reduced to functional hemoglobin. It has been clearly shown that heme is not added to globin until after its release from polyribosomes (Felicetti et al., 1966). A complete functional hemoglobin molecule contains four heme groups, each of which is bound to a separate globin-chain subunit. Minor hemoglobin components containing only one, two, or three heme groups per tetramer have been identified during experiments in which heme and globin are recombined in vitro (Winterhalter, 1966; Winterhalter and Glatthaar, 1971). One of these, IC_{II}, contains two hemes, both bound to α chains, and has been found in normal erythrocytes (Winterhalter and Glatthaar, 1971). Analysis of these partially heme-saturated tetramers has strongly supported the notion that heme has a higher affinity for α chains than for β chains (Winterhalter et al., 1971). Intermediates like IC_{II} have been shown to be important during the catabolism of some unstable hemoglobins (Winterhalter, 1966; Winterhalter et al., 1969). Winterhalter and Glatthaar (1971) have presented kinetic data suggesting that IC_{II} may be an intermediate in normal hemoglobin assembly.

Although the steps leading to the formation of a completely heme-saturated hemoglobin tetramer are poorly defined, the existence of partially saturated tetramers of globin clearly implies that heme-depleted globin chains can form dimers and tetramers with other heme-depleted or heme-saturated globin chains. Minute pools of heme-depleted free α chains, heme-containing free α chains, and $\alpha\beta$-chain dimers have been found in normal rabbit and human hemolysates (Baglioni and Campana, 1967; Shaeffer, 1967, Tavill et al., 1968, 1972; Zucker and Schulman, 1968; Winterhalter et al., 1969; Gill and Schwartz, 1973). Newly labeled α chains are first found in the free α-chain pool, later in the pool of $\alpha\beta$ dimers, and finally in complete hemoglobin molecules. The pool of free β chains is probably much more minute, since it is not detectable in normal hemolysates. Newly labeled β chains rapidly pass through the small pool of $\alpha\beta$ dimers into complete hemoglobin molecules (Tavill et al., 1968, 1972; Stamatoyannopoulos, 1972). These findings strongly suggest that $\alpha\beta$-chain dimers are physiologic intermediates in hemoglobin assembly.

Clinical and experimental heme-deficiency states, discussed in more detail later (see Heme Biosynthesis), cause newly synthesized globin chains to accumulate in the pools of free α chains and $\alpha\beta$-chain dimers. Repletion of these systems with heme decreases the sizes of these pools and "chases" the globin chains into complete hemoglobin tetramers (Felicetti et al., 1966; Tavill et al., 1968, 1972; Winterhalter et al., 1969). These findings suggest that the combination of globin chains to form tetramers and the combination of heme with each globin chain are interdependent even though tetramers can form before all globin chains are heme saturated, as noted above.

Complete hemoglobin molecules are several orders of magnitude more stable than free globin chains or globin dimers. Newly synthesized globin chains and dimers, present in low concentration, are rapidly and spontaneously assembled into complete tetramers. Similarly, $\alpha\alpha$ and $\beta\beta$ dimers are much less stable than $\alpha\beta$ dimers; homotetramers such as Hb H (β_4) are found only under grossly abnormal circumstances (Weatherall and Clegg, 1972). The information which directs the assembly process is built into the primary structure (amino acid sequence) of the globin chains themselves. Unstable mutant hemoglobins which have abnormal affinities for heme or abnormal assembly have been described (Tavill et al., 1968; White, 1971; Winterhalter and Glatthaar, 1971; Pagnier et al., 1974). These hemoglobins often have amino acid substitutions in one of the globin chains at or near the heme binding sites. The subject is discussed in more detail in Chapter 8.

In adult human erythrocytes, hemoglobin A is a heterogeneous compound. Several minor modified forms of hemoglobin A have been identified (Allen et al., 1958; Huisman and Meyering, 1960). These all have the same amino acid sequence as normal Hb A but carry carbohydrate or other modifying residues (see Chapter 1), which constitute post-translational modifications of the globin chains.

The most abundant minor modified hemoglobin component is Hb A_{Ic}. This component has a glucose residue attached to the N terminus of the β chain, by a peculiar Schiff base linkage (Bookchin and Gallop, 1968; Bunn et al., 1975a). Hb A_{Ic} is of interest because it is found in increased amounts in diabetes mellitus (Rahbar, 1968; Trivelli et al., 1971). The increase is due to the metabolic abnormality of the disease itself and not to other genetic factors (Koenig and Cerami, 1975; Tattersall et al., 1975; Koenig et al., 1976).

HEME BIOSYNTHESIS

Mechanism and Control of Heme Synthesis

Heme consists of divalent iron coordinately bound within a protoporphyrin 9 ring (Fig. 1–12); oxidized iron, when bound to protoporphyrin 9, forms oxidized heme (hemin). The porphyrin moiety of heme is synthesized by the complex metabolic pathway shown in Figure 4–5. Its biosynthesis begins with the condensation of glycine and succinyl CoA to form δ-amino levulinic acid (ALA). This reaction is catalyzed by the enzyme ALA synthetase in mitochondria of the developing erythroid cell. This enzymatic reaction requires pyridoxal phosphate and seems to be the rate-limiting step in the heme synthesis pathway. Heme synthesis then proceeds in the cell's cytoplasm by a series of extramitochondrial enzymatic reactions. However, the last two enzymatic reactions in the heme synthesis pathway are again localized to the cell's mitochondria: (1) the synthesis of PROTOgen 9 from COPROgen III, a reaction which is catalyzed by COPROgen oxidase; and (2) following the auto-oxidation of PROTOgen 9 to protoporphyrin 9 (PROTO 9), the synthesis of heme from protoporphyrin 9, which involves the binding of iron to the porphyrin ring, a reaction catalyzed by the enzyme heme synthetase (or ferrochelatase). It is not clear whether heme itself is produced initially or whether hemin is first produced and then reduced to heme by erythrocyte diaphorase enzymes.

It is most interesting that the initial and final enzymatic reactions in the heme synthesis pathway are localized in the cell's mitochondria, an anatomic arrangement well suited to allow heme to control its own synthesis by end-product inhibition. In fact the synthesis of heme is in great part controlled by the processes of end-product repression and feedback inhibition of the enzyme ALA

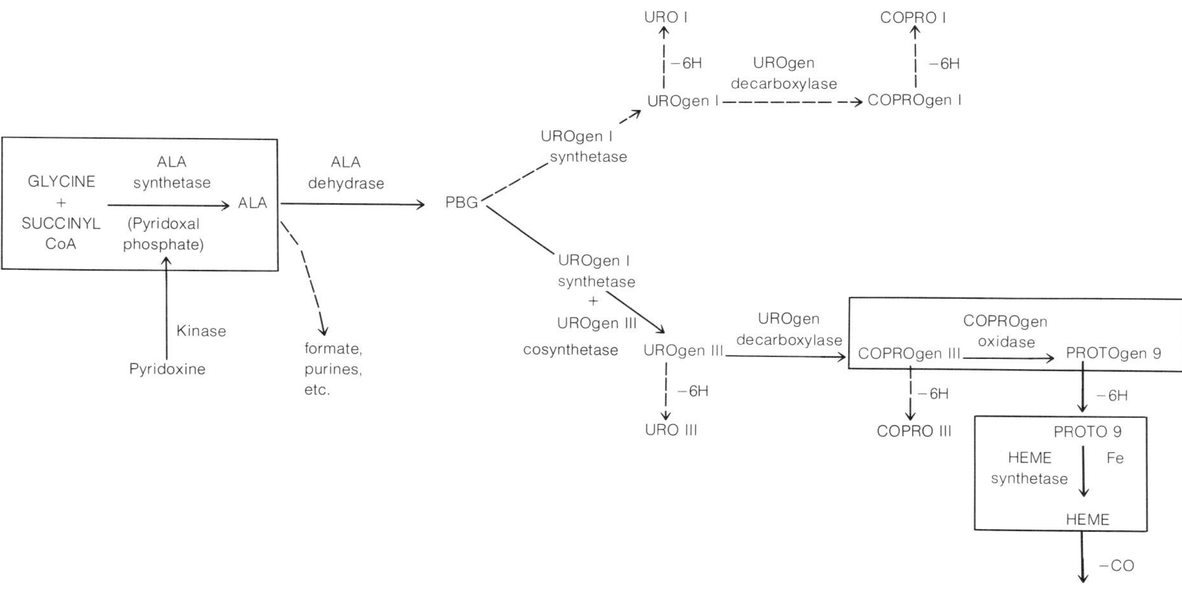

Figure 4–5. Biosynthesis of heme. Bold arrows show main pathway. Dashed arrows show by-pathways. Abbreviations: ALA, δ-aminolevulinic acid; PBG, porphobilinogen; UROgen, COPROgen, and PROTOgen, the porphyrinogens; URO, COPRO, and PROTO, the porphyrins. The reactions enclosed in boxes occur within mitochondria.

synthetase. Heme itself has two effects on this enzyme: first, it interacts directly with ALA synthetase and inactivates it (end-product inhibition); secondly, it decreases the synthesis of new enzyme (end product repression), and since ALA synthetase has a short half life, its cellular level rapidly decreases (Karibian and London, 1965; Granick and Kappas, 1967; Kappas and Granick, 1968). Similar mechanisms affecting the activity of heme synthetase may limit the formation of heme from protoporphyrin 9. Heme may also control (inhibit) heme synthesis by inhibiting the uptake or transfer of iron from transferrin into the reticulocyte (Ponka and Neuwirt, 1974). Heme synthesis is also controlled to some extent by globin synthesis: when protein synthesis in reticulocytes is inhibited by cycloheximide, heme synthesis is also rapidly and reversibly reduced (Grayzel et al., 1967). The onset of inhibition is too rapid to be due to decreased synthesis of enzymes responsible for heme production, and the inhibition is probably mediated via free heme which accumulates in the absence of globin synthesis (Ponka and Neuwirt, 1974). Heme synthesis is also abnormally reduced in thalassemia, presumably as a result of the primary decrease in globin synthesis which occurs in this disorder (see Chapter 5 and Weatherall and Clegg, 1972). The interaction between globin and heme synthesis will be discussed in greater detail in the section on Coordination of Heme and Globin Synthesis.

A number of humoral and pharmacological agents as well as environmental factors can affect heme synthesis. An adequate supply of iron, of course, is necessary for normal heme synthesis, and in some circumstances the availability of iron may be a limiting factor controlling the rate of heme synthesis at the heme synthetase step, where iron is essential. Iron deficiency results in decreased utilization of labeled glycine for heme synthesis. Although the levels of free protoporphyrin are increased in the erythrocyte in iron deficiency, total porphyrin content is decreased. There is some evidence that excess protoporphyrins in iron-deficient cells may exert feedback inhibition on earlier steps of the heme synthesis pathway (Heilmeyer, 1966).

A number of steroids, including naturally occurring compounds such as etiocholanolone and pregnanediol, are potent stimulators of heme synthesis and probably act by inducing the synthesis of ALA synthetase (Granick and Kappas, 1967; Kappas and Granick, 1968). Some of these compounds may play a physiological role in the stimulation of heme synthesis (Granick and Kappas, 1967).

Isoniazid (INH) and other antituberculous drugs such as cycloserine and pyrazinamide are inhibitors of heme synthesis and probably act via pyridoxine antagonism, thus secondarily inhibiting ALA synthetase activity. The inhibitory effect of these drugs can be reversed by pyridoxal phosphate. It is thought that these antituberculous drugs act by inhibiting pyridoxal phosphate as well as by interfering with the phosphorylation of pyridoxine to pyridoxal phosphate (Killam, 1957; McCormick and Snell, 1961). Lead inhibits the activity of multiple enzymes in the heme synthesis pathway: heme synthetase, ALA dehydrase, COPROgen oxidase, and possibly ALA synthetase (Goldberg, 1972). Ethanol also inhibits heme synthesis, probably by blocking phosphorylation of pyridoxine to pyridoxal phosphate (Hines and Cowan, 1970a; Hines and Grasso, 1970b; Ali and Brain, 1974) or by accelerating the degradation of pyridoxal phosphate (Lumeng and Li, 1974). All these inhibitors of heme synthesis can cause a clinically significant hematological disorder termed secondary sideroblastic anemia. This condition, which can also occur as a primary idiopathic disorder, is characterized by anemia, hypochromic red blood cells having a decreased intracellular hemoglobin content, and the presence of ringed sideroblasts in the marrow. Ringed sideroblasts are nucleated erythroid precursor cells that contain excessive deposits of iron in mitochondria which usually form a ring around the cell's nucleus. The marked increase in mitochondrial iron deposits probably results not only from passive accumulation of iron due to decreased utilization resulting from decreased heme synthesis, but also from increased cellular uptake of iron due to loss of inhibition of cellular iron uptake by heme (Ponka and Neuwirt, 1974).

Coordination of Heme and Globin Synthesis

As previously stated, disorders of reduced globin-chain synthesis secondarily inhibit heme synthesis. Conversely, various disorders of heme synthesis have inhibitory effects on globin-chain synthesis. Disorders of reduced heme synthesis which secondarily inhibit globin synthesis include iron deficiency, lead poisoning, isoniazid toxicity, and the primary sideroblastic anemias (Waxman and Rabinovitz, 1966; White et al., 1971; White and Harvey, 1972; Fuhr and Gengozian, 1973; White and Ali, 1973; White and Hoffbrand, 1974). Restoration of heme will usually reverse the inhibition of globin synthesis. In normal red cells and cell-free lysates, the addition of heme stimulates globin synthesis (Bruns and London, 1965; Grayzel et al., 1966; Waxman et al., 1967; Adamson et al., 1968; Zucker and Schulman, 1968). All these observations point to the existence of control mechanisms which closely coordinate the synthesis of heme and globin during hemoglobin biosynthesis. However, the precise mechanisms which insure that heme and globin are produced in roughly equal amounts remain obscure. The effect of heme on globin synthesis may be partially mediated by complex interactions between heme and the small pool of free α chains which is present in normal red cells. Erythroid cells or cell-free systems which are heme-deficient accumulate larger amounts of free α chains and $\alpha\beta$ dimers which are then rapidly "chased" into complete hemoglobin molecules when the heme supply is replenished (Zucker and Schulman, 1967; Tavill et al., 1968, 1972). In human reticulocytes affected by various defects of heme synthesis, α-chain synthesis is more severely inhibited than β-chain synthesis (White and Hoffbrand, 1974). This imbalance is partially corrected by the addition of heme. These observations indicate that heme deficiency produces a defect in hemoglobin assembly which secondarily inhibits globin synthesis. This inhibition may be mediated by the accumulation of free α chains and $\alpha\beta$ dimers which may in turn depress globin-chain synthesis by feedback mechanisms similar to those proposed for the coordination of α- and β-chain synthesis (see previous section in this chapter).

In summary, the mechanisms which coordinate heme and globin synthesis are complex and poorly understood. The physiological role of heme in the control of globin synthesis in intact erythroid cells may or may not be related to the mechanism of action of heme or hemin in the control of initiation of protein synthesis in cell-free reticulocyte lysates, which is discussed in the next section.

Effect of Hemin on Initiation of Polypeptide-Chain Synthesis

Cell-free systems prepared from unfractionated rabbit reticulocyte hemolysates synthesize globin actively (about 25 per cent of the rate of intact cells) for about 5 minutes and then abruptly stop producing globin. Concomitantly, polyribosomes disappear and inactive 80S monoribosomes accumulate (Adamson et al., 1968, 1969; Zucker and Schulman, 1968; Maxwell and Rabinovitz, 1969; Howard et al., 1970; Maxwell et al., 1971). The inactivation of these lysates is now known to be due to a rapid loss of the lysates' ability to initiate new rounds of globin synthesis (Gross and Rabinovitz, 1972a, 1972b; Hunt et al., 1972).

If heme (in the form of hemin) is added to the lysates at the beginning of the incubation, inactivation is considerably delayed. Globin synthesis, polyribosome integrity, and initiating capacity are all preserved for an additional 15 to 20 minutes. The initial rate of globin synthesis is not altered, but active synthesis persists for a longer time, resulting in a net increase in the total amount of globin synthesized.

Both the hemin effect and the inactivation occurring in lysates not supplemented with hemin are mediated by the postribosomal supernatant fraction. Fresh lysates can be inactivated by supernatants preincubated without hemin, while inactivated ribosomes can be reactivated if incubated with fresh supernatant. Numerous experiments indicate that lysates incubated without hemin accumulate a reversible inhibitor of initiation, the action of which can be blocked by hemin. This inhibitor has been called the heme-controlled repressor, or "HCR". This reversible inhibitor can, on prolonged incubation of the lysates, be transformed into an irreversible inhibitor which is not affected by hemin (Maxwell et al., 1971; Adamson et al., 1972; Gross and Rabinovitz, 1972b; Legon et al., 1973; Gross, 1974). The HCR has been isolated: it is a protein with a molecular weight of 300,000 to 500,000 (Adamson et al., 1972; Gross and Rabinovitz, 1972a, 1973; Mizuno et al., 1972).

The inhibitory effect of HCR can be overcome by the addition of initiation factors, and it is thought that one of the main effects of hemin is to activate an essential initiation factor (Adamson et al., 1972; Kaempfer and Kaufman, 1972; Kaempfer, 1974; Raffel et al., 1974). The addition of cyclic AMP to lysates also reverses the inhibitory effect of hemin deficiency (Legon et al., 1974), and evidence indicates that the activity of the HCR is associated with a protein kinase that is involved in the phosphorylation of a specific initiation factor (Levin et al., 1975, 1976; Kramer et al., 1976).

The effect of hemin on the initiation of globin synthesis in cell-free reticulocyte lysates is therefore well established. A number of arguments have been presented to attribute to this specific hemin effect and the HCR physiological roles in the control of hemoglobin synthesis in intact erythroid cells (Gross, 1974; Schulman, 1975). The finding of hemin-reversible repressor, without preincubation, in mature human erythrocytes which have ceased synthesizing hemoglobin has also been proposed as evidence that HCR is a physiological regulator (inhibitor) of globin synthesis (Freedman et al., 1974). However, it is also possible that the hemin effect which is observed in cell-free reticulocyte lysates is simply a nonspecific phenomenon without physiological importance for the control of globin synthesis in intact erythroid cells. The hemin effect is not specific for globin synthesis but also extends to the synthesis of nonglobin proteins in various cell-free systems (Beuzard et al., 1973; Mathews et al., 1973). However, in certain other cell-free systems, hemin has little or no effect on globin-mRNA translation (Gilbert and Anderson, 1970; Mathews et al., 1972). This topic continues to be controversial.

Although heme no doubt has significant effects and a physiological role in the control of globin synthesis in intact erythroid cells, these physiological functions may be fulfilled by its interaction with free α-chain and $\alpha\beta$-chain dimer pools in the course of hemoglobin assembly rather than by a specific effect on globin-chain initiation.

HEMOGLOBIN SYNTHESIS DURING ERYTHROPOIESIS

Hemoglobin is synthesized primarily in nucleated erythroid precursor cells in the bone marrow during the 6- to 8-day period of erythroid cell differentiation. Its synthesis continues at a low level for 1 to 2 days in the circulating anucleate reticulocyte, but mature erythrocytes synthesize no protein. Mature erythrocytes contain almost exclusively complete hemoglobin molecules (Winterhalter and Glatthaar, 1971); pools of free heme α chains, non-α chains, and globin dimers are minute (Baglioni and Campana, 1967; Gill and Schwartz, 1973). These findings imply that strict regulation must occur throughout erythropoiesis so that balanced synthesis of each hemoglobin component is assured and so that no one component accumulates in significant excess. The possible molecular bases of these control phenomena have been discussed earlier in this chapter.

The mechanisms which commit the primitive pluripotential stem cells in bone marrow to erythropoiesis are poorly understood. Much work has been done to study the role of erythropoietin, the polypeptide hormone which is the physiological mediator for stimulating erythropoiesis. Many changes in macromolecular synthesis have been reported from studies of bone marrow cells exposed to erythropoietin. However, it appears that this hormone acts primarily upon an early, but already committed, population of erythroid stem cells. The uncommitted pluripotential stem cells appear to be unaffected by its action. Moreover, most of the molecular events which follow erythropoietin stimulation have proved to be quantitative increases in the synthesis of heme, protein, DNA, and RNA which can be fully accounted for by the increased number of active erythroid cells appearing after erythropoietin exposure (Marks and Rifkind, 1972; Krantz, 1973) rather than by specific changes in genetic expression within individual cells induced by the hormone. On the other hand, recent evidence suggests that intracellular increases in globin messenger RNA in erythroid precursor cells may occur as a result of erythropoietin stimulation (Terada et al., 1972; Conkie et al., 1975; Ramirez et al., 1975a; Forget et al., 1976a).

The exact onset of globin gene expression in the early committed erythroid precursor cells has not yet been definitively identified. The most primitive recognizable erythroid precursors (pronormoblasts and basophilic normoblasts) already contain low but significant levels of cytoplasmic globin messenger RNA despite the absence of significant levels of globin-chain synthesis in the same cells (Harrison et al., 1973; Harrison et al., 1974a; Forget et al., 1976a). On the other hand, others have found insignificant levels of globin mRNA in similarly immature erythroid precursor cells (Terada et al., 1972; Ramirez et al., 1975a). Despite these apparently contradictory results (perhaps due to differences in methodology and in the systems studied) it is generally accepted that the major control of globin gene expression during erythroid cell differentiation is at the level of transcription of globin gene DNA into mRNA. Nevertheless, some translational control of globin mRNA activity may be present very early in erythroid cell maturation.

The coordination of heme and globin synthesis has also been studied during erythroid differentiation in separated populations of erythroid cells at different stages of maturation (Glass et al., 1975; Forget et al., 1976a). These studies indicate that heme synthesis is maximal in cells at an earlier stage of maturation than that at which globin synthesis is maximal. It appears, therefore, that there is a certain degree of asynchrony between heme and globin synthesis during erythroid cell differentiation.

Considerable insight into mechanisms governing globin gene expression during erythroid differentiation has been gained by studies of cultured murine erythroleukemia cells transformed by Friend leukemia virus (Friend et al., 1971; Ostertag et al., 1972a). These cells are poorly differentiated, resemble pronormoblasts, and contain virtually no globin mRNA. In the presence of dimethyl sulfoxide (DMSO), these cells are induced to differentiate into more mature erythroid cells with concomitant accumulation of globin mRNA and hemoglobin. The exact mechanism of action of DMSO in this process is unknown and may be nonspecific; other agents affecting membrane permeability can also induce differentiation of these cells in culture. Erythropoietin, on the other hand, does not induce differentiation of these cells, and thus this system may not be an accurate model for the physiological events which are responsible for, and accompany, normal erythroid cell differentiation.

A number of interesting observations have been made, however, concerning the process of differentiation in Friend erythroleukemia cells. Although most of the cell lines contain insignificant levels of globin mRNA in the uninduced state (Ross et al., 1972b, 1974; Harrison et al., 1973; Preisler et al., 1973; Conkie et al., 1974), a certain number of variant cell lines have been described in which significant levels of globin mRNA are present but not translated (Gilmour et al., 1974; Harrison et al., 1974b). Other workers have reported the finding of a translational repressor in extracts of Friend leukemia cells which inhibits the translation of globin mRNA (Cimadevilla and Hardesty, 1975; Cimadevilla et al., 1975). The mechanism of action of this repressor is different from that of the heme-controlled repressor of reticulocyte lysates previously described in this chapter (see Effect of Hemin on Initiation of Polypeptide-Chain Synthesis).

After exposure of the usual type of Friend cells to DMSO, there is roughly a 48-hour lag period; levels of globin mRNA then increase dramatically between 48 and 72 hours. However, significant hemoglobin synthesis and erythroid differentiation are observed only 4 to 5 days after the exposure to DMSO. Differentiation and globin mRNA accumulation can be prevented by addition of inhibitors of DNA transcription such as actinomycin D and bromodeoxyuridine. The globin chains synthesized by these erythroleukemia cells are structurally normal. There is usually equal synthesis of α and β chains but in some cell lines there can be excess synthesis of one chain over the other (Ostertag et al., 1972a).

The relative amounts of α and β mRNA present during the various stages of DMSO-induced differentiation have been measured by sensitive RNA-cDNA hybridization assays (Orkin et al., 1975). It was found that very early in the induction process, α-chain mRNA is present in a three- to fourfold excess over β-chain mRNA, but as mRNA accumulation approaches the levels found in more mature normal erythroid precursor cells, the α mRNA content is equal to or in only a 1.2- to 1.3-fold excess over β mRNA content.

These and future studies utilizing Friend erythroleukemia cells may provide important information on the various mechanisms which regulate hemoglobin synthesis during maturation in erythroid cells. However, many features of Friend erythroleukemia cells suggest that at least some of the results obtained with these cells may not necessarily be applicable to normal erythroid cells and may be due to specialized processes which have little relevance to the physiology of normal erythropoiesis.

CONCLUSIONS

The molecular biology of mammalian hemoglobin synthesis is exceedingly complex. The mechanisms by which globin mRNA is translated into globin chains in the cell cytoplasm have been thoroughly investigated, and many steps in the process have been described in great detail. Yet the precise control mechanisms which insure that the proper kinds and amounts of globin chains and heme are produced in erythroid cells remain largely unknown. Similarly, few details are known of the processes which control the synthesis, processing, and transport of globin mRNA during the intranuclear phase of its biogenesis. In this chapter, we have attempted to summarize the understanding of the various processes involved in the biosynthesis of hemoglobin: the synthesis, processing, and translation of globin mRNA; the assembly of hemoglobin from globin and heme; and the regulatory phenomena which may reflect the types of control mechanisms operating in erythropoietic tissue.

It is clear at the present time that the basic mechanisms of protein synthesis are similar in microorganisms, plants, animals, and humans (Watson, 1970). The processes involved in the synthesis of globin appear to reflect the universal mechanism used in nature for the expression of genetic information. Despite their limitations, hemoglobin synthesizing systems should continue to be useful models for the study of the molecular genetics of normal and abnormal protein synthesis in many different tissues.

Chapter 5

THE THALASSEMIAS

DEFINITION

The thalassemia syndromes are a group of hereditary disorders in which there is a defect in the synthesis of one or more of the normal polypeptide chains of hemoglobin. This defect causes absent or decreased synthesis of the affected chain. As a result, the erythrocytes have a low intracellular hemoglobin content (hypochromia) and are smaller than normal (microcytosis). In addition, the continued normal synthesis of the unaffected globin chain leads to the accumulation of unstable aggregates of these unmatched chains. These aggregates precipitate within the red blood cell, damage its membrane, and cause its premature destruction in the peripheral circulation or at an earlier stage in the bone marrow. In α thalassemia, synthesis of the α chain of normal adult hemoglobin (Hb A: $\alpha_2\beta_2$) is impaired, whereas in β thalassemia, it is the synthesis of β chains which is reduced or absent.

INCIDENCE AND POPULATION GENETICS

Thalassemia primarily affects people of Mediterranean, African, and Asian ancestry. However, sporadic cases have been reported in many varied ethnic groups. It is believed that malaria has exerted a selective pressure for the propagation of the thalassemia genes (Weatherall and Clegg, 1972), although the scientific basis for the proposed protection of the thalassemia heterozygote against malaria is unknown.

The actual incidence of thalassemia in various populations can be estimated only on the basis of limited surveys. In Southern

Italian, Sicilian, and Greek populations approximately 10 per cent of individuals are heterozygotes for β thalassemia. On certain Greek islands and in some villages of Sardinia the incidence can reach 20 to 30 per cent. In blacks, fewer than 5 per cent are affected with α or β thalassemia. In Thailand as many as 20 per cent of the population carry the trait for one or another type of thalassemia (Wasi et al., 1969). In Thailand α thalassemia is much more common than β thalassemia, but in other Oriental populations α and β thalassemia are probably equally prevalent.

Genetics of the Thalassemia Syndrome

Alpha and beta thalassemia are inherited as autosomal dominant traits. The location of the α and β thalassemia genes is not known with certainty, but there is good evidence that they are closely linked to the structural genes for the α and β globin chains, respectively. This conclusion is confirmed by the study of the interaction of α and β thalassemia with α and β globin chain structural variants: the genes for β-chain structural variants and β thalassemia behave as alleles, as do the genes for α-chain structural variants and α thalassemia (Weatherall and Clegg, 1972).

There has been no convincing evidence of crossing over between the β-thalassemia and β-structural genes. The study of families in which genes for both β thalassemia and a δ-chain variant coexist makes it possible to evaluate the proximity of these two genes: in four such families, providing 31 opportunities for crossing over between β-thalassemia and δ-structural genes, there is indeed evidence of two likely instances of such a crossover (Pearson et al., 1965; Thompson et al., 1965b). On the other hand, there has been no evidence of recombination, in 50 opportunities, between β-structural and δ-structural genes (Weatherall and Clegg, 1972). These findings suggest that the β-thalassemia gene is located farther away from the δ-structural gene than is the β-structural gene. Further family studies are necessary to confirm this conclusion.

There are only two families which provide genetic evidence for the linkage of the α-thalassemia and α-chain structural loci: in four offspring of two individuals doubly heterozygous for α thalassemia and an α-chain structural variant (Hb I or Hb G-Philadelphia) no crossing over occurred, indicating close linkage of the α-thalassemia to the α-chain structural gene(s) (Atwater et al., 1960; Rieder et al., 1976).

The genetics of α-thalassemia are otherwise quite confusing (reviewed in Weatherall and Clegg, 1972), and much of the confusion centers on whether or not the α-chain locus is duplicated in man and, if it is duplicated, whether the two genes are linked or independent. The evidence for and against α-chain locus duplication was reviewed in Chapter 4. Study of various α-thalassemia syndromes and the interaction of α thalassemia with α globin chain structural variants has not definitively resolved the issue (see later section in this chapter). However, the genetics of α thalassemia, especially in association with Hb Constant Spring, can be most easily explained if one accepts the presence of duplicated α-chain loci, at least in the Asian population in which α thalassemia is most prevalent. The detailed evidence for this conclusion will be reviewed in the section of this chapter dealing with the various α-thalassemia syndromes.

Molecular Pathology of the Thalassemia Syndromes

As stated in the introduction to this chapter, the thalassemia syndromes are all characterized by absent or decreased synthesis of one or more of the globin chains of human hemoglobin. In those cases where some of the affected globin chain is synthesized, the resulting globin chain is structurally normal (Guidotti, 1962; Baglioni, 1963; Jones and Schroeder, 1963). In this respect, the thalassemia syndromes differ from the other hemoglobinopathies, such as sickle cell anemia, in which a structurally abnormal globin chain is synthesized. The molecular basis of most structural hemoglobin variants is well understood and is discussed in Chapter 6. The precise molecular basis for the quantitative defect in globin-chain synthesis in thalassemia, on the other hand, has not been established in most cases. Nevertheless, a great deal of information has been obtained which clearly implicates certain molecular mechanisms in the pathogenesis of thalassemia. This information will now be reviewed.

Studies of Globin Synthesis in Intact Thalassemic Erythroid Cells

The thalassemic defect—the imbalance of globin-chain synthesis—was first directly demonstrated in thalassemic cells by three different laboratories between 1964 and 1966 (Heywood et al., 1964, 1965; Weatherall et al., 1965; Bank and Marks, 1966). The technique which was used consists of incubating peripheral blood reticulocytes for 1 to 2 hours in the presence of a radioactive amino acid precursor, usually leucine or valine. Globin is then prepared from the total cell lysate or from the Hb A purified from the lysate by column chromatography. The globin is fractionated by carboxymethyl-cellulose column chromatography in the presence of 8 molar urea, which separates the α, β, and γ globin chains. An example of a chromatogram obtained with globin isolated from normal nonthalassemic peripheral

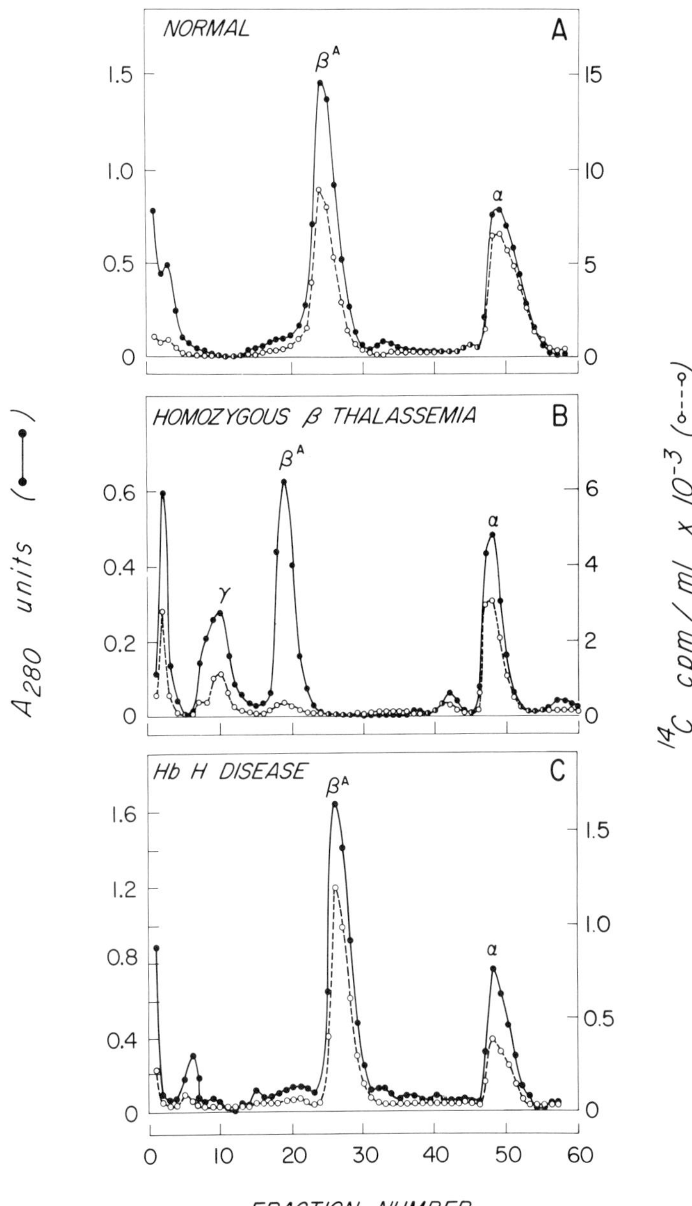

Figure 5–1. Globin synthesis in reticulocytes of patients with nonthalassemic hemolytic anemia, homozygous beta thalassemia, and Hb H disease. Peripheral blood was incubated with ^{14}C-leucine; globin then was prepared from the red cells and fractionated by carboxymethylcellulose column chromatography.
●——● represents optical density of globin chains.
○– – –○ represents radioactivity incorporated into newly synthesized globin chains.

reticulocytes is shown in Figure 5–1*A*. It can be seen that roughly equal amounts of radioactive, newly synthesized α and β chains are found under the α and β globin chain optical density peaks. One can thus obtain a quantitative ratio of β to α globin-chain synthesis (β/α synthetic ratio), which, in a normal cell, will be equal to 1.0. When applied to the study of thalassemic reticulocytes, the initial studies all demonstrated a decrease in incorporation of radioactivity into the β chain of hemoglobin A in β-thalassemic reticulocytes. Similar studies have since been repeated in a number of laboratories and the results of these studies all indicate marked decrease of β-chain synthesis relative to α-chain synthesis in β thalassemia (Bargellesi et al., 1967; Modell et al., 1969; Weatherall et al., 1969a; Conconi et al., 1970).

In the usual heterozygotes for β thalassemia, approximately half as much radioactivity is incorporated into β chains as into α chains, but in American blacks with β-thalassemia trait, the β/α ratio can be virtually normal (Friedman et al., 1972, 1973; Braverman et al., 1973). In homozygotes for β thalassemia, there is either total absence of β-chain radioactivity or a marked decrease in β-chain radioactivity with β/α ratios of 0.1 to 0.3 (Fig. 5–1*B*). It should be pointed out that this technique does not measure absolute rates of α- and β-chain synthesis but expresses only a ratio of one to another. An attempt has been made to express the data in terms of absolute rates (Bank et al., 1968), and the findings are consistent with a normal rate of α-chain synthesis in β thalassemia; therefore the low β/α ratio is due to decreased β-chain synthesis rather than to increased α-chain synthesis.

The same techniques have been applied to the study of α thalassemia (Weatherall et al., 1965; Clegg and Weatherall, 1967; Kan et al., 1968). In severe homozygous α thalassemia (hydrops fetalis with Hb Bart's) there is a total absence of α-chain synthesis (Weatherall et al., 1970). In Hb H disease, a less severe α-thalassemia syndrome, the globin synthesis profile reveals decreased incorporation of radioactivity into α chains compared to β chains (Fig. 5–1*C*), with an α/β ratio of 0.3 to 0.6 (Kan et al., 1968). When globin-chain synthesis is studied in α-thalassemia heterozygotes, a less striking imbalance in globin-chain synthesis is observed in comparison to the β-thalassemia heterozygotes (Kan et al., 1968). In the phenotypically obvious form of heterozygous α thalassemia (α-thal 1 trait), the α/β ratio is 0.70 to 0.80, whereas in the mild form of heterozygous α thalassemia (the "silent carrier" state or α-thal 2 trait), it is 0.80 to 0.95 (Kan et al., 1968). Alpha thalassemia in American blacks does not demonstrate as marked or as consistent an imbalance in globin-chain synthesis (Schwartz and Atwater, 1972).

The range of β/α ratios obtained in a large series of patients with various α- and β-thalassemia syndromes is shown in Figure 5–2.

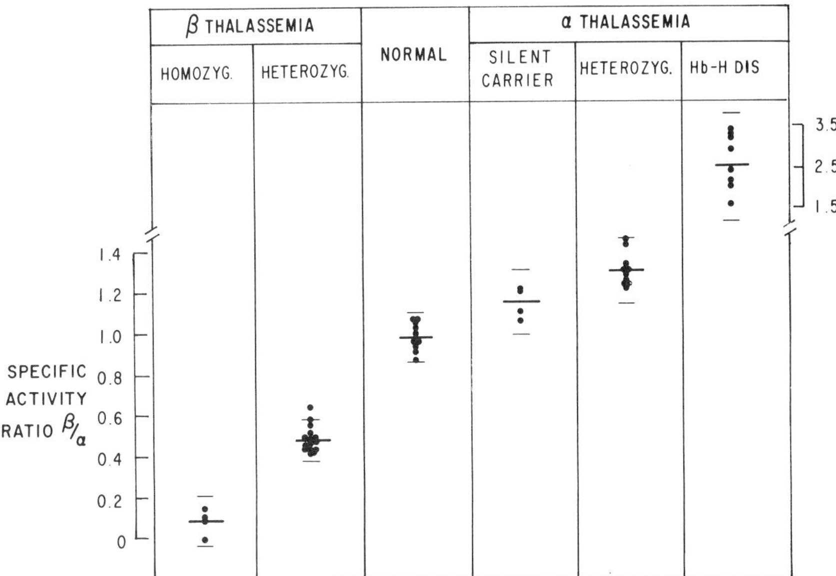

Figure 5–2. Range of values obtained for the ratio of β- to α-chain synthesis in nonthalassemic reticulocytes and in reticulocytes of patients with various α- and β-thalassemia syndromes. (From Nathan, D. G.: N. Engl. J. Med. *286*:586, 1972.)

When globin synthesis was studied in marrow of patients with β thalassemia, interesting observations were made. In homozygous β thalassemia, the β/α synthetic ratio was still abnormal but the value was closer to normal than in the peripheral blood of the same patient (Braverman and Bank, 1969; Friedman et al., 1972). Other workers have not been able to demonstrate such a striking difference between marrow and peripheral blood globin synthesis in β thalassemia (Bargellesi et al., 1967; Shchory and Ramot, 1972; Nienhuis et al., 1973). It is likely that some artifact in the technique is responsible for these discrepancies rather than some fundamental difference in the expression of the β-thalassemic defect between marrow and peripheral blood cells.

In heterozygous β thalassemia, an even more interesting observation has been made by Schwartz (1970). In the marrow of such persons, he found that the β/α synthetic ratio is very close to 1.0. This observation has been confirmed in a number of different laboratories (Clegg and Weatherall, 1972; Gill et al., 1972; Kan et al., 1972c; Shchory and Ramot, 1972; White et al., 1972; Natta et al., 1973a; Nienhius et al., 1973). The findings are difficult to interpret. It is unlikely that there is decreased β-chain synthesis only in reticulocytes and not in marrow, because over 90 per cent of globin-chain synthesis occurs in the marrow, and if decreased β-chain synthesis occurred only at the reticulocyte stage, then the β-thalassemic heterozygotes should not be anemic and their red cells should not be hypochromic and microcytic. Another possible explanation for hypochromia despite relatively equal amounts of α- and β-chain synthesis is that the α-chain synthesis as well as β-chain synthesis is decreased in the marrow cells of patients with heterozygous β thalassemia, whereas in the reticulocytes, the imbalance becomes manifest as α-chain synthesis returns to normal (Nathan, 1973).

There is as yet no experimental evidence to support this type of presumed feedback inhibition of synthesis of the nonaffected globin chain in thalassemia. Studies by Clegg and Weatherall (1972) on globin synthesis in heterozygous β-thalassemia marrow indicate that despite the β/α synthetic ratio of nearly 1.0, there is indeed imbalance between β and α globin chain synthesis in marrow, evidenced by the finding of a large pool of free α globin chains in such marrow cells. The authors postulate two explanations for the finding of β/α synthetic ratios close to 1.0: first, in marrow, nonglobin peptides may co-chromatograph with the β chain, thereby falsely increasing the radioactivity in the β-chain region; second, the authors also provide some evidence that, in vitro, α chains are more unstable in marrow as compared to those in peripheral blood and may undergo proteolysis in time, thereby falsely lowering the radioactivity found in the α-chain peak.

Studies by Wood and Stamatoyannopoulos (1975) failed to demonstrate a contaminating nonglobin peptide, but experiments using purified erythroid precursor cells did demonstrate increased free pools of α chains even in the most immature erythroid precursor cells in heterozygous β thalassemia. Their studies also provided convincing indirect evidence that turnover (? proteolysis) of α chains is the most likely explanation for the unexpected finding of a β/α synthetic ratio of 1.0 in heterozygous β-thalassemia marrow. A more recent report by Chalevelakis et al. (1975) has shown the presence of a minor nonglobin (? marrow granulocyte) protein contaminating the β-chain peak on CMC columns. More importantly, however, in short pulse-labeling experiments the authors demonstrated clearly that the β/α synthetic ratio in heterozygous β-thalassemia marrow changes with time, being abnormal (0.5) after short incubations and nearing unity after longer periods of incubation. Increased α-chain turnover is again implicated as the primary cause of the phenomenon. Assays of globin mRNA in purified nucleated marrow cells of patients with heterozygous β thalassemia have in fact demonstrated the expected deficiency of β mRNA (β/α mRNA content 0.4 to 0.6) (Pritchard et al., 1975).

Recently, cases of heterozygous β thalassemia of unusual severity have been reported in which the marrow β/α synthetic ratio ranges between 0.7 and 0.8 whereas the peripheral blood ratio remains at the usual level of 0.5 (Friedman et al., 1976a; Stamatoyannopoulos et al., 1974).

Molecular Basis of Thalassemia

The details of the normal process of protein and hemoglobin biosynthesis have been reviewed in Chapter 4 (see Figure 4–3). It is easy to see that, in the complex process of protein synthesis, a number of regulatory events could occur which would affect the rate of synthesis of a given protein and result in the presence of decreased amounts of an otherwise structurally normal protein in the cells. Various defects in the process of protein synthesis have been searched for to explain the decreased synthesis of structurally normal globin chains which occurs in thalassemia. This topic has been reviewed in detail elsewhere (Forget, 1974; Forget and Nathan, 1975; Benz and Forget, 1975) and will be summarized here.

If chain termination were defective (abnormally slow), less protein would accumulate in the cell. In thalassemia, however, there is no evidence for slow release of chains from ribosomes to cytoplasm (Clegg et al., 1968). At the level of chain elongation, decreased output of a structurally normal protein chain could result from a nucleotide sequence change (base substitution) in the messenger RNA, which results in its coding, not for a different amino acid, but for a different transfer RNA for the same amino acid; if the specific tRNA were in short supply in the cell, there would result an overall slowing of the rate of synthesis of the affected chain. This is the so-called modulation hypothesis to explain thalassemia (Ingram, 1964; Itano, 1965). However, there is good evidence that this phenomenon does not occur in thalassemia, since pulse-labeling experiments and peptide analysis (Dintzis' plots) of the nascent globin chains in β thalassemia have revealed normal rates of chain assembly and elongation of the β globin chain (Clegg et al., 1968; Rieder, 1972). At the level of initiation, decreased synthesis could occur if there is decreased initiation of the messenger RNA due to an abnormality in the messenger RNA, an abnormality of the ribosome, or abnormalities in the various initiation factors.

The following areas of study have revealed no abnormalities or differences in thalassemic cells compared to nonthalassemic cells: ribosome quantity and radioactive profile or polysomes (Burka and Marks, 1963); effect of added nonthalassemic ribosomal subunits to thalassemic ribosomes (Fuhr et al., 1969); translation by thalassemic ribosomes of synthetic mRNA (poly [U]) (Bank and Marks, 1966) and natural mRNA (rabbit globin mRNA) (Nienhuis et al., 1971); effect of added human and/or rabbit initiation factors to thalassemic ribosomes (Gilbert et al., 1970); the distribution of nascent α and β chains on thalassemic reticulocyte and marrow polysomes, as an index of specific chain initiation and elongation (Nathan et al., 1971; Cividalli et al., 1974b); and the specific mechanism of globin chain initiation (use of initiator tRNA) and initial dipeptide formation (Crystal et al., 1973).

All evidence therefore indicates the presence of a defect in the messenger RNA for the affected globin chain as the basis for the imbalanced globin-chain synthesis which occurs in the thalassemia syndromes. On the basis of the above evidence, the messenger RNA could be either quantitatively deficient or qualitatively (structurally) abnormal in its nontranslated portions. Such a structural defect of the mRNA might lead to more rapid degradation, and eventually concomitant quantitative deficiency of the mRNA, or it might lead to abnormal function of the mRNA such as absent or decreased binding to ribosomes without actual quantitative deficiency of the mRNA. The involvement of globin mRNA in the expression of the thalassemic defect has in fact been directly demonstrated in a number of laboratories (Benz and Forget, 1971; Nienhuis and Anderson, 1971; Benz et al., 1973; Dow et al., 1973; Grossbard et al., 1973; Natta et al., 1973a; Nienhuis et al., 1973)—messenger RNA isolated from thalassemic reticulocytes or marrow cells, when it is translated in a heterologous cell-free protein synthesizing system, will duplicate the imbalance of globin-chain synthesis, which is characteristic of the intact thalassemic reticulocyte. Although these observations demonstrate direct involvement of globin mRNA in the expression of the thalassemic defect, they still do not differentiate between overall quantitative or chemical deficiency of mRNA and simple deficiency of mRNA function. On the other hand, RNA-DNA hybridization studies (Housman et al., 1973; Kacian et al., 1973) and primary structure studies (Forget et al., 1974b; Marotta et al., 1974) of the messenger RNA isolated from thalassemic reticulocytes indicate that the messenger RNA for the affected (thalassemic) globin chain is indeed quantitatively deficient in these reticulocytes.

These latter observations were made possible by use of the RNA-dependent DNA polymerase (or reverse transcriptase) of RNA tumor viruses. This enzyme will synthesize, in vitro, a radioactive DNA copy (cDNA) of globin mRNA. The radioactive cDNAs of α and β mRNA can then be used as probes for the quantitation, in RNA-DNA hybridization experiments, of the relative chemical amounts of α and β mRNA in reticulocyte RNA of thalassemic patients. The cDNA can also be used as a template for RNA polymerase which will synthesize a highly radioactive ^{32}P-labeled RNA copy of the cDNA suitable for nucleotide sequence analysis by standard RNA sequencing techniques. Both of these general approaches were applied to the study of thalassemic mRNA, and both approaches demonstrated quantitative deficiency of β mRNA in β thalassemia and deficiency of α mRNA in α thalassemia (Housman et al., 1973, 1974; Kacian et al., 1973; Forget et al., 1974a, 1974b; Marotta et al., 1974). The results and interpretations of these studies have been reviewed in detail elsewhere (Forget, 1974; Forget and Nathan, 1975; Benz and Forget, 1975).

Subsequent studies have demonstrated even more directly quantitative deficiency of chain-specific globin mRNA in α and β thalassemia. It is possible to separate α from β globin mRNA by acrylamide-gel electrophoresis in the presence of formamide, a solvent which completely denatures nucleic acids. When nonthalassemic globin mRNA is fractionated by this technique, roughly equal amounts of α mRNA and β mRNA are revealed. On the other hand, when α- or β-thalassemic mRNAs are fractionated, marked deficiency of α and β mRNA, respectively, can be demonstrated (Forget et al., 1975a; Kazazian et al., 1975).

The demonstration of quantitative deficiency of globin mRNA in thalassemic reticulocytes and unfractionated marrow cells still leaves open the question of whether the messenger RNA is initially transcribed in abnormally low amounts from the DNA or whether it is transcribed initially in normal amounts but later becomes deficient owing to defects in mRNA processing or transport or to some structural defect which renders it unstable and susceptible to premature degradation. A defect at either the transcriptional or the post-transcriptional level could explain the deficiency of mRNA observed in thalassemia. Studies of globin-chain synthesis in purified β-thalassemic erythroid precursor cells before and after culture and differentiation in vitro indicate that the thalassemic imbalance of globin-chain synthesis is expressed at all stages of red cell maturation in homozygous β-thalassemia (Kim et al., 1976).

A different set of molecular mechanisms could be responsible for the cases of thalassemia in which there is totally absent synthesis of the affected globin chain (β^0 and α^0 thalassemia). A gene deletion and therefore total absence of mRNA could explain the findings, but other mechanisms must be ruled out. One such mechanism is a nonsense mutation in which there is a nucleotide base substitution in the mRNA which converts an amino acid codon into a chain termination codon. In such cases, only a short portion of the affected peptide chain is synthesized and then prematurely released. If this mechanism were responsible for β^0 or α^0 thalassemia, one should find within the cells α or β peptides corresponding to the incomplete chains, assuming there is no proteolytic destruction of the abnormally short chains (Baglioni et al., 1969). Such peptides have been sought but not found in both β^0 thalassemia of the Ferrara type (Dreyfus et al., 1972) and the α^0-thalassemia syndrome of hydrops fetalis with Hb Bart's (Weatherall et al., 1970).

In β^0 thalassemia of patients from Ferrara (Italy) there is evidence that β mRNA may be present in the cells, because β-chain synthesis can apparently be induced in a cell-free system by adding nonthalassemic (β^A or β^S) reticulocyte supernatant fraction to Ferrara-thalassemia ribosomes (Conconi et al., 1972; Rowley and Kosciolek, 1972). The results were interpreted as indicating the deficiency in these patients of a factor necessary for β mRNA translation

(Conconi and Del Senno, 1974). These authors have also reported experiments in which the transfusion of blood to patients with β^0 thalassemia of the Ferrara type apparently resulted in the synthesis in these patients of some β chains 10 to 15 days after the transfusion (Conconi and Del Senno, 1974; Conconi et al., 1975). More recently, RNA-cDNA hybridization assays have confirmed the presence of β-like mRNA in this disorder, but in reduced amounts compared to α mRNA (Ramirez et al., 1976; R. Williamson, personal communication).

Beta^0 thalassemia is probably genetically and biochemically heterogeneous. Studies of mRNA isolated from reticulocytes of various patients with β^0 thalassemia other than the Ferrara type have shown no evidence of β-chain mRNA activity when the mRNA was translated in various heterologous cell-free protein synthesizing systems (Dow et al., 1973; Nienhuis et al., 1973; Benz et al., 1975b; Kan et al., 1975e; Tolstoshev et al., 1976). On the other hand, RNA-cDNA hybridization studies have given variable results in β^0 thalassemia. In some cases, it is possible to demonstrate virtual absence of β mRNA in β^0 thalassemia (Forget et al., 1974c; Ottolenghi et al., 1975; Tolstoshev et al., 1976). However, in other cases, the hybridization assay does reveal the presence of a significant level of β or β-like mRNA in β^0 thalassemia (Kan et al., 1975e; Ramirez et al., 1976; Forget et al., 1976c). It is therefore unlikely that cases of β^0 thalassemia are due to gene deletions. Such cases may be due to defects in transcription or due to structurally and functionally abnormal β mRNA. In fact, studies of gene dosage by DNA-cDNA hybridization in a number of cases of homozygous β^0 thalassemia (some with absent β mRNA) have yielded results which are not consistent with the presence of β-globin gene deletions in these cases (Ottolenghi et al., 1975; Tolstoshev et al., 1976; Kan et al., 1975e; Ramirez et al., 1976; Forget et al., unpublished observations).

Gene quantitation has also been accomplished using DNA of cultured fibroblasts and lymphocytes from patients with homozygous hereditary persistence of fetal hemoglobin (HPFH) in which there is total absence of Hb A and Hb A_2 synthesis (see later section of this chapter). In contrast to the findings in homozygous β^0 thalassemia, these studies have demonstrated absence of β-chain genes (and presumably δ-chain genes) in the two cases studied (Kan et al., 1975d; Forget et al., 1976b). There was also total absence of β-chain mRNA in the one case in which it was measured (Forget et al., 1976b). It has also been shown that β- (and δ-) gene deletion exists in homozygous $\delta\beta$ thalassemia in which there is total absence of Hb A and Hb A_2 synthesis (Ottolenghi et al., 1976; Ramirez et al., 1976). Since both $\delta\beta$ thalassemia and HPFH appear to be associated with β-gene deletions, the difference in phenotypic expression between the two syndromes is not explained by this fact alone. It is possible that the extent of the chromosomal deletion, especially the involvement of intergene material between γ and δ genes, is different in both cases and that this material is involved in the differential expression of the γ genes in these two syndromes. This is pure speculation, however.

In the case of α^0 thalassemia, on the other hand, there is definitive evidence that the molecular basis of this disorder is deletion of the α globin chain loci. Incubation of α cDNA with liver DNA from hydropic infants with homozygous α thalassemia (Hb Bart's syndrome) reveals no significant hybridization, indicating deletion of the α globin chain genes (Ottolenghi et al., 1974; Taylor et al., 1974; Ramirez et al., 1975b). Subsequent hybridization studies utilizing DNA from the spleen of a patient with Hb H disease revealed deficiency of α globin genes to a level of approximately 25 per cent of normal (Kan et al., 1975a). These results are consistent with deletion of three of the α globin genes in Hb H disease and lend additional support to the presence of duplicated α-chain loci at least in the Asian population in which α thalassemia is prevalent: if the α-chain loci were not duplicated, the expected deficiency of α-chain genes would be 50 per cent (rather than 75 per cent) in Hb H disease (Kan et al., 1975a).

Thalassemia-like Disorders Associated with Structurally Abnormal Globin Chains

In the usual forms of thalassemia, the affected globin chain, which is synthesized in decreased amounts, is structurally normal, i.e., it shows no evidence of an amino acid substitution. There are two groups of thalassemia-like disorders, however, in which an abnormal globin chain is in fact synthesized: the Hb Lepore syndromes and the Hb Constant Spring syndromes.

THE HEMOGLOBIN LEPORE SYNDROMES. Hb Lepore is a structurally abnormal hemoglobin in which the abnormal globin chain is a hybrid or fused globin chain, having the N-terminal amino acid sequence of the normal δ chain and the C-terminal amino acid sequence of the normal β chain (Baglioni, 1962). The Lepore defect appears to have resulted from mispairing of δ and β loci during meiosis and subsequent nonhomologous crossing over of the chromosomes in the area of the mispaired δ and β loci (Baglioni, 1962). As illustrated in Figure 5–3A, such a crossover event would yield, on one chromosome, a fused $\delta\beta$ locus (without adjacent intact δ or β loci) and, on the other chromosome, a locus for a hybrid or fused globin chain having the N-terminal amino acid sequence of the β chain and the C-terminal sequence of the δ chain (an "anti-Lepore" chain) situated between a normal δ-chain locus and a normal β-chain locus. The Hb Lepore gene behaves as a β-thalassemic gene because there is only a low level of synthesis of its gene product (the $\delta\beta$ chain) and presumably absence of a normal β-chain locus on the affected chromosome. This latter assumption is confirmed by the find-

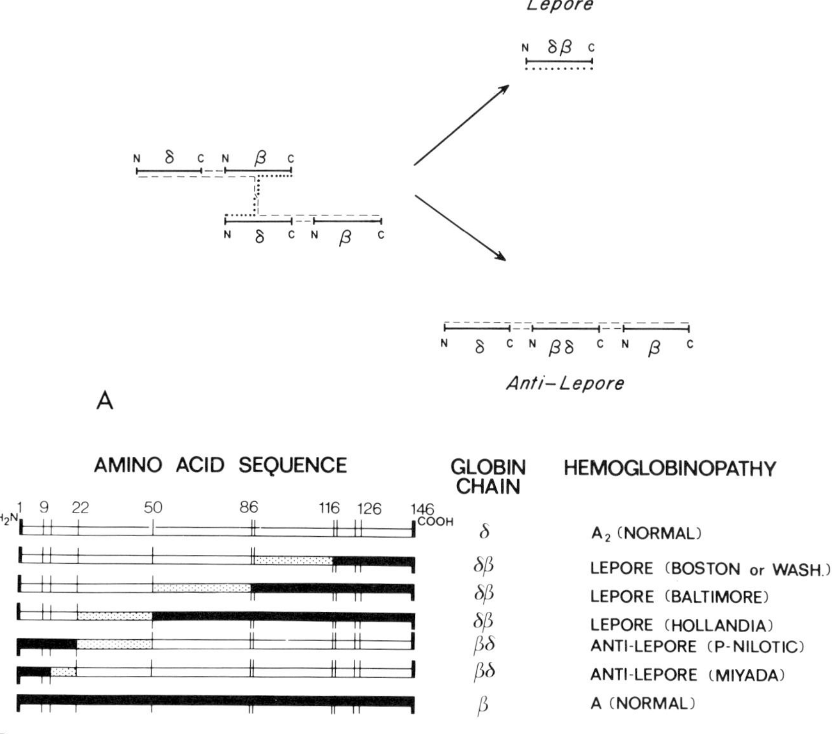

Figure 5–3. A, Origin of the Lepore and anti-Lepore globin chains by nonhomologous crossing over between δ- and β-globin genes. N and C refer to the extremities of the gene coding for the amino-terminal (N) and carboxy-terminal (C) ends of the globin chains. *B*, Different types of Lepore and anti-Lepore globin chains. The numbers refer to the position of amino acid residues in the globin chain: the 10 positions where δ and β sequences differ are indicated by the lighter vertical lines. The dotted area represents the region in which the δβ crossover occurred. (From Benz, E. J., and Forget, B. G.: *In* Brown, E. B. (ed.): Progress in Hematology. Vol. IX, New York, Grune & Stratton, 1975, p. 107.)

ings in patients homozygous for Hb Lepore, in which there is total absence of normal Hb A and Hb A_2 (Weatherall and Clegg, 1972). Three different types of Lepore chains have been described in which the transition from δ to β amino acid sequence occurs in different areas of the sequence (Fig. 5–3*B* and Table 6–2).

The reasons for the low level of synthesis of Hb Lepore are not known. There may be decreased synthesis because of relative instability of the mRNA for the Lepore chain: globin synthetic studies reveal that synthesis of the Lepore δβ chain, like that of the δ chain of the Hb A_2, occurs primarily in marrow cells and is virtually absent in peripheral blood reticulocytes (Rieder and Weatherall, 1965; Gill et al., 1972; Roberts et al., 1972; White et al., 1972a). Alternatively, transcription of the Lepore δβ gene may be reduced because of adjacent control genes which are responsible for the normally low level of expression of the δ gene. In either case, it is difficult to explain why Hb Lepore accumulates to a level of 10 to 15 per cent of the total Hb, whereas Hb A_2 is rarely increased to levels much greater than 5 per cent of the total Hb. The 5′-terminal sequences adjacent to the δ-chain gene cannot be the only factors regulating the expression of the Lepore δβ gene, otherwise Hb Lepore would accumulate only at a level similar to that of Hb A_2. The relative contributions of transcriptional versus post-transcriptional control in these phenomena are not known. Despite absence of Lepore-chain synthesis in peripheral blood cells, substantial amounts of mRNA for the Lepore chain can still be detected in these cells by molecular hybridization assays (Benz et al., 1975a).

The condition in which the δ, βδ, and β loci all occur on one chromosome is called the anti-Lepore syndrome, and its demonstration is important in confirming the nonhomologous crossover hypothesis for the origin of the Lepore δβ chain (Fig. 5–3*A*). Two instances of such an abnormal hybrid (N)βδ(C) chain have recently been demonstrated, in Hb P-Congo (Hb P-Nilotic) (Lehmann and Charlesworth, 1970; Badr et al., 1973) and Hb Miyada (Ohta et al., 1971) (Fig. 5–3*B*). The anti-Lepore syndromes do not resemble β thalassemia because the affected chromosome carries, in addition to the mutant gene, normal β and δ genes with normal output. There is therefore no overall deficit (or imbalance) in globin-chain synthesis and, consequently, no thalassemic phenotype.

The anti-Lepore hemoglobins accumulate in the red cell to approximately the same levels as do the Lepore hemoglobins. The synthesis of Hb Miyada is virtually limited to the bone marrow as is that of the Lepore hemoglobins (Roberts et al., 1973). This phenomenon has been interpreted as evidence of instability of the anti-Lepore globin mRNA and evidence that both the 5′- and 3′-terminal sequences of globin mRNA are important in maintaining its stability (Roberts et al., 1973; Clegg et al., 1974b). There could, however, also be effects of these mutations on the globin gene transcription process. The fact that the anti-Lepore hemoglobins are present at much lower levels than Hb A and at approximately the same levels as the Lepore hemoglobins indicates that the putative control genes at the 5′ extremity of the δ and β genes are not the sole factors regulating the expression of mutant fused δβ and βδ genes.

THE HEMOGLOBIN CONSTANT SPRING SYNDROMES. The second group of thalassemia-like conditions in which a structurally abnormal globin chain is synthesized are the hemoglobin Constant Spring syndromes (Clegg et al., 1971b; Milner et al., 1971). In Hb Constant Spring, an abnormally long α globin chain is synthesized, which is elongated at its C-terminal end by an additional 31 amino acids. This globin chain is produced in only small amounts and therefore the gene resembles an alpha-thalassemic gene. Red cells of patients heterozygous for Hb Constant Spring alone contain only 1 to 2 per cent of the mutant hemoglobin.

Three other similar hemoglobin variants have been described which have elongated α chains: Hb Icaria (Clegg et al., 1974a), Hb Koya Dora (DeJong et al., 1975), and Hb Seal Rock (Bradley et al., 1975). The three variants, like Hb Constant Spring, are also synthesized at very low levels. All four variants have different amino acids at portion 142 of their α chain (the first residue following the normal α-chain C-terminal residue at position 141). The following 30 amino acid residues, however, are the same in all four variants. These mutant hemoglobins probably arose by chain termination mutation (see Chapter 6).

The traits for Hb Constant Spring and Hb Icaria interact with heterozygous α thalassemia to give the more severe α-thalassemia syndrome, Hb H disease (see below). It is unclear how the chain termination mutation leads to the very low level of production of the elongated mutant globin chain. The synthesis of Hb CS, like that of Hb A_2, Hb Lepore, and Hb Miyada, is virtually limited to bone marrow cells and essentially absent in peripheral blood cells (Kan et al., 1974c). These findings suggest instability of the Hb Constant Spring mRNA but it is difficult to conceive how a single base substitution in the termination codon could lead in itself to instability of the mRNA. Other phenomena may be operative, such as decreased transcription and/or degradation of the mRNA during the "readthrough" process. Hb CS was not initially considered to be an unstable hemoglobin (Clegg et al., 1971b), but recent results suggest that the elongated chain is quickly degraded to shorter forms (Pootrakul et al., 1976).

PATHOPHYSIOLOGY OF THE ANEMIA

There are many primary and secondary causes for the anemia observed in thalassemia. It is easy to understand how reduced synthesis of one or another of the globin chains of hemoglobin A will result in an overall deficit of hemoglobin A synthesis and cause a hypochromic, microcytic anemia with a low mean corpuscular hemoglobin level of the red cells. This is true in both the heterozygous and homozygous states. In the homozygous state, however, another pathophysiological process worsens the anemia and is responsible for the major clinical manifestations of Cooley's anemia. The continued synthesis in normal amounts of the nonaffected globin chain results in the accumulation, within the red cells, of excessive amounts of these normal chains. Not finding complementary globin chains with which to bind, these chains form aggregates, precipitate within the cell, and become attached to the cell membrane (Bargellesi et al., 1968; Weatherall et al., 1969). These precipitates then lead to membrane damage (Gunn et al., 1972) and premature destruction of the red cell (Nathan and Gunn, 1966; Nathan et al., 1969). In β thalassemia, the resulting α-chain aggregates are called inclusion bodies or, perhaps improperly, Heinz bodies. In contrast to true Heinz bodies which are made up of total precipitated hemoglobin ($\alpha_2\beta_2$), these inclusion bodies have been shown, convincingly, to consist of only α globin chains (Fessas et al., 1966), which do have some attached heme, perhaps in the form of hemichromes (Rachmilewitz and Thorell, 1972). In α thalassemia, the resulting β_4 tetramers constitute Hb H, which is less insoluble than α-chain aggregates. In the neonatal and fetal periods, γ_4 tetramers occur in α thalassemia and constitute Hb Bart's. (Hemoglobin Bart's is seen in occasional adults with Hb H disease, particularly those with Hb Constant Spring.) The process of inclusion-body formation occurs in the erythroid precursors as well as in the mature red cells. It is responsible for the marked ineffective erythropoiesis and the hemolytic component seen in both the α- and β-thalassemia syndromes.

In β thalassemia, the role of thalassemic inclusions in the pathophysiology of the hemolytic anemia is manifested in the heterogeneous red cell population which is present in this disorder. Fetal hemoglobin is very heterogeneously distributed in the β-thalassemic red cells. Those cells which have the most fetal Hb are those which will have the least relative excess of α chains, since the γ chains combine with α chains to form Hb F. It has been demonstrated in β thalassemia that Hb A has a more rapid turnover (shorter half life) than Hb F (Gabuzda et al., 1963). This finding is consistent with the presence of different populations of red cells: those containing mainly Hb A are short lived and those containing much more Hb F have longer survival (Gabuzda et al., 1963). Indeed, differential centrifugation of red cells in β thalassemia reveals that the older, more rapidly sedimenting red cells contain much Hb F and have relatively few α-chain inclusions, whereas the younger, more slowly sedimenting cells are relatively deficient in Hb F and contain many α-chain inclusions (Loukopoulos and Fessas, 1965; Nathan and Gunn, 1966; Nathan et al., 1969). There is also a good positive correlation between the severity of the disease in β thalassemia and the size of the free α-chain pool and the degree of α to non-α globin chain imbalance (Bargellesi et al., 1968; Weatherall et al., 1969a).

These findings serve to emphasize the relationship of the α-chain inclusions to the hemolytic process and the beneficial role of γ-chain synthesis in lessening the imbalance of globin-chain synthesis, decreasing the formation of α-chain inclusions and thus increasing the red cells' survival. In β thalassemia, the α-chain inclusions are found in large quantities in the bone marrow erythroid precursors (Fessas, 1963; Yataganas and Fessas, 1969) and are probably the cause of the marked ineffective erythropoiesis or intramedullary destruction of erythroid cells which is observed in homozygous β

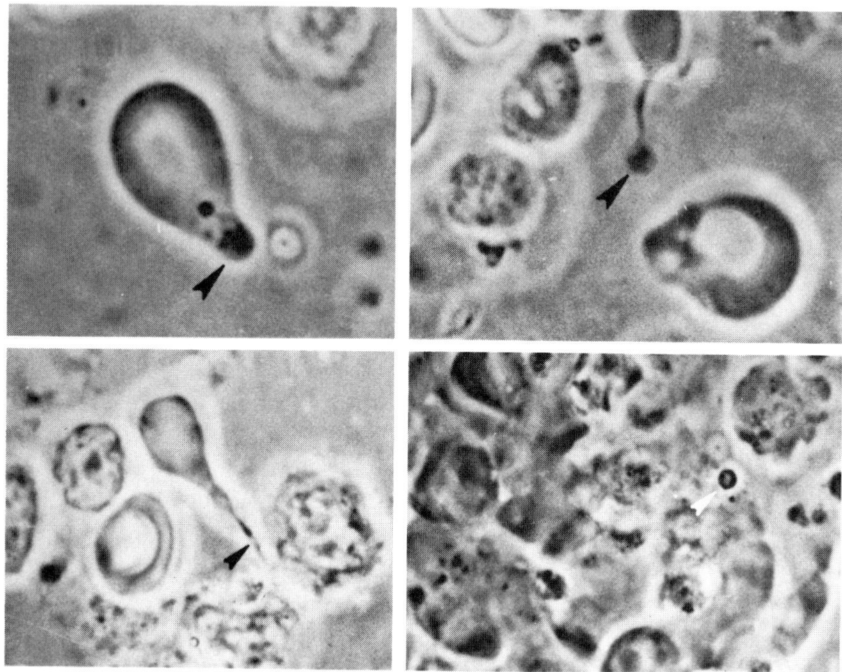

Figure 5–4 Phase microscopy of a wet preparation of scrapings from the spleen of a patient with homozygous beta thalassemia. Note alpha-chain inclusion bodies (arrows) within teardrop-shaped red cells, inclusions being pulled out or "pitted" from the red cell by reticuloendothelial cell action (lower left), and inclusions free in the splenic pulp (white arrow). (From Nathan, D. G.: N. Engl. J. Med. *286*:586, 1972.)

thalassemia (Finch et al., 1970). Prior to splenectomy, these inclusion bodies are practically never seen in peripheral red blood cells, but following splenectomy they appear in large numbers (Fessas, 1963). This observation correlates well with the demonstrated role of the spleen (and reticuloendothelial system) in removing inclusion bodies of the Heinz body type from red cells, thereby damaging and/or destroying these cells (Rifkind and Danon, 1965; Slater et al., 1968; Wennberg and Weiss, 1968). This phenomenon can be dramatically observed, under phase microscopy, in fresh wet preparations obtained from scrapings of β-thalassemic spleens removed at surgery (Fig. 5–4) and is probably the main basis of the hemolytic anemia observed in β thalassemia. In β thalassemia, the α-chain inclusions result from decreased β-chain synthesis. Another inclusion-body syndrome has recently been reported in which the inclusions apparently result from an absolute increase in α-chain production (Weatherall et al., 1973).

In the α-thalassemia syndrome of Hb H disease, the resulting β_4 tetramers (Hb H) are more stable than α-chain aggregates and precipitate more slowly. One does not observe, therefore, marked ineffective erythropoiesis and intramedullary destruction of erythroid cells as seen in β thalassemia, although some Hb H inclusions are seen in marrow normoblasts (Fessas and Yataganas, 1968). The β_4 inclusions form more gradually and occur mainly in mature red cells rather than in erythroid precursor cells. The spleen removes these inclusions and thus damages the red blood cells, as in β thalassemia (Rigas and Koler, 1961; Nathan and Gunn, 1966; Wennberg and Weiss, 1968; Nathan et al., 1969). Prior to splenectomy, no preformed Hb H inclusions are seen in the peripheral red blood cells, although soluble Hb H is present and can be made to precipitate in the form of small, stippled inclusions by in-vitro incubation of the blood with brilliant cresyl blue (BCB). After splenectomy, large, usually single, round, preformed inclusions are seen in the red cells by staining with BCB (as well as by methyl violet staining and by phase microscopy), in addition to the usual multiple, finely stippled inclusions (Nathan and Gunn, 1966; Weatherall and Clegg, 1972).

A number of secondary abnormalities also occur in thalassemia which can worsen the anemia. Excess iron stores accumulate because of repeated blood transfusions and increased gastrointestinal absorption (Erlandson et al., 1962; Bannerman et al., 1964; Necheles et al., 1969; Heinrich et al., 1973). This iron cannot be utilized owing to the decreased globin synthesis. It therefore accumulates in excess within the erythroid cells and is deposited in the mitochondria of these cells. This phenomenon may lead to decreased function of mitochondrial enzymes, including those which are necessary for heme synthesis. Decreased heme synthesis may contribute to an even further decrease in Hb A synthesis, but the more important cause of impaired heme synthesis is feedback inhibition due to accumulation of heme intermediates because of decreased globin synthesis (Bannerman, 1964).

The anemia of thalassemia may also be aggravated by folic acid deficiency which can easily develop in the thalassemic homozygote because of the high folic acid requirement resulting from the massive marrow erythroid hyperplasia and cellular turnover (Jandl and Greenberg, 1959; Luhby and Cooperman, 1961; Luhby et al., 1961). The splenomegaly invariably associated with homozygous thalassemia also contributes to the anemia by simply acting as a third space, by increasing intravascular volume and causing hemodilution (Prankerd, 1963), or by causing true hypersplenic destruction of red blood cells. After splenectomy the liver may act in a similar fashion but less effectively. Finally, since red cells containing fetal hemoglobin have high oxygen affinity (Chapter 3) there may exist actual tissue hypoxia at hemoglobin levels which would otherwise seem adequate to provide proper tissue oxygenation, if the hemoglobin were all normal adult Hb A (Maurer et al., 1970; DeFuria et al., 1974). In fact, thalassemic red cells appear to adapt poorly to anemia, as reflected by inappropriately low levels of red cell 2,3-DPG and relatively increased oxygen affinity (DeFuria et al., 1974; Pearson, 1975).

CLASSIFICATION OF THE THALASSEMIA SYNDROMES

The thalassemia syndromes are usually classified according to the type of the globin chain which is absent or present in decreased amount. The different types of thalassemia syndromes are listed in Table 5–1. Each type can occur in either the heterozygous or homozygous form. We will first consider the α-thalassemia syndromes. Heterozygous α thalassemia can occur in two forms: a phenotypically detectable form, referred to as α-thalassemia 1 trait, and a very mild defect, the α-thalassemia 2 trait, the existence of which is undectable, except by family studies and by its interaction with the α-thalas-

TABLE 5–1. *Classification of the Thalassemia Syndromes*

A. Alpha Thalassemia Syndromes
 1. Heterozygous alpha thalassemia 1
 2a. Heterozygous alpha thalassemia 2, or "silent carrier"
 2b. Hb Constant Spring trait
 3. Hb H disease: the combination of 1 with 2a or 2b
 4. Hydrops fetalis with Hb Bart's: homozygous alpha thalassemia 1

B. Beta Thalassemia Syndromes
 1. Heterozygous beta thalassemia
  a. With elevated Hb A_2 $\pm$ elevated Hb F (total absence of or reduced β-chain synthesis)
  b. With normal Hb A_2 and elevated Hb F: $\delta\beta$-thalassemia or F-thalassemia (total absence of β-chain synthesis)
  c. With normal Hb A_2 and Hb F (? "silent carrier")
  d. Hb Lepore trait
 2. "Homozygous" beta thalassemia or Cooley's anemia
  a. True homozygosity for one or another beta thalassemia gene
  b. Double heterozygosity for any two different beta thalassemia genes
  c. Thalassemia intermedia: certain doubly heterozygous combinations

C. Alpha + Beta Thalassemia
 1. Thalassemia of intermediate severity

D. Rare Forms of Thalassemia
 1. Gamma thalassemia
 2. Delta thalassemia

E. Interacting Thalassemia
 1. Alpha thalassemia + alpha chain variant
  a. Hb Q/alpha thalassemia
 2. Beta thalassemia + beta chain variant
  a. Sickle/beta thalassemia
  b. Hb C/beta thalassemia
  c. Hb E/beta thalassemia

F. Hereditary Persistence of Fetal Hemoglobin (not really a thalassemic disorder)
 1. Heterozygous
 2. Homozygous
 3. In association with beta chain structural variants

semia 1 gene. The latter is frequently referred to as the "silent carrier" state for α thalassemia. The heterozygous state for hemoglobin Constant Spring is phenotypically similar to α-thalassemia 2 trait or the silent carrier state, except that small amounts (1 to 2 per cent) of the abnormal hemoglobin are detectable. The homozygous state for the α-thalassemia 1 gene is the hydrops fetalis or hemoglobin Bart's syndrome. The doubly heterozygous state for the α-thalassemia 1 and α-thalassemia 2 genes is the less severe syndrome of hemoglobin H disease.

In the β-thalassemia syndromes, the heterozygous state for β thalassemia (thalassemia minor or minima) is quite heterogeneous, as indicated by the variations in the amounts of the minor components of hemoglobin present in the affected individual. The various heterozygous states include (1) high hemoglobin A_2-β thalassemia; (2) $\delta\beta$ thalassemia, or F thalassemia, characterized by normal hemoglobin A_2 but elevated hemoglobin F; (3) β-thalassemia trait with normal amounts of Hb F and Hb A_2 (? $\gamma\delta\beta$ thalassemia); and (4) hemoglobin Lepore trait, which is phenotypically similar to heterozygous β thalassemia but is characterized by normal levels of Hb A_2, the presence of small amounts (10 to 15 per cent) of the abnormal hemoglobin, and some elevation of Hb F. "Homozygous" β thalassemia (thalassemia major or Cooley's anemia) may result from the combination of any two of these genes. Occasionally, a child will inherit a β-thalassemia gene of standard severity from one parent and a mild gene (in some cases a "silent carrier" gene) from the other parent. The resulting syndrome is usually less severe clinically than in the usual cases of homozygous β thalassemia and is termed thalassemia intermedia. Finally, β and α thalassemia may interact with each other and with a variety of other hemoglobinopathies. These will all be discussed in the following section.

THE ALPHA THALASSEMIA SYNDROMES

Four clinical syndromes are associated with alpha thalassemia:

(1) Ordinary heterozygous α thalassemia: α-thalassemia 1.

(2a) Mild heterozygous α thalassemia: α-thalassemia 2, or "silent carrier."

(2b) Hb Constant Spring trait.

(3) Hemoglobin H disease: the result of combination of (1) and (2a) or (2b).

(4) Hydrops fetalis associated with hemoglobin Bart's: homozygosity for the α-thalassemia 1 gene.

Two alternate hypotheses have been proposed to explain the two types of α-thalassemia genes (Koler and Rigas, 1961; Wasi et al., 1964; Kattamis and Lehmann, 1970; Lehmann, 1970; Wasi, 1970;

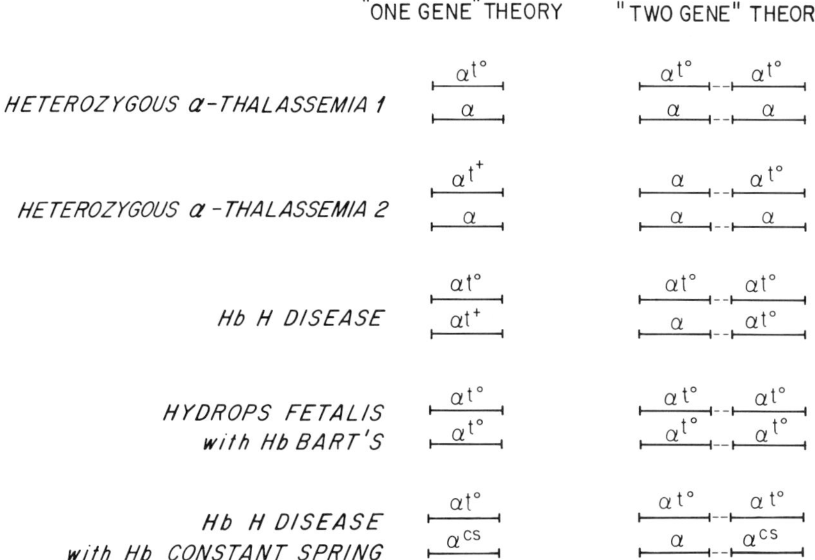

Figure 5–5. Genotypes of various α-thalassemia syndromes according to the "one gene" and "two linked genes" hypotheses. α, normal α-chain gene; α^{t0}, α-thalassemia gene with total absence of α-chain synthesis; α^{t+}, α-thalassemia gene with reduced α-chain synthesis; α^{CS}, gene for α-Constant Spring chain. The "one gene" hypothesis does not adequately explain the syndrome of Hb H disease with Hb Constant Spring (see text).

Koler et al., 1971; Weatherall and Clegg, 1972). In the first ("one gene") theory, it is believed that only one locus on each chromosome controls α-chain synthesis and that the two types of α-thalassemia genes are allelic but of different severity: one being associated with absent α-chain synthesis, the other with mildly decreased synthesis. In the alternate ("two gene") theory, duplication of the α-chain structural gene is postulated: in α-thalassemia 2, only one of the four genes would be affected, whereas in α-thalassemia 1, two genes, usually on the same chromosome (in cis), would be involved. Hemoglobin H disease, therefore, would be the result of α thalassemia affecting three of the four α-chain genes, and hydrops fetalis with Hb Bart's would be the result of α thalassemia affecting all four α-chain genes. The proposed genotypes of the various α-thalassemia syndromes, according to both theories, are diagrammatically illustrated in Figure 5–5.

Heterozygous Alpha Thalassemia

Heterozygosity for both types of α-thalassemia genes is benign. Affected patients are usually of Oriental or Mediterranean ancestry.

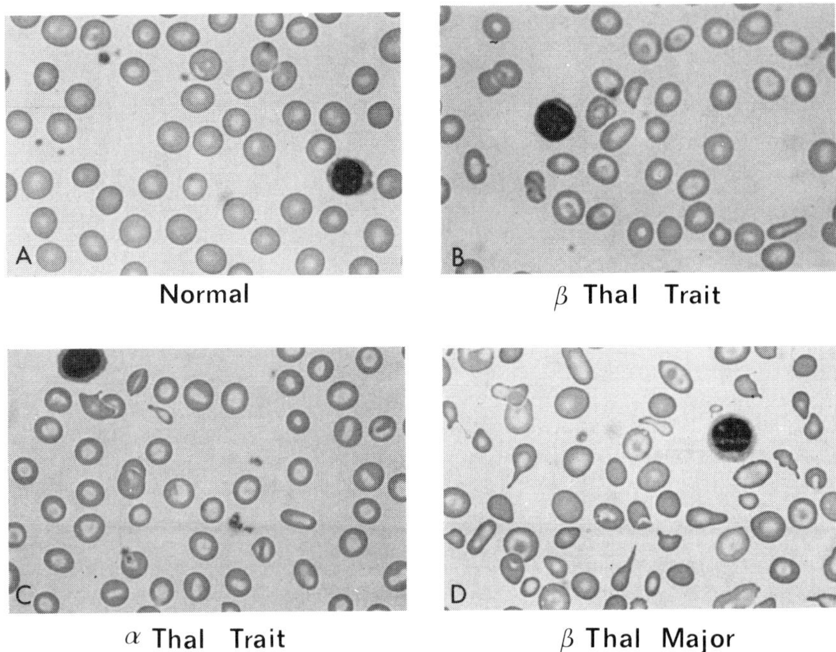

Figure 5–6. Peripheral blood smears of a normal individual (*A*) and patients with heterozygous β thalassemia (*B*), heterozygous α-thalassemia (*C*), and homozygous β thalassemia (*D*). This figure was prepared by Ms. Carola Kapff.

These carriers are detected usually on routine hematological examination, or during family studies of patients with the symptomatic thalassemic disorders. In α-thalassemia 1 trait, there is microcytosis and hypochromia of the red blood cells, with a mild degree of aniso- and poikilocytosis (Fig. 5–6). The hemoglobin level may be slightly depressed (10 to 12 g/100 ml) or near normal as a result of an elevated red cell count (greater than 5 million). Alpha-thalassemia 1 trait can be distinguished from beta-thalassemia trait by the presence of normal levels of hemoglobin A_2 and F. In the adult, the diagnosis is often difficult; iron deficiency and other causes of hypochromia and microcytosis must be ruled out before the diagnosis can be accepted. In some patients, incubation of the peripheral blood with 1 per cent brilliant cresyl blue (BCB) reveals occasional red cells (one in several thousand) bearing typical hemoglobin H inclusions similar to those shown in Figure 5–7A.

The hematological findings in patients heterozygous for α-thalassemia 2 are entirely normal. Diagnosis can only be inferred from family study.

During the neonatal period, the two types of heterozygous α thalassemia can be distinguished by the level of hemoglobin Bart's (γ_4) present in cord blood. This has been most thoroughly studied in

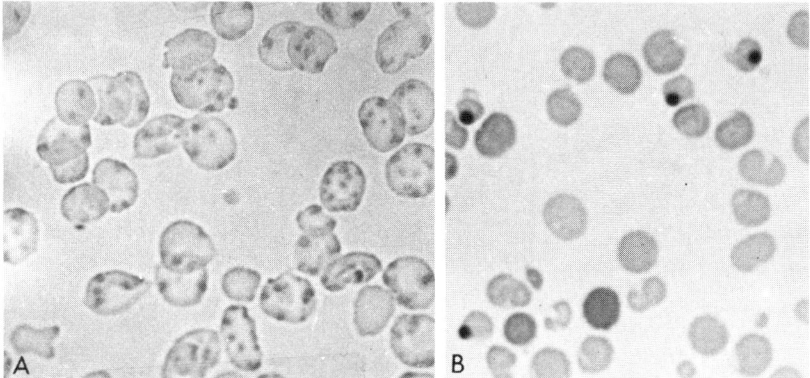

Figure 5–7. Red cell inclusions in Hb H disease. *A*, Inclusions induced by incubating peripheral blood in 1 per cent brilliant cresyl blue (BCB) and 0.4 per cent citrate for 30 minutes at 37° C (patient not splenectomized). *B*, Preformed inclusions, in peripheral blood of a splenectomized patient, stained by new methylene blue reticulocyte stain.

Thailand (Pootrakul et al., 1967b, 1970; Na-Nakorn et al., 1969; Na-Nakorn and Wasi, 1970). In patients with α-thalassemia 1 trait there is approximately 5 to 6 per cent hemoglobin Bart's, whereas in those with α-thalassemia 2 trait there is only 1 to 2 per cent hemoglobin Bart's. These components disappear by about the sixth month of life. Alpha-thalassemia 1 can also be detected with certainty in later life by the study of globin-chain synthesis in the peripheral blood reticulocytes of these individuals, as previously discussed in the section on globin synthesis in intact thalassemic erythroid cells. In α-thalassemia 1, there is approximately a 25 per cent reduction in α-chain synthesis relative to β-chain synthesis (Kan et al., 1968). A less significant decrease in α-chain synthesis can be detected by this technique in a group of patients with α-thalassemia 2, but the difference from normal is not great enough for precise identification of individual patients (Kan et al., 1968; Fig. 5–2).

It should be emphasized that the results obtained from analysis of Hb Bart's in cord blood and globin synthetic studies apply only to the α thalassemia found in the Mediterranean and Oriental populations. The findings in patients of African origin are much less well defined. Although α-thalassemia trait occurs in blacks, hemoglobin H disease is very rare, and when it occurs it is usually mild and has atypical features. Hydrops fetalis with Hb Bart's has never been described in blacks (and only once in a Mediterranean family [Diamond et al., 1965]). Hence, the existence of different types of α-thalassemia genes in different populations has been postulated (Lehmann, 1970; Schwartz and Atwater, 1972; Weatherall and Clegg, 1972). It has been proposed that in blacks the α-thalassemia gene is characterized by only slight reduction in α-chain synthesis and never total absence of α-chain synthesis. However, it is possible to propose a unified model for the causation of α thalassemia by gene deletion which in the context of the "two gene" theory can nevertheless account for the findings in blacks: blacks with the phenotype of "heterozygous" α thalassemia may have two deleted α-chain genes but with the deletions on different chromosomes (in trans) rather than on the same chromosome (in cis), as is apparently the case in the Oriental type of α thalassemia. Thus, because each chromosome bearing an α-thalassemia gene deletion would be linked to a second normal α-chain gene, it would be impossible, in a mating of two heterozygotes, for an offspring to inherit three or four deleted genes. Rare cases of Hb H disease in blacks would be due to rare crossing-over events leading to deletion of two α-chain genes on the same chromosome. There is no definitive evidence yet to favor this type of deletion model over the model proposing the presence of a nondeleted but low output α-chain gene in the black type of α thalassemia. Actual quantitation of gene numbers by molecular hybridization assays may soon resolve this question.

Hemoglobin H Disease

This condition is characterized by a chronic hemolytic anemia of variable severity (Rigas and Koler, 1961). Most patients have a hemoglobin level of approximately 8 to 10 g/100 ml, with moderate reticulocytosis (5 to 10 per cent). However, the variation is wide and one can see patients either with severe anemia or with very mild anemia. Mongoloid faces similar to that which is associated with homozygous beta thalassemia has occasionally been described. Splenomegaly is usually present and hepatomegaly is not uncommon. Anemia may become more severe during pregnancy, during infection, or after ingestion of oxidant drugs which accelerate the oxidation and precipitation of the Hb H (β_4). The peripheral blood smear typically shows hypochromia, microcytosis, poikilocytosis, polychromasia, and targeting of the red cells. Incubation of blood with 1 per cent brilliant cresyl blue (BCB) causes in-vitro precipitation of Hb H which is seen in the form of multiple speckled bodies (Fig. 5–7A). After splenectomy, large Hb H inclusion bodies, formed in vivo during red blood cell aging, can also be seen by supravital staining; they are usually single and round (Rigas and Koler, 1961; Nathan and Gunn, 1966) (Fig. 5–7*B*). The bone marrow typically shows erythroid hyperplasia. Punctate hemoglobin H inclusions can be demonstrated by BCB incubation in nucleated marrow precursor cells, but large, single, round, preformed inclusion bodies, though present in some late normoblasts (Fessas and Yataganas, 1968), are much less abundant than the numerous α-chain inclusion bodies found in homozygous β-thalassemic marrow cells.

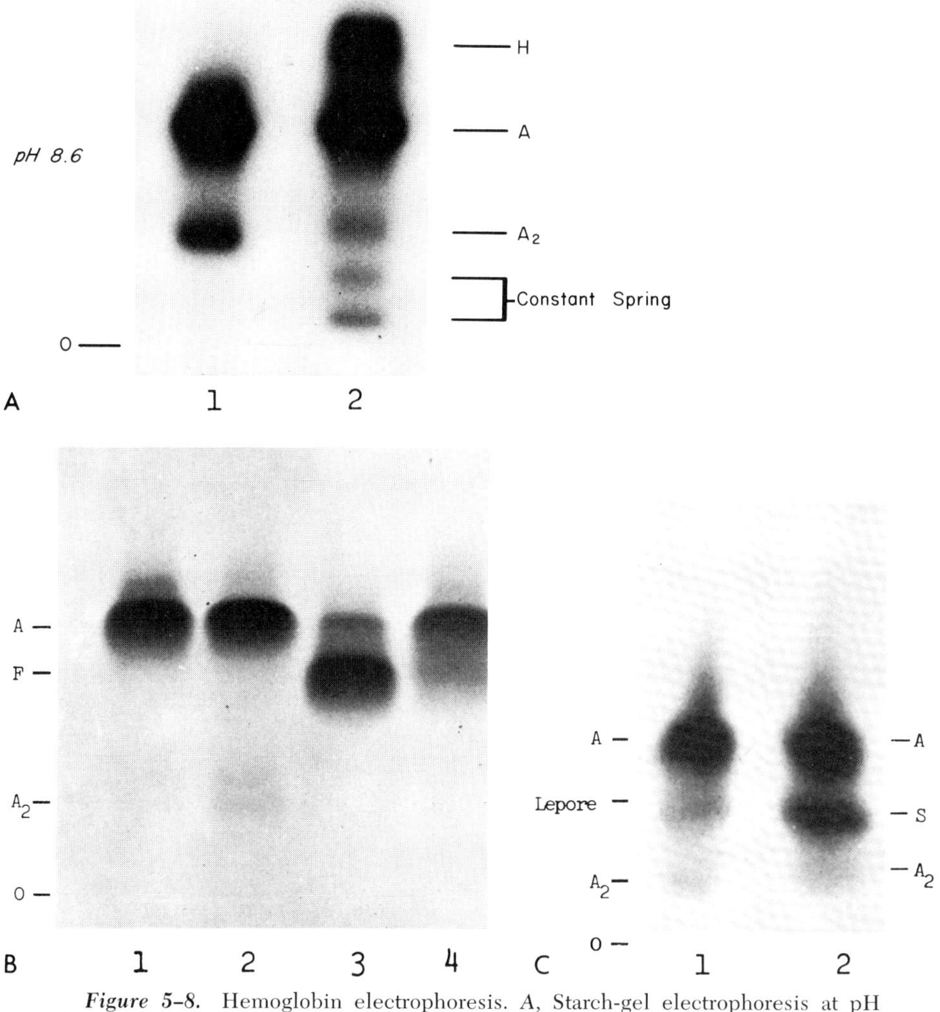

Figure 5–8. Hemoglobin electrophoresis. *A*, Starch-gel electrophoresis at pH 8.6; 1, Normal; 2, Hb H disease with Hb Constant Spring. *B*, Agarose electrophoresis at pH 8.6; 1, Normal; 2, β-thalassemia trait with increased Hb A_2; 3 and 4, homozygous β thalassemia with different relative amounts of Hb A and Hb F. *C*, Starch-gel electrophoresis at pH 8.6; 1, Hb Lepore trait; 2, sickle cell trait. (O indicates the origin and the anode is at the top.)

The diagnosis can be confirmed by hemoglobin electrophoresis (Fig. 5–8*A*). In the newborn, approximately 20 to 40 per cent hemoglobin Bart's (γ_4) is found. This is gradually replaced in older children and adults by hemoglobin H (β_4), the level of which varies between 5 and 30 per cent. Both Hb H and Hb Bart's migrate more rapidly than Hb A when electrophoresis is performed at pH 8.6. Hemoglobin A_2 is reduced to about 1 to 1.5 per cent. Biosynthetic studies have shown that in peripheral blood reticulocytes there is approximately a 50- to 75-per cent reduction in α-chain synthesis compared to β-chain synthesis (Clegg and Weatherall, 1967; Kan et al., 1968).

It is noteworthy that assays of globin mRNA isolated from reticulocytes of patients with Hb H disease reveal a much greater deficiency of α mRNA than expected on the basis of the β/α synthetic ratio in the same patient (Benz et al., 1973; Grossbard et al., 1973; Housman et al., 1973; Taylor et al., 1974; Forget et al., 1975a; Kazazian et al., 1975; Ottolenghi et al., 1975). In a thoroughly studied case, biosynthetic studies in intact cells revealed approximately 30 per cent as much α-chain synthesis as β-chain synthesis but there was only 10 to 15 per cent as much α mRNA as β mRNA when mRNA was studied by molecular hybridization, gel electrophoresis, and nucleotide sequence analysis (Housman et al., 1973; Forget et al., 1975a). These results suggest the possible presence of intracellular control mechanisms which can modulate the imbalance of globin-chain synthesis and partially compensate for the mRNA deficiency. Environmental factors can also affect the amount of Hb H which accumulates in red cells. In one of two brothers with Hb H disease, concomitant iron deficiency was asssociated with absence of Hb H (O'Brien, 1973). After therapy with iron, Hb H levels reached 16 per cent, a level similar to that present in the other brother.

Study of the families of patients with Hb H disease usually reveals that one parent has α-thalassemia 1 while the other is hematologically normal and presumably a "silent" carrier of the α-thalassemia 2 gene. Direct transmission of hemoglobin H disease to the offspring of an affected individual has rarely been observed, but in such cases the presence of an α-thalassemia 2 gene in the putatively normal spouse cannot be ruled out. Usually, the offspring of patients with Hb H disease inherit either α-thalassemia 1 trait or α-thalassemia 2 trait (confirmed by analysis of Hb Bart's in cord blood) (Na-Nakorn et al., 1969).

Hemoglobin H has also been described as an acquired defect, usually during the course of erythroleukemia or other myeloproliferative disorders (White et al., 1960; Beaven et al., 1963; Rosenzweig et al., 1968; Hamilton et al., 1971; Andre et al., 1972). In certain of these cases, the abnormality appears to be clonal, or limited to only a certain population of the red cells (Pagnier et al., 1972). The clinical manifestations associated with the primary myeloproliferative disorder easily distinguish this acquired defect from the hereditary variety of Hb H disease. The precise molecular basis of this interesting acquired abnormality remains unknown, but biosynthetic studies have confirmed the presumed decrease in α-chain synthesis relative to β-chain synthesis (Hamilton et al., 1971).

Pathophysiology of Hb H Disease

Deficiency of α-chain synthesis results in overall decreased synthesis of hemoglobin A, hence hypochromia and microcytosis. The excess β chains which accumulate form the β_4 tetramers of Hb H, which has a very high oxygen affinity and lacks the Bohr effect as well as heme-heme interaction (Chapter 1). Hence, it is a useless pigment for oxygen transport under physiologic conditions. In addition, hemoglobin H is an unstable tetramer; it is easily oxidized and tends to precipitate as the red cells age. These precipitates, which gradually form in vivo, are normally removed by the spleen and can be demonstrated most abundantly in peripheral blood cells after splenectomy. They cause disturbances in red cell metabolism and interfere with membrane function and deformability (Nathan and Gunn, 1966; Nathan et al., 1969). All these factors lead to shortened red cell survival and the hemolytic component of the disease. Shortened ^{51}Cr-labeled red cell survival and the apparent splenic trapping of ^{51}Cr-labeled red cells is observed in hemoglobin H disease but should be interpreted with caution: ^{51}Cr binds selectively to the β chain, and there is evidence that exchange of β chains can occur between hemoglobin A and Hb H (Gabuzda et al., 1965). The ^{51}Cr can pass from the labeled Hb A to Hb H which then precipitates and is removed from the red cells by the spleen without the cell being destroyed. Thus the cell loses its label without necessarily being destroyed, and this gives a false impression of the actual red cell life span and splenic sequestration (Gabuzda et al., 1965). More recent studies, however, indicate that ^{51}Cr may be a valid label for the determination of red cell life span in Hb H disease (Tso, 1972).

Hemoglobin Constant Spring Syndromes

In as many as 50 per cent of Oriental patients with hemoglobin H disease, hemoglobin electrophoresis shows, in addition to the usual findings, one or two more slowly migrating hemoglobin components, which amount to 3 to 5 per cent of the total hemoglobin (Clegg et al., 1971b; Milner et al., 1971) (Fig. 5–8*A*). This hemoglobin is called hemoglobin Constant Spring (Hb CS) and it has been found in patients of Greek (Sofroniadou et al., 1968), Thai (Pootrakul et al., 1970), and Chinese ancestry (Clegg et al., 1971b; Milner et al., 1971). Hemoglobin CS is made up of two normal β chains and two elongated α chains which have either 28 or 31 additional amino acid residues at their C-terminal ends. The shorter Hb CS chain presumably results from proteolytic digestion of the longer CS chain. Typically, one of the parents of a patient with Hb H–CS disease has α-thalassemia 1 trait, while the other appears to be hematologically normal, except that hemoglobin electrophoresis shows the presence of approximately 1 per cent hemoglobin Constant Spring. Therefore, heterozygotes for Hb Constant Spring are phenotypically similar to individuals with α-thalassemia 2 trait.

The fact that carriers of hemoglobin Constant Spring are phenotypically similar to persons with α-thalassemia 2 and not α-thalassemia 1 has been used to support the theory of α-chain gene duplication. Since the contribution of the α^{CS} gene to the total cell globin is negligible, the absence of hypochromia and other stigmata of thalassemia suggests that there must be more than only one other normal α-chain gene compensating for the deficiency of normal α chains due to the α^{CS} gene. Furthermore, it is difficult to postulate only a single pair of α-chain genes when Hb CS interacts with α-thalassemia 1 to give Hb H disease: there is total absence of α-chain synthesis from the α-thalassemia 1 locus (homozygotes totally lack Hb A and have the Hb Bart's hydrops fetalis syndrome). There must be, therefore, another normal α-chain locus in cis with the α^{CS} locus to account for the presence of some Hb A in these patients (see Figure 5–5). The "one gene" theory can explain the syndrome of Hb H disease associated with Hb CS only if one postulates that (1) the α-thalassemia gene in trans to the CS gene is an α-thalassemia 2 gene (which does not usually fit the clinical or genetic data); or (2) the chain termination mutation hypothesis for the origin of Hb CS is incorrect. An alternate hypothesis is that the abnormal chain arises because of the presence of a suppressor tRNA which reads the chain termination codon as the amino acid glutamine and allows translation to continue (Clegg et al., 1971b). The latter explanation is probably untenable, however, because if it were correct, one should observe other abnormally long proteins in these patients and not simply an abnormality limited to the α globin chain.

The syndrome of Hb H disease has also been described in association with a second α-chain termination mutant, Hb Icaria (Clegg et al., 1974a).

Hydrops Fetalis Associated with Hemoglobin Bart's

The homozygous state for α-thalassemia 1 results in the Hb Bart's hydrops fetalis syndrome. The affected fetus is usually delivered prematurely and either is stillborn or dies within an hour after birth, grossly hydropic with marked hepatosplenomegaly (Lie-Injo and Jo, 1960; Lie-Injo, 1962; Kan et al., 1967; Todd et al., 1967). For reasons yet unknown this syndrome occurs almost exclusively in individuals from Southeast Asia. With the exception of one case observed in a Greek Cypriot (Diamond et al., 1965), no other cases have been reported from the Mediterranean area, and none have been described in people of African ancestry.

The peripheral blood smear is characterized by hypochromia and large numbers of nucleated red blood cells. On hemoglobin electrophoresis, the predominant hemoglobin is hemoglobin Bart's

(γ_4) (Lie-Injo and Jo, 1960). In addition, one finds a smaller amount of Hb H and a minor component, hemoglobin Portland-1 ($\zeta_2\gamma_2$) (Todd et al., 1970; Weatherall et al., 1970). Hemoglobin Portland-1 is also found in lower (trace) amounts in normal cord blood (Capp et al., 1970). Studies of globin-chain synthesis in one case of Hb Bart's syndrome revealed total absence of α-chain synthesis (Weatherall et al., 1970).

Hemoglobin Bart's has a very high oxygen affinity similar to that of hemoglobin H. Thus, the bulk of the hemoglobin present in these infants cannot deliver oxygen effectively to the tissues. The cause of death is severe hypoxia. Delivery by cesarian section and exchange transfusion were attempted in one case but were not successful in prolonging life for more than a few hours (Weatherall et al., 1970).

Family studies in such cases usually show the presence of α-thalassemia 1 trait in both parents.

THE BETA THALASSEMIAS

HETEROZYGOUS BETA THALASSEMIA

The hallmark of heterozygous β thalassemia is microcytosis and hypochromia. With the increasing use of electronic cell counting equipment, the diagnosis may first be suspected by the discovery of a low MCV and MCH on routine blood counts (Pearson et al., 1973). Beta-thalassemia heterozygotes are usually not symptomatic and may not be anemic. However, mild anemia with hemoglobin levels of 10 to 11 g/100 ml is usually present in most patients; more pronounced anemia may be found in infancy and during pregnancy. The MCV and MCH are usually decreased well below normal with values of 55 to 70 μ^3 and 16 to 20 pg typically found. Despite the microcytosis, the MCHC is not usually as low as in iron deficiency. The peripheral blood smear typically shows microcytosis, hypochromia, aniso- and poikilocytosis with targeting and basophilic stippling of the red cells (see Figure 5–6). The bone marrow shows mild erythroid hyperplasia with many of the normoblasts showing poor hemoglobinization. Mild to moderate splenomegaly occurs in approximately one third of the cases.

The differential diagnosis between iron deficiency and β- (or α-) thalassemia trait can be difficult in practice. Table 5–2 lists the differentiating features.

In thalassemic heterozygotes, the MCV tends to be lower when related to the red cell count than in iron deficiency. This observation has led to the derivation of various formulas to differentiate thalassemia trait from iron deficiency on the basis of the red cell indices (Torlontano et al., 1972; England and Fraser, 1973; Mentzer, 1973)

TABLE 5–2. Differentiation of β-thalassemia Trait from Iron Deficiency Anemia (Hb 9 to 11 g/100 ml)

	β-THAL TRAIT	IRON DEFICIENCY ANEMIA
I. Definitive Tests		
A. Serum iron	Normal	Decreased
B. TIBC	Normal	Increased
C. % saturation	Normal	Decreased
D. Hb electrophoresis		
Hb A_2	Increased	Decreased
Hb F	± Increased	Normal
II. Associated Findings		
MCV/RBC*	< 13	> 13
RBC protoporphyrin	Normal	Increased
RBC morphology	3 to 4+ Abnormal	Tr-1+ Abnormal
Serum ferritin	Normal	Low
Dominant inheritance	+	0
Color of plasma	Straw-colored	Colorless

*See Mentzer, 1973.

(see Table 5–2). Although such findings are helpful, they do not provide conclusive evidence of the diagnosis. Precise diagnosis requires hemoglobin electrophoresis and measurement of the serum iron and iron binding capacity. Demonstration of absent stainable iron in bone marrow aspirates may be necessary to identify individuals with combined thalassemia trait and iron deficiency. This combination is quite common in early childhood and during pregnancy. Iron salts should not be withheld when iron deficiency complicates thalassemia trait.

It is noteworthy that the presence of iron deficiency may obscure the diagnosis of concomitant β-thalassemia trait. Iron deficiency causes a decrease in Hb A_2 synthesis in normals and in β-thalassemia trait as well; with iron deficiency, the usually elevated Hb A_2 levels in a β-thalassemic heterozygote may fall into the normal range (Wasi et al., 1968; Kattamis et al., 1972). Beta-thalassemia trait should therefore be suspected in cases in which anemia responds only partially and in which hypochromia and microcytosis persist after therapy for iron deficiency. The Hb A_2 levels will return to their normally elevated values in such patients after replenishment of iron stores.

Moderately severe anemia has occasionally been described in apparent heterozygous β thalassemia (McCarthy et al., 1968; Aksoy, 1970; Stamatoyannopoulos et al., 1974; Friedman et al., 1976a). However, severe anemia is unusual and when it occurs, one should look for associated secondary causes such as concomitant iron or folic acid deficiency. Such cases should also be distinguished by family studies from the milder forms of homozygous β thalassemia or double heterozygosity for β-thalassemia genes of different types and severity. The term thalassemia intermedia has been used to refer to either severe heterozygous β thalassemia or mild homozygous β thalassemia.

There are at least four different types of heterozygous β thalassemia which can be distinguished on the basis of hemoglobin electrophoresis.

1. Ordinary *beta thalassemia,* or high A_2-β thalassemia, by far the commonest variety, is characterized by an increased hemoglobin A_2 level of 4 to 6 per cent (see Figure 5–8*B*) and usually a normal level of hemoglobin F, although in approximately half the cases, a slightly elevated level of hemoglobin F (2 to 5 per cent) may be present (Pootrakul et al., 1973).

2. *In delta-beta thalassemia,* or F thalassemia, the Hb A_2 level is normal or slightly decreased, and the hemoglobin F is increased and varies between 5 and 20 per cent.

3. *Delta-beta thalassemia with normal levels of hemoglobins* A_2 *and F* (?$\gamma\delta\beta$ thalassemia). This type of heterozygous β thalassemia is difficult to distinguish clinically from heterozygous α thalassemia. It is usually suspected by the finding of a clinically significant beta-thalassemia syndrome in an offspring. Globin synthesis studies in peripheral blood reticulocytes may be the only laboratory means to make this diagnosis.

4. *Hb Lepore trait* is characterized by normal Hb A_2, slight elevation of Hb F, and the finding of 5 to 15 per cent Hb Lepore (see Figure 5–8*C*).

The clinical picture in all four types of heterozygous β thalassemia is rather similar except perhaps in types 2 and 3 where anemia and morphological abnormalities of the red blood cells may be minimal. The findings in type 3 may be virtually normal and the term "silent carrier" state has been applied to such cases.

The presence or absence of elevated Hb F in heterozygous A_2-β thalassemia is usually of no prognostic significance with regard to the severity of disease in a homozygous offspring. One exception to this rule is a rare variety of A_2-β thalassemia in which the heterozygote, in addition to an elevated Hb A_2 level, has an unexpectedly high Hb F level—5 to 15 per cent (Weatherall, 1964a; Schokker et al., 1966). The homozygous state for this rare disorder is much milder than homozygosity for the usual A_2-β thalassemia (Schokker et al., 1966).

The results of globin chain biosynthetic studies in heterozygous β thalassemia have been discussed in the section on the molecular pathology of thalassemia. The β/α synthetic ratio is 0.5 in the peripheral blood reticulocytes. In contrast, the ratio in the bone marrow is close to 1.0. As discussed previously, this finding of apparently balanced globin-chain synthesis in the bone marrow is not yet fully explained but it appears to be due to accelerated turnover (? proteolysis) of newly synthesized excess α chains.

The double inheritance of β thalassemia and a β-chain structural variant makes it possible to evaluate the amount of β^A-chain synthesis directed by the β-thalassemia gene. In high A_2-β thalassemia, there is some β^A-chain synthesis directed by the defective gene in approximately two thirds of the cases (β^+ thalassemia), whereas the other one third of the cases show totally absent β^A-chain synthesis (β^0 thalassemia). Total absence of β^Asynthesis is especially characteristic of the A_2-β thalassemia found in Ferrara, Italy (Bargellesi et al., 1967; Conconi et al., 1970) and in Thailand (Weatherall et al., 1969a). In $\delta\beta$ thalassemia, there is almost always total absence of β^A-chain synthesis directed by the $\delta\beta$-thalassemia gene.

Homozygous β Thalassemia (A_2-β Thalassemia)

Clinical Manifestations

The clinical course in most cases is severe. At birth, anemia is not evident, and examination of the peripheral blood smear shows only occasional hypochromic red cells. Diagnosis, however, can be established by study of globin-chain synthesis in the cord blood (Gaburro et al., 1970). Within a few months, hypochromic, microcytic hemolytic anemia develops, and a regular transfusion program must be undertaken to maintain an adequate hemoglobin level. The spleen and liver become progressively enlarged. A typical facies develops in many patients, with prominent frontal bossing, prominent cheek bones, and protruding upper jaw due to expansion of the marrow in the skull and facial bones. Skull x-ray demonstrates the typical "hair on end" appearance (Fig. 5–9*A*). The long bones may also become rarefied from the marrow expansion (Fig. 5–9*B*) and become subject to repeated pathologic fractures. Occasionally, the expanding marrow extrudes from ribs or vertebrae and forms large intrathoracic masses. Gallstones and leg ulcers are frequent complications, as they are in other severe hemolytic anemias.

Intercurrent infection is extremely common and, along with neglected anemia, is the most common cause of death in early childhood. With modern antibiotic therapy and proper transfusion therapy, these causes of death have become less frequent and many patients survive to their twenties. A benign form of pericarditis with pericardial effusion frequently occurs and is usually self-limited. Secondary hypersplenism may develop in some patients and cause thrombocytopenia, leukopenia, and rapid destruction of transfused red cells. This complication may pose a severe management problem, and splenectomy may be required to control it. However, the incidence of overwhelming infection (septicemia) following splenectomy is very high in thalassemic patients (Smith et al., 1962, 1964), and such patients should be observed carefully during febrile episodes.

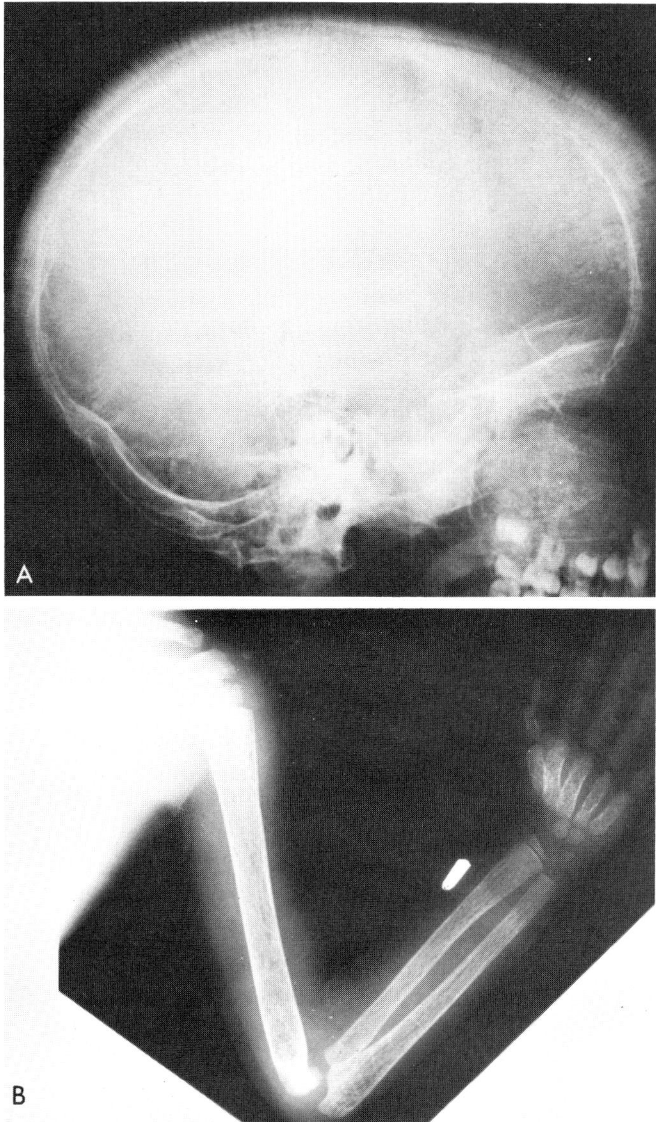

Figure 5–9. Bone changes in severe homozygous β thalassemia. *A*, Skull x-ray. (From Beck, W. S. (ed.): Hematology. 2nd ed. Boston, MIT Press, 1976.) *B*, X-ray of forearm and hand. (From Nathan, D. G.: N. Engl. J. Med. *286*:586, 1972.)

Physical growth and development of these children are usually below normal. Menarche and secondary sexual characteristics are usually absent, and the final stature of these patients tends to be short. This problem has been well reviewed by Logothetis et al. (1972). Growth retardation begins approximately at 4 years of age and reaches its most significant and noticeable levels at 9 to 10 years of age. There is no associated retardation in intellectual development. No good correlation exists between the degree of anemia (pretransfusion Hb level) and the degree of growth retardation. However, this finding does not rule out the possibility that the degree of anemia in the first few years of life may be related to the degree of growth retardation in later years. Although growth retardation is more pronounced in splenectomized patients, it is believed that this phenomenon simply reflects the correlation between severity of growth retardation and severity of the clinical course of the disease as manifested by hepatomegaly, cutaneous siderosis, and cephalofacial deformities (Logothetis et al., 1972).

Iron absorption is usually increased in thalassemia major (Erlandson et al., 1962; Bannerman et al., 1964; Necheles et al., 1969a; Heinrich et al., 1973). Additional iron overload is supplied by the frequent transfusions. Iron overload is probably responsible for damage to the heart, liver, pancreas, endocrine glands, and other organs. In addition, chronic anemia and hypoxia are believed to play an important role in contributing to the myocardial damage from hemosiderosis (Necheles et al., 1969b). Cardiac failure and arrhythmias are the most common causes of death as these patients survive to their twenties. Diabetes mellitus (Lassman et al., 1970) and hepatic insufficiency may also pose difficult management problems.

Some of the complications and associated manifestations of Cooley's anemia can be prevented or at least lessened by maintaining a near normal hemoglobin level in the children by a high transfusion regimen, as will be discussed in the section on management.

Although the preceding description applies to most patients with homozygous β thalassemia, a small number of patients have a much milder clinical course (so-called thalassemia intermedia) and may require few or no blood transfusions. This is especially true of homozygous β thalassemia in blacks, which appears to be a much milder disease.

Laboratory Findings

Anemia is severe, with marked hypochromia. The findings on peripheral blood smear are striking (see Figure 5–6): the red blood cells show severe hypochromia and microcytosis, marked anisocytosis and poikilocytosis with teardrop-shaped red cells, polychromasia, and basophilic stippling. Poorly hemoglobinized normoblasts are frequently found in the peripheral blood, and their number increases markedly following splenectomy. Even when anemia is severe, the reticulocyte count is usually not very high because of massive destruction of erythroid cells in the marrow, termed ineffective erythropoiesis.

The red cell osmotic fragility is decreased, a phenomenon explained by the marked hypochromia. The bone marrow is hypercellular with marked erythroid hyperplasia characterized by normoblasts which are poorly hemoglobinized (micronormoblastic). Storage cells resembling Gaucher cells are frequently found in the marrow (and spleen) (Beltrami et al., 1973). Examination of the marrow under phase microscopy or after supravital staining reveals the presence of many inclusion bodies (α-chain aggregates) in the normoblasts. This finding can be used as a diagnostic test for homozygous β thalassemia (Fessas, 1963; Yataganas and Fessas, 1969). The α-chain inclusions are also seen in peripheral blood red cells after splenectomy.

Increased nonconjugated bilirubin levels and other biochemical evidence of hemolysis can usually be found. Dipyrroles resulting from increased heme catabolism give the urine a dark brown color (Kreimer-Birnbaum et al., 1966b). The findings on hemoglobin electrophoresis vary from patient to patient and with the type of thalassemia (see Figure 5–8*B*). In the homozygous form of the usual variety of β thalassemia (high A_2-β^+ thalassemia) there is usually a variable amount of Hb A present. Hemoglobin F is usually elevated and may represent from 10 to 90 per cent of the patient's total hemoglobin and is heterogeneously distributed in the red cells. The total amount of circulating Hb A_2 may be low, normal, or increased, but the ratio of Hb A_2 to Hb A is usually higher than the normal ratio of 1 to 40, suggesting more efficient synthesis of Hb A_2 relative to Hb A in homozygous β thalassemia even if the absolute Hb A_2 level is below normal. Free α chains can also be seen in trace amounts as a slow moving component on the hemoglobin electrophoresis (Fessas and Loukopoulos, 1964). Hemoglobin A is totally absent in patients with homozygous β^0 thalassemia. Patients doubly heterozygous for high A_2-β thalassemia and $\delta\beta$ thalassemia in general have a higher level of Hb F and lower level of Hb A_2 than homozygotes for high A_2-β thalassemia. The former also tend to have a milder clinical course.

Delta-Beta Thalassemia or F Thalassemia

Heterozygous F thalassemia or $\delta\beta$ thalassemia is a condition characterized by mild hypochromia and microcytosis. The changes may be barely noticeable. Hemoglobin electrophoresis reveals low or normal Hb A_2 and elevation of Hb F (5 to 20 per cent). The condition is found mainly in Greeks (Stamatoyannopoulos et al., 1969), although it has also been found in blacks and in other racial groups. In association with the usual variety of high A_2-β thalassemia, a thalassemia intermedia syndrome usually results and is characterized by high levels of Hb F and only mild or moderate anemia and hemolysis (Kattamis et al., 1973). The homozygous form of $\delta\beta$ thalassemia is also a relatively mild disorder and may be barely symptomatic. The affected individuals usually have mild to moderate anemia (Hb 9 to 10 g/100 ml), mild or moderate splenomegaly, and no transfusion requirement. They have 100 per cent Hb F, with no Hb A or Hb A_2. The relatively benign nature of $\delta\beta$ thalassemia seems to be related to the fact that, although it is associated with totally absent β- and δ-chain synthesis, it is also associated with more efficient preservation of γ-chain synthesis than the usual form of β thalassemia: the overall degree of globin-chain imbalance (α vs. non-α) is not as pronounced (Mann et al., 1972) and therefore there is less α-chain inclusion-body formation and less hemolysis. Although $\delta\beta$ thalassemia is almost always associated with absent δ- and β-chain synthesis in cis, there is one black family in which double heterozygosity for $\delta\beta$ thalassemia and Hb S was associated with some β^A synthesis (Russo and Mollica, 1962). In a Chinese family with $\delta\beta$ thalassemia, the only type of γ chain found was $^G\gamma$ suggesting that, in that family, the thalassemia also affected the $^A\gamma$ gene (Mann et al., 1972).

Delta-Beta Thalassemia with Normal Levels of Hb A_2 and Hb F

In the study of parents of children with apparent homozygous β thalassemia, one occasionally encounters a parent in whom both Hb A_2 and Hb F levels are normal. Some of these cases may be heterozygous for the ordinary type of $\delta\beta$ or F thalassemia in which, for unknown reasons, the Hb F level is only at the upper limits of normal instead of constituting over 5 per cent of the total hemoglobin. Such cases have been well documented (Fessas, 1965), and the low level of Hb F is not usually constant within the family; other members in the family with thalassemia trait usually have the expected elevated Hb F levels (Stamatoyannopoulos et al., 1969a; Fessas, 1965).

There is a report of a family in which two children had β thalassemia of intermediate severity. One parent had typical A_2-β thalassemia trait, whereas the other parent was hematologically normal, having normal red cell morphology and normal levels of Hb A_2 and Hb F but an abnormal β/α synthetic ratio of 0.6 characteristic of mild heterozygous β thalassemia (Schwartz, 1969). This latter form of heterozygous β thalassemia was found in a number of relatives of the affected parent and has been termed the "silent carrier" state for β thalassemia.

Heterozygous β thalassemia with normal Hb A_2 and Hb F, however, may also be phenotypically similar to heterozygous high A_2-β thalassemia, and the offspring of such an individual and another individual with typical high Hb A_2-β thalassemia trait may have homozygous β thalassemia (thalassemia major) of usual severity instead of a milder thalassemia intermedia syndrome (Bernini et al., 1962; Aksoy and Erdem, 1969).

Finally, in another family a thalassemia-like disorder was observed in a neonate. A number of family members were found to have typical thalassemic red cell morphology, normal levels of Hb A_2 and Hb F, and a β/α synthetic ratio of 0.5 characteristic of heterozygous β thalassemia (Kan et al., 1972b). The findings suggest that the thalassemia defect in this family may involve the γ-, δ-, and β-chain genes on the same chromosome. Such an occurrence would explain the normal levels of Hb F as well as Hb A_2.

Hemoglobin Lepore Syndrome

Hemoglobin Lepore is composed of two α chains and two abnormal non-α chains which have the structure of the δ chain at their N terminus and that of the β chain at their C terminus (Baglioni, 1962). The Lepore chain is believed to have resulted from nonhomologous crossing over, at meiosis, of the δ and β loci, as previously discussed (see Figure 5–3*A*). At least three different Lepore hemoglobins have been described which vary by the point at which the crossing over occurred between the δ- and β-chain structural genes (see Figure 5–3*B* and Table 6–2).

Hemoglobin Lepore is produced at a markedly reduced rate and, in the heterozygote, it accounts for only about 5 to 15 per cent of the total hemoglobin. Hemoglobin Lepore is easily detected by standard hemoglobin electrophoresis and has approximately the same mobility as Hb S (see Figure 5–8*C*). Clinically, the peripheral blood findings are similar to those of heterozygous high A_2-β thalassemia. Hemoglobin electrophoresis, in addition to the finding of the abnormal hemoglobin, reveals low or normal Hb A_2 and slight elevation of Hb F. Homozygosity for Hb Lepore and the combination of heterozygous high A_2-β thalassemia with hemoglobin Lepore are clinically indistinguishable from true homozygous β thalassemia (Weatherall and Clegg, 1972). In homozygous Hb Lepore, there is no normal Hb A or Hb A_2, only Hb F (approximately 75 per cent) and Hb Lepore (10 to 20 per cent). These findings indicate that the chromosome bearing the Lepore gene has no normal δ or β gene associated with it and thus confirms the crossing-over hypothesis and the location of the δ gene to the N-terminal side of the β gene in the normal.

Mild Homozygous Thalassemia (Thalassemia Intermedia)

There is some evidence that certain forms of β thalassemia are milder and produce a less severe clinical syndrome in the homozygous state (Weatherall and Clegg, 1972). This is especially true of homozygous β thalassemia in the black, which is usually a mild disease (Weatherall, 1964a). The mild form of β thalassemia called the "silent carrier" state (Schwartz, 1969) results in a mild disease in association with the usual variety of A_2-β thalassemia. Homozygous $\delta\beta$ thalassemia (F thalassemia) also tends to be relatively mild because of the higher level of hemoglobin F synthesis in each cell resulting in less imbalance between α and non-α chains. Combination of $\delta\beta$ and high A_2-β thalassemia produces a disease of intermediate severity (Stamatoyannopoulos et al., 1969a; Kattamis et al., 1973). In addition, when a patient with homozygous β thalassemia also inherits an α-thalassemia gene, the disease will be milder because the associated α-thalassemia gene results in decreased synthesis of α chains and therefore less accumulation of free α chains. There will result less inclusion-body formation and less hemolysis (Kan and Nathan, 1970). The reverse is also true; a patient who has the α-thalassemia syndrome of hemoglobin H disease and who also inherits a β-thalassemia gene has much less hemolysis than patients with simple Hb H disease (Kan and Nathan, 1970; Knox-Macauley et al., 1972).

INTERACTION OF THALASSEMIA WITH ABNORMAL HEMOGLOBINS

When a patient acquires a thalassemia gene for a given globin chain on one chromosome and a gene for a structural variant of the same type of globin chain on the other chromosome, the percentage of the structurally abnormal hemoglobin observed is increased over the level found in a simple heterozygote for the structural variant, and the clinical severity of the condition approaches that of homozygosity for the abnormal hemoglobin (so-called interacting thalassemia). On the other hand, when a patient acquires the combination of thalassemia for one chain (i.e., β) and a structural variant for another globin chain (i.e., α), no increase in the abnormal hemoglobin is observed and the clinical severity of the condition is similar to that of the heterozygous state for the structural variant (noninteracting thalassemia). In fact, when α thalassemia is combined with a β-chain structural abnormality, the amount of the abnormal hemoglobin observed is sometimes less than in the simple heterozygous state. The precise molecular basis of this phenomenon is not understood. The common feature in all these syndromes is hypochromia and microcytosis of the red cells, as in thalassemia trait, in addition to the finding of the abnormal hemoglobin. Only the clinically important combinations will be briefly described here.

Beta Thalassemia in Association with Beta-Chain Structural Variants

Sickle Cell–β Thalassemia

This disease is described in detail in Chapter 7. S/β thalassemia primarily affects people of African, Italian, and Greek ancestry. The clinical picture resembles that of sickle cell anemia, but the disease in general tends to run a milder course. Splenomegaly is a common feature and is helpful in differentiating S/β thalassemia from sickle cell anemia in the older children and adults. Occasionally, the disease can be extremely mild, and the diagnosis may be discovered as an incidental finding.

Laboratory findings include targeting, hypochromia, and microcytosis of the red cells and a variable degree of anemia; occasional irreversibly sickled forms may be observed in the blood smear in the more severely affected cases. The hemoglobin electrophoresis reveals 60 to 90 per cent Hb S, 0 to 30 per cent Hb A, 1 to 20 per cent Hb F, and increased Hb A_2. The clinical severity of the disease cannot be correlated well with the level of hemoglobin A.

Hemoglobin C–β Thalassemia

This condition occurs mainly in blacks. A mild to moderate hemolytic anemia with splenomegaly is present.

Hemoglobin E–β Thalassemia

This is a common disease in Thailand. For reasons that are poorly understood, it is almost as severe as homozygous β thalassemia. Hemoglobin electrophoresis shows hemoglobin E, a high percentage of Hb F (approximately 50 per cent) and usually no hemoglobin A. The abnormal physico-chemical properties of Hb E (see Chapter 6) may be in part responsible for the severity of this syndrome.

Alpha Thalassemia in Association with Alpha-Chain Structural Variants

Hemoglobin Q–α Thalassemia

This condition is also found mainly in Thailand. The clinical picture is similar to that of Hb H disease. This syndrome is of interest mainly because of the associated hemoglobin electrophoresis findings. The affected individuals have total absence of Hb A. This finding is extremely difficult to explain if one assumes the presence of duplicated α-chain genes: one would expect some α-chain synthesis from the second α-chain gene in cis to the Hb Q, even if the two

α-chain genes of the other (α-thalassemia 1) chromosome are totally inactive. One must postulate, therefore, that the second α gene in cis with Hb Q is always affected by α thalassemia in the Hb Q heterozygote.

Hemoglobin G-Philadelphia and Hb I–α Thalassemia

The α-chain variant Hb G-Philadelphia has been found in a number of blacks, in the heterozygous state alone and in association with other Hb variants or α thalassemia. Heterozygotes for Hb G-Philadelphia show variability in the amount of the variant present in hemolysates: there is a trimodal distribution in the percentage of the variant in heterozygotes. Individuals have approximately 22, 30, or 41 per cent Hb G-Philadelphia (Baine et al., 1976). The differences have been attributed to two possible mechanisms: (1) the association of an $\alpha^{G\text{-Philadelphia}}$ gene with variable numbers (1, 2, or 3) of α^A loci due to heterogeneity in the duplication of α-chain loci in blacks, or (2) the association of an α-thalassemia gene in cis with $\alpha^{G\text{-Philadelphia}}$ in some individuals (Rucknagel and Winter, 1974; Rucknagel and Rising, 1975; Baine et al., 1976). In one study, biosynthetic studies revealed no imbalance between α- and β-chain synthesis in Hb G-Philadelphia heterozygotes (Baine et al., 1976), but in another study, heterozygotes for $\alpha^{G\text{-Philadelphia}}$ (alone or in association with Hb S or C) did manifest a deficit in α-chain synthesis compatible with an α-thalassemia–like syndrome (McCurdy et al., 1975). These findings, however, do not help distinguish between the two hypotheses (variable number of α-chain genes versus α thalassemia in cis with $\alpha^{G\text{-Philadelphia}}$). One black individual has been described, however, who is doubly heterozygous for $\alpha^{G\text{-Philadelphia}}$ and α thalassemia (Rieder et al., 1976). This individual has a syndrome analogous to Hb H disease. On hemoglobin electrophoresis there was 3.5 to 8 per cent Hb H and total absence of Hb A and Hb A_2; the α^G/β synthetic ratio was 0.63. The mother, two half-siblings, and one offspring had hematological evidence of heterozygous α thalassemia (without Hb G) with α/β synthetic ratios of 0.76 to 0.84. The father was not studied. This case illustrates definitely that, at least in some cases, $\alpha^{G\text{-Philadelphia}}$ is not associated with a functional α^A gene in cis, and that some forms of heterozygous α thalassemia in blacks are associated with totally absent α-chain synthesis from the chromosome bearing the α-thalassemia gene. In another black family, an individual inherited Hb G-Philadelphia from one parent and from the other parent Hb Seal Rock, a variant with an elongated α chain analogous to that of Hb Constant Spring (Bradley et al., 1975). The parent heterozygous for $\alpha^{G\text{-Philadelphia}}$ had 28 per cent Hb G-Philadelphia, whereas the doubly heterozygous individual had 39 per cent Hb G-Philadelphia, 2 per cent Hb Seal Rock, and the rest Hb A and Hb A_2, but had no Hb H. The α-thalassemia syndrome in this family is milder than in the previous one and the findings indicate that in this family either the $\alpha^{G\text{-}Philadelphia}$ gene or the $\alpha^{Seal\ Rock}$ gene (or both) is associated with a functional α^A gene in cis. Finally, one black individual has been described who inherited both α thalassemia and the α-chain variant Hb I (Atwater et al., 1960). This individual did not have Hb H and had 30 per cent Hb A.

These various family studies illustrate that α thalassemia in blacks is quite heterogeneous in the degree of suppression of α-chain synthesis and that there is probably heterogeneity in the number of α-chain loci in blacks.

GAMMA THALASSEMIA

An infant with hemolytic anemia at birth was found to have hypochromic microcytic red cells (Kan et al., 1972b). Heterozygous β thalassemia, with normal levels of hemoglobin A_2 and F, was found in the father and many of his relatives. Globin-chain synthesis studies revealed a decrease in γ- and β-chain synthesis in the reticulocytes of this infant. The disease became self-limited as the baby grew older. The hemolytic anemia disappeared, and the child developed the phenotype of simple heterozygous β thalassemia. It is believed that this child represents an example of heterozygous $\gamma\beta$ (+ δ) thalassemia. The disease should be suspected in cases of hypochromic hemolytic disease in the newborn. Homozygous γ thalassemia would probably not be compatible with life (Stamatoyannopoulos, 1971).

DELTA THALASSEMIA

Isolated delta thalassemia has been described as an incidental finding in both the heterozygous (Frazer et al., 1964) and homozygous (Ohta et al., 1970) forms. In the former, there is decreased Hb A_2; in the latter, total absence of Hb A_2 is noted. In neither situation are hypochromia, anemia, or red cell morphological changes observed. The doubly heterozygous state for δ thalassemia plus $\delta\beta$ thalassemia (Fessas and Stamatoyannopoulos, 1962) and δ thalassemia plus HPFH (Thompson et al., 1965a) have also been described and are clinically similar to simple heterozygosity for $\delta\beta$ thalassemia or HPFH except that there is total absence of Hb A_2.

HEREDITARY PERSISTENCE OF FETAL HEMOGLOBIN (HPFH) AND HB KENYA

HPFH is found primarily in blacks and in Greeks (Conley et al., 1963; Fessas and Stamatoyannopoulos, 1964). In blacks, there is absence of β- and δ-chain synthesis in cis to the HPFH gene. Heterozygous HPFH differs from heterozygous thalassemia in that non-α ($\gamma + \beta$) chain production is usually equal to α-chain synthesis (Sofroniadou et al., 1975; Natta et al., 1973b). There is no globin-chain imbalance and no microcytosis or hypochromia of the red blood cells. Furthermore, the most important difference is that the fetal hemoglobin is evenly distributed in all the red blood cells in contrast to the heterogeneous distribution of Hb F observed in thalassemic red cells. In most blacks with HPFH the fetal hemoglobin which is present has the typical adult ${}^{G}\gamma$:${}^{A}\gamma$ ratio of 2:3 (Huisman et al., 1971b). However, in some blacks with HPFH, all the Hb F present is of the ${}^{G}\gamma$ type and these individuals usually have a lower level of Hb F (15 per cent vs. 30 per cent) than other blacks with HPFH. In most Greeks with HPFH, all the Hb F is of the ${}^{A}\gamma$ type. Rare blacks with HPFH may also have predominantly Hb F of the ${}^{A}\gamma$ type (Huisman et al., 1971b). These findings indicate that the molecular defect leading to HPFH is quite heterogeneous.

In the heterozygous state, HPFH is asymptomatic. The hemoglobin F level is about 15 to 35 per cent of the total hemoglobin in the black and 10 to 20 per cent in the Greek type. Hemoglobin A_2 is decreased. The homozygous form of HPFH has been found only in the black (reviewed by Weatherall and Clegg, 1972). These individuals have 100 per cent fetal hemoglobin and have mild hypochromia, microcytosis, and red cell morphological changes but no anemia. In fact, mild erythrocytosis is present because of the high oxygen affinity of the blood resulting in relative tissue hypoxia. In two homozygous individuals globin synthesis has been studied and has revealed a mild to moderate deficit in γ-chain synthesis: γ/α 0.52 and 0.70 (Charache et al., 1975; Forget et al., 1976b). These individuals, therefore, have a degree of imbalanced globin-chain synthesis similar to that seen in β-thalassemia trait. Imbalance has also been observed in rare heterozygotes (Huisman et al., 1975; Friedman et al., 1976b).

In association with beta-chain structural variants, such as Hb S, HPFH gives hemoglobin electrophoresis findings similar to those found in Hb S/β^0 thalassemia or homozygous sickle cell anemia, but with an unusually high level of Hb F: absent Hb A, 65 to 85 per cent Hb S, and 15 to 35 per cent Hb F. Clinically, however, this disorder is benign with no anemia, hemolysis, hypochromia, or painful crises. The benign nature of this disorder is probably related to the fact that the Hb F is evenly distributed among the red cells, and it is known that Hb F inhibits the sickling of Hb S (see Chapter 7).

More recently, there have been reports of Hb S/HPFH in blacks in which there is synthesis of Hb A, presumably from an active β^A gene in cis to the HPFH gene (Huisman et al., 1975; Stamatoyannopoulos et al., 1975; Friedman and Schwartz, 1976). In two of these families the HPFH was of the ${}^{G}\gamma$ types. Similarly, in the Greek type

($^A\gamma$) of HPFH (Fessas and Stamatoyannopoulos, 1964), the British type (Weatherall et al., 1975a), and the Swiss type (Marti, 1963) there is convincing evidence for activity of the β-chain locus in cis to the HPFH gene (reviewed by Weatherall and Clegg, 1975).

As previously discussed, the ordinary type of HPFH in the black appears to be associated with gene deletion of β (and δ) structural genes. Obviously, the finding of some forms of HPFH with β-chain synthesis in cis indicates that the HPFH phenotype is not necessarily associated with δ- and β-*structural* gene deletions and that some other common feature must be present such as deletion of control gene elements situated between γ and δ or β structural loci. There is, however, no direct experimental evidence to support the latter hypothesis.

Hemoglobin Kenya is a newly discovered abnormal hemoglobin (Huisman et al., 1972b; Kendall et al., 1973) which is associated with an HPFH phenotype and has provided a more detailed understanding of the relationship between the $^G\gamma$-, $^A\gamma$-, δ-, and β-chain genes. The non-α chain of Hb Kenya consists of a fusion product containing the N terminus of the γ chain and the C terminus of the β chain, presumably the result of nonhomologous crossing over between a γ-chain gene and the β-chain gene (Fig. 5–10). The crossover from γ to β sequence occurred before position 136 (between residues 81 and 86) of the γ chain, so that it is not possible to tell whether it is an $^A\gamma$ or a $^G\gamma$ gene which is involved in the fusion product. However, individuals with Hb Kenya have increased levels of Hb F in their red cells and it is all of the $^G\gamma$ type. If one assumes that this Hb F comes from the γ-chain gene(s) in cis to the Kenya gene, and if the $^G\gamma\ ^g\gamma\ ^A\gamma\ ^a\gamma$ model of the γ-chain genes is correct (see Chapter 4), then the crossover must involve either the $^g\gamma$ or $^A\gamma$ genes. In addition, one must conclude from this finding that the $^A\gamma$ gene is situated to the N-terminal side of the δ- and β-chain genes and is closer to these genes than is the $^G\gamma$ chain gene. The arrangement of the non-α chain genes would therefore be (going from N- to C-terminal): $^G\gamma\ ^g\gamma\ ^A\gamma\ ^a\gamma\ \delta\ \beta$. The finding of Hb Kenya, however, does not rule out the possibility that the $^G\gamma$ (and $^g\gamma$) genes are situated to the C-terminal side of the β-chain gene.

Of additional importance is the fact that Hb Kenya, unlike Hb

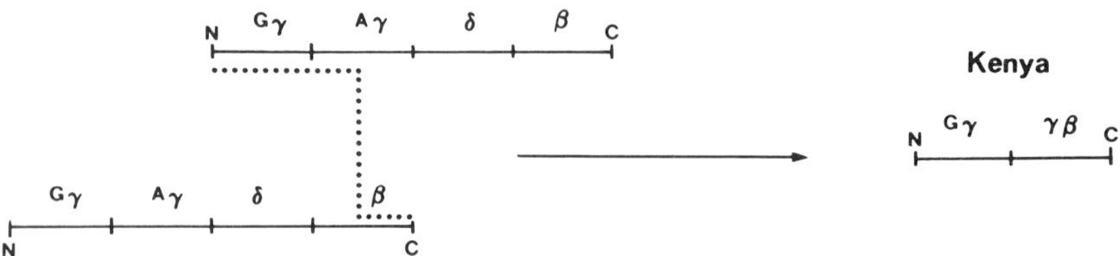

Figure 5–10. Origin of Kenya globin chain by nonhomologous crossing over between γ- and β-globin genes. N and C have the same designation as in Figure 5–3A.

Lepore, is not associated with a thalassemic phenotype, but rather an HPFH phenotype. Hemoglobin Kenya has been found in the simple heterozygous state as well as in association with Hb S (Kendall et al., 1973; Smith et al., 1973; Nute et al., 1976). In the simple heterozygote it makes up approximately 5 to 10 per cent of the total hemoglobin, but in association with Hb S it accounts for 17 to 19 per cent of the total. Rare simple heterozygotes have as much as 20 to 30 per cent Hb Kenya (Nute et al., 1976). All the patients are asymptomatic. There is no hypochromia or microcytosis and there are no morphological changes in the red cells. In all cases, the elevated fetal hemoglobin is uniformly distributed within the red cells and is of the $^{G}\gamma$ type (Kendall et al., 1973; Smith et al., 1973; Nute et al., 1976). Unlike the situation in the Hb Lepore and anti-Lepore syndromes, the synthesis of the Kenya fusion product is active in reticulocytes (Clegg et al., 1974b).

MANAGEMENT OF THE THALASSEMIA SYNDROMES

Prevention

An important step in the prevention of the occurrence of severely affected children with homozygous α or β thalassemia is the detection of the heterozygous state in adults. Physicians should be aware of the possibility of thalassemia trait occurring in individuals with hypochromic anemias which are refractory to iron therapy and should perform the necessary diagnostic studies to confirm the diagnosis. In areas where there is a high incidence of thalassemia trait, general population screening surveys could be established. Once identified, the affected individuals could be educated and counseled with respect to the disease process and its genetics. Two affected heterozygotes contemplating marriage and planning to have a family should be aware that chances of having a severely affected homozygous child are one in four.

Prenatal diagnosis of thalassemia is now feasible but is still considered an experimental procedure which is done only in a limited number of centers. The procedure involves obtaining a fetal blood sample and incubating it with radioactive leucine to determine the relative amounts of synthesis of γ, β, and α chains. The fetal blood sample can be obtained in one of two ways: (1) needle aspiration of a placental blood vessel without direct visualization, after localization of the placenta by ultrasound (Kan et al., 1974d); or (2) needle aspiration of a placental blood vessel (when the placenta is in a posterior or fundal position) under direct visualization using an amnioscope or fetoscope (Hobbins and Mahoney, 1974, 1975). Although fetal blood sampling has been successfully done a number of times by these techniques without fetal complications, the procedure cannot be considered totally safe: in a few cases fetal loss has occurred owing to infection, hemorrhage, premature labor, or undetermined causes (Alter et al., 1976b; Kan and Globus, 1976).

Another difficulty is obtaining a pure or relatively pure fetal sample. There may be variable contamination of the fetal blood with maternal placental blood. One can overcome the latter difficulty by various techniques which either concentrate and purify the fetal red cells by differential agglutination (Kan et al., 1974b) or correct for the maternal contamination by calculations based on differences in specific activity between fetal and maternal samples or by determining globin synthesis in various known mixtures of fetal plus maternal blood (Cividalli et al., 1974a; Chang et al., 1975). Another approach to the problem of maternal blood contamination is to transfuse the mother prior to the procedure in order to suppress erythropoiesis and thereby reduce the proportion of synthetically active reticulocytes in the maternal peripheral blood (Nathan and Alter, 1975). Finally, for the diagnosis of α-thalassemia syndromes due to gene deletions, prenatal diagnosis can be achieved by measurement of α-chain genes by molecular hybridization, using DNA obtained from cultured amniotic fluid fibroblasts (Kan and Globus, 1976; Kan et al., 1976a).

From the biochemical point of view, prenatal diagnosis of α and β thalassemia and structural hemoglobinopathies should pose no major obstacles. In the case of α thalassemia and α-chain structural variants, the detection of a quantitative or qualitative abnormality in α-chain synthesis should be feasible, since the α chain is normally fully expressed in the first trimester (see Figure 4–2). With respect to β thalassemia and β-chain structural variants, the β gene is normally expressed at only a very low level in the first and second trimesters (see Chapter 4), but there is still sufficient β-chain synthesis in utero to allow detection of an abnormal β chain or the determination, from the study of a large number of cases, of the range of normal fetal β-chain synthesis, below which β thalassemia should fall (Kazazian et al., 1973; Cividalli et al., 1974a; Chang et al., 1974, 1975). In fact, heterozygosity for Hb S (Kan et al., 1972a), α thalassemia (Kan et al., 1974a), and β thalassemia (Chang et al., 1975) has been diagnosed in studies of abortuses of pregnancies at risk. Prospective prenatal diagnosis attempts have been performed in a number of cases (Kan et al., 1975b and c; Nathan and Alter, 1975; Alter et al., 1976a, 1976b; Kan et al., 1976a, 1976b). Prospective diagnoses have been made of homozygous β thalassemia (Kan et al., 1975c), homozygous sickle cell anemia (Alter et al., 1976a; Kan et al., 1976b), heterozygous α and β thalassemia (Alter et al., 1976b; Kan et al., 1976a), and, incidentally, heterozygosity for Hb G-Philadelphia (Alter et al., 1976a). Some diagnostic errors, however, have occurred (Alter et al., 1976b).

It is not certain, however, that prenatal diagnosis will significantly reduce the incidence of homozygous individuals. Such cases will still arise in instances in which the parents are unaware, before the birth of their first affected child, that they have thalassemia trait. Furthermore, some parents may object to abortion yet wish to attempt having other (hopefully unaffected) children. In individual cases, however, the availability of precise prenatal diagnosis will be of great value.

SUPPORTIVE THERAPY

There is no specific therapy for the severely affected homozygous thalassemic patient. The treatment is mainly supportive and consists of a regular transfusion program to control the anemia. There are two general types of transfusion programs which can be undertaken. Until recently the standard program consisted of transfusing the patient in order to maintain a "safe" hemoglobin level. This usually meant transfusing the patient when his hemoglobin dropped to a level of 7 or 8 g/100 ml, hopefully before the patient became symptomatic.

The second type of transfusion program is the so-called high or hyper-transfusion (HT) regimen. This approach consists of transfusing the patients as frequently as necessary to maintain a "normal" hemoglobin level, which is not allowed to drop below a minimum of 10 g/100 ml. Such a program usually entails a transfusion of 2 to 3 units of packed red cells at intervals of every two to four weeks. The HT regimen has the obvious disadvantage that the patient receives a much larger total body burden of iron which cannot be naturally excreted by the body. Calculations of this excess infusion of iron, in comparison with a more standard transfusion regimen, give minimum values in the range of 1 to 2 grams of elemental iron per year for the net increment of iron accumulated (Necheles, 1969a; Piomelli et al., 1969). If one does not subtract iron removed by chelation therapy and the decreased iron absorbed from food, the increment may be as high as 3 to 4 grams of elemental iron per year in the HT regimen (Beard et al., 1969). Since the major cause of death in these children is related to the effects of iron overload in the second or third decade, many physicians have been reluctant to adopt this HT program. However, there is good evidence that children who are maintained on an HT regimen do as well as, if not better than, children maintained on a more standard regimen. The children in the HT group, in general, have fewer intercurrent illnesses and infections, are more active, and lead more normal and happy lives (Wolman, 1964; Wolman and Ortolani, 1969). There are fewer instances of cardiomegaly and hepatosplenomegaly and fewer bone changes and orthodontic problems (Beard et al., 1969; Piomelli et al., 1969). There is some dispute as to whether the HT regimen actually improves the growth and development of these children. Some studies claim that hypertransfusion does improve growth (Wolman, 1964; Beard et al., 1969; Piomelli et al., 1969; Kattamis et al., 1970), whereas other studies did not show improved growth (Johnston et al., 1966; Wolff and Luke, 1969; Wolman and Ortolani, 1969; Logothetis et al., 1972). One study even found some decrease in growth in the HT group (Brook et al., 1969). The discrepancy is probably related to the age at which HT is started: HT started after the first few years of life probably does not improve growth and development, but HT started in infancy may prevent growth retardation (Beard et al., 1969; Piomelli et al., 1969). The most recent follow-up studies on such patients have still not resolved the issue (Piomelli et al., 1974; Necheles et al., 1974).

It will be some time before one will be able to assess with certainty whether the HT program affects the longevity of the patients who receive it. Thus far, it appears that longevity may not be prolonged (Wolman and Ortolani, 1969) but is probably not shortened, and that the HT regimen seems to contribute to happier lives for the thalassemic children. Certainly one should not limit transfusions in thalassemic children for fear of iron overload. Because the HT regimen does not, in general, appear to shorten longevity, it seems reasonable generally to transfuse a child as frequently as necessary to maintain a minimum hemoglobin of 9 or 10 g/100 ml, if the facilities to do so are available. It seems important to institute such a program from an early age if one wishes to lessen the development of severe facial deformities, bone changes, cardiomegaly, and splenomegaly in these patients.

Any transfusion regimen, and especially the HT regimen, is associated with a certain incidence of transfusion-related complications. Hepatitis and other viral diseases, such as cytomegalovirus infections, are always a risk and are treated symptomatically. Isoimmunization to minor blood groups (Kell, Duffy, C, c, E), although relatively rare (Economidou et al., 1971), may cause difficulties in cross-matching and in survival time of the transfused red cells. This may be avoided by careful, full minor blood-group typing of the patient before the institution of transfusions and by careful selection of blood donors. Urticarial reactions usually respond to epinephrine or antihistamines and may be avoided in some cases by treatment with antihistamines prior to the transfusion. A more difficult problem is the febrile reaction due to prior sensitization of the patient to white blood cell or plasma protein antigens (Economidou et al., 1971). These may be avoided (or prevented) by use of white cell–free blood: frozen red cells or blood passed through Leuko-Pak[(R)] filters (Fenwal Laboratories). Antipyretics and occasionally steroids are necessary to treat severe febrile reactions.

Splenectomy

Splenectomy has an important place in the management of patients with homozygous β thalassemia. If a child is maintained on a good hypertransfusion regimen from an early age, marked splenomegaly may not develop (Beard et al., 1969; Piomelli et al., 1969) because of decreased production and thus decreased RE destruction of abnormal red cells. Even established splenomegaly may be reversible following institution of HT (O'Brien et al., 1972). However, many patients, in spite of adequate transfusions, do develop significant splenomegaly which may cause problems. Progressive splenomegaly usually aggravates the anemia and increases the transfusion requirement by causing a dilutional type of anemia due to the sequestration of transfused red cells in the large third space provided by the spleen's size.

Thalassemic children with splenomegaly have a greatly increased intravascular blood volume which can be reversed by splenectomy (Blendis et al., 1974). In addition, the patients may develop true hypersplenism, with evidence of destruction in the spleen of red cells and of other formed blood elements such as white cells and platelets. Rapid onset of splenomegaly and splenic destruction of transfused red cells may be triggered by isoimmunization to minor blood-group antigens. Such an occurrence is usually associated with difficulty in cross-matching the blood and development of a positive Coombs' test. In some instances, however, the only sign may be a sudden increase in the child's transfusion requirement and a sudden increase in spleen size. Splenomegaly, on the other hand, may be symptomatic simply by the sheer size of the spleen, causing pressure discomfort in the abdomen or pain from splenic infarcts. In cases in which splenomegaly is symptomatic or causes difficulty in maintaining adequate hemoglobin levels despite appropriate maintenance transfusions, splenectomy should be recommended. Splenectomy will usually result in a lessening of the transfusion requirement and, in combination with a good transfusion program, will usually make it possible to maintain the patient's hemoglobin at a near normal level much more easily than before splenectomy and thus achieve the maximum benefits of HT.

Splenectomy is rarely necessary before the child reaches the age of five or six years, but in certain instances splenectomy at an earlier age may be necessary. The decision to perform splenectomy may be aided by doing a chromium-51 tagged red cell survival study, with scanning of the spleen to demonstrate sequestration of labeled red cells. Splenectomy is rarely indicated before the age of three or four years, because of the demonstration of increased instances of rapidly fatal septicemia in children who have had splenectomy before that age (Eraklis et al., 1967). Thalassemic children, even those over the age of three or four, are particularly susceptible to this type of fatal gram-positive septicemia (Smith et al., 1962, 1964). The reasons for this high incidence are not known. The spleen and the reticuloendothelial (RE) system in general probably function as bacterial filters of the circulation. In the asplenic thalassemic individual, the loss of splenic filter function is probably aggravated, in addition, by some degree of RE system blockade due to the iron overload. A more recent study, however, did not show a high incidence of septicemia in a large series of thalassemic patients who had splenectomy after the age of two years (Englehard et al., 1975). The spleen probably has a function in antibody synthesis, the absence of which may also put the thalassemic patient at a disadvantage in handling infections. Indeed, immunoglobulin levels are low in some splenectomized thalassemic patients (Wasi et al., 1971) but not in all (Englehard et al., 1975). Because of the increased risk of infection, it is probably advisable, after splenectomy, to maintain thalassemic children on prophylactic doses of penicillin for at least two years (the time of peak incidence of postsplenectomy septicemia), if not indefinitely. Another postsplenectomy complication is the occasional development of marked thrombocytosis with thromboembolic phenomena which may require anticoagulation. Most patients, however, improve following splenectomy (Englehard et al., 1975) and some may even have improved growth and development (Blendis et al., 1974).

USE OF IRON-CHELATING AGENTS

Because of the marked iron overload which occurs in β thalassemia, it should be clinically advantageous to remove the excess iron stores, especially in patients maintained on high transfusion regimens, by the long-term administration of iron-chelating agents. There are two such agents which are currently available and have been extensively used in Britain and Europe. The first is desferrioxamine B, which is usually administered by intramuscular injection; the second is diethylenetriamine pentacetate (DTPA), which must be given by intravenous infusion, usually at the time of transfusion (Smith, 1962, 1964; Keberle, 1964). It should be theoretically possible to maintain a near balance of iron stores if one uses the following doses of the two agents concomitantly: 6 mg of I.V. DTPA with each transfusion and 0.5 to 1.0 g of desferrioxamine I.M. daily (Weatherall and Clegg, 1972).

The initial studies of urinary iron excretion in response to these drugs demonstrated that not all patients respond equally well. In some patients, concomitant use of vitamin C improved urinary iron excretion in response to desferrioxamine (Wapnick et al., 1969). However, the amount of iron excretion induced by desferrioxamine usually decreased in time and the drug became relatively ineffective (Smith, 1962, 1964; Beard et al., 1969). The reason for this loss of effectiveness is probably that desferrioxamine may only chelate iron which is in certain labile pools: the bulk of the storage iron may not be chelatable when desferrioxamine is administered in the usual manner (Lipschitz et al., 1971). Therefore, in practice, it is not usually possible to achieve a state of sustained negative iron balance in most thalassemic patients by administering desferrioxamine by daily intramuscular injections alone (Beard et al., 1969; Weatherall and Clegg, 1972). Exceptions may, however, exist: in a child with congenital hypoplastic anemia treated for 5 years with intramuscular desferrioxamine, 30 per cent of the amount of transfused iron was recovered in the urine (Lukens and Neuman, 1971). Desferrioxamine has rarely been associated with certain undesirable side effects: patients developed presumed allergic reactions (Beard et al., 1969) and the daily intramuscular injections caused local discomfort. Finally, cataracts have been described in experimental animals and in three individuals after long-term use of desferrioxamine. DTPA is generally considered quite toxic and its usefulness is very limited.

Subsequently, more optimistic reports have appeared on the use of desferrioxamine in thalassemia (Constantoulakis et al., 1974; Modell and Beck, 1974; O'Brien, 1974). These more recent studies have shown that with higher doses of desferrioxamine, including intravenous desferrioxamine at the time of transfusion, and with concomitant daily oral vitamin C, sustained high levels of urinary iron excretion and near normal iron balance can be achieved. More recently, preliminary studies have shown that slow continuous subcutaneous infusions of desferrioxamine (using portable devices) achieve significantly greater urinary iron excretion than single daily intramuscular injections (Propper et al., 1976). In general, however, significant iron excretion occurs only with increasing age and only after considerable iron overload has already occurred as determined by measurements of liver iron. It has not been demonstrated that desferrioxamine can actually prevent the occurrence of this initial iron accumulation: iron stores usually must reach levels nearly 10 times greater than normal before significant chelation is achieved. Although it appears that tissue siderosis cannot be totally prevented by chelation, it is possible that long-term chelation therapy may be of some benefit by eliminating additional increments of more reactive and potentially toxic iron, especially in patients on high transfusion regimens. Recently, Barry et al. (1974) demonstrated that liver iron stores stabilized and hepatic fibrosis failed to progress on long-term use of desferrioxamine. Growth and sexual development were also improved in these patients.

The role and mode of action of vitamin C in chelation therapy are not clear. Thalassemic patients are usually deficient in vitamin C (and E), both nonspecific and anti-oxidant substances, presumably because of the oxidant stress of iron overload. It seems, therefore, theoretically advantageous to replenish these vitamins in the thalassemic patient, both to counteract the tissue toxic oxidant stress of iron and to facilitate mobilization of iron. At one time there was some concern that vitamin C might act by increasing gastrointestinal tract absorption of iron, thus increasing the labile pool of chelatable iron and urinary excretion of iron. However, careful balance studies have ruled out this possibility (Nienhuis et al., 1975).

New iron-chelating drugs, especially orally effective agents, are being sought. One such agent, 2,3-dihydroxybenzoic acid, initially seemed to have some promise (Graziano et al., 1974); however, clinical trials in humans have failed to demonstrate substantial urinary iron excretion (Jones et al., 1975), although the drug seems to be effective as a free radical scavenger and thus may help counteract tissue iron toxicity (Graziano et al., 1976).

Other General Measures

The medical management of a child with homozygous β thalassemia otherwise involves good general pediatric and medical care, which includes a close relationship among physician, patient, and parents and education of parents and child with regard to seeking early medical attention for any illness, especially febrile episodes. Because of the propensity of these children to develop severe and frequently fatal infections, it is probably wise to treat any febrile illness, after taking appropriate cultures, with antibiotics until a specific diagnosis becomes apparent. In addition to the fatal septicemias, other infections which these patients develop include a *benign pericarditis*, believed to be of viral etiology (Engle, 1964); however, it may also be the result of streptococcal infection (Wasi, 1971) or due to an iron-induced pericardial irritation analogous to the arthritis of hemochromatosis. It usually subsides spontaneously, although pericardiocentesis may rarely be necessary to relieve tamponade. Other infections include *transfusion-related infections* such as hepatitis and cytomegalovirus infection, which must be treated symptomatically. The latter may be avoided by use of blood which is over 48 hours old.

Because of the marked marrow hyperplasia due to the hemolytic component of the disease, thalassemic children should be maintained on daily folic acid replacement (1 mg daily) to prevent the development of relative *folic acid deficiency* and a megaloblastic crisis, which may aggravate the anemia. Such a crisis may occasionally present as thrombocytopenia and a bleeding diathesis.

Certain children develop severe *cephalofacial deformities and malocclusion* because of marrow expansion in the maxilla. This complication can usually be avoided by proper transfusion from an early age and early splenectomy (Logothetis et al., 1971). Once the deformity is established, surgical management is possible (Jurkiewicz et al., 1969).

The consequences of *iron overload* must be treated as they develop: diabetes, with appropriate diet and insulin therapy; hepatic dysfunction, by dietary and other supportive means. Frequently, thalassemic children may have a prolonged prothrombin time which, despite its probable hepatocellular basis, may respond to vitamin K therapy. Some malabsorption of vitamin K may occur because of chronic pancreatic insufficiency due to pancreatic siderosis and fibrosis.

As previously discussed in the section on chelation therapy, vitamin C and vitamin E supplementation may be beneficial to counteract the oxidant effects of iron overload (Rachmilewitz et al., 1976).

The most serious and life-threatening complication is that of *cardiac hemosiderosis*, resulting in arrhythmia and chronic congestive heart failure (Engle, 1964). When these complications develop, the patients must be treated vigorously with low salt diet, digitalis, diuretics, and antiarrhythmic medications. Fatal Stokes-Adams attacks may occur from arrhythmias which are presumably due to iron deposition in the conducting system of the heart. In a child who develops recurrent arrhythmias, a cardiac pacemaker may be required to prevent a fatal arrhythmia.

Finally, androgen therapy (oxymetholone) has been reported to improve the anemia in a case of thalassemia intermedia (Craddock et al., 1972), although secondary causes may have contributed to the anemia in that particular case. Hormonal replacement therapy has been used in certain patients in an attempt to treat various *endocrine deficiencies*, presumably due to hemosiderosis, and improve development of secondary sexual characteristics. The therapy is not usually effective because sexual underdevelopment may be due in large part to target organ unresponsiveness (related to siderotic or hypoxic damage) rather than to hormonal deficiency.

Future Treatment

The future may offer more definitive forms of therapy for thalassemia. Two possible means of therapy may one day become available for the child with thalassemia major: (1) bone marrow transplantation, and/or (2) correction of the biochemical defect by genetic engineering and manipulation.

The art of bone marrow transplantation is being developed in a number of centers. It has been successfully carried out in the treatment of aplastic anemia and in certain cases of acute leukemia in relapse, using as a source of bone marrow that of an unaffected sibling who is histocompatible with the patient (Thomas et al., 1975). The major problem, however, is immunological: rejection of the graft by the recipient and graft-versus-host reaction have been difficult problems which have led to many failures and fatalities. In thalassemia, one would have to destroy the patient's own marrow before such a transplantation in order to prevent proliferation of the abnormal erythroid cells. This would be impossible to do without destroying the patient's own granulocyte precursors and megakaryocytes as well. Rejection of the marrow graft by the thalassemic patient is a very likely complication, even with proper immunosuppression and good histocompatibility, because of prior sensitization of the patient to various tissue antigens from the many previous blood transfusions. Rejection of the graft would leave the patient totally aplastic. If marrow engraftment is to be successful in thalassemic patients, transplantation should probably be done in infancy before transfusions are initiated. Finally, even if the transplanted marrow becomes engrafted, a graft-versus-host reaction could lead to a rapidly fatal outcome. Until the current problems of bone marrow transplantation are resolved, and one can offer the patient a good possibility of a successful outcome, bone marrow transplantation cannot be advised at this time in cases of thalassemia in which, with good medical management, the patient can be given some 20 or more years of useful life.

If one could suppress the excessive production of the normally produced globin chain in thalassemia, one would eliminate the precipitation of globin-chain aggregates which leads to much of the pathophysiology and disability in thalassemia. Research is proceeding in a search for drugs or other agents which might specifically inhibit the synthesis of one or another globin chain. In β thalassemia, if one could induce γ-chain synthesis, or prevent the neonatal γ to β chain switchover, one would increase the relative amount of γ chain in the thalassemic red cell. This would decrease the disability of the patients by decreasing or eliminating the formation of α-chain aggregates, which are so important in the development of the hemolytic component of the disease: the γ chains could combine with the excess α chains and balance would be achieved. Research is also under way in this area.

In the not too distant future, actual gene therapy for thalassemia may be feasible. Methods for isolating, purifying, and replicating eukaryotic genes are being rapidly developed as well as techniques for insertion of foreign DNA into eukaryotic cells. The technical scientific difficulties of such an approach are formidable but not insurmountable. A considerable amount of controversy exists, however, concerning the ethical and moral aspects of such an approach. A number of scientists and geneticists strongly oppose the idea of tampering with human genomes because of the potentially harmful consequences which could ensue. It is conceivable that the technical capability of gene therapy will be achieved before the ethical issues are resolved.

These types of therapeutic approaches are not imminent but remain likely future possibilities. Once the genetic defect is known more precisely at the messenger RNA and DNA levels, one may have more insight into ways to approach the treatment of thalassemia at the molecular level. In the meantime, the cornerstone of the treatment of thalassemia must remain good general medical care and proper supportive management of the patient in a center which is equipped to make this possible.

Chapter 6

HUMAN HEMOGLOBIN VARIANTS

To the nonspecialist, perhaps the most bewildering aspect of "hemoglobinology" is the number and variety of human hemoglobin variants. This topic continues to expand logarithmically. At present there are over 250 variants of known structure (Table 6–1). It is not surprising that the first human hemoglobin variants to be recognized were those that attracted clinical attention. Hörlein and Weber (1948) reported the first hemoglobinopathy. They studied a family with congenital cyanosis and demonstrated that affected family members had hemoglobin with abnormal spectral properties. Later, it was shown that they had one of the M hemoglobins. In the early 1950's, sickle cell anemia was found to be due to an electrophoretically abnormal hemoglobin having a single amino acid substitution in the β chain (β6 Glu→Val). Thereafter, electrophoresis became widely employed in the search for other human hemoglobin variants. Those having relatively high gene frequencies were discovered quite readily. Hemoglobins C, D, and E were identified within two years following the structural identification of hemoglobin S. Large-scale screening programs were initiated to find other abnormal hemoglobins. Initially, new variants were named by successive letters of the alphabet. By the time hemoglobin Q was encountered, it became apparent that the letters of the alphabet would soon be exhausted. To add to the confusion, some hemoglobins with identical electrophoretic properties were shown to have different structures. Gradually, investigators agreed to give new hemoglobins a specific name, most often reflecting the origin of the patient. Many colorful and provocative names have appeared in the literature, some exotic (Hb Aida), others chauvinistic (Hb Brigham), parochial (Hb

*TABLE 6–1. Human Hemoglobin Variants: 1976**

	Total	Unstable	Abnormal O_2 Affinity	Hbs M	No Clinical Manifestations
α Chain	80	9	4	2	65
β Chain	166	65	28	3	70
γ Chain	14	1			
δ Chain	9				
Total	269				

*Compiled from Table 6–2.

Riverdale-Bronx), or patriotic (Hb Abraham Lincoln). For a while the naming of hemoglobin variants was treated somewhat lightly because many believed the hemoglobin would be more often remembered by its structure rather than by its eponym. However, just as people naturally tend to call their friends by name rather than by social security number, the names of the variants have stuck. As Table 6–2 shows, the same variant (with a specific structural abnormality) is often "rediscovered" in different laboratories all over the world: $\alpha_2^{47\,Asp \rightarrow Gly}\beta_2$ has nine interesting names, but it is generally called Hb L-Ferrara, after the place where it was first described.

CLINICAL CLASSIFICATION

The large list of human hemoglobin variants shown in Table 6–2 is more readily comprehended if the variants are classified according to their clinical manifestations (Table 6–3). The majority of known variants are unassociated with any apparent clinical sequelae. Many of these were discovered accidentally or during the survey of large populations. Although they may be of genetic or anthropological interest, they have no apparent functional abnormalities.

The clinically significant human hemoglobin variants are classified in Table 6–3. Disorders due to the presence of sickle hemoglobin constitute the most important group both in the United States and worldwide. (The sickle syndromes are discussed in detail in Chapter 7.) Hb C is the second most commonly encountered variant. Like Hb S, Hb C has decreased solubility within the red cell. The pathogenesis of homozygous Hb C disease is discussed at the end of this chapter. Approximately 65 unstable hemoglobin variants have been described to date. They constitute an important form of congenital nonspherocytic hemolytic anemia. (This entity is discussed in Chapter 8.) Variants with abnormal oxygen binding are described in Chapter 9. This group has provided a considerable amount of relevant physiological and biochemical information. Individuals with congenital methemoglobinemia may have one of the so-called M he-

Text continued on page 210.

TABLE 6–2. *Human Hemoglobin Variants**

ALPHA CHAIN

Residue and Helical Number	Amino Acid Substitution	Name	Major Abnormal Property	Reference
5(A3)	Ala→Asp	Hb J-Toronto		1
6(A4)	Asp→Ala	Hb Sawara		2
11(A9)	Lys→Glu	Hb Anantharaj		3
12(A10)	Ala→Asp	Hb J-Paris-I, J-Aljezur		4,70
15(A13)	Gly→Asp	Hb I-Interlaken, J-Oxford, N-Cosenza		5,6
	Gly→Arg	Hb Ottawa, Siam		7,8
16(A14)	Lys→Glu	Hb I, I-Philadelphia, I-Texas, I-Burlington, I-Skamania		9
21(B2)	Ala→Asp	Hb J-Nyanza		10
22(B3)	Gly→Asp	Hb J-Medellin		11
23(B4)	Glu→Gln	Hb Memphis		12
	Glu→Lys	Hb Chad		13
	Glu→Val	Hb G-Audhali		14
27(B8)	Glu→Gly	Hb Fort Worth		15
27(B8)	Glu→Val	Hb Spanish Town		268
30(B11)	Glu→Lys	Hb O-Padova		16
	Glu→Gln	Hb G-Honolulu, G-Singapore, G-Chinese, G-Hong Kong		17
43(CE1)	Phe→Val	Hb Torino	Unstable; ↓ O_2 affinity	18
	Phe→Leu	Hb Hirosaki		19
47(CE5)	Asp→Gly	Hb L-Ferrara, Umi, Kokura, Michigan-I, Michigan-II, Yukuhashi-II, L-Gaslini, Tagawa-II, Beilinson, Mugino		20
	Asp→His	Hb Hasharon, Sinai, Sealy	Unstable	21,22
	Asp→Asn	Hb Arya	Slightly unstable	23
48(CE6)	Leu→Arg	Hb Montgomery		24
50(CE8)	His→Asp	Hb J-Sardegna		25
51(CE9)	Gly→Asp	Hb J-Abidjan		26
	Gly→Arg	Hb Russ		27
53(E2)	Ala→Asp	Hb J-Rovigo	Unstable	28
54(E3)	Gln→Arg	Hb Shimonoseki		29
	Gln→Glu	Hb J-Mexico, J-Paris-II, Uppsala		30
57(E6)	Gly→Arg	Hb L-Persian Gulf		31
	Gly→Asp	Hb J-Norfolk, Kagoshima, Nishik-I, II, III		32
58(E7)	His→Tyr	Hb M-Boston, M-Osaka, M-Gothenburg, M-Kiskunhalos	Ferri-Hb; ↓ O_2 affinity	33
60(E9)	Lys→Asn	Hb Zambia		34
61(E10)	Lys→Asn	Hb J-Buda	↓ O_2 affinity	35
64(E13)	Asp→Asn	Hb G-Waimanalo, Hb-Aida		36,37
	Asp→His	Hb Q-India		38
68(E17)	Asn→Asp	Hb Ube-2		39
	Asn→Lys	Hb G-Philadelphia, G-Knoxville-II, Stanleyville-I, G-Bristol, G-Uzuakoli, D-Baltimore, D-Washington, D-St. Louis		40
71(E20)	Ala→Glu	Hb J-Habana		41
72(EF1)	His→Arg	Hb Daneshgah-Teheran		42
74(EF3)	Asp→His	Hb Mahidol, G-Taichung, Q-Thailand		43,44
	Asp→Asn	Hb G-Pest		35
	Asp→Gly	Hb Chapel Hill	↑ O_2 affinity	280
75(EF4)	Asp→His	Hb Q-Iran		44
	Asp→Tyr	Hb Winnipeg		45
78(EF7)	Asn→Lys	Hb Stanleyville-II		46
80(F1)	Leu→Arg	Hb Ann Arbor	Unstable	47,48
84(F5)	Ser→Arg	Hb Etobicoke	Unstable	49
85(F6)	Asp→Asn	Hb G-Norfolk	↑ O_2 affinity	50,51
	Asp→Tyr	Hb Atago		52
	Asp→Val	Hb Inkster		53

*Kindly supplied by the Director of the International Hemoglobin Information Center, Augusta, Georgia.

Table continued on following page.

TABLE 6–2. Human Hemoglobin Variants—Continued

ALPHA CHAIN

Residue and Helical Number	*Amino Acid Substitution*	*Name*	*Major Abnormal Property*	*Reference*
87(F8)	His→Tyr	Hb M-Iwate, M-Kankakee, M-Oldenburg	Ferri-Hb; ↓ O_2 affinity	54
90(FG2)	Lys→Asn	Hb J-Broussais, Tagawa-I		55
	Lys→Thr	Hb J-Rajappen		56
92(FG4)	Arg→Gln	Hb J-Cape Town	↑ O_2 affinity	57
	Arg→Leu	Hb Chesapeake	↑ O_2 affinity	58,59
94(G1)	Asp→Tyr	Hb Setif	Unstable	60
	Asp→Asn	Hb Titusville	↓ O_2 affinity	61
95(G2)	Pro→Leu	Hb G-Georgia	↑ Dissociation	62,63
	Pro→Ser	Hb Rampa	↑ Dissociation	63,64
	Pro→Ala	Hb Denmark Hill	↑ O_2 affinity	65
	Pro→Arg	Hb St. Lukes	↑ Dissociation	66
100(G7)	Leu			
102(G9)	Ser→Arg	Hb Manitoba		67
112(G19)	His→Gln	Hb Dakar*	Unstable	68
	His→Asp	Hb Hopkins-2	Unstable; ↑ O_2 affinity	69
	His→Arg	Hb Strumica, Serbia		70,71
114(GH2)	Pro→Arg	Hb Chiapas		30
115(GH3)	Ala→Asp	Hb J-Tongariki		72
116(GH4)	Glu→Lys	Hb O-Indonesia, Buginese-X, Oliviere		73
118(H1)	Thr→Gly	Hb Hopkins-2-II		74
120(H3)	Ala→Glu	Hb J-Meerut (J-Birmingham)		75,76
127(H10)	Lys→Thr	Hb St. Claude		77
136(H19)	Leu→Pro	Hb Bibba	Unstable; ↑ dissociation	78
141(HC3)	Arg→Pro	Hb Singapore		79
	Arg→His	Hb Suresnes	↑ O_2 affinity	281

*Hb Dakar has recently been shown to be identical to Hb Grady rather than having the substitution shown above (see ref. 269).

BETA CHAIN

Residue and Helical Number	*Amino Acid Substitution*	*Name*	*Major Abnormal Property*	*Reference*
2(NA1)	His→Arg	Hb Deer Lodge		80
6(A3)	Glu→Val	Hb S	Sickling	81
	Glu→Lys	Hb C		82
	Glu→Ala	Hb G-Makassar		83
7(A4)	Glu→Gly	Hb G-San Jose		84
	Glu→Lys	Hb C-Siriraj		85
9(A6)	Ser→Cys	Hb Porto Alegre	Polymerization	86
10(A7)	Ala→Asp	Hb Ankara		87
14(A11)	Leu→Arg	Hb Sögn	Unstable	88
	Leu→Pro	Hb Saki	Unstable	89
15(A12)	Trp→Arg	Hb Belfast	Unstable	90
16(A13)	Gly→Asp	Hb J-Baltimore, J-Trinidad, J-Ireland, J-Georgia		91
	Gly→Arg	Hb D-Bushman		92
17(A14)	Lys→Glu	Hb Nagasaki		93
19(B1)	Asn→Lys	Hb D-Ouled Rabah		94
20(B2)	Val→Met	Hb Olympia	↑ O_2 affinity	95
	Val→Asp	Hb Strasbourg	Unstable	285
22(B4)	Glu→Lys	Hb E-Saskatoon		96
	Glu→Gly	Hb G-Taipei		97
	Glu→Ala	Hb G-Saskatoon, Hsin Chu, G-Coushatta, G-Taegu		98,99
	Glu→Gln	Hb D-Iran		100

TABLE 6–2. *Human Hemoglobin Variants*—Continued

BETA CHAIN

Residue and Helical Number	*Amino Acid Substitution*	*Name*	*Major Abnormal Property*	*Reference*
24(B6)	Gly→Arg	Hb Riverdale-Bronx	Unstable	101
	Gly→Val	Hb Savannah	Unstable	102
	Gly→Asp	Hb Moscva	Unstable; ↓ O_2 affinity	103
25(B7)	Gly→Arg	Hb G-Taiwan-Ami		104
26(B8)	Glu→Lys	Hb E		105
	Glu→Val	Hb Henri Mondor	Unstable	286
27(B9)	Ala→Asp	Hb Volga, Drenthe	Unstable	106,107
28(B10)	Leu→Gln	Hb St. Louis	Unstable; ferri-Hb	108
	Leu→Pro	Hb Genova	Unstable; ↑ O_2 affinity	109
30(B12)	Arg→Ser	Hb Tacoma	Unstable; ↓ Bohr; normal O_2 affinity	110
32(B14)	Leu→Pro	Hb Perth, Abraham Lincoln	Unstable	111,112
	Leu→Arg	Hb Castilla	Unstable	113
35(C1)	Tyr→Phe	Hb Philly	Unstable	114
37(C3)	Trp→Ser	Hb Hirose	↑ O_2 affinity	115
39(C5)	Gln→Lys	Hb Alabama		24
40(C6)	Arg→Lys	Hb Athens-Georgia	↑ O_2 affinity	116
41(C7)	Phe→Tyr	Hb Mequon	Unstable	117
42(CD1)	Phe→Ser	Hb Hammersmith, Chiba	Unstable; ↓ O_2 affinity	118
	Phe→Leu	Hb Louisville, Bucuresti	Unstable; ↓ O_2 affinity	119,120
43(CD2)	Glu→Ala	Hb G-Galveston, G-Port Arthur, G-Texas		121
46(CD5)	Gly→Glu	Hb K-Ibadan		122
47(CD6)	Asp→Asn	Hb G-Copenhagen		123
48(CD7)	Leu→Arg	Hb Okaloosa	Unstable; ↓ O_2 affinity	124
50(D1)	Thr→Lys	Hb Edmonton		125
51(D2)	Pro→Arg	Hb Willamette	Unstable; ↑ O_2 affinity	270
52(D3)	Asp→Asn	Hb Osu-Christiansborg		126
	Asp→Ala	Hb Ocho-Rios		127
56(D7)	Gly→Asp	Hb J-Bangkok, J-Meinung, J-Korat, J-Manado		58
	Gly→Arg	Hb Hamadan		128
57(E1)	Asn→Lys	Hb G-Ferrara		129
58(E2)	Pro→Arg	Hb Yukuhashi, Dhofar		130,131
59(E3)	Lys→Glu	Hb I-High Wycombe		132
	Lys→Thr	Hb J-Kaohsiung, J-Honolulu		133
61(E5)	Lys→Glu	Hb N-Seattle		134
	Lys→Asn	Hb Hikari		135
62(E6)	Ala→Pro	Hb Duarte	Unstable; ↑ O_2 affinity	136
63(E7)	His→Arg	Hb Zürich	Unstable; ↑ O_2 affinity	137
	His→Tyr	Hb M-Saskatoon, M-Emory, M-Kurumi, M-Hida, M-Radom, M-Arhus, M-Chicago, Leipzig, Hörlein-Weber, Novi Sad, M-Erlangen	Ferri-Hb; ↑ O_2 affinity	33
	His→Pro	Hb Bicetre	Unstable; ferri-Hb	282
64(E8)	Gly→Asp	Hb J-Calabria, J-Bari, J-Cosenza	Unstable	138
65(E9)	Lys→Asn	Hb Sicilia		139
	Lys→Gln	Hb J-Cairo		271
66(E10)	Lys→Glu	Hb I-Toulouse	Unstable; ferri-Hb	140
67(E11)	Val→Asp	Hb Bristol	Unstable	141
	Val→Glu	Hb M-Milwaukee-I	Ferri-Hb; ↓ O_2 affinity	33
	Val→Ala	Hb Sydney	Unstable	142
69(E13)	Gly→Asp	Hb J-Cambridge, J-Rambam		123
70(E14)	Ala→Asp	Hb Seattle	↓ O_2 affinity	143
71(E15)	Phe→Ser	Hb Christchurch	Unstable	144
73(E17)	Asp→Asn	Hb Korle-Bu, G-Accra		145,146
	Asp→Val	Hb Mobile		147
74(E18)	Gly→Val	Hb Bushwick		148
	Gly→Asp	Hb Shepherds Bush	Unstable; ↑ O_2 affinity	149
75(E19)	Leu→Pro	Hb Atlanta	Unstable	150
76(E20)	Ala→Asp	Hb J-Chicago		151
77(EF1)	His→Asp	Hb J-Iran		152

Table continued on following page.

TABLE 6–2. *Human Hemoglobin Variants*—Continued

Residue and Helical Number	*Amino Acid Substitution*	BETA CHAIN *Name*	*Major Abnormal Property*	*Reference*
79(EF3)	Asp→Gly	Hb G-Hsi-Tsou	↑ O_2 affinity	153,154
80(EF4)	Asn→Lys	Hb G-Szuhu, Gifu	↑ O_2 affinity	154
81(EF5)	Leu→Arg	Hb Baylor	Unstable; ↑ O_2 affinity	272
82(EF6)	Lys→Asn (Asp)	Hb Providence	↓ O_2 affinity	155,156
	Lys→Thr	Hb Rahere	↑ O_2 affinity	157
	Lys→Met	Hb Helsinki	↑ O_2 affinity	287
83(EF7)	Gly→Cys	Hb Ta-Li		158
	Gly→Asp	Hb Pyrgos		159
85(F1)	Phe→Ser	Hb Bryn Mawr, Buenos Aires	Unstable; ↑ O_2 affinity	160,161
87(F3)	Thr→Lys	Hb D-Ibadan		162
88(F4)	Leu→Arg	Hb Boräs	Unstable	163
	Leu→Pro	Hb Santa Ana	Unstable	164
89(F5)	Ser→Asn	Hb Creteil	↑ O_2 affinity	165
90(F6)	Glu→Lys	Hb Agenogi	↓ O_2 affinity	166
91(F7)	Leu→Pro	Hb Sabine	Unstable	167
	Leu→Arg	Hb Caribbean	Unstable; ↓ O_2 affinity	283
92(F8)	His→Tyr	Hb M-Hyde Park, M-Akita	Normal O_2; ferri-Hb	168
	His→Gln	Hb Istanbul, Hb-St. Etienne	Unstable; ↑ O_2 affinity; ↑ dissociation	169,170
	His→Asp	Hb J-Altgeld Gardens	Normal O_2 affinity	171
	His→Pro	Hb Newcastle		172
95(FG2)	Lys→Glu	Hb N-Baltimore, Hopkins-I, Jenkins, N-Memphis, Kenwood		173
97(FG4)	His→Gln	Hb Malmö	↑ O_2 affinity	174
	His→Leu	Hb Wood	↑ O_2 affinity	175
98(FG5)	Val→Met	Hb Köln, San Francisco (Pacific), Ube-I	Unstable; ↑ O_2 affinity	176
	Val→Gly	Hb Nottingham	Unstable; ↑ O_2 affinity	177
	Val→Ala	Hb Djelfa	Unstable	178
99(G1)	Asp→Asn	Hb Kempsey	↑ O_2 affinity	179
	Asp→His	Hb Yakima	↑ O_2 affinity	180
	Asp→Tyr	Hb Ypsilanti (Ypsi)	↑ O_2 affinity	181
100(G2)	Pro→Leu	Hb Brigham	↑ O_2 affinity	182
101(G3)	Glu→Gln	Hb Rush	Unstable	183
	Glu→Lys	Hb British Columbia	↑ O_2 affinity	273
	Glu→Gly	Hb Alberta	↑ O_2 affinity	274
102(G4)	Asn→Lys	Hb Richmond	Asymmetrical hybrids	184
	Asn→Thr	Hb Kansas	↓ O_2 affinity; ↑ dissociation	185
	Asn→Ser	Hb Beth Israel	↓ O_2 affinity	186
103(G5)	Phe→Leu	Hb Heathrow	↑ O_2 affinity	187
104(G6)	Arg→Ser	Hb Camperdown	Slightly unstable	188
106(G8)	Leu→Pro	Hb Casper	↑ O_2 affinity	189
	Leu→Pro	Hb Southampton		190
	Leu→Gln	Hb Tübingen		191
107(G9)	Gly→Arg	Hb Burke	Unstable; ↓ O_2 affinity	284
108(G10)	Asn→Asp	Hb Yoshizuka	↓ O_2 affinity	192
109(G11)	Val→Met	Hb San Diego	↑ O_2 affinity	193
111(G13)	Val→Phe	Hb Peterborough	Unstable; ↓ O_2 affinity	194
113(G15)	Val→Glu	Hb New York		195
115(G17)	Ala→Pro	Hb Madrid	Unstable	196
117(G19)	His→Arg	Hb P-Galveston		197
119(GH2)	Gly→Asp	Hb Fannin-Lubbock	Unstable	288, 289
120(GH3)	Lys→Glu	Hb Hijiyama		198
	Lys→Asn	Hb Riyadh		275
121(GH4)	Glu→Gln	Hb D, D-Chicago, D-Punjab, D-North Carolina, D-Los Angeles, D-Portugal, Oak Ridge	↑ O_2 affinity	199
	Glu→Lys	Hb O-Arab, Egypt		73
	Glu→Val	Hb Beograd		200
124(H2)	Pro→Arg	Hb Khartoum	Unstable	79
126(H4)	Val→Glu	Hb Hofu		201
127(H5)	Gln→Glu	Hb Hacettepe		202

TABLE 6–2. *Human Hemoglobin Variants*—Continued

BETA CHAIN

Residue and Helical Number	Amino Acid Substitution	Name	Major Abnormal Property	Reference
129(H7)	Ala→Asp	Hb J-Taichung		203
	Ala→Glu or Asp	Hb K-Cameroon		122
130(H8)	Tyr→Asp	Hb Wien	Unstable	204
131(H9)	Gln→Glu	Hb Camden, Tokuchi		205,206
132(H10)	Lys→Gln	Hb K-Woolwich		122
135(H13)	Ala→Pro	Hb Altdorf	Unstable	276
136(H14)	Gly→Asp	Hb Hope	Unstable	207
141(H19)	Leu→Arg	Hb Olmsted		174
143(H21)	His→Arg	Hb Abruzzo	↑ O_2 affinity	208
	His→Gln	Hb Little Rock	↑ O_2 affinity	209
	His→Pro	Hb Syracuse	↑ O_2 affinity	210
144(HC1)	Lys→Asn	Hb Andrew-Minneapolis	↑ O_2 affinity	211
145(HC2)	Tyr→His	Hb Bethesda	↑ O_2 affinity	212
	Tyr→Cys	Hb Rainier	↑ O_2 affinity; alkali resistant	212
	Tyr→Asp	Hb Fort Gordon, Osler, Nancy	↑ O_2 affinity	213,214
	Tyr→Term	Hb McKees Rocks	↑ ↑ O_2 affinity	215
146(HC3)	His→Asp	Hb Hiroshima	↑ O_2 affinity	216
	His→Pro	Hb York	↑ O_2 affinity	217
	His→Arg	Hb Cochin, Port Royal		218

DELTA CHAIN

Residue and Helical Number	Amino Acid Substitution	Name	Reference
2(NA2)	His→Arg	Hb A_2-Sphakiá	219
12(A9)	Asn→Lys	Hb A_2-NYU	220
16(A13)	Gly→Arg	Hb $A_2'(B_2)$	221
20(B2)	Val→Glu	Hb A_2-Roosevelt	277
22(B4)	Ala→Glu	Hb A_2-Flatbush	222
43(CD2)	Glu→Lys	Hb A_2-Melbourne	223
69(E13)	Gly→Arg	Hb A_2-Indonesia	224
116(G18)	Arg→His	Hb A_2-Coburg	225
136(H14)	Gly→Asp	Hb A_2-Babinga	226

GAMMA CHAIN

Residue and Helical Number	Amino Acid Substitution	Name	Reference
1(NA1)	Gly→Cys (136 Gly)	Hb F-Malaysia	227
5(A2)	Glu→Lys (136 Ala)	Hb F-Texas-I	228,229
6(A3)	Glu→Lys	Hb F-Texas-II	230
7(A4)	Asp→Asn	Hb F-Auckland	231
12(A9)	Thr→Lys	Hb F-Alexandra	232
22(B4)	Asp→Gly (136 Ala)	Hb F-Kuala Lumpur	233
61(E5)	Lys→Glu (136 Ala)	Hb F-Jamaica	234
75(E19)	Ile→Thr	Hb F-Sardinia	235
80(EF4)	Asp→Tyr (136 Ala)	Hb F-Victoria Jubilee	236
97(FG4)	His→Arg	Hb F-Dickinson	237
117(G19)	His→Arg (136 Gly)	Hb F-Malta-I	238
121(GH4)	Glu→Lys (136 Ala)	Hb F-Hull	239
125(H3)	Gly→Ala	Hb F-Port Royal	240
130(H8)	Trp→Gly (136 Gly)	Hb F-Poole	241

Table continued on following page.

TABLE 6–2. *Human Hemoglobin Variants*—Continued

FUSION HEMOGLOBINS

	A6	A9	B4	D1	F2	F3	G18	G19	H2	H4	*Reference*
	9	12	22	50	86	87	116	117	124	126	
δ Chain →→→→→→→→→→	Thr	Asn	Ala	Ser	Ser	Gln	Arg	Asn	Gln	Met	
β Chain →→→→→→→→→→	Ser	Thr	Glu	Thr	Ala	Thr	His	His	Pro	Val	
Lepore-Hollandia			δ	β							242
Lepore-Baltimore				δ	β						243
Lepore-Washington-Boston						δ	β				244
Miyada		β	δ								130
P-Congo			β				δ				245
P-Nilotic			β	δ							246

	NA1	EF4	EF5	F2	F3	HC3	
	1	80	81	86	87	146	
γ Chain →→→→→→→→→→	Gly	Asp	Leu	Ala	Gln	His	
β Chain →→→→→→→→→→	Val	Asn	Leu	Ala	Thr	His	
Kenya			γ	β			247

DELETED RESIDUES

Residue Number	*Amino Acid Substitution*	*Name*	*Major Abnormal Property*	*Reference*
β6 or 7	Glu→0	Hb Leiden	Unstable; slightly ↑ O_2 affinity	255
β17-18	(Lys-Val)→0	Hb Lyon	↑ O_2 affinity	256
β23	Val→0	Hb Freiburg	↑ O_2 affinity	257
β42-44 or 43-45	(Phe-Glu-Ser)→0 or (Glu-Ser-Phe)→0	Hb Niteroi	↓ O_2 affinity; unstable	258
β56-59	(Gly-Asn-Pro-Lys)→0	Hb Tochigi	Unstable; not known	259
β74-75	(Gly-Leu)→0	Hb St. Antoine	Unstable; normal O_2 affinity	260
β87	Thr→0	Hb Tours	↑ O_2 affinity; unstable	260
β91-95	(Leu-His-Cys-Asp-Lys)→0	Hb Gun Hill	Unstable; ↑ O_2 affinity	261
β131	Gln→0	Hb Leslie, Deaconess	Unstable; normal O_2 affinity	262,263
β141	Leu→0	Hb Coventry	Unstable	278
β145-146	(Tyr-His)→0	Hb McKees Rock	↑ O_2 affinity	279

MORE THAN ONE POINT MUTATION IN THE SAME POLYPEPTIDE CHAIN

Residue and Helical Number	*Amino Acid Substitution*	*Name*	*Major Abnormal Property*	*Reference*
β6(A3)	Glu→Val, 73 Asp→Asn	Hb C-Harlem, G-Georgetown	Normal O_2 affinity	264
	Glu→Lys, 95 Lys→Glu	Hb Arlington Park	Not done	265
α78(EF7)	Asn→Asp 79 Ala→Gly	Hb J-Singapore	Not done	266
β6(A3)	Glu→Val 58 Pro→Arg	Hb C-Ziguinchor		267

TABLE 6–2. *Human Hemoglobin Variants* – Continued

	Extended Chains Residue	Name	Major Abnormal Property	Reference
α141	140 (31 additional residues) Tyr-Arg-Gln-Ala-Gly-Ala-Ser- 150 Val-Ala-Val-Pro-Pro-Ala-Arg-Trp-Ala-Ser-Gln-Arg-Ala- 160 170 Leu-Leu-Pro(His,Ser,Leu)-Arg-Pro-Phe-Leu-Val-Phe-Glu	Hb Constant Spring		248
α141	31 additional residues – identical to Hb Constant Spring except for residue 142, which is lysine instead of glutamine	Hb Icaria		249
α141	Probably 31 additional residues – identical to Hb Constant Spring except for residue 142, which is serine instead of glutamine	Hb Koya Dora		250
α139–141	140 Thr-Ser-Asn-Thr-Val-Lys-Leu-Glu-Pro-Arg (Frame shift)	Hb Wayne		251
β145	144 Lys-Ser-Ile-Thr-Lys-Leu-Ala-Phe-Leu-Leu-Ser-Asn-Phe- 157 Tyr-COOH (Frame shift)	Hb Cranston	Unstable; ↑ O_2 affinity	252
β147	144 Lys-Tyr-His-Thr-Lys-Leu-Ala-Phe-Leu-Leu-Ser-Asn-Phe- 157 Tyr-COOH (Frame shift)	Hb Tak	↑ O_2 affinity	253
α115–118	115 116 117 118 119 Ala-Glu-Phe-Thr-*Glu-Phe-Thr*-Pro (Insertion)	Hb Grady	Normal	254

REFERENCES FOR TABLE 6–2

1. Crookston, J. H., Beale, D., Irvine, D., and Lehmann, H.: Nature (London) *208*:1059, 1965.
2. Sumida, I., Ohta, Y., Imamura, T., and Yanase, T.: Biochim. Biophys. Acta *322*:23, 1973.
3. Pootrakul, S., Kematorn, B., Na-Nakorn, S., and Suanpan, S.: Biochim. Biophys. Acta *405*:161, 1975.
4. Rosa, J., Maleknia, N., Vergoz, D., and Dunet, R.: Nouv. Rev. Fr. Hematol. *6*:423, 1965.
5. Marti, H. R., Pik, C., and Mosimann, P.: Acta Haematol. *32*:9, 1964.
6. Liddell, J., Brown, D., Beale, D., Lehmann, H., and Huntsman, R. G.: Nature (London) *204*:269, 1964.
7. Vella, F., Casey, R., Lehmann, H., Labossiere, A., and Jones, T. G.: Biochim. Biophys. Acta *336*:25, 1974.
8. Pootrakul, S., Srichiyanont, S., Wasi, P., and Suanpan, S.: Humangenetik *23*:199, 1974.
9. Beale, D., and Lehmann, H.: Nature (London) *207*:259, 1965.
10. Kendall, A. G., Barr, R. D., Lang, A., and Lehmann, H.: Biochim. Biophys. Acta *310*:357, 1973.
11. Gottlieb, A. J., Restrepo, A., and Itano, H. A.: Fed. Proc. *23*:172, 1964.
12. Kraus, A. P., Miyaji, T., Iuchi, I., and Kraus, L. M.: J. Lab. Clin. Med. *66*:886, 1965.
13. Boyer, S. H., Crosby, E. F., Fuller, G. F., Ulenurm, L., and Buck, A. A.: Am. J. Hum. Genet. *20*:570, 1968.
14. Marengo-Rowe, A. J., Beale, D., and Lehmann, H.: Nature (London) *219*:1164, 1968.
15. Schneider, R. G., Brimhall, B., Jones, R. T., Bryant, R., Mitchell, C. B., and Goldberg, A. I.: Biochim. Biophys. Acta *243*:164, 1971.
16. Vettore, L., DeSandre, G., Dilorio, E. E., Winterhalter, K. H., Lang, A., and Lehmann, H.: Blood *44*:869, 1974.
17. Swenson, R. T., Hill, R. L., Lehmann, H., and Jim, R. T. S.: J. Biol. Chem. *237*:1517, 1962.
18. Beretta, A., Prato, V., Gallo, E., and Lehmann, H.: Nature (London) *217*:1016, 1968.
19. Ohba, Y., Miyaji, T., Matsuoka, M., Yokoyama, M., Numakura, H., Nagata, K., Takebe, Y., Izumi, Y., and Shibata, S.: Biochim. Biophys. Acta *405*:155, 1975.
20. Bianco, J., Modiano, G., Bottini, E., and Lucci, R.: Nature (London) *198*:395, 1963.
21. Halbrecht, I., Isaacs, W. A., Lehmann, H., and Ben-Porat, F.: Isr. J. Med. Sci. *3*:827, 1967.
22. Ostertag, W., and Smith, E. W.: Humangenetik *6*:377, 1968.
23. Rahbar, S., Mahdavi, N., Nowzari, G., and Mostafavi, I.: Biochim. Biophys. Acta *386*:525, 1975.
24. Brimhall, B., Jones, R. T., Schneider, R. G., Hosty, T. S., Tomlin, G., and Atkins, R.: Biochim. Biophys. Acta *379*:28, 1975.
25. Tangheroni, W., Zorcolo, G., Gallo, E., and Lehmann, H.: Nature (London) *218*:470, 1968.
26. Cabannes, R., Renaud, R., Mauran, A., Pennors, H., Charlesworth, D., Price, B. G., and Lehmann, H.: Nouv. Rev. Fr. Hematol. *12*:289, 1972.
27. Reynolds, C. A., and Huisman, T. H. J.: Biochim. Biophys. Acta *130*:541, 1966.
28. Alberti, R., Mariuzzi, G. M., Artibani, L., Bruni, E., and Tentori, L.: Biochim. Biophys. Acta *342*:1, 1974.
29. Miyaji, T., Iuchi, I., Takeda, I., and Shibata, S.: Acta Haematol. Jap. *26*:531, 1963.
30. Jones, R. T., Brimhall, B., and Lisker, R.: Biochim. Biophys. Acta *154*:488, 1968.
31. Rahbar, S., Kinderlerer, J. L., and Lehmann, H.: Acta Haematol. *42*:169, 1969.
32. Baglioni, C.: J. Biol. Chem. *237*:69, 1962.
33. Gerald, P. S., and Efron, M. L.: Proc. Nat. Acad. Sci. (Wash.) *47*:1758, 1961.
34. Barclay, G. P. T., Charlesworth, D., and Lehmann, H.: Brit. Med. J. *4*:595, 1969.
35. Brimhall, B., Duerst, M., Hollán, S. R., Stenzel, P., Szelényi, J., and Jones, R. T.: Biochim. Biophys. Acta *336*:344, 1974.
36. Blackwell, R. Q., Jim, R. T. S., Tan, T. G. H., Weng, M.-I., Liu, C.-S., and Wang, C. L.: Biochim. Biophys. Acta *322*:27, 1973.

37. Ramot, B., Kinderlerer, J. B., and Lehmann, H.: Cited in WHO Technical Report Series No. 509, Annex 1, Geneva, 1972.
38. Sukumaran, P. K., Merchant, S. M., Desai, M. P., Wiltshire, B. G., and Lehmann, H.: J. Med. Genet. 9:436, 1972.
39. Miyaji, T., Iuchi, I., Yamamoto, K., Ohba, Y., and Shibata, S.: Clin. Chim. Acta *16*:347, 1967.
40. Baglioni, C., and Ingram, V. M.: Biochim. Biophys. Acta *48*:253, 1961.
41. Colombo, B., Vidal, H., Kamuzora, H., and Lehmann, H.: Biochim. Biophys. Acta *351*:1, 1974.
42. Rahbar, S., Nowzari, G., and Daneshmand, P.: Nature [New Biol.] *245*:268, 1973.
43. Pootrakul, S., and Dixon, G. H.: Canad. J. Biochem. *48*:1066, 1970.
44. Lorkin, P. A., Charlesworth, D., Lehmann, H., Rahbar, S., Tuchinda, S., and Lie-Injo, L. E.: Brit. J. Haematol. *19*:117, 1970.
45. Vella, F., Wiltshire, B. G., Lehmann, H., and Galbraith, P.: Clin. Biochem. *6*:66, 1973.
46. Van Ros, G., Beale, D., and Lehmann, H.: Brit. Med. J. *4*:92, 1968.
47. Rucknagel, D. L., Brandt, N. J., and Spencer, H. H.: Proc. First Inter-American Symp. Hemoglobins, Caracas, 1969.
48. Adams, J. G., III, Winter, W. P., Rucknagel, D. L., and Spencer, H. H.: Science *176*:1427, 1972.
49. Crookston, J. H., Farquharson, H. A., Beale, D., and Lehmann, H.: Canad. J. Biochem. *47*:143, 1969.
50. Lorkin, P. A., Huntsman, R. G., Ager, J. A. M., Lehmann, H., Vella, F., and Darbre, P. D.: Biochim. Biophys. Acta *379*:22, 1975.
51. Cohen-Solal, M., Manesse, B., Thillet, J., and Rosa, J.: FEBS Lett. *50*:163, 1975.
52. Fujiwara, N., Maekawa, T., and Matsuda, G.: Int. J. Pept. Protein Res. *3*:35, 1971.
53. Reed, R. E., Winter, W. P., and Rucknagel, D. L.: Brit. J. Haematol. *26*:475, 1974.
54. Miyaji, T., Iuchi, I., Shibata, S., Takeda, I., and Tamura, A.: Acta Haematol. Jap. *26*:538, 1963.
55. DeTraverse, P. M., Lehmann, H., DeCoquelet, M. L., and Isaacs, W. A.: Compt. R. Scéanc. Soc. Biol. *160*:2270, 1966.
56. Hyde, R. D., Kinderlerer, J. L., Lehmann, H., and Hall, M. D.: Biochim. Biophys. Acta *243*:515, 1971.
57. Botha, M. C., Beale, D., Isaacs, W. A., and Lehmann, H.: Nature (London) *212*:792, 1966.
58. Clegg, J. B., Naughton, M. A., and Weatherall, D. J.: J. Mol. Biol. *19*:91, 1966.
59. Charache, S., Weatherall, D. J., and Clegg, J. B.: J. Clin. Invest. *45*:813, 1966.
60. Wajcman, H., Belkhodja, O., and Labie, D.: FEBS Lett. *27*:298, 1972.
61. Schneider, R. G., Atkins, R. J., Hosty, T. S., Tomlin, G., Casey, R., Lehmann, H., Lorkin, P. A., and Nagai, K.: Biochim. Biophys. Acta *400*:365, 1975.
62. Huisman, T. H. J., Adams, H. R., Wilson, J. B., Efremov, G. D., Reynolds, C. A., and Wrightstone, R. N.: Biochim. Biophys. Acta *200*:578, 1970.
63. Smith, L. L., Plese, C. L., Barton, B. P., Charache, S., Wilson, J. B., and Huisman, T. H. J.: J. Biol. Chem. *247*:1433, 1972.
64. DeJong, W. W. W., Bernini, L. F., and Khan, P. M.: Biochim. Biophys. Acta *236*:197, 1971.
65. Wiltshire, B. G., Clark, K. G. A., Lorkin, P. A., and Lehmann, H.: Biochim. Biophys. Acta *278*:459, 1972.
66. Bannister, W. H., Grech, J. L., Plese, C. F., Smith, L. L., Barton, B. P., Wilson, J. B., Reynolds, C. A., and Huisman, T. H. J.: Eur. J. Biochem. *29*:301, 1972.
67. Crookston, J. H. Farquharson, H., Kinderlerer, J., and Lehmann, H.: Canad. J. Biochem. *48*:911, 1970.
68. Rosa, J., Oudart, J. L., Pagnier, J., Belkhodja, O., Boigne, J. M., and Labie, D.: 12th Congress Internat. Soc. Haemat., New York, 1968, Abstracts, p. 72.
69. Charache, S., and Ostertag, W.: Blood *36*:852, 1970.
70. Niazi, G. A., Efremov, G. D., Nikolov, N., Hunter, E., Jr., and Huisman, T. H. J.: Biochim. Biophys. Acta *412*:181, 1975.
71. Beksedic, D., Rajevska, T., Lorkin, P. A., and Lehmann, H.: FEBS Letters *58*:226, 1975.
72. Gajdusek, D. C., Guiart, J., Kirk, R. L., Carrell, R. W., Irvine, D., Kyn-

och, P. A. M., and Lehmann, H.: J. Med. Genet. *4*:1, 1967.
73. Baglioni, C., and Lehmann, H.: Nature (London) *196*:229, 1962.
74. Ostertag, W., von Ehrenstein, G., and Charache, S.: Nature [New Biol.] *237*:90, 1972.
75. Blackwell, R. Q., Wong, H. B., Wang, C.-L., Weng, M.-L., and Liu, C.-S.: Biochim. Biophys. Acta *351*:7, 1974.
76. Kamuzora, H., Lehmann, H., Griffiths, K. D., Mann, J. R., and Raine, D. N.: Ann. Clin. Biochem. *11*:53, 1974.
77. Vella, F., Galbraith, P., Wilson, J. B., Wong, S. C., Folger, G. C., and Huisman, T. H. J.: Biochim. Biophys. Acta *365*:318, 1974.
78. Kleihauer, E. F., Reynolds, C. A., Dozy, A. M., Wilson, J. B., Moores, R. R., Berenson, M. P., Wright, C.-S., and Huisman, T. H. J.: Biochim. Biophys. Acta *154*:220, 1968.
79. Clegg, J. B., Weatherall, D. J., Wong, H. B., and Mustafa, D.: Nature (London) *222*:379, 1969.
80. Labossiere, A., Vella, F., Hiebert, J., and Galbraith, P.: Clin. Biochem. *5*:46, 1972.
81. Ingram, V. M.: Biochim. Biophys. Acta *36*:402, 1959.
82. Hunt, J. A., and Ingram, V. M.: Biochim. Biophys. Acta *42*:409, 1960.
83. Blackwell, R. Q., Oemijati, S., Pribadi, W., Weng, M.-I., and Liu, C.-S.: Biochim. Biophys. Acta *214*:396, 1970.
84. Hill, R. I., Swenson, R. T., and Schwartz, H. C.: J. Biol. Chem. *235*:3182, 1960.
85. Tuchinda, S., Beale, D., and Lehmann, H.: Brit. Med. J. *1*:1583, 1965.
86. Bonaventura, J., and Riggs, A.: Science *158*:800, 1967.
87. Arcasoy, A., Casey, R., Lehmann, H., Cavdar, A. O., and Berki, A.: FEBS Lett. *42*:121, 1974.
88. Monn, E., Gaffney, P. J., and Lehmann, H.: Scand. J. Haematol. *5*:353, 1968.
89. Beuzard, Y., Basset, P., Braconnier, F., Gammal, H. E., Martin, L., Oudard, J. L., and Thillet, J.: Biochim. Biophys. Acta *393*:182, 1975.
90. Kennedy, C. C., Blundell, G., Lorkin, P. A., Lang, A., and Lehmann, H.: Brit. Med. J. *4*:324, 1974.
91. Baglioni, C., and Weatherall, D. J.: Biochim. Biophys. Acta *78*:637, 1963.
92. Wade, P. T., Jenkins, T., and Huehns, E. R.: Nature (London) *216*:688, 1967.
93. Maekawa, M., Maekawa, T., Fujiwara, N., Tabara, K., and Matsuda, G.: Int. J. Pept. Protein Res. *II*: 147, 1970.
94. Elion, J., Belkhodja, O., Wajcman, H., and Labie, D.: Biochim. Biophys. Acta *310*:360, 1973.
95. Stamatoyannopoulos, G., Nute, P. E., Adamson, J. W., Bellingham, A. J., Funk, D., and Hornung, S.: J. Clin. Invest. *52*:342, 1973.
96. Vella, F., Lorkin, P. A., Carrell, R. W., and Lehmann, H.: Canad. J. Biochem. *45*:1385, 1967.
97. Blackwell, R. Q., Yang, H. J., and Wang, C. C.: Biochim. Biophys. Acta *175*:237, 1969.
98. Vella, F., Isaacs, W. A., and Lehmann, H.: Canad. J. Biochem. *45*:351, 1967.
99. Bowman, B. H., Barnett, D. R., and Hite, R.: Biochim. Biophys. Acta *26*:466, 1967.
100. Rahbar, S.: Brit. J. Haematol. *24*:31, 1973.
101. Ranney, H. M., Jacobs, A. S., Udem, L., and Zalusky, R.: Biochim. Biophys. Acta *33*:1004, 1968.
102. Huisman, T. H. J., Brown, A. K., Efremov, G. D., Wilson, J. B., Reynolds, C. A., Uy, R., and Smith, L. L.: J. Clin. Invest. *50*:650, 1971.
103. Idelson, L. I., Didkovskii, N. A., Casey, R., Lorkin, P. A., and Lehmann, H.: Nature (London) *249*:768, 1974.
104. Blackwell, R. Q., and Liu, C.-S.: Biochem. Biophys. Res. Commun. *30*:690, 1968.
105. Hunt, J. A., and Ingram, V. N.: Biochim. Biophys. Acta *49*:520, 1961.
106. Idelson, L. I., Didkovskiĭ, N. A., Filippova, A. V., Casey, R., Kynoch, P. A. M., and Lehmann, H.: FEBS Lett. *58*:122, 1975.
107. Kuis-Reerink, J. D., Jonxis, J. H. P., Niazi, G. A., Wilson, J. B., Bolch, K. C., Gravely, M., and Huisman, T. H. J.: Biochim. Biophys. Acta. *439*:63, 1976.
108. Cohen-Solal, M., Seligmann, M., Thillet, J., and Rosa, J.: Abstract 408, 14th Int. Congress of Hematology, Sao Paulo, Brazil, 1972. FEBS Lett. *33*:37, 1973.

109. Sansone, G., Carrell, R. W., and Lehmann, H.: Nature (London) *214*:877, 1967.
110. Brimhall, B., Jones, R. T., Baur, E. W., and Motulsky, A. G.: Biochemistry *8*:2125, 1969.
111. Jackson, J. M., Yates, A., and Huehns, E. R.: Brit. J. Haematol. *25*:607, 1973.
112. Honig, G. R., Green, D., Shamsuddin, M., Vida, L. N., Mason, R. G., Gnarra, D. J., and Maurer, H. S.: J. Clin. Invest. *52*:1746, 1973.
113. Garel, M. C., Blouquit, Y., and Rosa, J.: FEBS Lett. *58*:145, 1975.
114. Rieder, R. F., Oski, F. A., and Clegg, J. B.: J. Clin. Invest. *48*:1627, 1969.
115. Yamaoka, K.: Blood *38*:730, 1971.
116. Brown, W. J., Niazi, G. A., Jayakalshmi, M., Abraham, E. C., and Huisman, T. H. J.: Biochim. Biophys. Acta. *437*:70, 1976.
117. Burkert, L. B., Sharma, V. S., Piscotta, A. V., Ranney, H., and Bruckheimer, P.: Blood *48*:645, 1976.
118. Dacie, J. V., Shinton, N. K., Gaffney, P. J., Jr., Carrell, R. W., and Lehmann, H.: Nature (London) *216*:663, 1967.
119. Keeling, M. M., Ogden, L. L., Wrightstone, R. N., Wilson, J. B., Reynolds, C. A., Kitchens, J. L., and Huisman, T. H. J.: J. Clin. Invest. *50*:2395, 1971.
120. Bratu, V., Lorkin, P. A., Lehmann, H., and Predescu, C.: Biochim. Biophys. Acta *251*:1, 1971.
121. Bowman, B. H., Oliver, C. P., Barnett, D. R., Cunningham, J. R., and Schneider, R. G.: Blood *23*:193, 1964.
122. Allan, N., Beale, D., Irvine, D., and Lehmann, H.: Nature (London) *208*:658, 1965.
123. Sick, K., Beale, D., Irvine, D., Lehmann, H., Goodall, P. T., and MacDougall, S.: Biochim. Biophys. Acta *140*:231, 1967.
124. Charache, S., Brimhall, B., Milner, P., and Cobb, L.: J. Clin. Invest. *52*:2858, 1973.
125. Labossiere, A., Hill, J. R., and Vella, F.: Clin. Biochem. *4*:114, 1971.
126. Konotey-Ahula, F. I. D., Kinderlerer, J. L., Lehmann, H., and Ringelhann, B.: J. Med. Genet. *8*:302, 1971.
127. Beresford, C. H., Clegg, J. B., and Weatherall, D. J.: J. Med. Genet. *9*:151, 1972.
128. Rabhar, S., Nowzari, G., Haydari, H., and Daneshmand, P.: Biochim. Biophys. Acta *379*:645, 1975.
129. Tentori, L., Bruni, E., and Marinucci, M.: Int. Istanbul Symposium on Abnormal Hemoglobins and Thalassemia. M. Aksoy, Ed. Ankara.
130. Yanase, T., Hanada, M., Seita, M., Obya, I., Ohta, Y., Imamura, T., Fijimura, T., Kawasaki, K., and Yamaoka, K.: Jap. J. Hum. Genet. *13*:40, 1968.
131. Marengo-Rowe, A. J., Lorkin, P. A., Gallo, E., and Lehmann, H.: Biochim. Biophys. Acta *168*:58, 1968.
132. Boulton, F. E., Huntsman, R. G., Lehmann, H., Lorkin, P., and Romero Herrera, A.: Brit. J. Haematol. *20*:671, 1971.
133. Blackwell, R. Q., Liu, C.-S., and Shih, T.-B.: Biochim. Biophys. Acta *229*:343, 1971.
134. Jones, R. T., Brimhall, B., Huehns, E. R., and Motulsky, A. G.: Biochim. Biophys. Acta *154*:278, 1968.
135. Shibata, S., Miyaji, T., Iuchi, I., Ueda, S., and Takeda, I.: Clin. Chim. Acta *10*:101, 1964.
136. Beutler, E., Lang, A., and Lehmann, H.: Blood *43*:527, 1974.
137. Muller, C. J., and Kingma, S.: Biochim. Biophys. Acta *50*:595, 1961.
138. Tentori, L.: Int. Symp. Abnormal Hemoglobins and Thalassemia. Istanbul, Turkey, Abstracts 68, 1974.
139. Ricco, G., Pich, P. G., Massa, U., Rossi, G., Ajmar, F., Arese, P., and Gallo, E.: FEBS Lett. *39*:200, 1974.
140. Rosa, L., Labie, D., Wajcman, H., Boigne, J. M., Cabannes, R., Bierme, R., and Ruffie, J.: Nature (London) *223*:190, 1969.
141. Steadman, J. H., Yates, A., and Huehns, E. R.: Brit. J. Haematol. *18*:435, 1970.
142. Carrell, R. W., Lehmann, H., Lorkin, P. A., Raik, E., and Hunter, E.: Nature (London) *215*:626, 1967.
143. Kurachi, S., Hermodson, M., Hornung, S., and Stamatoyannopoulos, G.: Nature [New Biol.] *243*:275, 1973.
144. Carrell, R. W., and Owen, M. C.: Biochim. Biophys. Acta *236*:507, 1971.
145. Konotey-Ahulu, F. I. D., Gallo, E., Lehmann, H., and Ringelhann, B.: J. Med. Genet. *5*:107, 1968.

146. Boi-Doku, F. S., Kinderlerer, J., and Lehmann, H.: Atlas of Protein Sequence and Structure, May, 1972, Vol. 5.
147. Schneider, R. G., Hosty, T. S., Tomlin, G., Atkins, R., Brimhall, B., and Jones, R. T.: Biochem. Genet. *13*:411, 1975.
148. Rieder, R. F., Wolf, D. J., Clegg, J. B., and Lee, S. L.: Nature (London) *254*:725, 1975.
149. White, J. M., Brain, M. C., Lorkin, P. A., Lehmann, H., and Smith, M.: Nature (London) *225*:939, 1970.
150. Hubbard, M., Winton, E., Lindeman, J. G., Dessauer, P. L., Wilson, J. B., Wrightstone, R. N., and Huisman, T. H. J.: Biochim. Biophys. Acta *386*:538, 1975.
151. Romain, P. L., Schwartz, A. D., Shamsuddin, M., Adams, J. G., III, Mason, R. G., Vida, L. N., and Honig, G. R.: Blood *45*:387, 1975.
152. Rahbar, S., Beale, D., Isaacs, W. A., and Lehmann, H.: Brit. Med. J. *1*:674, 1967.
153. Blackwell, R. Q., Shih, T.-B., Wang, C.-L., and Liu, C.-S.: Biochim. Biophys. Acta *257*:49, 1972.
154. Blackwell, R. Q., Yang, H. T., and Wang, C.-C.: Biochim. Biophys. Acta *188*:59, 1969.
155. McCurdy, P. R., Fox, J., and Moo-Penn, W.: Am. J. Hum. Genet. *27*:62a, 1975.
156. Charache, S., McCurdy, P., and Fox, J.: 18th Ann. Meeting Am. Soc. Hemat., Dallas, Texas, December, 1975.
157. Lorkin, P. A., Stephens, A. D., Beard, M. E. J., Wrigley, P. F. M., Adams, L., and Lehmann, H.: Brit. Med. J. *4*:200, 1975.
158. Blackwell, R. Q., Liu, C.-S., and Wang, C.-L.: Biochim. Biophys. Acta *243*:467, 1971.
159. Tatsis, B., Sofroniadou, K., and Stergiopoulos, K.: Ann. Meeting Am. Soc. Hemat., Miami, Florida, 1972, Abstract 168.
160. Bradley, T. B., Wohl, R. C., Murphy, S. B., Oski, F. A., and Bunn, H. F.: Ann. Meeting Am. Soc. Hemat., Miami, 1972, Abstract 67.
161. DeWeinstein, B. I., White, J. M., Wiltshire, B. G., and Lehmann, H.: Acta Haematol. *50*:357, 1973.
162. Watson-Williams, E. J., Beale, D., Irvine, D., and Lehmann, H.: Nature (London) *205*:1273, 1965.
163. Hollender, A., Lorkin, P. A., Lehmann, H., and Svensson, B.: Nature (London) *222*:953, 1969.
164. Opfell, R. W., Lorkin, P. A., and Lehmann, H.: J. Med. Genet. *5*:292, 1968.
165. Cohen-Solal, M., Blouquit, Y., Carel, M. C., Reyes, F., Thillet, J., Carburi, J., Beuzard, Y., and Rosa, J.: Int. Symp. Abnormal Hemoglobins and Thalassemia, Istanbul, Turkey, Abstracts 5, 1974.
166. Miyaji, T., Suzuki, H., Ohba, Y., and Shibata, S.: Clin. Chim. Acta *14*:624, 1966.
167. Schneider, R. G., Satoshi, U., Alperin, J. B., Brimhall, B., and Jones, R. T.: N. Engl. J. Med. *280*:739, 1969.
168. Heller, P., Coleman, R. D., and Yakulis, V.: J. Clin. Invest. *45*:1021, 1966.
169. Aksoy, M., Erdem, S., Efremov, G. D., Wilson, J. B., Huisman, T. H. J., Schroeder, W. A., Shelton, J. R., Shelton, J. B., Ulitin, O. N., and Müftüoglu, A.: J. Clin. Invest. *51*:2380, 1972.
170. Beuzard, Y., Courvalin, J. C., Cohen-Solal, M., Carel, M. C., Rosa, J., Brizard, C. P., and Gibaud, A.: FEBS Lett. *27*:76, 1972.
171. Adams, J. G., III, Przywara, K. P., Shamsuddin, M., and Heller, P.: 18th Ann. Meeting Am. Soc. Hemat., Dallas, Texas, December, 1975.
172. Finney, R., Casey, R., Lehmann, H., and Walker, W.: FEBS Lett. *60*:435, 1975.
173. Clegg, J. B., Naughton, M. A., and Weatherall, D. J.: Nature (London) *207*:945, 1965.
174. Lorkin, P. A., Lehmann, H., Fairbanks, V. F., Berglund, G., and Leonhardt, T.: Biochem. J. *119*:68, 1970.
175. Taketa, F., Huang, Y. P., Libnoch, J. A., and Dessel, B. H.: Biochim. Biophys. Acta *400*:348, 1975.
176. Carrell, R. W., Lehmann, H., and Hutchison, H. E.: Nature (London) *210*:915, 1966.
177. Gordon-Smith, E. C., Dacie, J. V., Blecher, T. E., French, E. A., Wiltshire, B. G., and Lehmann, H.: Proc. Roy. Soc. Med. *66*:507, 1973.
178. Gacon, G., Wajcman, H., and Labie, D.: FEBS Lett. *58*:238, 1975.
179. Reed, C. S., Hampson, R., Gordon, S., Jones, R. T., Novy, M. J., Brimhall, B., Edwards, M. J., and Koler, R. D.: Blood *31*:623, 1968.

180. Jones, R. T., Osgood, E. E., Brimhall, B., and Koler, R. D.: J. Clin. Invest. *46*:1840, 1967.
181. Glynn, K. P., Penner, J. A., Smith, J. R., and Rucknagel, R. L.: Ann. Intern. Med. *69*:769, 1968.
182. Lokich, J. J., Mahoney, C., Bunn, H. F., Bruckheimer, S. M., and Ranney, H.: J. Clin. Invest. *52*:2060, 1973.
183. Adams, J. B., Winter, W. P., Tausk, K., and Heller, P.: Blood *43*:261, 1974.
184. Efremov, G. D., Huisman, T. H. J., Smith, L. L., Wilson, J. B., Kitchens, J. L., Wrightstone, R. N., and Adams, H. R.: J. Biol. Chem. *244*:6105, 1969.
185. Bonaventura, J., and Riggs, A.: J. Biol. Chem. *243*:980, 1968.
186. Nagel, R. L., Lynfield, J., Johnson, J., Landau, L., Bookchin, R. M., and Harris, M. B.: N. Engl. J. Med. *295*: 125, 1976.
187. White, J. M., Szur, L., Gillies, I. D. S., Lorkin, P. A., and Lehmann, H.: Brit. Med. J. *3*:665, 1973.
188. Wilkinson, T., Ching Geh Chua, Carrell, R. W., Robin, H., Exner, T., Kit Ming Lee, and Kronenberg. Biochim. Biophys. Acta *393*:195, 1975.
189. Koler, R. D., Jones, R. T., Bigley, R. H., Litt, M., Lovrien, E., Brooks, R., Lahey, M. E., and Fowler, R.: Am. J. Med. *55*:549, 1973.
190. Hyde, R. D., Hall, M. D., Wiltshire, B. G., and Lehmann, H.: Lancet *2*:1170–1172, 1972.
191. Kleihauer, E., Waller, H. D., Benöhr, H. C., Kohne, E., and Gelinsky, P.: Klin. Wochenschr. *48*:651, 1971.
192. Imamura, T., Fujita, S., Ohta, Y., Hanada, M., and Yanase, T.: J. Clin. Invest. *48*:2341, 1969.
193. Nute, P. E., Stamatoyannopoulos, G., Hermodson, M. A., Roth, D., and Hornung, S.: J. Clin. Invest. *53*:320, 1974.
194. King, M. A. R., Wiltshire, B. G., Lehmann, H., and Morimoto, H.: Brit. J. Haematol. *22*:125, 1972.
195. Ranney, H. M., Jacobs, A. S., and Nagel, R. L.: Nature (London) *213*:876, 1967.
196. Outeirino, J., Casey, R., White, J. M., and Lehmann, H.: Acta Haematol. *52*:53, 1974.
197. Schneider, R. G., Alperin, J. B., Brimhall, B., and Jones, R. T.: J. Lab. Clin. Med. *73*:616, 1969.
198. Miyaji, T., Oba, Y., Yamamoto, K., Shibata, S., Iuchi, I., and Hamilton, H. B.: Science *159*:204, 1968.
199. Baglioni, C.: Biochim. Biophys. Acta *59*:437, 1962.
200. Efremov, G. D., Duma, H., Ruvidic, R., Rolovic, Z., Wilson, J. B., and Huisman, T. H. J.: Biochim. Biophys. Acta *328*:81, 1973.
201. Miyaji, T., Ohba, Y., Yamamoto, K., Shibata, S., Iuchi, I., and Takenaka, H.: Nature (London) *217*:89, 1968.
202. Altay, C., Altinoz, N., Wilson, J. B., Bolch, K. C., and Huisman, T. H. J.: Biochim. Biophys. Acta. *434*: 1, 1976.
203. Blackwell, R. Q., Yang, H.-J., and Wang, C.-C.: Biochim. Biophys. Acta *194*:1, 1969.
204. Lorkin, P. A., Pietschmann, H., Braunsteiner, H., and Lehmann, H.: Acta Haematol. *51*:351, 1974.
205. Wade Cohen, P. T., Yates, A., Bellingham, A. J., and Huehns, E. R.: Nature [New Biol.] *243*:467, 1973.
206. Shibata, S.: Personal communication.
207. Minnich, V., Hill, R. J., Khuri, P. D., and Anderson, M. E.: Blood *25*:830, 1965.
208. Tentori, L., Carta Sorcini, M., and Buccella, C.: Clin. Chim. Acta *38*:258, 1972.
209. Bromberg, P. A., Alben, J. O., Bare, G. H., Balcerzak, S. P., Jones, R. T., Brimhall, B., and Padilla, F.: Nature [New Biol.] *243*:177, 1973.
210. Jensen, M., Oski, F. A., Nathan, D. G., and Bunn, H. F.: J. Clin. Invest. *55*:469, 1975.
211. Zak, S. J., Brimhall, B., Jones, R. T., and Kaplan, M. E.: Blood *44*:543, 1974.
212. Hayashi, A., Stamatoyannopoulos, G., Yoshida, A., and Adamson, J.: Nature [*New Biol.*] *230*:264, 1971.
213. Kleckner, H. B., Wilson, J. B., Lindeman, J. G., Stevens, P. D., Niazi, G., Hunter, E., Chen, C. J., and Huisman, T. H. L.: Biochim. Biophys. Acta *400*:343, 1975.
214. Charache, S., Brimhall, B., and Jones, R. T.: Johns Hopkins Med. J. *136*:132, 1975.
215. Winslow, R. M., Swenberg, M., Gross, E., Chervenick, P., Buchman, R. R., and Anderson, W. F.: Am. J. Hum. Genet. *27*:95a, 1975.
216. Perutz, M. F., del Pulsinelli, P., Ten Eyck, L., Kilmartin, J. V., Shibata, S., Iuchi, I., Miyaji, T., and Ham-

ilton, H. B.: Nature [New Biol.] *232*:147, 1971.

217. Bare, G. H., Bromberg, P. A., Alben, J. O., Brimhall, B., Jones, R. T., Mintz, S., and Rother, I.: Nature *259*:155, 1976.

218. Wajcman, H., Kilmartin, J. V., Najman, A., and Labie, D.: Biochim. Biophys. Acta *400*:354, 1975.

219. Jones, R. T., Brimhall, B., Huehns, E. R., and Barnicot, N. A.: Science *151*:1406, 1966.

220. Ranney, H. M., Jacobs, A. S., Ramot, B., and Bradley, T. B., Jr.: J. Clin. Invest. *48*:2057, 1969.

221. Ball, E. W., Meynell, M. J., Beale, D., Kynoch, P., Lehmann, H., and Stretton, A. O. W.: Nature (London) *209*:1217, 1968.

222. Jones, R. T., and Brimhall, B.: J. Biol. Chem. *242*:5141, 1967.

223. Sharma, R. S., Harding, D. L., Wong, S. C., Wilson, J. B., Gravely, M. E., and Huisman, T. H. J.: Biochim. Biophys. Acta *359*:233, 1974.

224. Lie-Injo, L. E., Pribada, W., Boerma, F. W., Efremov, G. D., Wilson, J. B., Reynolds, C. A., and Huisman, T. H. J.: Biochim. Biophys. Acta *229*:335, 1971.

225. Sharma, R. S., Williams, L., Wilson, J. B., and Huisman, T. H. J.: Biochim. Biophys. Acta *393*:379, 1975.

226. DeJong, W. W. W., and Bernini, L. F.: Nature (London) *219*:1360, 1968.

227. Lie-Injo, L. E., Kamuzora, H., and Lehmann, H.: J. Med. Genet. *11*:25, 1974.

228. Jenkins, G. C., Beale, D., Black, A. J., Huntsman, G. R., and Lehmann, H.: Brit. J. Haematol. *13*:252, 1967.

229. Ahern, E. E., Wiltshire, B. G., and Lehmann, H.: Biochim. Biophys. Acta *271*:61, 1972.

230. Larkin, I. L. M., Baker, T., Lorkin, P. A., Lehmann, H., Black, A. J., and Huntsman, R. G.: Brit. J. Haematol. *14*:233, 1968.

231. Carrell, R. W., Owen, M. C., Anderson, R., and Berry, E.: Biochim. Biophys. Acta *365*:323, 1974.

232. Loukopoulos, D., Kaltsoya, A., and Fessas, P.: Blood *33*:114, 1969.

233. Lie-Injo, L. E., Wiltshire, B. G., and Lehmann, H.: Biochim. Biophys. Acta *322*:224, 1973.

234. Ahern, E. J., Jones, R. T., Brimhall, B., and Gray, R. H.: Brit. J. Haematol. *18*:369, 1970.

235. Grifoni, V., Kamuzora, H., Lehmann, H., and Charlesworth, D.: Acta Haematol. *53*:347, 1975.

236. Ahern, E. J., Holder, W., Ahern, V., Serjeant, G. R., Serjeant, B. E., Forbes, M., Brimhall, B., and Jones, R. T.: Biochim. Biophys. Acta *393*:188, 1975.

237. Schneider, R. G., Haggard, M. E., Gustavson, L. P., Brimhall, B., and Jones, R. T.: Brit. J. Haematol. *28*:515, 1974.

238. Cauchi, M. N., Clegg, J. B., and Weatherall, D. J.: Nature (London) *223*:311, 1969.

239. Sacker, L. S., Beale, D., Black, A. J., Huntsman, R. G., Lehmann, H., and Lorkin, P. A.: Brit. Med. J. *3*:531, 1967.

240. Brimhall, B., Vedvick, T. S., Jones, R. T., Ahern, E. J., Palomino, L., and Ahern, V.: Brit. J. Haematol. *27*:313, 1973.

241. Lee-Potter, J. P., Deacon-Smith, R. A., Simpkiss, M. J., Kamuzora, H., and Lehmann, H.: J. Clin. Path. *28*:317, 1975.

242. Barnabas, J., and Muller, C. J.: Nature (London) *194*:931, 1962.

243. Ostertag, W., and Smith, E. W.: Eur. J. Biochem. *10*:371, 1969.

244. Baglioni, C.: Proc. Nat. Acad. Sci. (Wash.) *48*:1880, 1962.

245. Lehmann, H., and Charlesworth, D.: Biochem. J. *119*:43, 1970.

246. Badr, F. M., Lorkin, P. A., and Lehmann, H.: Nature [New Biol.] *242*:107, 1973.

247. Huisman, T. H. J., Wrightstone, R. N., Wilson, J. B., Schroeder, W. A., and Kendall, A. G.: Arch. Biochem. Biophys. *153*:850, 1972.

248. Clegg, J. B., Weatherall, D. J., and Milner, P. F.: Nature (London) *234*:337, 1971.

249. Clegg, J. B., Weatherall, D. J., Contopolou-Griva, I., Caroutsos, K., Poungouras, P., and Tsevrenis, H.: Nature (London) *251*:245, 1974.

250. DeJong, W. W. W., Meera Khan, P., and Bernini, L. F.: Am. J. Hum. Genet. *27*:81, 1975.

251. Seid-Akhaven, M., Winter, W. P., Abramson, R. K., and Rucknagel, D. L.: Ann. Meeting Am. Soc. Hemat., Miami, Florida, 1972, Abstract 9.

252. Bunn, H. F., Schmidt, G. J., Haney, D. N., and Dluhy, R. G.: Proc. Nat. Acad. Sci. (USA) *72*:3609, 1975.
253. Flatz, G., Kinderlerer, J. L., Kilmartin, J. V., and Lehmann, H.: Lancet 10:732, 1971.
254. Huisman, T. H. J., Wilson, J. B., Gravely, M., and Hubbard, M.: Proc. Nat. Acad. Sci. (USA) *71*: 3270, 1974.
255. DeJong, W. W. W., Went, L. N., and Bernini, L. F.: Nature (London) *220*:788, 1968.
256. Cohen-Solal, M., Blouquitt, Y., Garel, M. G., Thillet, J., Gaillard, L., Creyssel, R., Gibaud, A., and Rosa, J.: Biochim. Biophys. Acta *351*:306, 1974.
257. Jones, R. T., Brimhall, B., Huisman, T. H. J., Kleihauer, E., and Betke, K.: Science *154*:1024, 1966.
258. Praxedes, H., and Lehmann, H.: Proc. 14th Int. Congress of Hematology, Sao Paulo, Brazil, 1972.
259. Shibata, S., Miyaji, T., Ueda, S., Matsuoka, M., Iuchi, I., Yamada, K., and Shinkai, N.: Proc. Jap. Acad. *46*:440, 1970.
260. Wajcman, H., Labie, D., and Schapira, G.: Biochim. Biophys. Acta *295*:495, 1973.
261. Bradley, T. B., Wohl., R. C., and Rieder, R. F.: Science *157*:1581, 1967.
262. Lutcher, C. L., and Huisman, T. H. J.: Blood *47*:99, 1976.
263. Moo-Penn, W. F., Jue, D. L., Bechtel, K. C., Johnson, M. H., Bemis, E., Brosious, E., and Schmidt, R. M.: Biochem. Biophys. Res. Commun. *65*:8, 1975.
264. Bookchin, R. M., Nagel, R. L., and Ranney, H. M.: J. Biol. Chem. *242*:248, No. 2., 1967.
265. Adams, J. G., and Heller, P.: Blood *42*:990, 1973.
266. Blackwell, R. Q., Wong, H. B., Liu, C.-S., and Weng, M.-L.: Biochim. Biophys. Acta *278*:482, 1972.
267. Goossens, M., Garel, M. C., Auvinet, J., Basset, P., Gomes, P. F., and Rosa, J.: FEBS Lett. *58*:149, 1975.
268. Ahern, E., Ahern, V., Holder, W., et al.: Biochim. Biophys. Acta *427*:530, 1976.
269. Garel, M. C., Goosens, M., Oudart, J. L., Blouquit, Y., Thillet, J., and Rosa, J.: Biochim. Biophys. Acta *453*:459, 1976.
270. Jones, R. T., Koler, R. D., Duerst, M. L., and Dhindsa, D. S.: Hemoglobin *1*:45, 1976.
271. Garel, M. C., Hassan, W., Coquelet, M. T., et al.: Biochim. Biophys. Acta *420*:97, 1976.
272. Schneider, R. G., Hettig, R. A., Bilunos, M., and Brimhall, B.: Hemoglobin *1*:85, 1976.
273. Jones, T. R., Brimhall, B., and Gray, G.: Hemoglobin *1*:171, 1976.
274. Mant, M. J., Salkie, M. L., Cope, N., et al.: Hemoglobin *1*:183, 1976.
275. El-Hazmi, M. A. F., and Lehmann, H.: Hemoglobin *1*:59, 1976.
276. Marti, H. R., Winterhalter, K. W., di Iorio, E. E., et al.: FEBS Lett. *63*:193, 1976.
277. Rieder, R. F., Clegg, J. B., Weiss, H. J., et al.: Biochim. Biophys. Acta *439*:501, 1976.
278. Casey, R., Lang, A., Lehmann, H., and Shinton, N. K.: Brit. J. Haemat. *33*:143, 1976.
279. Winslow, R. M., Swenberg, M.-L., Gross, E., et al.: J. Clin. Invest. *57*:772, 1976.
280. Orringer, E. P., Wilson, J. B., and Huisman, T. H. J.: FEBS Lett. *65*: 297, 1976.
281. Poyart, C., Krishnamoorthy, R., Bursaux, E., Gacon, G., and Labie, D.: FEBS Lett. *69*:103, 1976.
282. Wajcman, H., Krishnamoorthy, R., Gacon, G., Elion, J., Allard, C., and Labie, D.: J. Mol. Med. *1*:187, 1976.
283. Ahern, E., Ahern, V., Hilton, T., Serjeant, G. R., Serjeant, B. E., Seakins, M., Lang, A., Middleton, A., and Lehmann, H.: FEBS Lett. *69*:99, 1976.
284. Turner, J. W., Jones, R. T., Brimhall, B., DuVal, M. C., and Koler, R. D.: Biochem. Genet. *14*:577, 1976.
285. Garel, M. C., Blouquit, Y., North, M. L., Arous, N., and Rosa, J.: FEBS Lett. *72*:1, 1976.
286. Blouquit, Y., Arous, N., Machado, P. E. A., Perrone, F., and Garel, M. C.: FEBS Lett. *72*:5, 1976.
287. Ikkala, E., Koskela, J., Pikkarainen, P., et al.: Acta Haemat. *56*:257, 1976.
288. Schneider, R. G., Berkman, N. L., Brimhall, B., and Jones, R. T.: Biochim. Biophys. Acta *453*:478, 1976.
289. Moo-Penn, W. F., Bechtel, K. C., Johnson, M. H., Jue, D. L., Therrell, B. L., Morrison, B. Y., and Schmidt, R. M.: Biochim. Biophys. Acta *453*:472, 1976.

TABLE 6–3. Clinically Important Hemoglobin Variants

I. The Sickle Syndromes
  A. Sickle cell trait
  B. Sickle cell disease
    1. SS
    2. SC
    3. SD_{Punjab}
    4. SO_{Arab}
    5. S/Thal
II. The Unstable Hemoglobins (Congenital Heinz Body Anemia)
  (Approx. 70 variants)
III. Hemoglobins with Abnormal Oxygen Affinity
  A. High affinity (familial erythrocytosis)
    (Approx. 30 variants)
  B. Low affinity (Hb Kansas, Hb Beth Israel → familial cyanosis)
IV. The M Hemoglobins (Familial Cyanosis)
  (5 variants)
V. Structural Variants which result in a Thalassemic Phenotype
  A. Lepore hemoglobins (β-thalassemia phenotype)
  B. Chain termination mutants (i.e., Hb Constant Spring: α-thalassemia phenotype)

moglobins. The five M hemoglobins encountered thus far have very interesting properties, which are described in Chapter 10. There are three different Lepore-type hemoglobins which result in a β-thalassemia phenotype (see Chapter 5) and four different α-chain termination mutants which cause α thalassemia (Chapter 5).

GENETIC BASIS OF THE HEMOGLOBIN VARIANTS

Mendelian Inheritance

As Chapter 4 explains, the α and non-α globin polypeptide chains are products of separate genes. Thus, a mutant hemoglobin involves a structural abnormality of a specific globin subunit. Hemoglobin variants are inherited as co-dominant traits, according to classic Mendelian genetics. Figure 6–1 shows two pedigrees. If both parents have sickle trait (AS) (left-hand panel), half of these children will be AS, while one fourth will be AA and the remaining fourth will be homozygotes (SS). If one parent has sickle trait and the other C trait, one fourth of the offspring will be AA, one fourth will be AS, one fourth will be AC, and the remaining fourth will be double heterozygotes (SC).

As Table 6–1 shows, variants have been encountered for each of the four globin chains (α,β,γ, and δ) that are found in human red cells in postnatal life. The relatively small number of γ-chain variants is due in part to the fact that hemoglobin F is barely detectable after the first six months of life. Likewise, δ-chain variants may often escape detection, since they are present in small amounts (1 to

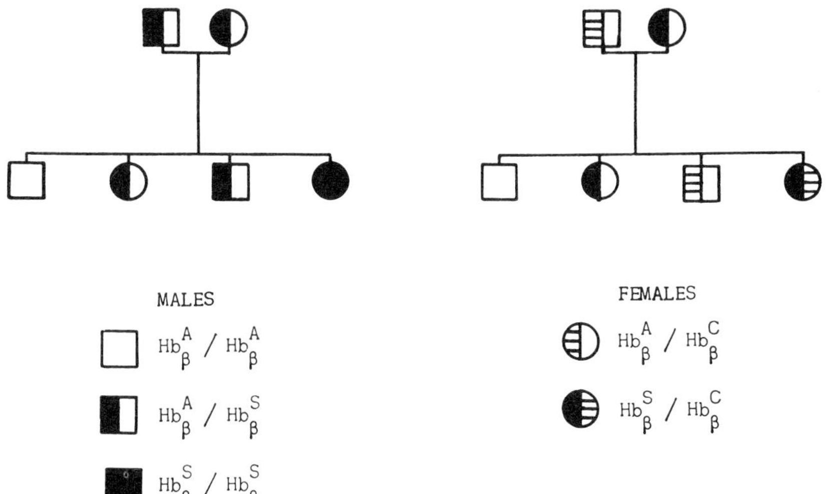

Figure 6–1. Pedigrees showing the inheritance of homozygous sickle cell anemia (SS) (*left*) and Hb SC disease (*right*). (From Rucknagel, D., and Laros, R. K.: Clin. Obst. Gynec. *12*:49, 1969.)

3 per cent). No functional significance has been ascribed to any of the γ-chain variants that have been reported with the exception of Hb F-Poole, an unstable fetal hemoglobin causing hemolytic anemia in the neonatal period (Lee-Potter et al., 1975). Occasionally, individuals may inherit more than one hemoglobin variant. A heterozygote for both an α-chain variant and a β-chain variant will have four major hemoglobin bands on electrophoresis ($\alpha_2^A\beta_2^A$, $\alpha_2^X\beta_2^A$, $\alpha_2^A\beta_2^Y$, and $\alpha_2^X\beta_2^Y$). Figure 6–2 shows an electrophoretic pattern of an individual who has an α-chain variant (HB I) and a β-chain variant (Hb S).

SINGLE BASE SUBSTITUTIONS

Of the 269 variants listed in Tables 6–1 and 6–2, the vast majority (238) are single amino acid substitutions in a globin polypeptide chain. The structural alteration can be explained by a single base substitution in the corresponding triplet codon of the globin gene DNA (and its corresponding mRNA).* For example, hemoglobins Rainier ($\alpha_2\beta_2{}^{145\ \mathrm{Tyr}\rightarrow\mathrm{Cys}}$), Bethesda ($\alpha_2\beta_2{}^{145\ \mathrm{Tyr}\rightarrow\mathrm{His}}$), and Fort Gordon

*For descriptive purposes, in the following discussions the mutations are described in terms of the nucleotide sequence changes created in the transcription product of the gene: the globin messenger RNA (mRNA). The actual mutation, of course, occurs in the complementary DNA sequence of the gene at the appropriate corresponding position.

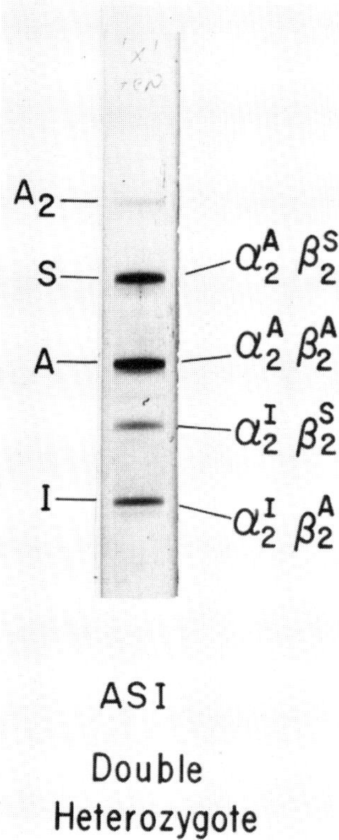

Figure 6–2. Gel electrofocusing pattern of individual doubly heterozygous for an α-chain variant (Hb I) and a β-chain variant (Hb S).

($\alpha_2\beta_2$ $^{145\ \mathrm{Tyr}\longrightarrow\mathrm{Asp}}$) can all be explained by single base substitutions in the triplet UAU, which is thought to code for tyrosine 145 (Table 6–4).

A few variants have amino acid substitutions at two different sites on the same subunit. These include hemoglobins C-Harlem (β6 Glu→Val, 73 Asp→Asn), Arlington Park (β6 Glu→Lys, 95 Lys→Glu), J-Singapore (α78 Asn→Asp, 79 Ala→Gly), and C-Ziguinchor (β6 Glu→Val, 58 Pro→Arg). These variants also presumably arose by the same mechanism of single base substitutions in the involved triplet codons of the globin gene DNA (and thence the mRNA).

It is presumed that there exist unique "normal" mRNA sequences for the α and β globin chains. This hypothesis is supported by the fact that all the amino acid substitutions thus far described in human hemoglobins can be explained by single nucleotide base substitutions in a single corresponding codon of the normal mRNA, as illustrated in Table 6–4. In fact, the occurrence of multiple variants with different amino acid substitutions at the same site has permitted the hypothetical assignment of specific nucleotide bases in certain positions of many mRNA codons, the full sequence of which

TABLE 6–4. Single Base Substitutions in Hemoglobin Variants

β-Chain Variants		Residue Number 144	145	146	Termination Codon
β^A	Base sequence	AAG -	UAU -	CAC -	UAA*
	Amino acid sequence	Lys -	Tyr -	His-	COOH
β Rainier	Base sequence	AAG -	UGU -	CAC -	UAA
	Amino acid sequence	Lys -	Cys -	His-	COOH
β Bethesda	Base sequence	AAG -	CAU -	CAC -	UAA
	Amino acid sequence	Lys -	His -	His-	COOH
β Fort Gordon	Base sequence	AAG -	GAU -	CAC -	UAA
	Amino acid sequence	Lys -	Asp -	His-	COOH

*The nucleotide sequence for this segment of mRNA was proposed by Marotta et al. (1974) on the basis of direct nucleotide sequence studies of normal globin mRNA.

could not otherwise be predicted (Fitch, 1974). Thus far, direct studies of the sequence of normal globin mRNA has not uncovered any contradictions in this general theory (Forget et al., 1974b; Marotta et al., 1974).

There is one possible exception, however, to this general scheme. Three different variants have been described with amino acid substitutions at β-chain residue number 67: Hb Sydney ($\alpha_2\beta_2{}^{67\ \text{Val}\rightarrow\text{Ala}}$), Hb M-Milwaukee-1 ($\alpha_2\beta_2{}^{67\ \text{Val}\rightarrow\text{Glu}}$), and Hb Bristol ($\alpha_2\beta_2{}^{67\ \text{Val}\rightarrow\text{Asp}}$). As illustrated in Table 6–5, Hb M-Milwaukee-1 and Hb Bristol could not arise by a single nucleotide base substitution in a single common normal valine codon: the former must arise from a GUG or GUA valine codon, whereas the latter must arise from a GUC or GUU valine codon. Direct nucleotide sequence analysis of human globin mRNA suggests that the normal codon for $\beta^{67\ \text{Val}}$ in the indi-

TABLE 6–5. Hemoglobin Variants Affecting Residue β^{67}

Variant	Possible Mutant Codons	Corresponding Normal Valine Codons
Hb Sydney ($\beta^{67\ \text{Val}\rightarrow\text{Ala}}$)	GCU	GUU
	GCC	GUC
	GCA	GUA
	GCG	GUG
Hb M-Milwaukee ($\beta^{67\ \text{Val}\rightarrow\text{Glu}}$)	GAA	GUA
	GAG	GUG
Hb Bristol ($\beta^{67\ \text{Val}\rightarrow\text{Asp}}$)	GAU	GUU
	GAC	GUC

Note that Hb Bristol and Hb M-Milwaukee cannot originate by a single base substitution in a common normal valine codon.

viduals thus far studied is in fact GUG (Marotta et al., 1977). Hemoglobin Bristol could have arisen through a double nucleotide base substitution—GUG→GAU (or GAC)—or perhaps as a mutation in a "normal" gene that had a silent polymorphism (base substitution) in the $\beta^{67\,Val}$ codon—GUC or GUU instead of GUG. The globin mRNA of only a small number of individuals has thus far been studied, and it is certainly feasible that silent polymorphisms may in fact exist in the mRNA sequences of normal α and β mRNA in different individuals or in different ethnic groups. A second example of probable polymorphism has recently been identified at β codon number 20 (see Table 6–2).

Elongated Subunits: Termination Errors

A second general class of abnormal hemoglobins is that in which the mutant globin chain is abnormally long or short. These seem to have resulted from a variety of different genetic mechanisms. Hb Constant Spring (CS) has abnormally long α chains carrying 28 or 31 extra amino acids at the C-terminal end of the α chain, the sequence of the first 141 amino acid residues being normal (Clegg et al., 1971b; Milner et al., 1971). The shorter form of the α^{CS} chain probably results from post-translational proteolytic cleavage of the last three amino acids of the chain (Clegg et al., 1971b). One can account for the abnormally long α^{CS} chain by a single base substitution in the normal termination codon of the α-chain mRNA (Clegg et al., 1971b). Mutation of the UAA or UAG termination codon of the α-chain mRNA to a CAA or CAG would result in a codon which codes for glutamine, and glutamine is precisely the amino acid in position 142 of the α^{CS} chain (i.e., the first amino acid of the abnormal segment of the α^{CS} chain). In the case of Hb CS, then, a simple base substitution would abolish the termination signal and allow the translation of normally untranslated sequences of the mRNA, which are known to exist (see Chapter 4 and Figure 6–3).

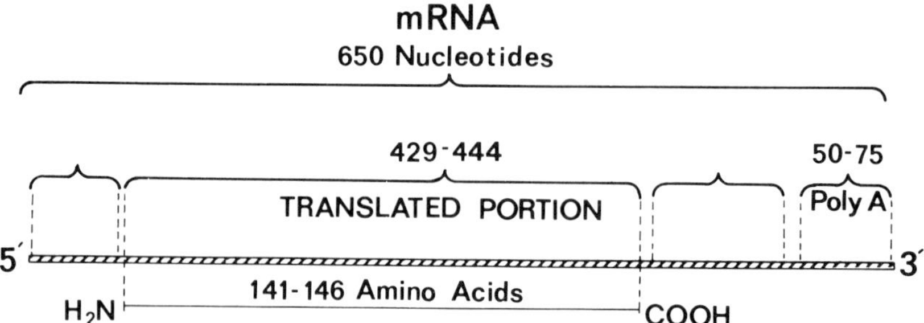

Figure 6–3. Schematic diagram showing the translated and untranslated portions of globin mRNA. Included in the translated portion are the six nucleotides of the initiation and termination codons.

The hypothesis of chain termination mutation as the basis for Hb CS has been strengthened by the finding of three other variants with elongated α chains: Hb Icaria (Clegg et al., 1974a), Hb Seal Rock (Bradley et al., 1975), and Hb Koya Dora (DeJong et al., 1975). These variants both have the same number of extra residues at the C-terminal end of the α chain and they differ only in the nature of the amino acid at position number 142; the other 30 additional C-terminal residues are the same in all four variants. The amino acid present at position 142 is lysine in Hb Icaria, glutamic acid in Hb Seal Rock, and serine in Hb Koya Dora. The presence of these residues can be explained, just as in Hb CS, by base substitutions in the termination codon: UAA (or UAG) to AAA (or AAG) in Hb Icaria, UAA (or UAG) to GAA (or GAG) in Hb Seal Rock, and UAA (or UAG) to UCA (or UCG) in Hb Koya Dora. In fact, direct nucleotide sequence analysis of normal globin mRNA has confirmed the presence of untranslated nucleotide sequences in the mRNA, and some of these nucleotide sequences can be matched to amino acid sequences in the elongated α-chain sequence of Hb CS (Forget et al., 1974b; Marotta et al., 1974). These various findings all support the hypothesis that chain termination mutations can be the cause of certain variant hemoglobins.

ELONGATED SUBUNITS: FRAME-SHIFT MUTATIONS

Hb Wayne (Seid-Akhavan et al., 1972, 1976) also has an abnormally long α chain with extra amino acids at its C terminus, but it probably arose by a different mechanism. The α chain of Hb Wayne has the normal α-chain amino acid sequence through position 138; then a totally new sequence of eight amino acids is present at the C-terminal end of the α chain. The mechanism of mutation in this case was probably a single nucleotide base deletion which caused a "frame shift," or change in the mRNA reading phase or frame. It can be described as follows: the normal α-chain mRNA sequence coding for the C-terminal α-chain amino acids (numbers 137 to 141) is thought to have been identified (Forget et al., 1974b; Marotta et al., 1974). This mRNA sequence is

137	138	139	140	141	142	143
(ACC)	(UCC)	(AAA)	(UAC)	(CGU)	(UAA)	(GCN).
Thr	Ser	Lys	Tyr	Arg	term.	

In the mRNA of the Hb Wayne α chain, one of the A's of codon 139 (or one of the C's of codon 138) is presumed deleted. The mutant sequence would then be read in the following order:

137	138	139	140	141	142
(ACC)	$(\text{UC}^{\text{C}}_{\text{A}})$	(AAU)	(ACC)	(GUU)	(AAG).
Thr	Ser	Asn	Thr	Val	Lys

Because the translational apparatus can only decode the mRNA by reading successive intact triplet codons, the apparatus cannot detect or correct for deletions. It is readily apparent that a single base deletion will disrupt the normal decoding phase or triplet punctuation built into the mRNA, and as a result the UAA will no longer be read as an intact termination codon. The "U" is now read as part of the codon for position 141 and the "AA", as part of the codon for position 142. Consequently, translation of the mRNA continues until a new stop signal is encountered, and an abnormally long α chain is synthesized.

The nucleotide sequence of the untranslated portion of normal human α-chain mRNA, which is located just distal to (to the 3′ side of) the termination codon, can be predicted by comparing the amino acid sequences of the α Constant Spring and α Wayne chains with reference to the genetic code (Laux et al., 1973). A unique nucleotide sequence of 26 base residues can be derived which contains a new "in phase" termination codon, UAG, at the predicted position to terminate the α Wayne chain. Some of these nucleotide sequences predicted for α-chain mRNA have in fact been found by direct nucleotide sequence analysis of normal human α-chain mRNA (Forget et al., 1974b; Marotta et al., 1974). This finding supports the hypothesis that the α^{CS} and α^{Wayne} chains arose by the mechanisms outlined above.

Two hemoglobins with abnormally long β globin chains have been described: Hb Tak (Flatz et al., 1971) and Hb Cranston (Bunn et al., 1975b). The amino acid sequence of the β^{Tak} chain is normal through position 146, the normal β-chain C-terminal residue, just as the α-chain sequence of hemoglobin Constant Spring is normal through position 141, the normal α-chain C-terminal residue. However, the β^{Tak} chain is not likely to have arisen by the same type of mutation which produced the α^{CS} chain. The first "extra" (147th) amino acid in the β^{Tak} chain is threonine. None of the threonine codons (ACN) can be formed from any of the termination codons (UAA, UAG, or UGA) by a single base substitution: a double base substitution must be postulated. The first two nucleotide bases following the normal β-chain termination codon are thought to be GC– (Forget et al., 1974b; Marotta et al., 1974) (see also Table 6–6). GCN must code for alanine and not lysine, which is the amino acid found in position 148 of the β^{Tak} chain and which must have as its codon

TABLE 6–6. Frame-Shift Mutations of β-Chain mRNA Giving Rise to Hb Tak and Hb Cranston

SEQUENCE	GLOBIN CHAIN
144 145 146 Lys - Tyr - His - Term AAG - UAU - CAC - UAA - GCN	β^{A}
144 145 146 147 148 149 Lys - Ser - Ileu - Thr - Lys - Leu AAG AGU AUC ACU AAG CUN	$\beta^{Cranston}$
144 145 146 147 148 149 Lys - Tyr - His - Thr - Lys - Leu AAG UAU CAC ACU AAG CUN	β^{Tak}

The nucleotide sequence of normal β mRNA was determined by Marotta et al. (1974) and Forget et al. (1975); N indicates any of the four nucleotides. The frame shift results from reduplication of the underlined dinucleotides in the normal sequence: AG in codon 144 for $\beta^{Cranston}$, and AC in codon 146 for β^{Tak} (Fitch, 1974; Bunn et al., 1975b; Forget et al., 1975b).

AAG or AAA. It is therefore unlikely that Hb Tak arose by simple chain termination mutation (single base substitution in the termination codon of the β mRNA).

Studies of Hb Cranston provide further insight into the probable molecular basis of Hb Tak. The amino acid sequence of the $\beta^{Cranston}$ chain is normal through residue number 144, where it changes to a different amino acid sequence for 13 additional residues (Bunn et al., 1975b). The sequence of the first five new amino acids can be reconciled to the previously proposed nucleotide sequence for this portion of the normal β-chain mRNA (Forget et al., 1974b; Marotta et al., 1974) by postulating a frame-shift mutation resulting from duplication of the last two nucleotide bases of the codon for amino acid 144, AAG-AGU (Table 6–6 and Bunn et al., 1975b). Such a frame shift would account for the new residues in positions 145 to 147 and result in read-through beyond the normal termination codon (Table 6–6).

Fitch (1974), on the basis of the normal β mRNA sequence, proposed a similar mechanism for the origin of the β^{Tak} chain: duplication of the last two nucleotide bases of the codon for amino acid 146, CAC-ACU, resulting in a frame shift which allows read-through of the normal termination codon and translation of normally untranslated portions of the β mRNA.

The type of frame shifts proposed for the origins of the β^{Tak} and $\beta^{Cranston}$ chains could have arisen through nonhomologous crossing over of chromosomes at meiosis, with resulting insertion of repeated nucleotide base pairs, although other defects of DNA replication, excision, and repair could result in the same type of mutation.

If Hbs Tak and Cranston arose by the mechanisms just proposed, they should have identical sequences from residue number 148 onward, because this portion of the sequence would result from the read-through (in the same "frame" or order) of the same untranslated portion of the β mRNA. The completed structural analysis of Hb Tak shows that this is indeed true (Lehmann et al., 1975).

Again direct nucleotide sequence analysis of normal globin mRNA has provided support for these hypotheses. Nucleotide sequences have been identified in normal β mRNA which can be correlated to almost the entire elongated amino acid sequence of the β^{Cranston} and β^{Tak} chains, and one long, normally untranslated nucleotide sequence provides a new chain termination codon in the predicted position following the C-terminal Tyr codon (Forget et al., 1975).

Hemoglobin Grady: Crossover in Phase

One last elongated globin chain has been described. In Hb Grady (Huisman et al., 1974) the α chain contains three additional amino acids but the additional residues are not located at the C terminus of the affected globin chain. The α^{Grady} chain contains a "repetition" of the tripeptide sequence normally found at positions 116 to 118; then its sequence continues as the normal α-chain sequence:

114 115 116 117 118 119 120
Pro-Ala-<u>Glu-Phe-Thr</u>-<u>Glu-Phe-Thr</u>-Pro-Ala- etc.

This hemoglobin variant may have arisen by nonhomologous crossing over of complementary globin chain genes, with insertion (reduplication) of three adjacent codons (Huisman et al., 1974). On the other hand, the new codons could have resulted from some other defect in DNA replication or repair.

Shortened Subunits

A few mutant hemoglobins have abnormally short globin chains (Table 6–2). In all cases described, one or a few adjacent amino acids are missing from the abnormal chains. The remainder of the subunit is normal. These variants probably involve deletion of one or more intact codons (of the mRNA) which code for the missing amino acids. If an entire codon is deleted, then no frame shift will result and the remainder of the amino acid sequence will not differ from normal. Such codon deletions could arise by nonhomologous crossing over of complementary globin chain genes or by other mechanisms of faulty

DNA replication, which have been previously alluded to. These variants are generally unstable and are associated with congenital Heinz body hemolytic anemia (see Chapter 8).

One hemoglobin variant, Hb McKees Rocks, has a shortened β subunit that is probably due to a nonsense mutation (Winslow et al., 1976). The β chain of the variant has a structure identical to β^A chains through residue 144, but lacks the two C-terminal residues (-Tyr-His). This mutant hemoglobin may have arisen because of a substitution of A or G for U, at the third base of the codon UA$\underline{U}$ for tyrosine at position 145, thus producing a termination codon (UAA or UAG). However, the same structure could have resulted from a frame shift or a deletion.

Fusion Subunits

The final class of mutant hemoglobins to be considered are the hemoglobins with fused or hybrid globin chains. Hemoglobin Lepore, for example, contains normal α chains and abnormal non-α chains. These non-α chains have a normal length but an abnormal sequence: the first 50 to 80 amino acids have the normal N-terminal amino acid sequence of δ chains, while the last 60 to 90 residues have the normal C-terminal amino acid sequence of β chains. The Lepore chain is thus a fusion or hybrid NH_2-$\delta\beta$-COOH chain. Three different Lepore chains have been described, in which the switch from δ to β sequences occurs at different points of the sequence (Fig. 5–2*B*). Hemoglobin Kenya is analogous except that the abnormal hybrid chain contains γ and β sequences (NH_2-$\gamma\beta$-COOH) (see Chapter 5).

Hemoglobin Lepore appears to have arisen through nonhomologous crossing over between part of the δ locus on one chromosome and part of the β locus on the complementary chromosome, as illustrated in Figure 2–2A. This phenomenon occurs as a consequence of misalignment of a chromosome pair during meiosis, resulting in the pairing of a β gene with a δ gene instead of with its homologous β gene. Such an event should give rise to two abnormal chromosomes: the first, the Lepore chromosome, has no normal intact β or δ loci but has instead only the fused $\delta\beta$ Lepore gene. Because of the absence of a normal β locus in cis and the low output of the Lepore gene product, heterozygous Hb Lepore patients should have the clinical features of β-thalassemia trait while homozygous Hb Lepore syndrome should mimic β thalassemia major. This prediction has proved to be true (see Chapter 5 and Weatherall and Clegg, 1972). The second abnormal chromosome arising from a $\delta\beta$-gene nonhomologous crossing-over event should be an "anti-Lepore" chromosome, which carries normal β and δ loci as well as a gene for an NH_2-$\beta\delta$-COOH anti-

Lepore globin chain (see Figure 5–3*A*). Because of the presence of a normal β locus in cis, patients with this chromosome should be clinically normal except for the presence of the anti-Lepore hemoglobin. Such patients have recently been identified and two different anti-Lepore hemoglobins have been characterized: Hb Miyada and Hb P-Nilotic (see Figure 5–3*B*). The discovery of these anti-Lepore hemoglobins strongly supports the model of nonhomologous crossing over for the origin of Hb Lepore.

Hb Kenya seems to have arisen by nonhomologous crossing over between γ and β loci, giving an NH_2-$\gamma\beta$-COOH fusion product (see Figure 5–10). Because the γ loci are less homologous to the β loci and are situated farther away from the β loci than are the δ loci, the Kenya crossover must have required a greater degree of mispairing during meiosis. Only one type of Hb Kenya has been described so far. The "anti-Kenya" gene has not been identified. The occurrence of both Hb Lepore and Hb Kenya provides strong support for the hypothesis that the γ, δ, and β loci are closely linked on the same chromosome in the order NH_2-$\gamma\delta\beta$-COOH (see Chapter 4).

PATTERN OF SYNTHESIS OF HEMOGLOBIN VARIANTS

From the previous discussions, one can conclude that abnormal hemoglobins probably arise by many different types of mutations in the globin genes which result in the synthesis of a globin mRNA with an abnormal nucleotide sequence. Most of these hemoglobins are made in reduced amounts. It is readily apparent that any of the steps in mRNA metabolism could result in reduced synthesis of the abnormal globin chain. The mutant mRNA could be transcribed, processed, or transported less efficiently. Alternatively, the abnormal mRNA could be unstable and degraded rapidly or translated more slowly than normal because it contains an abnormal codon which requires a transfer RNA which is in short supply in the cell (so-called modulation; see Chapter 5). Finally, the mutant globin chain could be synthesized normally but be structurally unstable or unable to associate normally with other chains to form tetramers; as a result, the abnormal chain could be preferentially lost owing to precipitation or catabolism. All these processes would result in reduced amounts of the abnormal hemoglobin.

White (1971) has reviewed the many studies done to distinguish among the above possibilities. In most cases, the abnormal globin chain is synthesized at a normal rate but is preferentially lost or degraded because of increased catabolism or because of the inadequate capacity of the mutant chain to participate in tetramer assembly. In most cases for which decreased synthesis has been alleged to exist, these post-translational phenomena have not been completely ruled out, nor has the precise mechanism of presumed decreased synthesis been elucidated. Abnormal translation (elongation) times have not been found in such cases. In Hb Gun Hill (Rieder, 1971), the abnormal β chain seems to accumulate 20 to 50 per cent faster than normal, but the assembly time of the chain is normal. This entire area remains poorly understood.

Hemoglobins with abnormal α chains tend to be present in heterozygotes as an even smaller percentage (10 to 25 per cent) of the total hemoglobin than hemoglobins with mutant β chains (35 to 50 per cent) (Fig. 6–4). This is best explained by the independent evidence for duplication of the α-chain loci (see Chapter 2 and Wasi, 1973). A mutant α-chain locus would then constitute only 1 of 4 α-chain loci in the diploid heterozygous state, whereas mutant β-chain loci would constitute 1 of 2 β-chain loci.

The synthesis of Hb Lepore, the anti-Lepore hemoglobins, and Hb Constant Spring (like that of normal Hb A_2) appears to be confined almost entirely to bone marrow and is virtually absent from circulating reticulocytes. The molecular mechanisms responsible for this observation are obscure, but instability of the mRNA has been suggested (see Chapter 5).

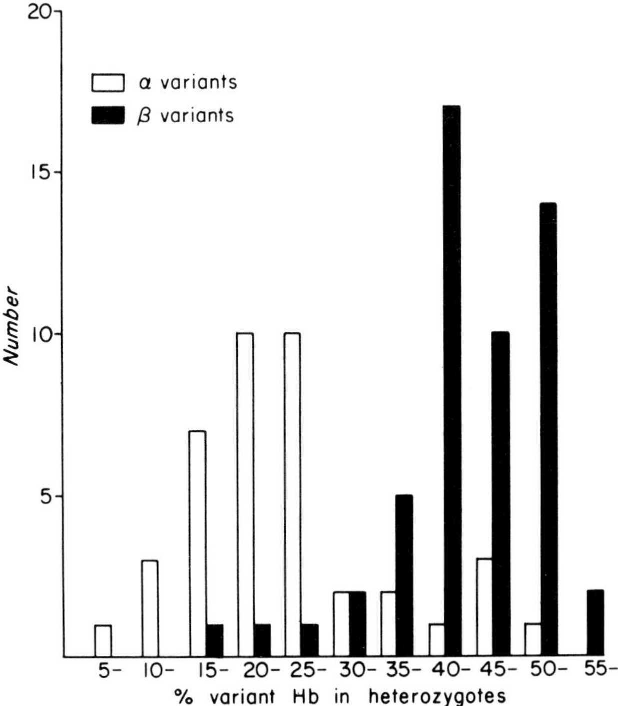

Figure 6–4. Distribution of variant hemoglobins in humans heterozygous for α-chain and β-chain mutant hemoglobin. (From Nute, P., et al.: Ann. N.Y. Acad. Sci. *241*: 39, 1974a.)

Finally, the reasons for the extremely low output of the abnormally long α-chain variants (Wayne, Seal Rock, Icaria, Koya Dora, and Constant Spring) are not understood. These variants constitute only 1 to 3 per cent of the total hemoglobin, and it is not immediately obvious why these frame-shift and chain-termination mutants should be present in such low amounts. Simple translation of normally untranslated sequences of the mRNA cannot be the only factor. The two β-chain frame-shift mutants accumulate in much greater amounts (25 to 40 per cent of the total hemoglobin). The observed low yields of the Lepore and anti-Lepore hemoglobins are also difficult to understand (see Chapter 5).

In summary, the molecular mechanisms by which mutant hemoglobins arise have been reasonably well delineated, but the effects of these mutations on the ultimate amounts of the mutant hemoglobins finally accumulated in the cell remain poorly understood at the molecular level.

COMMON HEMOGLOBIN VARIANTS

Hb S $(\alpha_2\beta_2{}^{6\ \mathrm{Glu}\rightarrow\mathrm{Val}})$

Hb S is the most common human hemoglobin variant. The sickle syndromes are an important group of disorders and are discussed in detail in Chapter 7. Representative blood films of the sickle syndromes and some of the other common hemoglobinopathies are shown in Figure 6–5.

Hb C $(\alpha_2\beta_2{}^{6\ \mathrm{Glu}\rightarrow\mathrm{Lys}})$

Hb C was the second variant to be identified electrophoretically (Itano and Neel, 1950) and structurally (Hunt and Ingram, 1960). The replacement of lysine for glutamic acid at the sixth position of the β chain (the same site as the substitution in hemoglobin S) gives Hb C a relatively high positive charge. Accordingly, it has slow mobility upon zone electrophoresis at alkaline pH, identical to that of Hb A_2. However, hemoglobins A_2 and C can be separated by column chromatography (Huisman, 1972). Hb C is found primarily in blacks. In areas of West Africa, the gene frequency (and therefore, the incidence of C trait) may be as high as 28 per cent. About 2 per cent of black Americans are AC heterozygotes, while approximately $0.02 \times 0.02 \times 0.25$, or 1 out of 10,000 are CC homozygotes. Hb C is probably the second most commonly encountered variant worldwide.

Individuals who have *Hb C trait* (AC) lack any clinical manifestations. Red cell life span is normal (Prindle and McCurdy, 1969). The red cells contain about 30 to 40 per cent Hb C, 50 to 60 per cent

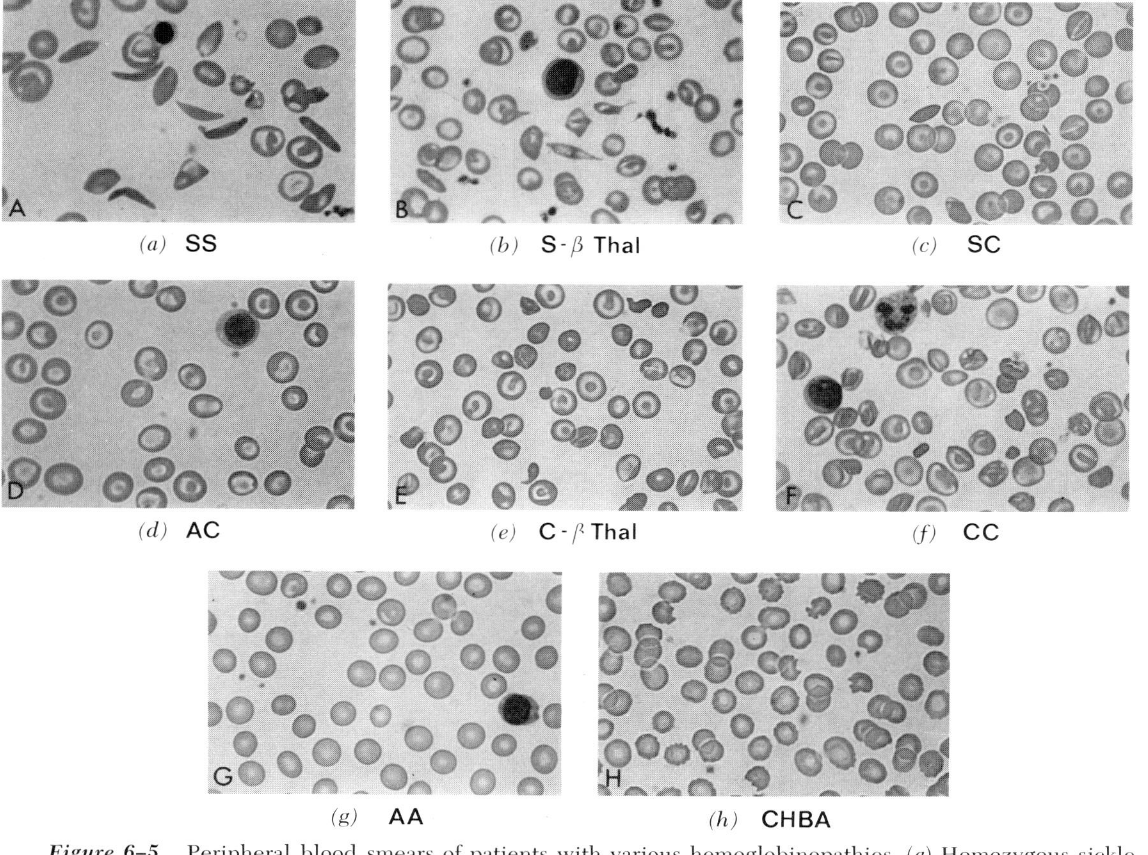

Figure 6–5. Peripheral blood smears of patients with various hemoglobinopathies. (*a*) Homozygous sickle cell anemia; (*b*) sickle/β thalassemia; (*c*) hemoglobin SC disease; (*d*) hemoglobin C trait; (*e*) hemoglobin C/β thalassemia; (*f*) homozygous hemoglobin C disease; (*g*) normal; (*h*) congenital Heinz body hemolytic anemia. (This figure was prepared by Ms. Carola Kapff.)

Hb A, and slightly increased amounts of Hb A_2 (Huisman, 1972). If α thalassemia is also present, the proportion of Hb C will be reduced (Weatherall et al., 1973). Stained films of AC blood show increased numbers of target cells, but these are much fewer in number than what is seen in homozygotes (Fig. 6–5*d*).

Patients who are doubly heterozygous for Hb C and Hb S have a disease of moderate severity. Hb C participates with Hb S in sickling more readily than does Hb A. Hb SC disease is discussed in detail in Chapter 7.

Patients who are *homozygous for Hb C* have a mild to moderate congenital hemolytic anemia (Ranney, 1953; Spaet et al., 1953; Singer, 1954; Terry et al., 1954; Hartz and Schwartz, 1955; Jensen et al., 1957; Smith and Krevans, 1959; Redetski et al., 1968). They are usually asymptomatic, although ill-defined arthralgia and abdominal pain and, rarely, hemorrhagic manifestations have been reported. Splenomegaly is generally present. As in other chronic hemolytic disorders, cholelithiasis and "aplastic crises" may occur. Packed cell volume generally ranges between 25 and 37 per cent, accompanied by a moderate reticulocytosis (4 to 8 per cent). Red cell survival is decreased with splenic sequestration (Singer, 1954; Jensen et al., 1957). Erythropoiesis is not sufficient to maintain a normal red cell mass (Jensen et al., 1957; Prindle and McCurdy, 1969). Mean corpuscular hemoglobin is normal but hemoglobin concentration per cell is increased (Murphy, 1968). The majority of erythrocytes on a dried stained blood film are target cells (Fig. 6–5*f*). These are plumper and of smaller diameter than the target cells seen in liver disease or biliary obstruction. Hb CC erythrocytes do not appear targeted when examined in a wet preparation (Murphy, 1968). However, their increased resistance to osmotic hemolysis indicates that these red cells have an increased ratio of surface area to volume (Charache et al., 1967). The mechanism by which red cells containing Hb C (or for that matter Hb S, D, or E) assume a target appearance and have abnormal osmotic fragility is not known. On electrophoresis, Hb C constitutes over 90 per cent of the total. Hb F may be slightly increased. No Hb A is seen.

The shortened life span of CC erythrocytes is probably based on the fact that they are abnormally rigid and therefore may traverse capillaries less readily than normal red cells. Hb CC blood and cell suspensions have increased viscosity and decreased filterability (Charache et al., 1967; Murphy, 1968). This is particularly true of microspherocytes which make up a minor population of CC red cells. The increased viscosity of CC red cells may be due in part to a marked increase in cell water bound to hemoglobin (Murphy, 1968). Deoxy Hb C is less soluble than deoxy Hb A (Charache et al., 1967), although this difference is much less than that for Hb S. The amino acid substitution (β6 Glu$\rightarrow$Lys) may favor intracellular aggregation of

Hb molecules. Hb CC cells will form intracellular crystals when suspended in a hypertonic medium (Kraus and Diggs, 1956; Wheby et al., 1956). A concentration of about 48 per cent Hb C is required for crystallization (Charache et al., 1967). Formation of these crystals is enhanced if the cells are deoxygenated (Charache et al., 1967). There is ultrastructural evidence that hemoglobin aggregation adjacent to the membrane precedes the formation of intracellular crystals (Lessin et al., 1969). This increased cellular rigidity probably does not require the presence of morphologically demonstrable inclusions.

The oxygen saturation curve of dilute solutions of Hb C is normal. Furthermore, Hb C has normal reactivity to 2,3-DPG and CO_2 (Bunn, 1972). However, the whole blood oxygen affinity of Hb C is reduced (Bellingham and Huehns, 1968). This may be explained in part by increased red cell 2,3-DPG due to decreased mean red cell age. The fact that CC red cells have a decrease of solvent water (Murphy, 1968) may affect intracellular pH and thus oxygen affinity. In addition, the aggregation of Hb C at high concentration, if oxygen-linked, may also influence intracellular oxygen affinity.

Hb D

Itano (1951) encountered a new hemoglobin variant which co-migrated with Hb S on moving-boundary electrophoresis but failed to sickle. It was labeled Hb D and was subsequently found to have the structure $\alpha_2\beta_2{}^{121\ \mathrm{Glu}\rightarrow\mathrm{Gln}}$ (Hb D-Punjab or D-Los Angeles) (Baglioni, 1962). Since that time, other variants have been found which also co-migrate with Hb S when electrophoresis is run at an alkaline pH. A number of these have been named with the prefix D followed by the locale where they were discovered (e.g., D-Ibadan [$\alpha_2\beta_2{}^{87\ \mathrm{Thr}\rightarrow\mathrm{Lys}}$], D-Iran [$\alpha_2\beta_2{}^{22\ \mathrm{Glu}\rightarrow\mathrm{Gln}}$], etc.) or the prefix G (e.g., G-Galveston [$\alpha_2\beta_2{}^{43\ \mathrm{Glu}\rightarrow\mathrm{Ala}}$], G-San Jose [$\alpha_2\beta_2{}^{7\ \mathrm{Glu}\rightarrow\mathrm{Gly}}$], etc.). None of these hemoglobins sickle, yet when they co-exist with Hb S in the doubly heterozygous state, they can affect sickling to a varying degree. For example, Hb S/D-Punjab is a much more severe condition than Hb S/D-Ibadan (Watson-Williams et al., 1965). The interaction of S and D hemoglobins is covered in detail in Chapter 7. Note that all the D (and G) hemoglobins involve an increase in one unit of positive charge per affected subunit: either a substitution of a neutral for a negatively charged amino acid or a substitution of a positively charged residue for a neutral one. Although they co-migrate with Hb S under standard electrophoretic conditions at alkaline pH, most of them can be separated from Hb S by electrophoresis on agar gel at pH 6.0 to 6.5. In addition to their failure to sickle, these hemoglobins also differ from Hb S in their solubility properties. Thus, heterozygotes for Hb D (or G) will have negative solubility tests for Hb S.

Hb D-Punjab (D-Los Angeles) is by far the most commonly encountered of the "D" hemoglobins (Vella and Lehmann, 1974). Among Sikhs of the Punjab region of India, Hb D has an incidence of 2 to 3 per cent. A number of homozygotes have been reported from various parts of the world (Bird and Lehmann, 1956; Chernoff, 1958; Stout et al., 1964; Ozsoylu, 1970). These individuals have normal hemoglobin values with no evidence of hemolysis. Red cell indices are generally within normal limits. Some individuals have had target cells and decreased osmotic fragility. Hemoglobin electrophoresis shows 95 per cent Hb D and normal amounts of Hb A_2. Tests for sickling are negative. This condition must be distinguished from the double heterozygous state Hb D/β_0 thalassemia. Appropriate family studies and careful measurement of red cell indices and Hbs A_2 and F are important in establishing the diagnosis. Individuals doubly heterozygous for Hb D and β thalassemia usually have mild anemia and minimal hemolysis (Rieder, 1976) in contrast to those with E/β thalassemia (see below) and S/β thalassemia (see Chapter 7).

Hb E ($\alpha_2\beta_2^{26\ Glu \rightarrow Lys}$)

Hb E is the third most prevalent hemoglobin variant worldwide. It is found primarily in Orientals, although it has also been reported in blacks (Bunn et al., 1976). The gene frequency in Thailand and Burma is approximately 15 per cent. The maintenance of such a high gene frequency may be a reflection of some type of balanced polymorphism, in which AE heterozygotes have improved fitness. Hb E co-migrates with Hb A_2 and Hb C on electrophoresis.

AE heterozygotes are commonly encountered. They have no hematological abnormalities. Hemoglobin electrophoresis reveals about 30 per cent Hb E; the remainder is Hb A. As in AS and AC heterozygotes, the proportion of Hb E decreases significantly in individuals who also have α thalassemia (Tuchinda et al., 1964; Wasi et al., 1969). In addition, the relative amount of Hb E in AE heterozygotes may decrease if they become iron-deficient (Wasi et al., 1968). Patients who are doubly heterozygous for Hb E and β thalassemia have an anemia which is variable in its severity but is generally more severe than in patients with Hb S/β thalassemia (Sturgeon et al., 1955; Chernoff, 1956).

Individuals homozygous for Hb E may have a mild anemia with somewhat reduced red cell survival. Others have normal hemoglobin levels with no evidence of hemolysis (Lehmann et al., 1956). Most of these individuals have significantly reduced mean corpuscular volume (Lehmann et al., 1956). Red cell indices may be difficult to interpret because both iron deficiency and the thalassemias are very prevalent in Southeast Asia. Target cells are seen on dried peripheral smears and, in keeping with this observation, there is increased resistance to osmotic lysis (Chernoff, 1955; Lehmann et al., 1956). The basis for these morphological abnormalities is unknown. It is curious that homozygotes for hemoglobins S, C, D, and E all have target cells and reduced osmotic fragility, although there are significant differences in red cell indices among these conditions.

Whole blood oxygen dissociation curves of EE homozygotes are shifted slightly to the right (Kolatat, 1964; Bellingham and Huehns, 1968), probably owing to increased red cell 2,3-DPG (Gacon et al., 1974). Purified Hb E has normal oxygen affinity, Bohr effect, and reactivity to 2,3-DPG (Bunn et al., 1972b; Gacon et al., 1974). Hemoglobin E appears to be relatively unstable to an oxidant stress (Frischer and Bowman, 1975) and may behave abnormally in subunit association (Pagnier et al., 1974). However, these phenomena probably have no clinical significance.

Hb G-Accra (Korle-Bu) ($\alpha_2\beta_2{}^{73\ \mathrm{Asp}\rightarrow\mathrm{Asn}}$)

Hemoglobin Korle-Bu is encountered quite frequently in central Africans. There are no clinical or hematological manifestations associated with either the heterozygous or the homozygous state (Lehmann and Huntsman, 1966). It is interesting that red cells from an individual homozygous for Hb Korle-Bu had a perfectly normal appearance on blood smear. No target cells were seen (Lehmann and Huntsman, 1968). This variant is of additional interest because of its interaction with Hb S. As discussed in detail in Chapter 7, Hb Korle-Bu behaves like Hb F in its failure to participate in the gelation of Hb S (Bookchin et al., 1970). Thus, individuals who are doubly heterozygous for Hb S and Hb Korle-Bu have a mild form of Hb "SD" disease.

Hb H (β_4)

Hb H is a tetramer composed of four normal β chains. This abnormal hemoglobin is seen in some individuals with α thalassemia (see Chapter 5).

Hb I ($\alpha_2{}^{16\ \mathrm{Lys}\rightarrow\mathrm{Glu}}\beta_2$)

Hb I is probably the most commonly encountered α-chain variant (Schneider et al., 1966). It has been found in individuals of various racial backgrounds. They have no apparent clinical or hematological abnormalities. Heterozygotes have about 25 per cent Hb I and 75 per cent Hb A. This proportion is similar to other α-chain variants (Fig. 6–4) and provides indirect evidence that each parent contributes two α-chain genes (see above). Biosynthetic studies of an AI heterozygote confirm that the reduced amount of Hb I in the red cell is due to a relative decrease in synthesis rather than preferential destruction of Hb I (Esan et al., 1970). The amino acid substitution in Hb I is in one of the invariant residues. Nevertheless, Hb I has perfectly normal functional properties (McDonald et al., 1974).

Chapter 7

SICKLE CELL ANEMIA AND RELATED DISORDERS

Sickling of red blood cells was first described in 1910 by Herrick who observed unusual shapes of red cells in blood smears of a black student. The dependence of sickling and unsickling on deoxygenation and reoxygenation was noted by Hahn and Gillespie in 1927. During the ensuing years this phenomenon was observed not only in patients with chronic hemolytic anemia and recurrent episodes of painful crises, but also in the blood cells of some normal, healthy individuals. According to Konotey-Ahulu (1974), the characteristics and familial incidence of recurrent severe painful crises were recognized for many years in Ghana, where the lowland incidence of sickle cell trait exceeds 20 per cent.

In the late 1940's, interrelationships among the asymptomatic healthy carriers, the severely anemic individuals who had recurrent painful crises, and the less commonly encountered patients who exhibited clinical syndromes intermediate between sickle cell trait and sickle cell anemia were largely clarified by family studies and by analysis of the hemoglobin of affected individuals. Neel (1947, 1949) and Beet (1949) presented formal genetic evidence which indicated that sickle cell trait represented the heterozygous state for a gene which in the homozygous state was manifest as sickle cell anemia.[1]

In-vitro studies by Ham and Castle (1940) established the relationship between sickling and increasing viscosity with decreasing oxygen tension. In the same year, I. J. Sherman demonstrated that

[1]In 1946, Accioly presented a brief but correct genetic analysis in an obscure Brazilian journal (see Azevêdo, 1973).

upon deoxygenation, sickle cells became birefringent. Castle reported these observations to Linus Pauling during a historic train ride in 1948. The following year Pauling, Itano, Singer, and Wells (1949) demonstrated that hemoglobin S differed electrophoretically from normal hemoglobin.

Pauling and his associates showed that most of the hemoglobin of individuals with sickle cell anemia was of the abnormal "S" type, with a greater net positive charge than normal hemoglobin (Hb A). Of the hemoglobin prepared from red cells of asymptomatic individuals with sickle cell trait, about 35 per cent was found to be of the S type while the remainder was normal Hb A. The introduction of zone electrophoresis and its adaptation to use in clinical laboratories led to the delineation of intermediate forms of sickling which resulted from the simultaneous presence of heterozygosity for Hb S and for another abnormal but nonsickling hemoglobin, e.g., Hb C or Hb D; similar syndromes of intermediate severity could also be attributed to the simultaneous presence of single genes for Hb S and for β thalassemia.

In 1950, Harris showed that deoxygenation of a concentrated solution of Hb S resulted in the formation of liquid crystals (or tactoids) accompanied by a marked increase in viscosity. Harris concluded that the sickling of red cells was due to polymerization of the abnormal hemoglobin into elongated fibers. Proof of the structural abnormality of sickle hemoglobin was provided by Ingram (1956, 1959), who demonstrated that Hb S differed from Hb A by the substitution of valine for glutamic acid in the sixth position of the β chain.

THE MOLECULAR BASIS OF SICKLING

The growing knowledge of the stereochemistry of hemoglobin function has allowed a more thorough understanding of how the sickling phenomenon takes place at the molecular level. The primary questions which need to be resolved are (1) What is the structure of the sickle polymer and how are Hb S molecules oriented within the polymer? (2) What is the sequence of events in the formation of the polymer? In order to approach these problems, it is necessary to derive a model which is in agreement with a number of experimental observations.

STRUCTURE OF THE SICKLE FIBER

Nature of Intermolecular Bonding

The sickling phenomenon must be explained ultimately by the substitution of the hydrophobic valine residue for glutamic acid at the sixth position of the β chain. This is probably due to a local alteration on the surface of the molecule at this site rather than to any widespread conformational changes. In dilute solution, hemoglobin S has entirely normal functional properties including oxygen affinity, heme-heme interaction, Bohr effect, and reactivity with 2,3-DPG and CO_2 (Allen and Wyman, 1954; Bunn, 1972; Rossi-Bernardi et al., 1975).

The early studies by Murayama (1966) indicated that the aggregation of sickle hemoglobin molecules involved hydrophobic bonding. Evidence supporting this conclusion included the demonstration of a negative temperature coefficient of gelation and the ability of nonpolar molecules such as propane and urea to disrupt sickling. Later studies by Bookchin and Nagel (1973b) showed that electrostatic bonds were also important in the polymerization of sickle hemoglobin molecules in the formation of the sickle fiber. They found that the minimum concentration of deoxygenated S hemoglobin required for gelling decreased progressively at ionic strengths below 0.15. Thus, salt exerted some degree of inhibition upon the aggregation of the hemoglobin molecules. Taken together, these results indicate that the polymerization of sickle hemoglobin is complex and cannot be explained by a simple two-point interaction between neighboring molecules.

Studies on the *interaction of sickle and nonsickle hemoglobins* have provided more specific information about the contact points between neighboring molecules in the sickle polymer. The early studies of Singer and Singer (1953) established that the presence of hemoglobin F increased the minimum concentration of total hemoglobin required for gelation (MGC). In fact, these MGC results suggested that hemoglobin F failed to participate at all in the sickling phenomenon. The Singers (1953) also demonstrated that hemoglobins A and C participated in gelling to an increasing degree, and that these interactions correlated with the clinical severity of the heterozygous states SA and SC.

Bookchin, Nagel, and Ranney extended this experimental approach to other hemoglobin variants having known amino acid substitutions (1967, 1970). They demonstrated that Hb C-Harlem ($\alpha_2\beta_2^{6\ Glu \rightarrow Val,\ 73\ Asp \rightarrow Asn}$) sickled less readily than hemoglobin S. Furthermore, hemoglobin Korle-Bu ($\alpha_2\beta_2^{73\ Asp \rightarrow Asn}$) participated in gelation with hemoglobin S less readily than did hemoglobin A (Bookchin et al., 1970). These observations, summarized in Table 7–1, indicated that the aspartate residue at position 73 of the beta chain is probably an important site in the polymerization of sickle hemoglobin. Subsequently, interaction of other hemoglobin variants with hemoglobin S has also been shown to be different from that of hemoglobin A. For example, hemoglobin O-Arab ($\alpha_2\beta_2^{121\ Glu \rightarrow Lys}$) and hemoglobin D-Punjab ($\alpha_2\beta_2^{121\ Glu \rightarrow Gln}$) both interact strongly with sickle hemoglo-

TABLE 7–1. Effect of Non-S Hemoglobins and Chemical Modifications on the Gelling of Sickle Hemoglobin

Experiment	MGC* (g/100 ml)	Reference
I. *Interaction of S and non-S Hbs (all deoxy)*		
100% S	24	Singer and Singer; 1953; Bookchin et al.; 1970
50% S, 50% O-Arab	21	Milner et al., 1970
50% S, 50% D-Punjab	24	Charache and Conley, 1967
50% S, 50% C	27	Singer and Singer, 1953
50% S, 50% A	30	Singer and Singer, 1953; Bookchin et al., 1970
50% S, 50% Korle-Bu	36	Bookchin et al., 1970
50% S, 50% F	36	" " " "
II. *Asymmetrical Hybrids (all deoxy)*		
40% S, 60% A: half hybrid ($\alpha_2\beta^S\beta^A$)	30	Bookchin et al., 1975
40% S, 60% A: no hybrid	30	" " "
40% S, 60% F: half hybrid ($\alpha_2\beta^S\gamma$)	39	" " "
40% S, 60% F: no hybrid	31	" " "
III. *Valency Hybrids*		
100% deoxy S (no hybrids)	24	Bookchin and Nagel, 1971
50% deoxy S, 50% CNMet-S (no hybrids)	30	" " " "
$\alpha_2^{CNMet}\beta_2^S$	34	Bookchin and Nagel, 1973a
$\alpha_2\beta_2^{S\text{-}CNMet}$	34	" " " "
$\alpha_2^{CNMet}\ \beta_2^{S\text{-}CNMet}$	No Gel	" " " "
IV. *Chemical Modifications (all deoxy)*		
Native Hb S ($\alpha_2\beta_2^S$)	23	Benesch et al., 1974
Pyridoxal derivatives:		
$\alpha_2^P\beta_2^S$	30	" " "
$\alpha_2\beta_2^{S\text{-}P}$	26	" " "
Native Hb S ($\alpha_2\beta_2^S$)	24	Nigen et al., 1974
Carbamylated derivatives:		
$\alpha_2^{CNO}\beta_2^S$	24	" " "
$\alpha_2\beta_2^{S\text{-}CNO}$	29	" " "
$\alpha_2^{CNO}\beta_2^{S\text{-}CNO}$	29	" " "

*Minimum concentration required for gelation (MGC) measured by method of Singer and Singer (1953) in 0.15 M phosphate, pH 7.35.

bin (McCurdy, 1960; Milner et al., 1970). Thus, β121 Glu may be another important contact point between neighboring molecules in the sickle polymer. The fact that hemoglobin Memphis ($\alpha_2^{23\ Glu \rightarrow Gln}\beta_2^{6\ Glu \rightarrow Val}$) gels less readily than does hemoglobin S (Kraus et al., 1966) indicates that this site on the alpha chain contributes to the polymerization of sickle hemoglobin molecules. Data on several different α-chain variants (Benesch et al., 1976) suggest that other nearby sites on the surface of the α chain are also involved in the aggregation of Hb S.

It is likely that non-S hemoglobins can participate in gelation by the formation of asymmetrical hybrid tetramers such as $\alpha_2\beta^S\beta^A$ (Moffat, 1974; Bookchin et al., 1975; Goldberg et al., 1975; Table 7–1). X-ray crystallographic data of Wishner et al. (1975) (described below) indicate that only one of the two β chains has an intermolecular contact at β6.

Optical Studies

Perutz and Mitchison (1950) studied the absorption of sickled erythrocytes with polarized light. Their results, when interpreted in terms of the later x-ray structural information, indicated that the dyad axis of the hemoglobin tetramers in the sickle hemoglobin fiber lay perpendicular to the fiber axis. More recent optical data of Hofrichter et al. (1973) confirm this early conclusion. Their measurements further indicate that the long molecular axis of the tetramer (65 Å dimension) is within 22 degrees of the fiber axis. These results impose an important constraint on the orientation of the hemoglobin molecule within the fiber lattice.

Ultrastructural Studies

A number of investigators have studied the ultrastructure of deoxygenated sickle hemoglobin, both in intact red cells and in concentrated solutions (Stetson, 1966; Murayama, 1966; White, 1968; Bertles and Döbler, 1969; Edelstein et al., 1973; Finch et al., 1973; Josephs et al., 1976). Electron micrographs demonstrate bundles of long straight fibers whose axis is parallel to the long axis of the sickled erythrocyte. Ultrastructural examination of a gel of deoxyhemoglobin S revealed fibers that each have a diameter of approximately 170 Å, with spacing between fibers ranging between 180 and 240 Å (Finch et al., 1973). A representative electron micrograph is shown in Figure 7–1 (Finch et al., 1973).

From a consideration of the dimensions of the tetrameric hemoglobin molecule (65 × 55 × 50 Å), Murayama (1966) and others concluded that the hemoglobin fiber is a helical polymer consisting of six strands (i.e., six molecules per cross-sectional area) (Fig. 7–2*A*). The detailed structure of the helix, including the pitch and the orientation of the hemoglobin molecules within the helix, is not entirely clear. X-ray diffraction data of Magdoff-Fairchild and coworkers (1972) were interpreted to support a six-stranded helical structure. However, other preparations of hemoglobin S have yielded a different morphological appearance on electron microscopy. Recent data of Josephs et al. (1976) obtained on intact sickled cells indicate that most of the Hb S fibers have helical structures (200 Å diameter) consisting of eight strands, with adjacent strands staggered by half a molecule (Fig. 7–2*B*).

Wishner et al. (1975, 1976) have done *x-ray diffraction analyses* of crystals of deoxyhemoglobin S grown in 10 to 15 per cent polyethylene glycol. The unit cell consists of two tetrameric molecules with the dimensions 63 × 184 × 52 Å. At both 5 Å and 3 Å resolution, there were no significant differences between the crystals of deoxy Hb S and deoxy Hb A in the regions around the $\beta 6$ residues. As dis-

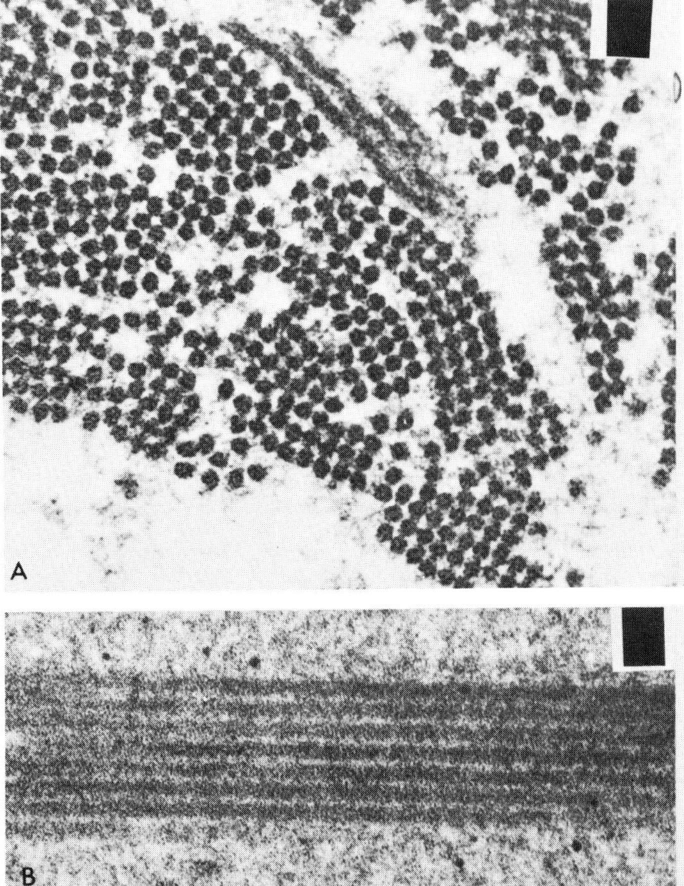

Figure 7-1. Electron micrographs of centrifuged pellet of deoxyhemoglobin S (× 325,000). *A*, Transverse section showing bundles of Hb S fibers. *B*, Longitudinal section showing parallel alignment of fibers. (From Finch, J. T., et al.: Proc. Natl. Acad. Sci. U.S.A. *70*:718, 1973.)

cussed in the section above on the interaction of sickle and nonsickle hemoglobins, a number of specific residues are known to affect the gelling behavior of sickle hemoglobin. These include β6 Val, β73 Asp, β121 Glu, and α23 Glu. The x-ray data of Wishner et al. indicate that these residues are all at sites of intermolecular contact, including interactions between molecules of the same strand and between molecules of adjacent strands. This is shown diagrammatically in Figure 7–3. Only one of the β6-valines is involved in an intermolecular interaction. These x-ray results indicate that adjacent interlocking strands are out of register by 32 Å (half the repeat distance) and rotated by half a turn. Such a structure does not fit the fiber model proposed by Finch et al. (1973) (Fig. 7–2A) but is compatible with the recent electron microscopic results of Josephs et al. (1976)

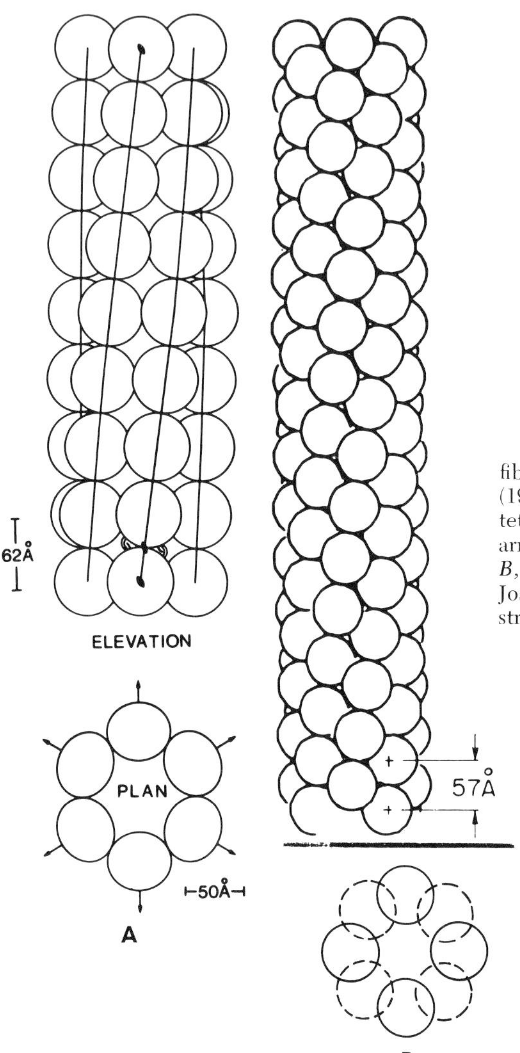

Figure 7–2. *A*, Model of Hb S fiber proposed by Finch et al. (1973) showing individual Hb S tetramers (represented as spheres) arranged in a six-stranded helix. *B*, Model of Hb S fiber proposed by Josephs et al. (1976) showing eight-stranded helix.

described above (Fig. 7–2*B*). It should be emphasized that the crystals analyzed by Wishner et al. (1975, 1976) were prepared under nonphysiological conditions and may not reflect the spatial orientation of molecules of deoxyhemoglobin S within the sickled red cell.

Participation of Small Molecules in the Sickling Phenomenon

In order to understand the sickling of red cells in vivo, it is necessary to determine how various intracellular mediators of hemoglobin function affect the polymerization of deoxy sickle hemoglobin.

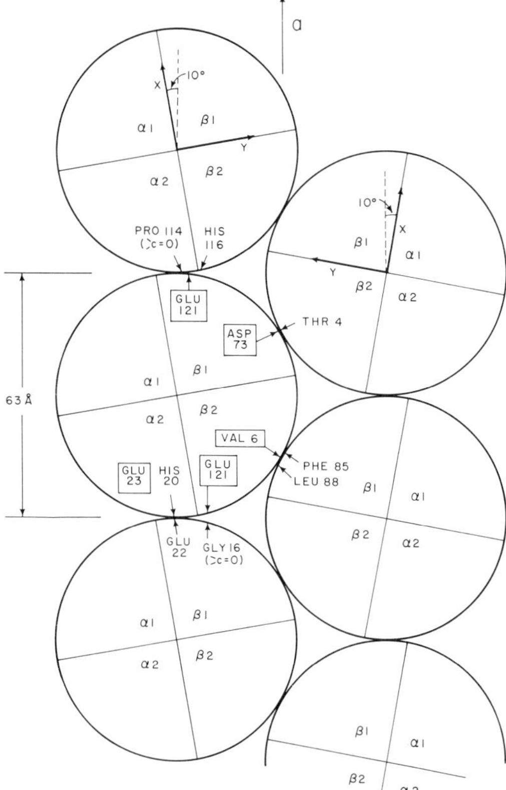

Figure 7–3. Intermolecular contacts between neighboring strands of Hb S. This model was constructed from x-ray crystallographic data of Wishner et al. (1975).

These factors include pH, ionic strength, organic phosphates (particularly 2,3-DPG), and PCO_2. The influence of these variables on sickling had not been studied until recently.

As pointed out in Chapters 2 and 3, 2,3-DPG is an important mediator of intracellular hemoglobin function. It has been demonstrated recently that 2,3-DPG facilitates the sickling phenomenon. Using analytical ultracentrifugation and viscosity measurements, Briehl and Ewert (1973) showed that the aggregation of deoxyhemoglobin S was enhanced by decreasing pH and increasing concentrations of 2,3-DPG. The promotion of sickling by 2,3-DPG has also been confirmed by measurements of viscosity (Paniker et al., 1972) and gelation (Nagel and Bookchin, 1974a) of Hb solutions and by intact cell preparations (Jensen et al., 1973a). X-ray diffraction data of Arnone (1972) indicate that there is a small, but significant, change in the three-dimensional structure of the N-terminal end of the β chain when 2,3-DPG is bound to hemoglobin. This alteration in the three-dimensional configuration may enhance sickling by an alteration at the primary binding site in the vicinity of β6-valine.

Water plays a complex role in the sickling phenomenon. Careful measurements of cell volumes indicate that, during sickling, the red cell loses osmotically active water (Masys et al., 1974). This phenomenon can be explained by a decrease in oncotic pressure due to hemoglobin polymerization. In addition, water molecules become incorporated into the fiber lattice. Transverse water proton relaxation times show a progressive increase in tumbling time for irrotationally bound water during the deoxygenation of sickle hemoglobin and its accompanying polymerization (Cottam et al., 1974; Chuang et al., 1975; Zipp et al., 1976).

Chemically Modified Sickle Hemoglobin

The gelation or polymerization of sickle hemoglobin has been studied following the chemical modification of the molecule at a number of sites. There has been a considerable amount of work done on the effects of cyanate on the sickling phenomenon both in vitro and in vivo following the introduction of sodium cyanate by Cerami and Manning (1971) as a potential form of therapy in sickle cell anemia. Nigen and his associates (1974) have shown that when sickle hemoglobin is selectively carbamylated at the N terminus of the α chain, there is little effect on minimum gelling concentration, whereas hemoglobin S carbamylated only on the β chain showed a decreased tendency to polymerize (Table 7–1). Recently, Benesch et al. (1974) reacted hemoglobin S selectively at the N terminus of the β chain with pyridoxal phosphate and found that this modification had a small effect on sickling. In contrast, they showed that selective blocking of the α-chain N-terminal amino group with pyridoxal sulfate caused a more marked increase in minimum gelling concentration (Table 7–1). These two sets of results seem to be in conflict. The effect of selective modifications at the N termini of α and β chains must be strongly dependent on the nature of the blocking groups. Recently, Roth and his associates (1974) found that nitrogen mustard, a potent alkylating agent, reacted specifically at β2-histidine (the second residue of the β chain) and caused a marked inhibition of sickling without a significant alteration in the functional properties of the molecule, such as oxygen affinity. Since this modification is close to the site of the primary amino acid substitution in sickle hemoglobin, it probably has a direct steric effect on the primary binding site. In contrast, selective chemical modification at the β93-sulfhydryl group appears not to have a profound effect on the polymerization of sickle hemoglobin (Yamaoka et al., 1974).

Effect of Conformation on Sickling

Since the early experiments of Hahn and Gillespie, it has been known that deoxygenation favors the sickling of red cells. Harris

(1950) subsequently demonstrated in cell-free solutions that the deoxy form of hemoglobin S was a prerequisite for the formation of liquid crystals (tactoids). Since hemoglobin undergoes a marked change in quaternary conformation upon deoxygenation, it has been assumed that this structural transition opens up one or more binding sites on the hemoglobin S molecule necessary for its aggregation. Bookchin and Nagel (1971) have found that the T quaternary conformation is not required for the participation of non-S hemoglobins in gelling. For example, mixtures of cyanmethemoglobin A (R structure) and deoxyhemoglobin S gel equally as readily as mixtures containing equivalent amounts of deoxyhemoglobin A and deoxyhemoglobin S. Further studies by Bookchin and Nagel (1973a) have been designed to assess the importance of the tertiary conformation of the subunits in the hemoglobin tetramers participating in aggregation. They examined hemoglobin hybrids in which either the α or the β chain of hemoglobin S was locked in the r tertiary structure by converting the heme to cyanmet. They observed that these hybrid hemoglobins, $\alpha_2^{CNMet}\beta_2^{S}$ and $\alpha_2\beta_2^{S\text{-}CNMet}$, both gelled at a hemoglobin concentration approximately 50 per cent higher than $\alpha_2\beta_2$ (see Table 7–1). These findings were unexpected because they implied that the tertiary conformation of the β^S chain was not essential in the sickling process. These studies are somewhat hard to interpret, since electron exchange probably occurs following preparation and incubation of these mixed liganded hemoglobin hybrids. This is a very difficult phenomenon to measure or to control. By this means, some of the hybrids would be converted into homogeneous tetramers, $\alpha_2\beta_2^S$ and α_2^{CNMet} $\beta_2^{S\text{-}CNMet}$. Such a phenomenon would blunt any intrinsic difference in the sickling of the two hybrids.

Deoxyhemoglobin is not the only form of hemoglobin which is capable of undergoing a transition to the T quaternary structure. Perutz (1974) has found that methemoglobin, particularly at low pH and in the presence of organic phosphates, can assume a T-like structure. Briehl and Ewert (1974) have presented ultracentrifugation data showing that concentrated solutions of methemoglobin S can polymerize in the presence of organic phosphates. The binding of nitric oxide (NO) to the heme groups of hemoglobin also results in a species which is capable of assuming the T conformation (Salhany et al., 1974). Briehl and Salhany (1975) have also found that NO-hemoglobin S, under appropriate conditions, can polymerize into a gel. Both ultracentrifugation data and the demonstration of birefringence support this conclusion.

Sequence of Events in Sickling

Until recently the great majority of experimental studies on the polymerization of sickle hemoglobin have been assumed to be equilibrium measurements. However, the sickling phenomenon is markedly affected by kinetic considerations. The polymerization of deoxyhemoglobin S is very strongly concentration-dependent, so that above a critical concentration there is a concerted transition from hemoglobin sol to hemoglobin gel. This phenomenon was shown quite convincingly by ultracentrifugation studies (Williams, 1973; and Briehl and Ewert, 1973). Malfa and Steinhart (1974), Harris and Bensusan (1975), and Hofrichter et al. (1974) have found that the polymerization of a solution of sickle hemoglobin can appear abruptly after a delay of up to several hours under appropriate incubation conditions. It has been estimated by Hofrichter and his associates (1974) that the rate of aggregation of sickle hemoglobin varies as the 30th power of hemoglobin concentration:

$$1/t_d = k(C/C_s)^n$$

where t_d = delay time, C = hemoglobin concentration, C_s = solubility (see below), and $n \cong 30$. Note that the delay time is markedly affected by small changes in hemoglobin concentration or solubility.

From their experimental observations, Hofrichter et al. (1973, 1974) proposed that sickling occurs in stages, as shown in Figure 7–4: nucleation followed by fiber growth and alignment of adjacent fibers. The last process is entropically driven and proceeds relatively slowly.

In some experimental systems, notably ultracentrifugation (Williams, 1973; Briehl and Ewert, 1973), no small aggregates are observed in solutions in equilibrium with the sickle gel. In contrast, Wilson et al. (1974) obtained quasi-elastic light scattering, data indicating demonstrable pregelation aggregation. Concerted gel formation implies an equilibrium between fibers or filaments and single

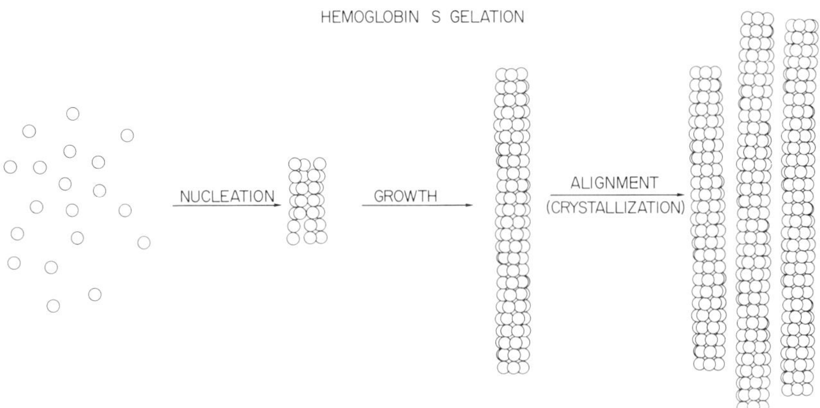

Figure 7–4. Model for the polymerization of deoxyhemoglobin S into aligned fibers. (From Hofrichter, J., et al.: Proc. Natl. Acad. Sci. U.S.A. *70*:3604, 1973.)

molecules of deoxyhemoglobin S, whereas the results of light-scattering experiments suggest that hemoglobin S molecules are bifunctional and that any size aggregate can combine with any other size aggregate in a linear array. Moffat and Gibson (1974), whose studies were based on changes in turbidity with temperature jump, favor a rate-limiting formation of nuclei containing a minimum of 15 deoxy Hb S molecules, followed by polymerization of the nuclei to one another or (more likely) by the addition of individual molecules to the nuclei. Aggregates of hemoglobin S adjacent to the membrane of the intact red cell may provide an initial site for nucleation. Sundin and Williams (1976) have shown that the addition of "inside out" red cell ghosts to concentrated solutions of deoxyhemoglobin S shortens the delay time. The lack of definitive information about the molecular structure of filaments of deoxyhemoglobin S and the different methods used to observe pregelation events make the detailed interpretation of the kinetic data uncertain.

Because of the complex kinetic factors discussed above, the commonly used determinations of sickling such as minimum gelling concentration and viscosity are not true equilibrium measurements. It is likely that at equilibrium there is a simple biphasic system consisting of sickle fiber (containing at least 30 molecules) and free tetramers. If so, sickling can be measured most precisely and directly by a determination of *solubility* (Hofrichter et al., 1976). This can be done by centrifugation, separating the dense gel from the sol. The hemoglobin concentration of the supernatant (sol phase) provides a measure of solubility. The slow transition from isotropic (randomly oriented) to anisotropic (aligned) fibers probably has little effect on solubility.

It is apparent that the sickling phenomenon in the intact red cell must be largely dependent upon kinetic considerations because the extent of deoxygenation during circulation through the capillary bed is strongly time-dependent. This subject is considered in detail in the next section and in a recent review by Eaton et al. (1975).

This large body of experimental information represents a considerable advance in the understanding of the molecular basis of the sickling phenomenon. However, the orientation of the individual sickle hemoglobin tetramers within the fiber is not yet established. Thus, the specific intermolecular contacts are not known. Such information would be useful in designing a suitable drug for the inhibition of sickling in vivo.

CELLULAR BASIS OF SICKLING

The growing body of information on the molecular basis of sickling, summarized in the previous section, provides only a partial understanding of the mechanisms underlying the clinical manifestations of sickle cell anemia. The *cellular* basis of sickling is dependent upon a number of additional factors such as the composition and concentration of the hemoglobin within the red cell, the age of the cell, the integrity of its membrane, the rate of extent of oxygen release as well as alterations or abnormalities in the microcirculation. In common with other types of hemolytic anemia, sickled red cells are unduly rigid and, as a result, have a shortened life span. In addition, plugging of the microvasculature by sickled red cells leads to tissue ischemia. All Hb S-containing cells will acquire the classic sickle-shape deformity upon deoxygenation because of the intracellular polymerization of hemoglobin (see Figures 7–5 and 7–6). This process is ordinarily reversible upon reoxygenation of the cell. However, repeated sickling induces sufficient membrane damage to certain susceptible cells that the rigidity and sickle shape persist, even after the cell has been reoxygenated. It is likely that both processes contribute to the various clinical findings encountered in the sickle syndromes.

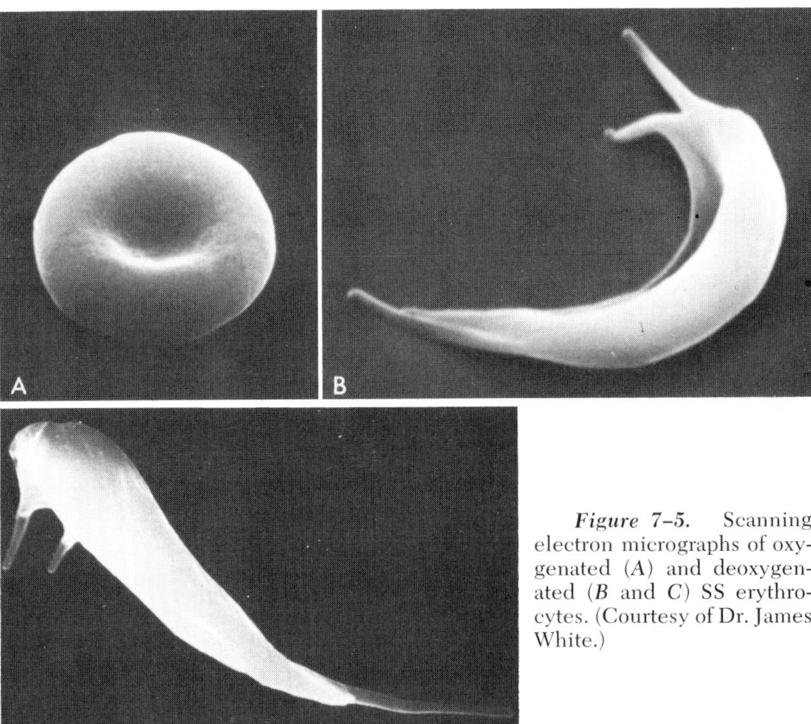

Figure 7–5. Scanning electron micrographs of oxygenated (*A*) and deoxygenated (*B* and *C*) SS erythrocytes. (Courtesy of Dr. James White.)

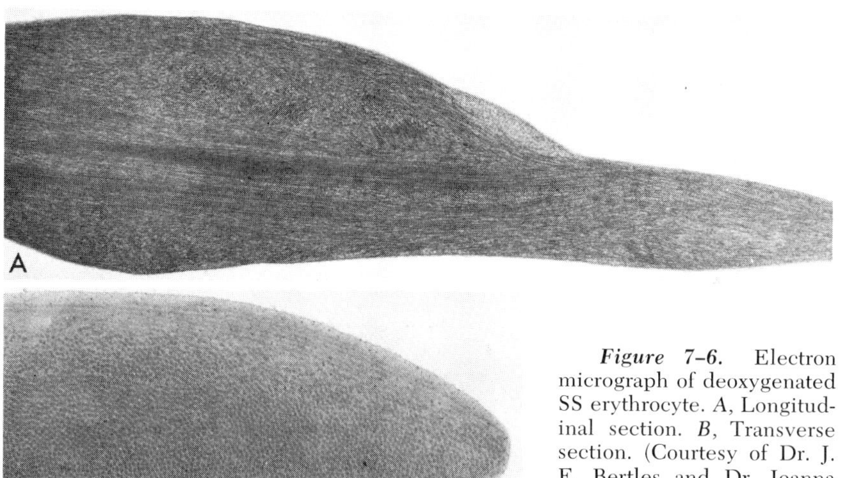

Figure 7–6. Electron micrograph of deoxygenated SS erythrocyte. *A*, Longitudinal section. *B*, Transverse section. (Courtesy of Dr. J. F. Bertles and Dr. Joanna Döbler.)

The "Sickle Cycle"

When the oxygen tension of the Hb S-containing red cell is lowered to a critical point, intracellular polymerization of hemoglobin occurs, leading to the formation of the classic sickle shape (see Figure 7–5). This phenomenon can be monitored by direct morphological examination or by indirect measurements such as viscosity or filterability. The oxygen saturation at which a given cell sickles is determined by a number of factors. As Figure 7–7 shows, the presence of non-S hemoglobin has a profound effect on cellular sickling comparable to its influence on gelation of a cell-free solution (Table 7–1). Griggs and Harris (1956) showed that, under physiologic conditions, the sickling of red cells from homozygotes was first noted at O_2 saturations below 85 per cent. Sickling was nearly complete at 38 per cent O_2 saturation. A progressive increase in whole blood viscosity paralleled the appearance of sickled cells. In contrast, no sickling of AS red cells was observed until the O_2 saturation fell below 40 per cent. These in-vitro studies provide a crude assessment of the sickling phenomenon in vivo. SS homozygotes would be expected to have a significant amount of sickling at oxygen tensions normally encountered in the capillary and venous circulation. However, kinetic considerations discussed below make such predictions unreliable. The fact that AS heterozygotes rarely have clinical manifestations is not surprising in view of the severe and nonphysiologic degree of hypoxemia necessary to induce the sickling deformity.

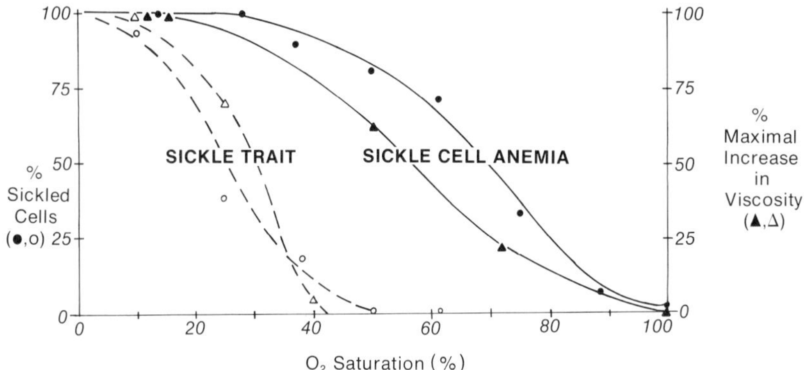

Figure 7–7. Measurement of viscosity and percentage of sickled forms in SS and AS red cell suspension at different oxygen saturations. (Figure prepared from data of Griggs and Harris [1956].)

The precise chain of events which initiates vaso-occlusive crises is not well understood. It is likely that rigid sickled cells (deformed by deoxygenation or irreversibly sickled) obstruct blood at the capillary level. The resulting stasis promotes local hypoxia, deoxygenation of red cells, and further sickling. In this way, the area of vaso-occlusion is amplified (Harris et al., 1956). Local anatomical and physiological factors such as distribution of blood vessels and rate of blood flow help to determine where and when this vicious cycle will occur. Of equal importance is the relationship between the rate of sickling of a partially deoxygenated red cell and the duration of its flow through the microcirculation. In the past few years, a variety of elegant techniques have been applied to this problem. If oxygen is rapidly and exhaustively removed by chemical means, such as addition of dithionite, sickling is very rapid. Zarkowsky and Hochmuth (1975) observed the characteristic deformities of SS red cells within 2 seconds of deoxygenation. However, the rate of sickling of partially deoxygenated cells is a more physiologically relevant consideration (Allison, 1956; Charache and Conley, 1964).

A number of investigators have noted an intermediate phase prior to the assumption of the classic "holly leaf" sickle shape. Padilla et al. (1973) observed a loss of the flicker phenomenon, indicating an increase in cell rigidity that preceded the shape change. Messer and Harris (1970) documented this intermediate phase of cell rigidity by filtration measurements of rapidly deoxygenated SS red cells. Rampling and Sirs (1973) also noted nonspecific abnormalities that preceded true sickling. Recently, Messer et al. (1975) have correlated the rheological properties of deoxygenated SS red cells with serial electron micrographs. They found that during the intermediate phase in which increased rigidity was first detected, there was no ultrastructural evidence of aligned fibers. In contrast, the formation of the classic elongated sickle shape was accompanied by the presence of parallel fibers similar to those shown in Figure 7–5. This intermediate cellular phase of sickling may be closely analogous to the intermediate phase of gelation mentioned above, in which the sickle fibers are randomly oriented.

The mean in-vivo capillary circulation time varies widely from one tissue to another but it ranges between 0.5 and 2.0 seconds. Most SS cells will not have enough time to assume the sickle shape during their rapid passage through capillaries. Jensen et al. (1960) and Serjeant et al. (1973) found that the percentage of sickled forms in venous blood from various sites correlated inversely with the oxygen saturation of the blood sample. However, most if not all of this sickling probably occurred following the transit of blood through capillaries. Beyond that point, the rigid cell should pose no threat to the perfusion of the tissue. The fact that sickle infarcts rarely occur in the myocardium despite its very large oxygen extraction is probably due to rapid circulation through this tissue. Because of these kinetic considerations it is unlikely that the transformation of red cells into sickled forms is the initial event that triggers a vaso-occlusive crisis. However, it is plausible that red cells in the intermediate phase of sickling are sufficiently rigid that they could impede blood flow and initiate the "vicious sickle cycle."

Irreversibly Sickled Cells

Upon examination of peripheral blood films of patients with sickle cell anemia, anywhere from 2 to 30 per cent of the red cells have the characteristic elongated sickle deformity (see Figure 6–5). The presence of such cells is surprising, since the red cells in a peripheral blood smear are fully oxygenated and therefore would not be expected to sickle. Electron microscopy of such cells fails to reveal any aligned sickle fibers so characteristic of deoxygenated sickle cells (Bertles and Döbler, 1969). Thus, these cells have a permanently sickled shape even in the absence of any intracellular polymerization of hemoglobin. These observations indicate that such cells have a damaged membrane which is no longer capable of assuming the normal biconcave disc shape upon reoxygenation.

Irreversibly sickled cells (ISC's) are unduly rigid. Indeed, the presence of these cells explains why oxygenated SS blood has a higher viscosity than normal blood having a comparable packed cell volume (Chien et al., 1970). As mentioned above, these cells may be responsible in part for the plugging of capillaries and, perhaps, the initiation of vaso-occlusive crises. Because of their rigidity, ISC's have a markedly shortened life span (Bertles and Milner, 1968) and contribute significantly to the hemolytic anemia of patients with SS disease. The percentage of ISC's in the peripheral blood provides no insight concerning the *turnover* of these cells. Because of their high MCHC, these cells are dense and can readily be separated from other red cells by centrifugation. Bertles and Milner (1968) have shown that these cells have a relatively low content of Hb F. It is likely that cells that are not well endowed with Hb F are at a distinct disadvantage from the time they emerge from the bone marrow. Without the protection provided by Hb F, these cells have a high probability of repeated sickling and within a few days become ISC's.

Shen et al. (1949) were able to generate ISC's in vitro by prolonged incubation of deoxygenated blood from a patient with sickle cell anemia. Tosteson et al. (1956) showed that such treatment induces a membrane lesion, with enhanced leakage of potassium ion from the cell. Deoxygenation of SS red cells also results in a significant loss of cell water (Masys et al., 1974). In addition to changes in cation permeability, sickling also causes disruption in the anatomical integrity of the red cell membrane. With the use of phase-optic cinematography, Padilla et al. (1973) showed that repetitive sickling can lead to fragmentation and loss of small segments of membrane (microspherules) in excess of hemoglobin. This phenomenon may explain why a small population of SS red cells has increased osmotic fragility, even though the majority of cells are less fragile than normal (Harris et al., 1956). Repeated injury to the red cell membrane eventually leads to the formation of an irreversibly sickled cell.

Recently, a number of investigators have attempted to unravel the physico-chemical factors which put the ISC membrane into rigor mortis. Normal red cells lose their pliability and become rigid echinocytes when depleted of ATP (Weed et al., 1969). Furthermore, stiffening of red cell ghosts is also correlated with accumulation of membrane-bound calcium. Weed et al. (1969) proposed that red cell ATP may serve to chelate calcium, thereby preserving the pliability of the membrane. Jensen et al. (1973c) observed a similar relationship when ISC's were artificially generated during in-vitro incubations. They found a close relationship between the decline of red cell ATP and the generation of ISC's. Furthermore, the formation of ISC's was markedly inhibited by omission or chelation of Ca^{++} during the incubation. Subsequently, low levels of ATP (Glader et al., 1976) and high levels of membrane-bound calcium (Eaton et al., 1973; Palek, 1973) were demonstrated in naturally occurring ISC's. Upon deoxygenation, the influx of extracellular Ca^{++} into SS red cells was markedly enhanced, while deoxygenation had no effect on calcium leak into normal red cells (Eaton et al., 1973).

The precise role of calcium in the pathogenesis of ISC's is controversial. The fact that a calcium ionophore can induce a temporary retention of the sickled shape after reoxygenation (Eaton et al., 1975) implies that Ca^{++} may be directly responsible for the generation of

ISC's. However, Palek et al. (1975) found that the rate of transformation of SS red cells into ISC's was not influenced by either intracellular ATP or extracellular calcium. They have pointed out the difficulties in distinguishing between Ca^{++}-loaded stiff echinocytes and naturally formed ISC's. It is likely that the primary membrane lesion in ISC's is induced by intracellular polymerization of hemoglobin and that enhanced Ca^{++} influx, like K^{+} efflux, is a secondary phenomenon. In support of this conclusion, Clark and Shohet (1976) have found that normal red cell ghosts reconstituted with Hb S were able to form irreversibly sickled forms even in the absence of calcium.

The direct interaction of Hb with the inner surface of the red cell membrane may also affect the rheology of SS red cells. Red cell membranes are capable of binding more Hb S than Hb A (Fischer et al., 1975). Furthermore, in AS reticulocytes, newly synthesized β^{S} chains are more adherent to red cell stroma than are β^{A} chains (Bank et al., 1974) and, in some cases, have a faster turnover rate compatible with membrane binding (DeSimone et al., 1974a; Shaeffer et al., 1976). These phenomena may account for the presence of dense precipitates of hemoglobin adherent to the membranes of both SS and AS red cells which have been observed by dark-field and phase microscopy (Schneider et al., 1972). The inclusions from AS red cells were found to contain more Hb S than Hb A.

Irrespective of the sequence of steps leading to its formation, the ISC's owe their increased rigidity to a permanently altered membrane protein lattice. Lux and John (1975) observed that the sickled shape of ISC's was preserved even after hemoglobin-free ghosts had been extracted with triton, which removed membrane lipid and the majority of membrane protein. The remaining protein was shown to be composed primarily of spectrin and red cell actin.

Oxygenation of Sickle Blood

Since the sickling phenomenon depends on the formation of deoxyhemoglobin S, it is important to define the oxygen binding properties of sickle red cells. As mentioned above, Hb S in dilute solution has normal oxygen equilibria. However, SS blood has markedly decreased oxygen affinity (Bromberg and Jensen, 1967b). Like patients with other types of anemia, SS homozygotes have elevated red cell 2,3-DPG (Charache et al., 1970). However, P_{50} values of SS blood are higher than would be predicted from red cell 2,3-DPG values, and there is not a significant correlation between P_{50} and red cell 2,3-DPG (Seakens et al., 1973). In view of the intracellular polymerization of deoxyhemoglobin S, Allen and Wyman (1954) predicted, from thermodynamic principles, that high concentrations of Hb S would have low oxygen affinity, but they did not have adequate methods to test their prediction. Recently, May and Huehns (1972b) showed that the P_{50} of SS red cells suspended in artificial media rose sharply when the MCHC was increased from 10 g/100 ml to 30 g/100 ml, while the oxygen affinity of AA red cells was nearly unaffected. Seakens et al. (1973) found that SS red cells having the highest MCHC (irreversibly sickled cells) had the highest P_{50} values. As Rossi-Bernardi et al. (1975) have pointed out, the decreased oxygen affinity of SS red cells is a two-edged sword. On the one hand, the right-shifted curve greatly facilitates oxygen unloading (see Chapter 3) and helps to explain why SS homozygotes tolerate severe degrees of anemia surprisingly well when they are free of crises or infection. On the other hand, decreased oxygen affinity promotes the formation of deoxyhemoglobin and, as a result, promotes sickling.

EPIDEMIOLOGY OF SICKLING

Sickle cell syndromes are found among Africans, Greeks, Italians, Saudis, Israeli Arabs, and the Veddoids of Southern India. Most of the sickle cell anemia found in the New World is of African origin, but sickle cell thalassemia is far commoner in Americans of Greek or Italian origin than is sickle cell anemia.

The sickle cell gene is found largely in the tropical parts of Africa in which malaria parasites flourished over past centuries. Prevalence of sickle trait is as high as 30 per cent in some areas of Africa. During the early surveys of sickling in Africa, it was stated that sickle cell anemia was rare or absent despite the high frequencies of sickle cell trait. The laboratory evaluations which formed the basis for these statements were incomplete: in populations affected with hookworm and with malaria, anemia and splenomegaly were frequent, and the diagnosis of sickling was based solely on sickle cell preparations. Presumably the severely affected sicklers died in childhood, and the laboratory methods used did not permit the identification of mild sicklers. A large loss of Hb S genes from the gene pool due to the loss of homozygotes would be expected in populations with high gene frequency for Hb S. The maintenance of such high gene frequencies implies a selective advantage for heterozygotes for hemoglobin S. Allison (1954, 1957a) suggested that a balanced polymorphism was based upon a selective advantage possessed by individuals heterozygous for hemoglobin S, as compared with normal individuals, with respect to infections with falciparum malaria. The protection conferred by sickle cell trait appears to reduce the mortality rate of children with cerebral malaria. Parasitemia can be demonstrated in sickle cell trait or anemia with falciparum malarial infections but the degree of parasitemia appears to be somewhat lower in sickle cell trait than in individuals with normal hemoglobin. In-vitro studies by Luzzato et al. (1970) provide information on the mechanism by which sickle trait provides protection against malaria. Once an AS cell is parasitized, it is more likely to sickle. This rigid cell is then removed from the circulation and destroyed. Power's (1975) detailed analysis of this model offers an explanation for the restriction of this protection to children with falciparum malaria. With the declining incidence of malaria, the selective advantage of heterozygotes in resistance to infection no longer affects gene frequencies.

SICKLE CELL TRAIT

Sickle cell trait is found in high incidence in many populations of African ancestry; about 8 per cent of American blacks and up to 30 per cent of certain African populations are affected.

Clinical Features

The presence of sickle cell trait is rarely associated with clinical manifestations. While spontaneous hematuria or splenic infarction at high altitudes occurs in AS individuals, such an association should not be regarded as unequivocal evidence of the pathogenicity of sickle cell trait under ordinary circumstances. The occurrence of spontaneous hematuria in sickle cell trait is so rare that the coexistence of another condition, such as an anomaly in the renal microcirculation, in affected individuals is very likely. Diminished vasa recta in the renal medulla have been reported (Statius van Eps et al., 1970). Most individuals with sickle cell trait have an impairment in the ability to make concentrated urine (Schlitt and Keitel, 1960) due to small medullary infarcts. However, renal acidification is normal (Oster et al., 1976).

Reports of sudden death following severe muscular exercise in individuals with sickle cell trait have lacked pertinent information concerning other potential but undetected illnesses in the patients. Observation that sickle cell trait is found with the expected frequency among black professional football players suggests that the tolerance of individuals with sickle cell trait for severe muscular exertion is not impaired (Murphy, 1973). Flying at high altitudes in unpressurized aircraft has apparently resulted in splenic infarctions in a few individuals with sickle trait. Nearly all the vaso-occlusive phenomena seen in SS disease have been described in individuals with sickle trait. (For references see Harris and Kellemeyer, 1970.) However, the significance of these anecdotal reports is difficult to assess in view of the very large group of AS individuals at risk. It is safe to conclude that vaso-occlusive complications are extremely rare in those with sickle trait. Nevertheless, it would seem prudent for individuals with sickle cell trait to avoid exposure to potentially low ambient oxygen, e.g., high altitude flying without pressurization[2] or scuba diving. If general anesthesia is properly administered, AS individuals are not subject to any added risk (Searle, 1972). However, there may be increased morbidity in the application of a tourniquet to an injured extremity of an individual with sickle trait (Stein and Urbaniak, 1975). Data are now being accumulated about the relationship between sickle cell trait and a variety of other diseases (Heller, 1974). It is not possible to make firm statements on the basis of evidence at hand. Certainly, the denial of employment or of life insurance to individuals with sickle cell trait on the grounds of increased risk of illness or of early death is not justified.

Diagnosis

Individuals with sickle trait have normal blood counts. Red cell morphology is usually normal, although some AS individuals may have occasional target cells. The diagnosis of sickle trait is established by the combination of a positive test for sickling (such as the metabisulfite slide test or solubility test [Sickledex]) and a characteristic pattern on hemoglobin electrophoresis. If performed properly, the metabisulfite test is highly reliable, but since it requires a microscope and a skilled observer it is not suitable for large-scale screening or field studies. Several solubility tests are commercially available in kit form. They are easy to perform and quite reliable, but occasional false positives have been noted in individuals with unstable hemoglobins (Fairbanks and Pettit, 1972). Hemoglobin electrophoresis reveals about 60 per cent Hb A, 35 per cent Hb S, and normal amounts of Hb A_2. The proportion of Hb S in AS individuals may be diminished in the presence of folic acid deficiençy (Heller et al., 1963b), iron deficiency (Levere et al., 1964), or α thalassemia (De Simone et al., 1974b; Steinberg et al., 1974).

Screening Programs

The advisability of screening programs has become a controversial issue. Certainly the appropriate tests should be available to all individuals who want to know if they or their children have a sickling disorder. Occasionally screening clinics detect individuals with clinically significant disorders such as SS, SC, or S/thalassemia.

---

[2]Even pressurized cabins in commercial airplanes flying at high altitudes (40,000 ft) have a relatively low atmospheric PO_2 (120 mm Hg) corresponding to an alveolar PO_2 of 66 mm Hg (normal = 107 mm Hg) (Liebman et al., 1976).

Few people derive any obvious benefit from the knowledge that they have sickle trait unless they are engaged in occupations that may confer increased risk. In addition, establishing the diagnosis of sickle trait may be useful to some individuals who are planning families. If screening programs are employed, it is very important that confidentiality be preserved and that affected individuals have the benefit of adequate education and counseling. Such services are now being provided in a number of Sickle Centers in various urban areas in the United States.

SICKLE CELL DISEASE

The term sickle cell disease generally includes the symptomatic forms of sickling: sickle cell anemia (SS disease, homozygosity for Hb S), sickle cell–hemoglobin D disease (SD disease/$\alpha_2^A\beta^S\beta^{121\ Gln}$), sickle cell–hemoglobin O disease (SO disease/$\alpha_2^A\beta^S\beta^{121\ Lys}$), sickle cell–hemoglobin C disease (SC disease), and sickle cell–β thalassemia of either the S/β^0 or S/β^+ type. Other rarer forms of sickle cell disease may also be found. The approximate order of decreasing severity is SS, SD, SO, SC; the variable severity of sickle β thalassemia probably reflects the type of thalassemia present. Since β thalassemia is itself so heterogeneous in its clinical severity, the wide spectrum of clinical expression of S/β thalassemia might be expected: the disorder may be as severe as sickle cell anemia or nearly asymptomatic, detected in the course of hospitalization for other illnesses. However, the possibility remains that other factors, e.g., altered primary structure of Hb S, or different hemoglobin-membrane interactions, might influence the manifestations of sickle β thalassemia in different individuals. The presence of α thalassemia probably ameliorates sickle cell anemia (Van Enk et al., 1972).

While some clinical features of the genetic variants of sickling may differ from those of sickle cell anemia (e.g., the frequency of severe retinal lesions of SC disease), in general the differences in symptoms between sickle cell anemia and the genetic variants of sickling are in the severity and frequency of the manifestations of sickling. Powars (1975) has emphasized the observation that the deaths in young children associated with infection are nearly confined to patients with sickle cell anemia.

The manifestations of sickle cell disease may be considered in four major groups:

(1) Chronic hemolytic anemia.

(2) Systemic manifestations, including impairment of growth and development and increased susceptibility to infections.

(3) Vaso-occlusive or painful "crises"–episodes of pain of varying severity which come on over a few minutes or hours and last for a

few hours or several days. The pain may involve one or more sites; pleural, abdominal, and bone or muscular pain are common. The pain is attributed to the occlusion of small vessels by sickled cells with release of kinins and, in many instances, microinfarctions.

(4) Organ damage which is the consequence of multiple microvaso-occlusive events and of chronic anemia. Organ damage is to some extent cumulative, and adults with severe sickle cell anemia have greater or lesser impairment of a number of different organ systems; cardiac, pulmonary, renal, skeletal, cerebral, and hepatic damage may all be evident.

Anemia of Sickle Cell Disease

The anemia of sickle cell disease is due to accelerated red cell destruction, which is independent of red cell age. The populations of red cells which have the greatest proportions of fetal hemoglobin do, however, appear to survive longer than do the red cells which contain little or no fetal hemoglobin (Bertles and Milner, 1968). Patients with sickle cell anemia are usually jaundiced, but this finding is not a constant feature of the other sickling disorders.

The marked shortening of red cell survival places a high demand on erythropoiesis. Temporary decline in erythropoiesis consequent to infection results in a more severe anemia. If the initial clinical observations on the patient are made as the infection is subsiding, a remarkable reticulocytosis (up to 50 per cent) may be observed. This recovery phase from temporary bone marrow suppression is probably more common than a true hyperhemolytic crisis, although the latter may be observed, particularly in children. Glucose-6-phosphate dehydrogenase (G-6-PD) deficiency is found in the expected frequency in patients with sickle cell anemia, and some examples of hyperhemolytic crises have been associated with this deficiency (Smits et al., 1969). In other patients an increasingly severe anemia probably represents an episode of acute splenic sequestration.

The greatly increased erythropoiesis of sickle cell anemia leads to a significant increase in requirements for folic acid, and evidence of folate deficiency is sometimes encountered. In patients who have a good dietary intake, it is doubtful whether supplemental folic acid is necessary, but in the presence of infection or when dietary intake is poor, the administration of 1 or 2 mg per day of folic acid is often recommended. The high folic acid content of milk usually prevents folic acid deficiency in children. Iron deficiency is occasionally and unexpectedly encountered in sicklers (Peterson et al., 1974a). Medicinal iron should not be given, however, unless the diagnosis of iron deficiency is firmly established, since iron overload may develop in later life.

SYSTEMIC MANIFESTATIONS OF SICKLE CELL DISEASE

The two outstanding manifestations which might be classed as systemic are (a) increased susceptibility to infections, particularly bacterial infections, and (b) impaired growth and development.

Powars (1975) has recently described the clinical findings of sickle cell disease in a series of 422 patients who resided in the Los Angeles area during the preceding 20 years. The diagnosis was well established in this large group of patients. Firm distinctions between sickle cell disease and sickle β^0 thalassemia can be made with the usual laboratory tests on the blood of the affected child (excluding tests of in-vitro synthesis of β polypeptide chains) when the patient is above 6 months of age. Studies of the parents may of course permit earlier diagnosis.

Susceptibility to Infection

The clinical manifestations during the early years, particularly the first year of life, deserve particular attention. Evidence of accelerated red cell destruction is apparent by age 3 months, but growth and development are usually normal in infancy. Powars (1975) and others (Jenkins et al., 1960; Pearson, 1974) have called attention to the frequency of sudden death in infants with sickle cell anemia and the relationship of sudden deaths to infections, particularly pneumococcal sepsis (Seeler et al., 1972). Sudden death in early childhood in patients with sickle cell anemia is probably most frequently caused by bacterial infection (Seeler et al., 1972): the concomitant intravascular sickling may be less impressive on autopsy examination than is intravascular sickling in adults who have died in sickle cell crises. Nearly all the patients in whom sudden death has been related to pneumococcal sepsis have had SS disease, rather than the other sickling disorders.

The relationship of recognizable bacterial infection to mortality in sickle cell disease is also reflected in the morbidity. *Diplococcus pneumoniae* is much more frequently isolated in young children with pulmonary symptoms and fever (Barrett-Connor, 1971; Powars, 1975) than in adult SS homozygotes with the same symptoms.

Both Powars (1975) and Pearson (1974) have called attention to the frequency of pneumococcal infections, including sepsis and meningitis in American children with sickle cell disease, an association noted earlier by Janet Watson (Robinson and Watson, 1966). In her detailed survey of infections in Dade County, Florida, Barrett-Connor (1971) reported a greatly increased incidence of bacterial infections, including pneumococcal meningitis and *Haemophilus influenzae* meningitis, in children with sickle cell anemia as compared with the black population of that county; Salmonella, Shigella, and tuberculous infections were also more frequent but their incidence was less striking than that of pneumococcal infections. Ward and Smith (1976) also noted a high incidence of *H. influenzae* sepsis in children with SS disease. In another series (Robinson and Halpern, 1974; Robinson, 1974), *Escherichia coli* constituted the second most frequently encountered pathogen in children with sickle cell disease, many of whom had urinary tract infections. In Ghana, the increased susceptibility to infection is reflected in malaria and typhoid rather than pneumococcal infections (Ringelhann, 1973).

The pathophysiological basis for the increased susceptibility to infection of infants with sickle cell anemia has recently been reviewed by Johnston (1974). This phenomenon is at least partially related to altered reticuloendothelial function, particularly in the spleen. Pearson and O'Brien (1974) have shown that at age 9 to 12 months, a time when the spleen is regularly palpable in infants with sickle cell anemia, the phagocytic function of the spleen as measured by uptake of isotopes is impaired. The presence of Howell-Jolly bodies also attests to the presence of functional asplenia. As a result of successive infarctions, the spleen slowly decreases in size and is usually not palpable in children with sickle cell anemia after the age of 7. Children with sickle cell anemia are prone to the same kinds of life-threatening bacterial infections as other asplenic children. In young children the spleen appears to play a major role in host defense, a role that appears to diminish with advancing age. Alternatively, decreasing incidence of infections with age may reflect immunity induced by previous infection. While repeated infections occurred in several children in the series of Barrett-Connor (1971) and Ward and Smith (1976), recurrences were nearly absent in Powars' group (1975).

The basis of the increased susceptibility of young children with sickle cell anemia to infection is probably related in part to the reticuloendothelial blockage by sickled cells and cell fragments. The role of the spleen as a site of synthesis of proteins important in host defenses in young children has not been fully evaluated. A functioning spleen may be necessary for the formation of antibodies to particulate antigens. Schwartz and Pearson (1972) found that SS children failed to develop a normal rise in heterophil antibody titer following the intravenous injection of sheep red cells. A deficiency of pneumococcal serum opsonizing activity found in some children with sickle cell disease (Winkelstein and Drachman, 1968) appears to be related to an abnormality in the properdin pathway with impaired fixation of the third component of complement (C_3) to the pneumococci (Johnston et al., 1973).

A defect in neutrophil kinetics and delayed chemotaxis has also been demonstrated by Boggs et al. (1973).

Improved clinical care has resulted in longer survival for patients with sickle cell anemia in Africa (Konotey-Ahulu, 1973, 1974) as well as in America. The greatest risk for severe bacterial infection appears to be in children 7 years of age or younger. In Powars' study (1975) the peak morbidity occurred between the second and third year of life, and except for hospital admissions for pregnancy and complications thereof, morbidity as measured by hospital admissions was essentially the same between ages 7 and 30. Children who appear to constitute an exception are those who have had cerebrovascular accidents: many have repeated episodes and resulting neurological impairment. Powars (1975) found the death rate during the first decade of life to be 10 per cent, with a rate of 5 per cent or less during any of the subsequent decades.

Patients with SC disease do not appear to share the susceptibility to bacterial infections in childhood, but patients with either SC or S/β thalassemia have crises, particularly the chest syndrome, and bone infarcts in childhood.

Growth and Development

Impairment of growth and development correlates fairly well with the severity of the anemia and symptoms of sickle cell disease. No abnormalities in growth are encountered until late infancy. Thereafter, growth is probably slower in many patients with SS disease, but delayed puberty allows for continuing growth. Consequently, most adult patients with SS disease do not differ appreciably from their siblings in height or appearance. A few patients with severe sickle cell anemia form "a subset," with severely retarded growth and delayed puberty. The "tower skull" of chronic hemolytic anemia is occasionally seen; Konotey-Ahulu (1974) has called attention to gnathopathy, an overgrowth of the maxillary portion of the skull which occurs frequently in Ghanian patients with sickle cell anemia but is not commonly encountered in America.

Coagulation in Sickle Cell Disease

Among other "systemic" manifestations of sickle cell disease are abnormalities in coagulation. This topic has been reviewed by Rickles and O'Leary (1974). Haut et al. (1973) demonstrated a significant, although transient, shortening of platelet survival in three patients during sickle crises. A modest fall in platelet count has also been observed during painful crises (Gordon et al., 1974). Freedman and Karpatkin (1975) have reported elevated platelet counts in patients with SS disease with significant decline in numbers of circulatory platelets during vaso-occlusive crises. There are conflicting reports on platelet function during crises. Although fibrinogen levels are often elevated, particularly during crisis (Gordon et al., 1974), fibrinogen turnover is enhanced (Mattii et al., 1973). Furthermore, the presence of increased amounts of plasma high molecular weight fibrinogen complexes in SS patients may reflect enhanced rates of in vivo fibrin formation (Alkjaersig et al., 1976). The levels of these complexes decreased toward normal after patients were treated with antiplatelet drugs (aspirin and dipyridamole).

Sickle Cell Crisis

While sickle cell crisis in young children is often associated with evident bacterial or presumed viral infections, clear evidence for infection is frequently absent in older children or adults. Overall, about one-third of acute painful crises in adults are probably associated with a concurrent or preceding infection. A shortening in survival of SS red cells has been noted for a few days after the induction of pyrexia (Basu and Woodruff, 1963). An associated enhancement of sickling may be responsible for precipitating a vaso-occlusive crisis.

The frequency and severity of painful crises vary considerably among patients and even in a given patient. Crises may occur rather infrequently in some patients, while in others recurrent episodes of painful crises interfere with schooling or steady employment. Common experience is documented by Powars' (1975) observation that in any group of sicklers, a few patients account for most of the hospital admissions. While cerebral thrombosis carries grave implications for recurrence with continuing or progressive disability, particularly in children, and recurrent bone infarctions may lead to bone changes by x-ray (which are generally asymptomatic except in the hips), the organ damage of adult patients does not correlate very well with the observed frequency or severity of sickle crises in childhood.

The effects of recurrent episodes of severely painful crises on the mental state of the affected patient and on the structure of the family are variable in the extreme. Some patients with little chronic disability are psychologically incapacitated and others with similar histories of painful crises have succeeded in attending school and have had permanent employment thereafter. That such contrasts can be observed in two affected siblings reflects some unknown variation in the disease or in the reactions of affected individuals.

Chest Crises

The "chest syndrome" is one of the frequent manifestations of sickling vaso-occlusive crises. Since the pathogenesis of the symptoms is not entirely clear, we have retained the designation "chest syndrome." Affected patients have sudden onset of pleural pain with fever. X-ray findings may be absent initially or evanescent, or areas of possible infarction or infection may be demonstrated. The obvious problem is the difficulty in distinguishing pulmonary infection, infarction due to sickling in situ, or pulmonary embolism.

The susceptibility of young children with sickle cell anemia to bacterial infections, particularly to pneumococcal infections, has been referred to earlier. Barrett-Connor (1973) has called attention to the prolonged course of bacteriologically proven pneumococcal pneumonia in patients with sickle cell disease. In addition, severe bouts of Mycoplasma pneumonia are frequently encountered in these patients (Shulman et al., 1972). Etiological agents are less frequently identified in adults with pulmonary symptoms, but in all age groups the "chest syndrome" appears to be the commonest diagnosis for sicklers admitted to the hospital. Pulmonary vascular occlusion has been demonstrated in sickle cell anemia as well as in its genetic variants. While vascular occlusion may occasionally be caused by marrow or fat emboli from infarcted bone, it is generally believed to represent thrombosis of sickled cells in situ rather than embolization of blood or marrow clots (Moser and Shea, 1957; Diggs, 1969). Infection and infarction of the lung in these patients share so many clinical features (fever, leukocytosis, pleurisy with or without pleural effusion) that it may be difficult to distinguish firmly between the two pathological processes (Barrett-Connor, 1973). Since infection may be accompanied by microinfarctions, and thrombosis by superimposed infection, the distinction in clinically severe examples of the chest syndrome may be somewhat academic. The frequency of episodes of chest pain in the last trimester of pregnancy in patients with SC disease has been noted by many hematologists, and chronic pulmonary occlusion with pulmonary hypertension and cor pulmonale has been noted in SS and SC patients. It may be that the viscosity of the higher hematocrit plus sickling carries an increased risk in SC patients for pulmonary as well as for ocular (see below) disability. Anticoagulation has been of no demonstrated value in the chest syndrome.

Musculoskeletal Crises

Musculoskeletal crises occur in all age groups. An erroneous diagnosis of acute rheumatic fever is occasionally made at the time of the initial crisis. The frequency of objective findings such as swelling and tenderness appears to be higher in children. Dactylitis may be the initial symptom of SS disease in infants. It is characterized by the rather sudden onset over hours to a day or two of painful swelling of the dorsum of both hands and feet. Usually at least two

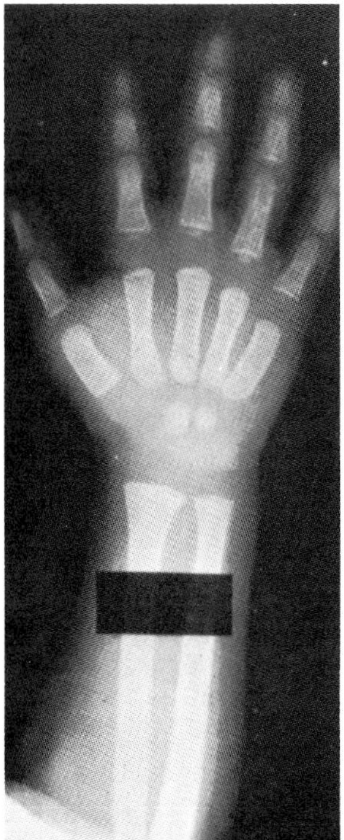

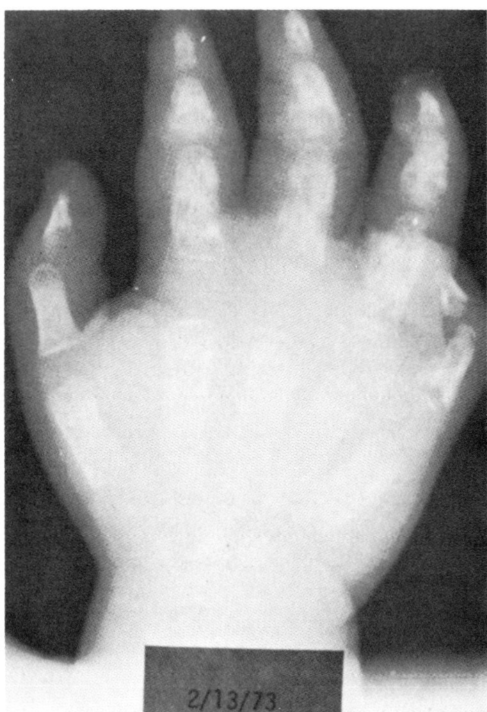

Figure 7–8. X-ray of child's hand during (left) and two weeks following (right) an attack of dactylitis. Note the development of destructive bony lesions (From Nathan, D. G., and Oski, F. A.: Hematology of Infancy and Childhood, W. B. Saunders Co., 1974.)

and frequently all four extremities are involved. Dactylitis may occur before the first year of age and generally does not occur after the age of 5. Children with dactylitis usually have fever and, as might be expected, irritability. A single episode may last for one to two weeks and may recur one or more times during the next several months or years. X-rays may show no abnormalities, but evidence of cortical thinning and marked bone destruction with healing may be seen (Fig. 7–8). Most episodes subside without sequelae, but deformity of hands due to infarction and destruction of the carpal or metacarpal bones may rarely occur. A shortened digit secondary to infarcted bone has been reported (Serjeant and Ashcroft, 1971).

The age predilection of dactylitis is thought to result from the rapid growth of bone which has a limited blood supply. The occlusion of a vessel by sickled cells may not be easily compensated for by a collateral blood supply in bone. The regular features of symmetrical local swelling and involvement of more than one extremity are admittedly not so readily explained. The growing bones appear to be a site at which sickling is particularly likely to occur once the proportion of sickle hemoglobin in the infant has greatly exceeded that of Hb F. The absence of dactylitis in older children or adults may be due either to lower growth rate of bones after the age of 5 or to greater osseous vascularity.

Powars (1975) has found that patients who have had skeletal crises as children are more likely to have bone deformities as adults. The painful crises with localization of pain to a small area of bone may be difficult to distinguish from osteomyelitis, particularly if the patient has fever and leukocytosis. Bone infarctions can sometimes be demonstrated by aspiration (Charache and Page, 1967) or by x-ray (Reynolds, 1965) but not until several days have elapsed after onset of pain. Recently, ^{99m}Tc-sulfur colloid scans have been used to localize bone infarction due to sickling (Alavi et al., 1974), but similar abnormalities are seen in osteomyelitis. In known sicklers, it is usually advisable to wait for a day or two to observe the progress of symptoms of sudden onset isolated to a single bony site rather than to undertake a long course of probably unnecessary antibiotic therapy for osteomyelitis.

Occasional musculoskeletal vaso-occlusive crises begin suddenly with back pain, which is followed by pain in other areas of the body. Such a sequence of symptoms may reflect an initial infarct in the spine, particularly in the lumbosacral spine, followed by fat embolization. Fat emboli have been described in a few patients, but it is not known how often such emboli occur in nonfatal crises.

Sometimes, a sickle crisis may present as an acute monarticular or polyarticular arthritis. The elbows and knees are most often involved. The presence of signs of inflammation and joint effusion may mimic rheumatoid arthritis, gout, or acute septic arthritis (Schumacher et al., 1973). Examination of the joint fluid is helpful in this differential diagnosis. If the effusion is due to sickling, the synovial fluid will be clear and yellow with normal viscosity. Microscopic examination reveals a low white cell count ($\sim$100 to 1000/mm^3) with a predominance of mononuclear cells and an absence of bacteria or uric acid crystals. Synovial biopsy may show sickled erythrocytes in the lumen of small vessels. SS patients have a higher incidence of gout than normal individuals (Ball and Sorenson, 1970), although this complication is less common than sickle arthropathy.

Splenic Sequestration Crises

The frequent "autosplenectomy" which results in the absence of splenic function in older children and adults with sickle cell anemia was referred to earlier. Only a few patients with sickle cell anemia retain splenomegaly. In contrast, over half the patients with SC disease and S/β thalassemia have enlarged spleens. Splenic calcifications are sometimes visualized roentgenographically in a few SS patients with splenomegaly.

Rarely, again usually in children, the presence of continuing splenomegaly seems to predispose to life-threatening episodes of so-called "sequestration crises" (Pearson, 1969; Seeler and Schwiaki, 1972). In such crises, the already enlarged spleen rapidly enlarges over several hours as the child becomes progressively more anemic. A child with splenic sequestration is usually admitted to the hospital with impending or actual shock, grossly enlarged spleen, and severe anemia. The sequence of events suggests that blood has collected in the spleen. Prompt transfusion and supportive measures are necessary. There is some uncertainty as to whether a single episode of splenic sequestration is an indication for splenectomy when the patient's condition has stabilized. A history of a single episode of sequestration implies an increased risk for a second episode.

Abdominal Crises

When the sole manifestations of sickle cell crises are abdominal symptoms and signs, the differential diagnosis may include many causes of the acute abdomen. Gallstones occur with increased frequency in sickle cell disease (Barrett-Connor, 1968) and causes of acute abdominal pain other than crises must be considered. Patients with sickle crises may have classic rebound tenderness. The presence of bowel sounds favors the diagnosis of sickle crisis rather than an acute process requiring surgical intervention. The white count and differential and the leukocyte alkaline phosphatase levels are not helpful in making this differential diagnosis. Because of these uncertainties, SS patients have often undergone unnecessary abdominal surgery. After the age of 10, many patients have similar pain patterns with recurrent crises, and the perceptive patient's assessment of his or her pain is frequently helpful. The hepatobiliary manifestations of sickle cell disease are discussed below.

Crises with Neurological Manifestations

Occlusion of vessels in the brain by sickle cells may be manifest either by seizures or by sudden onset of neurological deficits, including hemiplegia. Such occlusive events, although not common, occur in young individuals; dramatic improvement in the initial symptoms may be seen over the course of days or weeks, although Powars (1975) has pointed out that affected children may have continuing or recurring neurological deficits. Recent studies which suggest that exchange transfusion should be employed in the treatment of neurological manifestations need to be verified with larger numbers of patients in both treated and control groups (Russell et al., 1974, 1976; see pp. 266 and 267).

Sudden Death

Death of patients with sickle cell anemia is frequently sudden, occurring within minutes or hours following symptoms of crisis. The information that the patient died suddenly at home or on the way to the hospital is frequently obtained when efforts are made to secure information about patients who have failed to keep appointments with physicians. Sometimes the historical sequence of events suggests that the patient had an infection followed by occlusion of cardiac or cerebral vessels. Autopsy findings of massive occlusion of vessels by sickled cells are difficult to interpret, since post-mortem sickling will lead to similar findings. Probably in most of these patients, particularly in young children, pneumococcal sepsis or other infection is the commonest precipitating cause of the fatal outcome.

Chronic Organ Damage in Sickle Cell Disease

Manifestations of specific organ damage appear in SS patients after mid-childhood and constitute significant aspects of the illness of adult sicklers. Many different organs may be affected; the heart, lungs, kidneys, liver, skin, and skeletal, ocular, and central nervous systems all bear the scars of the disease (Diggs, 1973).

Cardiovascular Manifestations

The cardiovascular manifestations of sickle cell anemia are generally related to anemia, with a hyperdynamic state, and to the pulmonary abnormalities which follow occlusion of pulmonary vessels by sickled cells. Klinefelter (1942), in an attempt to distinguish sickle crisis with musculoskeletal symptoms from acute rheumatic fever, concluded that the auscultatory findings in sickle cell disease might indeed closely mimic those of rheumatic heart disease. The degree of anemia in children with sickle cell anemia would be expected to result in a sustained increase in cardiac output (Varat et al., 1972; Lindsay et al., 1974), which increases even further on exercise. Arterial hypoxemia, related in part to pulmonary disease, probably causes a further demand on the heart in older patients. The pulmonary disease (see below) is only slowly cumulative, but pulmonary hypertension is occasionally found. The chronicity and severity of sickle cell anemia find few counterparts in other diseases and most of the findings are probably related to the long-standing anemia. Hemosiderosis of remarkable degree is more common in thalassemia and indeed is likely to be more significant, in the authors' experience, in sickle thalassemia than in sickle cell anemia.

The symptoms of cardiac origin are those of dyspnea on exertion and, in a few patients, symptoms of overt congestive heart failure. An enlarged, hyperactive heart, with a loud systolic murmur, is commonly encountered, and in perhaps a third of the cases a diastolic murmur is heard. Structural mitral stenosis may be distinguished by echocardiography. While it was originally believed that rheumatic heart disease was very uncommon in sickle cell disease, there have been numerous examples of the coexistence of rheumatic valvular disease (as well as congenital heart disease) and sickle cell anemia. There is no evidence for the existence of a sickle cell cardiomyopathy. In view of the very low O_2 tensions in the coronary sinus, which might in theory favor sickling, clinical evidence of coronary artery insufficiency is strikingly absent.

Pulmonary Involvement

Since sickling occurs in deoxygenated red cells containing hemoglobin S, the development of impaired pulmonary function is particularly troublesome in patients with sickle cell disease. In adults with sickle cell disease, gas exchange is frequently abnormal even during the stable noncrisis state (Bromberg, 1974). Resting arterial PO_2 is usually decreased in adult patients with sickle cell anemia, S thalassemia, and SC disease, although it is seldom at dangerously low levels. Since the oxygen affinity of the blood in sickle cell anemia is shifted to the right, the reduction in arterial PO_2 usually produces lowered oxygen saturation of the arterial blood. Most patients with sickle cell disease have arterial unsaturation (Sproule et al., 1958). In compensation for the anemia, larger volumes of oxygen per red cell must be delivered to the tissues than is the case in nonanemic individuals. Curiously, the values for pulmonary arterial oxygen saturation have been found to be higher than would be expected from systemic arterial PO_2 values in SS patients, suggesting peripheral arteriovenous shunting (Sproule et al., 1958).

The calculated alveolar-arterial (A-a) PO_2 differences in these patients, which may range upward of 20 mm Hg, resemble or exceed those in patients with comparable degrees of anemia of other cause (Bromberg and Jensen, 1967a). The widened alveolar-arterial PO_2 difference apparently reflects a large contribution of intrapulmonary shunting, since such gradients were observed in patients breathing 100 per cent oxygen (Sproule et al., 1958). Inequality in ventilation and perfusion appears to play a significant role in some of the patients. Decreased oxygen diffusion does not appear to be a major factor in the etiology of the oxygen unsaturation, although some impairment in gas diffusion can usually be demonstrated. (Reduction of diffusing capacity as measured by CO methods is generally demonstrable in anemia of any cause; the observed reduction is attributed to the reduction of the numbers of red cells in capillaries.) In most patients with sickle cell disease, tissue oxygen supply on exercise is limited by cardiac output rather than by impaired pulmonary function. Cor pulmonale is distinctly unusual in sickle cell disease, and pulmonary vascular resistance is generally normal.

Despite the absence of evidence for remarkable pulmonary abnormalities in most patients with sickle cell disease, it appears logical to consider the observed arterial oxygen unsaturation a significant factor in the morbidity of sickle cell disease. Hypoxemia may well promote the formation of irreversibly sickled cells (ISC) and the sequence of microthrombi that may be initiated by the trapping of ISC's.

Hepatobiliary Involvement

The chronic jaundice of patients with sickle cell anemia reflects accelerated red cell destruction. Hepatic injury in sickle cell disease frequently occurs as a result of transfusion-induced hepatitis. In addition, these patients may develop hepatic infarcts, which occasionally become infected, resulting in hepatic abscess (Brittain et al., 1966). If a significant portion of hepatic parenchyma becomes infarcted, fibrosis and deterioration of liver function may result (Green, 1953).

Like patients with other types of congenital hemolytic anemia, patients with sickle cell disease have a high incidence of cholelithiasis (Barrett-Connor, 1968). Although about one-third of these patients have gallstones, only 10 per cent develop symptoms that can be attributed to biliary disease. On occasion, sicklers are subject to attacks of cholestatic jaundice in which very high serum bilirubin and alkaline phosphatase levels suggest choledocholithiasis (Klion et al., 1964). However, such episodes are difficult to distinguish from hepatic crises due to sickling. Both usually resolve uneventfully. The decision to recommend cholecystectomy in sickle cell disease must be individualized: the existence of asymptomatic gallstones in a severely anemic patient is probably of no great moment, while significant symptoms of gallbladder disease (e.g., recurring attacks of cholecystitis) would constitute a strong indication for surgical intervention.

Genitourinary Manifestations

The involvement of the kidney in sickle cell disease is rather constant if the loss of the ability to produce a concentrated urine is considered renal involvement. The impairment in renal concentrating capacity appears in childhood in sickle cell trait. Since the concentrating defect in children is reversed following transfusions of normal blood, the pathogenic mechanism must be secondary to the abnormal red blood cells (Keitel et al., 1958; Statius van Eps et al., 1967). In the hypertonic environment of the renal medulla, red cells sickle even with normal O_2 tensions (Perillie and Epstein, 1963). A disorder of the countercurrent distributor in the medullary circulation has been proposed as the etiological factor for the concentrating defect. However, as Buckalew and Someren (1974) have pointed out, the mechanism by which the decreased medullary blood flow would produce the isosthenuria is not clear. By injection at autopsy of kidneys of patients with sickle cell disease Statius van Eps et al. (1970) demonstrated decreased filling of medullary vasa recta, dilated capillaries, and extravasation of contrast material from ruptured capillaries. The renal concentrating defect of sicklers is unusual because tubular reabsorption of free water appears to be normal or decreased only slightly (Heinemann and Cheung, 1957). Lief et al. (1969) have shown in rats after papillectomy that tubular reabsorption of free water is normal in spite of a marked defect in maximum urine osmolality. Buckalew and Someren (1974) have suggested that the concentrating defect is due to decreased perfusion of nephrons with long loops of Henle extending into the papillae. The preservation of tubular reabsorption of free water reflects normal function of the shorter ascending loops of Henle in the outer medulla which are not affected by the damage to papillae.

HEMATURIA. Hematuria occurs in patients with sickle cell anemia and in those with the genetic variants of sickling, including some patients with sickle cell trait. Diggs (1973) indicated that the anatomical lesion is a papillary necrosis with formation of a papillary ulcer. Peritubular extravasation of blood in kidneys surgically removed for hematuria has also been observed. Again, the evidence suggests a papillary lesion secondary to impaired blood supply as in the concentrating defect. While, in the authors' experience, hematuria has been rather common in patients with sickle cell/Hb C disease, it is distinctly uncommon in sickle cell trait when one considers the number of individuals at risk in each of the two groups. The possibility of causes of painless hematuria other than sickling should be carefully evaluated in such patients. In some sicklers with hematuria, blood loss continuing over many weeks may lead to iron deficiency anemia. The therapeutic maneuver of oral iron administration should not be overlooked in the frustration of both physician and patient concerning the prolonged hematuria. The use of diuretic agents to decrease medullary hypertonicity has been recommended and should be used in the attempt to stop prolonged hematuria. Occasionally renal bleeding has been so extensive and prolonged that nephrectomy was performed (Mostofi et al., 1957; Lucas and Bullock, 1960). However, nephrectomy has largely been abandoned because, in many patients, bleeding has occurred on separate occasions from each kidney. Epsilon-aminocaproic acid (EACA) may be useful (Bilinski et al., 1969); however, it should be used with caution, since it may prevent the dissolution of clots in the renal pelvis.

RENAL FAILURE AND THE NEPHROTIC SYNDROME. Morphological renal changes are found in patients with sickle cell anemia in the absence of clinical signs of renal disease. The glomerular capillaries, afferent arterioles, interlobular arteries, and small medullary vessels are distended with erythrocytes, some of which appear sickled (Buckalew and Someren, 1974). Enlarged glomeruli (Bernstein and Whitten, 1960) may have electron-dense material in the mesangial cytoplasm (Pitcock et al., 1970). Similar changes were found on electron microscopy by McCoy (1969) and Antonovych (1971) in renal sections of patients with sickle cell anemia and the nephrotic syndrome. It was suggested by McCoy (1969) that the electron-dense deposits represent some form of iron which remains from phagocytosis of red cells or hemoglobin by mesangial cells. Since iron is frequently found in renal tissues in patients with hemolytic anemia (primarily in proximal tubular cells), it is difficult to attribute renal insufficiency to the presence of the metal. Pardo et al. (1975) have proposed that the glomerular lesion in SS disease is due to an immune complex composed of renal tubular epithelial antigen and antibody directed toward that antigen.

Frank renal failure, sometimes following the nephrotic syndrome, occurs in a relatively small number of patients with sickle cell anemia. Patients who become uremic develop an increased transfusion requirement which can be reduced by hemodialysis (Friedman et al., 1974). In patients with sickle cell anemia who have survived to the fourth and fifth decades, mild nitrogen retention is common. Some of the patients have elevated levels of uric acid due to increased purine turnover (Walker and Alexander, 1971; Diamond et al., 1976); but uric acid stones are rare. It is likely that renal insufficiency of variable degree will be encountered more frequently as longer average life span leads to an older population with sickle cell anemia.

PRIAPISM. Male patients with sickle cell disease occasionally develop spontaneous and painful engorgement of the penis. This distressing symptom accounted for 3 to 5 per cent of admissions of male SS patients in two series from the southern United States (Campbell and Cummins, 1951; Hasen and Raines, 1962). Priapism occurs with about equal frequency in prepubertal and postpubertal patients, although the latter are more difficult to treat and may develop impotence following the acute episode. While a number of approaches to therapy have been employed, conservative management is recommended (Karayalcin et al., 1972). As with other types of sickle crises, the patient should be given sedation, analgesia, and adequate intravenous fluids. Seeler (1973) has treated 6 boys with packed red cell transfusion. Twenty-four hours after doubling the hematocrit, a marked decrease in pain was noted, followed by a resolution of priapism over the next several days. Surgical intervention such as incision and drainage or irrigation is only indicated when conservative measures fail. It is uncertain whether surgery decreases (Grace and Winter, 1968) or increases (Karayalcin et al., 1972) the likelihood of impotence.

Ocular Abnormalities

Impressive changes in the eyes may accompany sickle cell anemia and its genetic variants. These changes were reviewed recently by Armaly (1974). Condon and Serjeant (1972a and 1972b) compared the incidence of a variety of ocular manifestations in 70 patients with SC disease and 76 patients with SS disease. Whitened peripheral retina (88 per cent), peripheral vessel disease (96 per cent), tortuosity of vessels (11 per cent), and peripheral arteriovenous anomalies (28 per cent) were found in about equal frequency in SS and SC disease, but the ocular lesions leading to the greatest disability are found primarily in SC disease. In SC disease the following lesions were found: vitreous hemorrhages (16 per cent) and retinitis proliferans (33 per cent). Retinal detachment occurs more frequently in patients with SC disease. The reason for the higher incidence of major ocular disability in SC disease than in SS disease is not understood; since lesions follow vessel occlusion by sickled cells, it may be that the higher packed cell volume in SC disease plus sickling leads to large changes in viscosity, with capillary plugging in the microvasculature of the eye. The early diagnosis of retinal lesions in SS and SC disease is important, since retinal detachment may be prevented by laser beam therapy (Ryan and Goldberg, 1971).

Musculoskeletal Manifestations

The great variety of bony changes that result from infarctions of bone and from the marrow hyperplasia consequent to accelerated red cell destruction have been described in the monograph by Reynolds (1965). Calvarial thickening is frequent, but the "hair-on-end" appearance so often encountered in thalassemia is uncommon in sickle cell disease. X-rays of the spine may reveal sclerosis consequent to old infarcts as well as the nearly pathognomonic biconcave deformity of the vertebrae, called "fishmouth vertebrae" (Fig. 7–9). This abnormality is generally encountered in older patients with sickle cell disease and is distinguished from a similar nonspecific deformity of a number of skeletal disorders by the flat "floor" or "roof" on the depressed area, sparing the peripheral bone, and by the coarse bony trabeculae of sickle cell disease. Bony changes may be seen in any of the long bones but the most symptomatic changes occur in the hip,

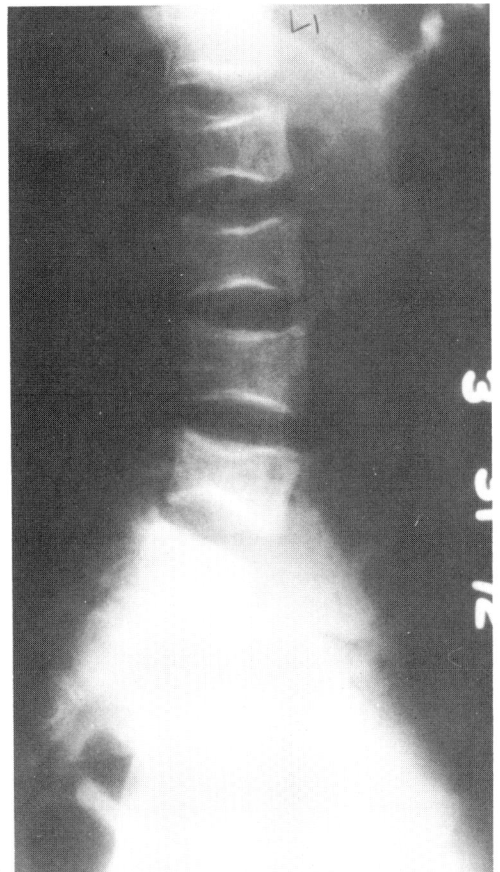

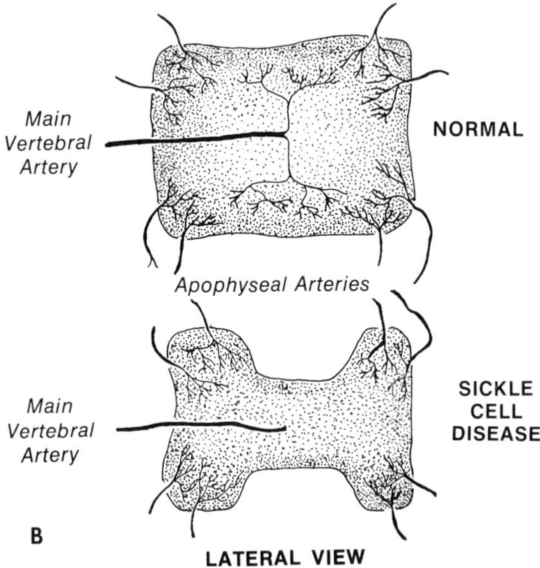

***Figure* 7–9.** *A*, X-ray of lumbosacral spine of patient with SS anemia. Note classic fishmouth deformity. (Courtesy of Dr. Charles Peterson.) *B*, Pathogenesis of fishmouth deformity. The central depression of the vertebral end plates is caused by local inhibition of bone growth from ischemia. The central portion of the growth plate suffers ischemic damage owing to impaired circulation through the main vertebral artery. In contrast, the ring epiphyses and outer portion of the vertebral plates are spared because of numerous perforating apophyseal arteries.

where avascular necrosis of the femoral head may lead to disability, requiring surgical correction. Some patients may require a total hip prosthesis. Aseptic necrosis of the femoral head occurs both in SS disease and in the genetic variants. The suggested higher incidence in patients with the genetic variants is not convincing when patients of similar age are compared.

Osteomyelitis has been found in sickle cell disease of all types. Staphylococcus is the commonest etiological agent. In addition, SS and S/β thalassemia patients have a peculiar susceptibility to develop Salmonella osteomyelitis. Chronic osteomyelitis in sickle cell disease appears to be less common than formerly, probably because of the administration of effective antibiotics earlier in the course of the disease. The infection probably begins in a nidus of infarcted bone.

Skin Ulcers

One of the most troublesome problems of many patients with sickle cell disease is the recurrent chronic skin ulcers of the lower extremities. This subject has been reviewed by Serjeant (1974). The lesions usually begin around the ankle and may become very large. The ulcers appear to be more common in the patients with more severe anemia. Similar lesions have been described, admittedly rarely, in patients with thalassemia and in other types of congenital hemolytic anemia. Most of the leg ulcers are found in patients with SS disease or with S/β thalassemia. The finding of scars of healed ulcers on the lower extremities of young black patients strongly suggests one of the sickling diseases. Unfortunately, the ulcers are very slow to heal, and healing is not infrequently followed by the appearance of another ulcer months or years thereafter. Leg ulcers may be more frequent in tropical areas, but both the frequency and the chronicity may reflect difficulty in keeping the ulcer clean.

Some ulcers heal fairly well with frequent simple clean dressing changes or with weekly application of supportive paste (Unna) boots. If these measures are ineffective, transfusions may be added to the regimen to reduce the circulating Hb S to less than 50 per cent. Rarely, skin grafting is necessary. Skin grafting should be undertaken only after conservative measures (including transfusion) have failed, since both prolonged elevation and transfusions are usually used as adjuncts to grafting, and the simpler measures make the graft unnecessary. The oral administration of zinc sulfate may hasten the healing of leg ulcers (Serjeant et al., 1970).

Neurological Complications of Sickle Cell Disease

There is a significant incidence of neurological complications in sickle cell disease, but the actual incidence is not known because of the paucity of prospective studies. Portnoy and Herion (1972) found that 26 per cent of 89 patients with sickle cell disease had neurological complications; the commonest manifestation, hemiplegia, occurred in 17 per cent of patients with sickle cell anemia. Coma, convulsions, and visual disturbances were the next most common symptoms. A few of these patients (3 of the 23 in the series of Portnoy and Herion) had recurrent cerebrovascular incidents with spastic quadriplegia and disability. Two additional patients died promptly after the onset of hemiplegia. The potentially ominous significance of neurological manifestations is also noted by Powars (1975). However, in 15 of the episodes of hemiplegia, improvement occurred, while 6 showed little neurological improvement.

In the series of Portnoy and Herion, convulsions occurred in 11 of the patients (12 per cent) and constituted an isolated manifestation in 7 patients. Coma occurred as an isolated finding or associated with other non-neurological findings, e.g., sepsis.

Thrombosis, hemorrhage, and berry aneurysms have been described in sickle cell disease. Thrombosis appears to be the more common lesion. In 6 of 7 patients with neurological manifestations on whom angiograms were done (Russell et al., 1974), 3 had complete occlusion of vessels, and 2 had small aneurysms. Three of the patients who were transfused for one year had improved or stable angiograms, while in two who were not transfused the vascular lesions appeared to progress over the same period. This study suggests the need for further data on the potential benefit of transfusions in children with neurological manifestations.

Differential Diagnosis

The diagnosis of moderate or severe forms of sickle cell anemia is usually quite straightforward. Such patients will have recurrent painful crises, marked anemia, fixed sickle forms on peripheral smear, and >80 per cent Hb S on routine hemoglobin electrophoresis. However, as Table 7–2 shows, these findings may also be present in patients with S/D-Punjab. Agar-gel electrophoresis at low pH is required to separate these two variants. Severe cases of S/β thalassemia may present the same clinical findings, but microcytosis is evident on blood smears in this genetic variant.

In patients who have milder clinical manifestations, other forms of the "sickle syndrome" must be considered. Some of these entities are listed in Table 7–2 and are discussed at the end of the chapter. If the diagnosis remains in doubt after the routine hematological evaluation is completed, it may be necessary to perform structural analysis of the patient's hemoglobin. In addition, studies of family members can provide important additional information which may prove vital in establishing the diagnosis.

TABLE 7–2. *Differential Diagnosis of SS Disease*

Diagnosis	Clinical Severity	Hematocrit	RBC Morphology	Electrophoresis	Distribution of Hb F
SS	Marked	18 to 30	Targets; 2 to 30% ISC's	80 to 95% S 2 to 20% F 2 to 4% A_2	Uneven
S/D-Punjab	Moderate to Marked	20 to 30	Targets; frequent ISC's	~50% S ~50% D*	
S/β^0 Thal	Moderate to Marked	20 to 35	Hypochronic; microcytic; targets; rare ISC's	50 to 85% S 10 to 30% A 3 to 6% A_2	Uneven
S/β^+ Thal	Mild to Moderate	25 to 40	Slightly microcytic; targets; rare ISC's	55 to 75% S 10 to 30% A 5 to 20% F 3 to 6% A_2	Uneven
S/HPFH	Mild	38 to 48	Targets	70 to 80% S 20 to 30% F 1 to 3% A_2	Even

*Agar-gel electrophoresis.

TREATMENT OF SICKLE CELL DISEASE

The improved prognosis in sickle cell disease which has attended better living conditions, nutrition, and medical care (including antibiotics) has been observed not only in the United States (Powars, 1975) but also in some parts of Africa (Konotey-Ahulu, 1973). The serious acute complications mostly occur in the youngest age group: the life-threatening infections, sepsis and meningitis, the sequestration crises, and the sudden collapse and death which may also be related to infection occur with diminishing frequency in older patients.

Supportive Therapy

Infections

Since patients with sickle cell disease have increased susceptibility, antibiotics should be administered at the earliest sign of infection, particularly to children, in whom bacterial infections constitute a major hazard. In some centers, children are given prophylactic penicillin. Antimalarial prophylaxis is indicated in endemic areas.

In the vaso-occlusive crisis—the most common reason for hospital admission of adults—evidence of bacterial infection is frequently absent. However, the slow resolution of the chest syndrome following the administration of antibiotics cannot constitute evidence against bacterial infection.

Anemia

Patients with sickle cell anemia usually tolerate anemia quite well. Worsening of anemia because of folic acid deficiency is readily prevented by administering a daily supplement of this vitamin. Androgen treatment results in a significant increase in red cell mass (Lundh and Gardner, 1970; Alexanian and Nadell, 1975) and may be indicated in selected patients who appear to be symptomatic because of severe anemia. The rise in red cell 2,3-DPG and decrease in oxygen affinity during androgen therapy (Chapter 3) would theoretically enhance sickling. However, treatment had no significant effect on red cell survival (Lundh and Gardner, 1970; Alexanian and Nadell, 1975). The possible benefits from long-term oral androgen therapy must be weighed against adverse effects, chief among which is hepatotoxicity. Furthermore, male sicklers have a tendency to develop priapism during treatment (Lundh and Gardner, 1970).

Blood transfusions are seldom indicated in the treatment of the anemia of sickle cell disease. However, vaso-occlusive complications can be prevented by exchange transfusions. Charache (1974c) has described this procedure in detail. In order to be effective, at least 50 per cent of the patient's red cells should be of donor origin. This clinical impression is supported by whole blood viscosity measurements by Charache and Conley (1975). Exchange transfusion should not be undertaken lightly, since it entails a considerable commitment of time and resources as well as the familiar risks of hepatitis, red cell sensitization, and iron overload. Nevertheless, such a program may be indicated in selected patients, particularly if they are going through a period of increased risk such as major surgery or pregnancy. It is important to match the patient's blood carefully, particularly for red cell antigens which have a relatively low frequency in blacks.

Painful Crises

The management of the painful vaso-occlusive crisis is best achieved by vigorous hydration, analgesics, and appropriate antibiotics if there is any evidence of infection. Because of their inability to produce concentrated urine, SS patients have an increased fluid requirement and are prone to dehydration. Careful attention should also be paid to the patient's acid-base status. Acidosis should be promptly corrected, since it can trigger a painful crisis (Greenberg and Kass, 1958). However, alkali therapy does not appear to be effective either in the treatment of acute painful crises (Cooperative Urea Trials Group, 1974) or in their prevention (Mann and Stuart, 1974). Oxygen is usually administered during acute painful crises but its efficacy is doubtful unless the patient has a significant ventilatory hypoxia. In contrast, hyperbaric oxygen may be an effective albeit cumbersome form of treatment (Reynolds, 1971). Prompt and adequate relief of pain is of prime importance. Unfortunately, many patients who have frequent painful crises become dependent upon, if not addicted to, a variety of narcotics and analgesics. Nevertheless, such an individual deserves the benefit of the doubt. Blood transfusion has been recommended in the management of acute painful crises (Brody, 1970) but the efficacy of this treatment is doubtful. In contrast, exchange transfusion is effective in the prevention of painful crises.

Surgery

Since patients with sickle cell disease may not tolerate major surgery very well, hematologists are conservative in recommending surgical procedures. Close attention should be paid to maintenance of adequate hydration and acid-base balance as well as to optimal oxygenation before, during, and after surgery (Flye and Silver, 1973;

Searle, 1972). If extensive surgery is planned on an elective basis, such as a total hip replacement, it is reasonable to prepare the patient with exchange transfusion.

Pregnancy

The management of sickle cell disease in pregnancy has been the subject of considerable discussion. There is an increased risk of fetal wastage, but with appropriate management the maternal risk is probably not greatly increased. This statement does not apply in patients who do not receive antenatal care; such patients have a much higher risk of serious complications. (Diggs [1973] cites a maternal mortality of 6 per cent and fetal mortality of 50 per cent for these patients.) In the antenatal period, folic acid should be administered daily. A superimposed physiologic anemia of pregnancy may appear to increase the anemia. Most of the serious complications occur in the last trimester, and in some clinics regular transfusions of normal red cells are given during the last three months. Regular prophylactic exchange transfusion is not usually necessary, but the occurrence of serious complications just before or after delivery is not predictable. Pritchard et al. (1971) has found that this treatment resulted in a lower incidence of fetal wastage. Transfusions should be given in any pregnant patient with sickle cell disease in whom markedly increased anemia or crises have occurred in the final trimester. Whether to interrupt an early pregnancy is ultimately dependent on the patient's informed decision. The risks should be defined as clearly as our limited knowledge makes possible.

ANTI-SICKLING AGENTS

During the past 20 years, a variety of agents have been proposed for the treatment of sickle cell anemia. Many of these are listed in Table 7–3. Usually, an initial wave of enthusiasm has been followed by the sober realization that the drug was either ineffective or in some cases unsafe. Currently, none of the anti-sickling agents appear to be of clinical value.

Present-day knowledge of the molecular bases of sickling should enable the design of specific anti-sickling agents. The ligand-dependent polymerization of molecules of sickle hemoglobin suggests that agents which would (1) shift the oxygen dissociation curve to the left (i.e., increase the oxygen affinity), thereby favoring the oxy conformation of the tetramer, or (2) interfere with the intermolecular contacts involved in polymerization of deoxyhemoglobin S would be beneficial in sickle cell disease. Cyanate, which carbamylates the N-terminal residues of proteins, was extensively investigated by Cerami

TABLE 7–3. *Agents Which Have Been Proposed for the Treatment of Sickle Cell Anemia*

Agents	Proposed	Efficacy Contested
Priscoline	Smith (1953)	
Cobalt	Gross et al. (1955)	
Met Hb	Beutler (1961)	
Anticoagulants		Salvaggio et al. (1963)
CO	Sirs (1963) Beutler (1975)	Perruganan and McElfresh (1964)
Alkali		Schwartz and McElfresh (1964)
Dextran	Watson and Williams (1963) Barnes et al. (1965)	Oski et al. (1965)
Carbonic Anhydrase Inhibitors	Hilkowitz (1957)	dosSantos and Lehmann (1959) Finney and Hatch (1965)
Phenothiazines	Hatborn and Lewis (1966)	Pearson and Noyes (1967) Oski et al. (1968)
Androgens	Isaacs, Hayhoe (1967)	Raper et al. (1970)
Urea	Nalbandian (1970)	Cooperative Urea Trials Group (1974)
Cyanate	Gilette et al. (1974)	Harkness and Roth (1975)

and his associates (Gillette et al., 1973; Peterson et al., 1974b). Patients treated with cyanate in low doses generally exhibited prolongation of the red cell life span and a higher circulating hemoglobin with increased oxygen affinity. Unfortunately, the appearance of reversible peripheral neuropathy in patients treated with cyanate made it impossible to evaluate the effects of higher doses of this carbamylating agent on incidence of crises or on the long-term course of sickle cell disease in a large number of patients (Peterson et al., 1974c; Charache et al., 1975c). It is likely that orally administered sodium cyanate has a low therapeutic index. In a double-blind crossover study, Harkness and Roth (1975) found that patients on oral cyanate for six months had the same incidence of painful crises as when they received a placebo. Extracorporeal carbamylation of the patient's blood may be a reasonable alternative. This approach permits more extensive chemical modification of the hemoglobin without risk of toxic side effects. Diederich et al. (1976) found that a small number of patients derived considerable clinical benefit from extracorporeal carbamylation. Such an approach may be potentially useful for the administration of other anti-sickling agents, such as nitrogen mustard (Roth et al., 1972), that cannot be administered systemically.

A number of other anti-sickling drugs are now being investigated, and a safe pharmacological approach to sickle cell disease may emerge in the next decade. Some agents, such as zinc (Brewer and Oelschlegel, 1974) and procaine (Baker et al., 1974), appear to prevent sickling by interacting with the red cell membrane. Other agents, such as alkyl ureas (Roth et al., 1974), dimethyladipimidate (Lubin et al., 1975), and dichloromethane (Milosz and Settle, 1975), penetrate through the membrane and interfere with the polymerization of sickle hemoglobin.

Prognosis

In many of the early reviews on sickle cell anemia the assessment of prognosis has been unduly pessimistic. This has been due in part to case selection. Only patients with relatively severe disease tend to require frequent emergency room visits and hospital admissions. There is a surprisingly large group of SS homozygotes who remain relatively symptom-free and who do not solicit medical attention. Furthermore, during the past 30 years there has been a marked improvement in the care of patients with sickle cell anemia. Infections are treated more promptly with increasingly effective antibiotics. More careful attention is devoted to the maintenance of fluid balance and the prevention of dehydration, and blood transfusions are used for more severe anemia secondary to complications of sickling. It also appears that maternal mortality of SS patients has decreased in recent years. In underdeveloped nations, the mortality in sickle cell anemia remains high. A recent survey from Nigeria reports an alarmingly high death rate, particularly in children from rural areas (Attah and Ekere, 1975).

No single factor is a consistent predictor of prognosis in SS disease. The section on molecular pathogenesis of sickling discusses the impairment of the polymerization of deoxyhemoglobin S by hemoglobin F. One might expect that those SS homozygotes who have relatively high levels of hemoglobin F should have a decreased tendency to sickle and milder clinical manifestations. Although this relationship appears to be true when a large group of patients are analyzed statistically (Jackson et al., 1961), the level of hemoglobin F is not of prognostic value in any given patient. Steinberg et al. (1973) have reported a mean Hb F of 5.4 per cent in a group of 21 patients with relatively mild disease (compared to a mean value of 3.2 per cent in 12 patients with severe sickle cell disease). The group with mild disease did have significantly higher hematocrits. The percentage of irreversibly sickled cells in blood smears is also not useful as an indicator of prognosis.

Considerable variation in the severity of sickle cell disease has been reported among different ethnic and geographical groups. Patients from Jamaica were initially considered to have relatively mild disease (Serjeant et al., 1968). However, it is now conceded that the spectrum of clinical severity in Jamaica does not differ significantly from that in the United States. In contrast to the United States, virtually every SS homozygote in Jamaica is registered and followed by physicians who have an interest and expertise in sickle cell disease. In the United States, mild cases would often escape attention.

There are small ethnic groups of SS homozygotes who appear to have a genuinely milder form of the disease. A group of Shi Arabs from Saudi Arabia have been found to have a very benign form of

TABLE 7–4. *Sickling Disorders**

	Genotype Adult Hb	Hemoglobins Present	Clinical Expression
Group I. Homozygous for Hb S			
A. Without other Hb abnormality (sickle cell anemia)	$\alpha\alpha\beta^S\beta^S$	S, F(2–20%), A_2	Severe anemia, vaso-occlusive crises and complications
B. With α thalassemia	$\alpha^{Thal^1}, \alpha^{Thal^2}\beta^S\beta^S$ $\alpha^{Thal}\alpha\beta^S\beta^S$	S, F(43%), Bart's, A_2 S, F(27%), A_2	Mild anemia in childhood Doubtful
C. With α-chain structural varient			
1. With Hb Memphis	$\alpha\alpha^{23\ Gln}\beta^S\beta^S$	S, F, A_2, Memphis/S	Mild course, with hemolytic anemia and few crises
2. With Hb G-Philadelphia	$\alpha\alpha^{68\ Lys}\beta^S\beta^S$	S, G/S, F, A_2, G_2	Like severe sickle cell anemia
3. With Hb Stanleyville-II	$\alpha\alpha^{76\ Lys}\beta^S\beta^S$	S, Stanleyville/S F, A_2, Stanleyville$_2$	Like severe sickle cell anemia
Group II. Heterozygous for Hb S			
A. Without other Hb abnormality	$\alpha\alpha\beta^A\beta^S$	A, S, A_2	Asymptomatic; rare complications
B. With α thalassemia	$\alpha\alpha^{Thal}\beta^A\beta^S$	A, S(<30%), A_2	Asymptomatic; RBC microcytic, hypochromic
C. With β thalassemia (1)	$\alpha\alpha\beta^S\beta^{Thal^0}$	S, F, A_2(increased)	Moderate to severe anemia and crises; RBC microcytic; may be mistaken for SS
(2)	$\alpha\alpha\beta^S\beta^{Thal+}$	A(10–30%), S, F, A_2 (increased)	Ranges from mild to severe
(3)	$\alpha\alpha\beta^s(\delta\beta)^{Thal}$	S, F (10-25%) A_2(decreased)	Mild anemia without crises

D. With hereditary persistence of Hb F	$\alpha\alpha\beta^{S}$ –	S, F(20–30%), A_2 (decreased)	Hb F homogeneously distributed in RBC
E. With β-chain structural variants			
1. Hb C**	$\alpha\alpha\beta^{S}\beta^{6\ Lys}$	C, S, A_2**	Moderate anemia, occasional crises
2. Hb G-San Jose†	$\alpha\alpha\beta^{S}\beta^{7\ Gly}$	G†, S, A_2	Asymptomatic
3. Hb J-Baltimore	$\alpha\alpha\beta^{S}\beta^{16\ Asp}$	J, S, A_2	Asymptomatic
4. Hb E**	$\alpha\alpha\beta^{S}\beta^{26\ Lys}$	S, E, A_2**	Moderate to severe anemia
5. Hb K-Ibadan	$\alpha\alpha\beta^{S}\beta^{46\ Glu}$	K, S, A_2	Asymptomatic
6. Hb Osu-Christianborg†	$\alpha\alpha\beta^{S}\beta^{52\ Asn}$	Osu-Christianborg†, S, A_2	Asymptomatic
7. Hb Ocho-Rios†	$\alpha\alpha\beta^{S}\beta^{52\ Ala}$	Ocho-Rios†, S, A_2	Asymptomatic
8. Hb Korle-Bu†	$\alpha\alpha\beta^{S}\beta^{73\ Asn}$	Korle-Bu†, S, A_2	Asymptomatic
9. Hb D-Ibadan†	$\alpha\alpha\beta^{S}\beta^{87\ Lys}$	D†, S, A_2	Asymptomatic
10. Hb Richmond	$\alpha\alpha\beta^{S}\beta^{102\ Lys}$	Richmond, S, A_2	Asymptomatic
11. Hb D-Punjab†	$\alpha\alpha\beta^{S}\beta^{121\ Gln}$	D†, S, A_2	Moderate anemia, crises
12. Hb O-Arab**	$\alpha\alpha\beta^{S}\beta^{121\ Lys}$	O, S, A_2**	Moderate to severe anemia, crises
13. Hb K-Woolwich	$\alpha\alpha\beta^{S}\beta^{132\ Gln}$	K, S, A_2	Asymptomatic
14. Hb Lepore†	$\alpha\alpha\beta^{S}\beta^{\delta\times\beta}$	S, F, Lepore†, A_2	Mild to severe anemia
15. Hb C-Harlem	$\alpha\alpha\beta^{S}\beta^{6\ Val,\ 73\ Asn}$	S, C-Harlem	Moderate to severe anemia, crises

*Modified from Milner, 1974.
**Hb C, Hb O Arab, and Hb E are not separated from Hb A_2 on routine alkaline electrophoresis.
†Not separated from Hb S on routine alkaline electrophoresis.

sickle cell disease (Brown et al., 1972). Appropriate genetic and laboratory studies have documented that these individuals are SS homozygotes. This group has very high levels of hemoglobin F (15 to 30 per cent). It is not surprising that these patients have a much lower incidence of cholelithiasis than those with more severe sickle cell disease (Perrine, 1973). A similar form of SS disease with elevated hemoglobin F encountered among the Veddoids of India has recently been studied by Brittenham and his associates (1974).

Associated genetic factors may be important determinants of the overall clinical severity of sickle cell anemia. The coexistence of α thalassemia may result in a significantly lower mean corpuscular hemoglobin concentration and, consequently, a decreased tendency to sickle (Van Enk et al., 1972). Piomelli and his colleagues (1972) reported that glucose-6-phosphate dehydrogenase deficiency was more common in SS homozygotes than in the general Afro-American population. Such an association could be interpreted to mean that this enzyme deficiency might improve the fitness and survival rate of patients with SS disease. However, two subsequent studies have failed to confirm this finding (Beutler et al., 1974a; Steinberg and Dreiling, 1974).

Prevention

Genetic counseling can play an important role in the prevention of sickle cell anemia. If both marital partners are known to be AS heterozygotes, they may elect not to have children, knowing that there is a 25 per cent chance that their offspring will be homozygous.

The antenatal diagnosis of sickle cell anemia can now be made early in the second trimester of pregnancy by the testing of a very small sample of fetal blood obtained from the placenta (Kan et al., 1976b; Alter et al., 1976a). If it is established that the fetus is an SS homozygote, the parents may decide to interrupt the pregnancy. Antenatal diagnosis is discussed in detail on page 183.

SICKLING DISORDERS OTHER THAN SICKLE CELL ANEMIA

As might be expected of a gene with the high frequency of Hb S, sickle cell hemoglobin is frequently encountered in association with other genetically determined abnormalities of the α or β polypeptide chains (Table 7–4).

Hemoglobin SC Disease

Hemoglobin C trait is found in about 3 per cent of Afro-Americans (Motulsky, 1973), and hemoglobin SC disease is the commonest of the genetic variants of sickling in populations of African ancestry. Indeed, in older adults, patients with Hb SC disease probably outnumber SS homozygotes since SC disease is milder and leads to fewer lethal complications in the younger age groups. Typically, patients with Hb SC disease have infrequent crises and a hemolytic anemia of a milder degree than that usually found in sickle cell anemia (McCurdy et al., 1975). Examination of the peripheral blood reveals numerous target cells and occasional plump sickled cells (see Figure 6–5). Sometimes intracellular crystals can be seen (Diggs and Bell, 1965). Most of the complications described under sickle cell anemia may be seen in Hb SC disease, and a few manifestations seem to be at least as common in SC as in SS disease: (1) serious eye lesions (Condon and Serjeant, 1972a and b; see above); (2) hematuria, presumably from renal papillary lesions; (3) avascular necrosis of the heads of the femora; and (4) acute "chest syndromes," particularly in the last trimester of pregnancy. The increased viscosity of the venous blood in Hb SC disease (as compared to SS blood) results from the presence not only of deoxygenated sickle cells but also of a higher packed red cell volume than in sickle cell anemia. Sickle cell hemoglobin C disease is quite variable in its clinical manifestations, and many patients are first detected in adult life. The most common complaint in childhood is generally musculoskeletal or growing pains. Splenomegaly is present in about 60 per cent of patients (Milner, 1974).

Sickle Cell Thalassemia

Sickle cell thalassemia is next in frequency to Hb SC disease among the genetic variants of sickling. Since β thalassemia is common in Greece and in Italy, and sickle cell trait is found generally in lower incidence in some of these populations, the genetic variant, sickle cell–β thalassemia, is the most common form of the sickle syndrome in individuals of Mediterranean ancestry. Beta thalassemia is also found in Africans, and the expression of S/β thalassemia in Africans is generally milder than in the Mediterranean populations. (This difference probably reflects the observed clinical differences in thalassemia in the two groups: thalassemia major generally is an incapacitating disease in Greeks and Italians, and while severe thalassemia has been described in Africans, the usual manifestations of homozygosity for thalassemia in the latter group are considerably milder—sometimes designated thalassemia intermedia [see Chapter 5].)

It is sometimes difficult to distinguish between sickle cell anemia and S/β thalassemia (Table 7–2). The finding of an enlarged spleen in an older patient may be useful in the differential diagnosis. Splenomegaly is much more likely to be encountered in patients (>6

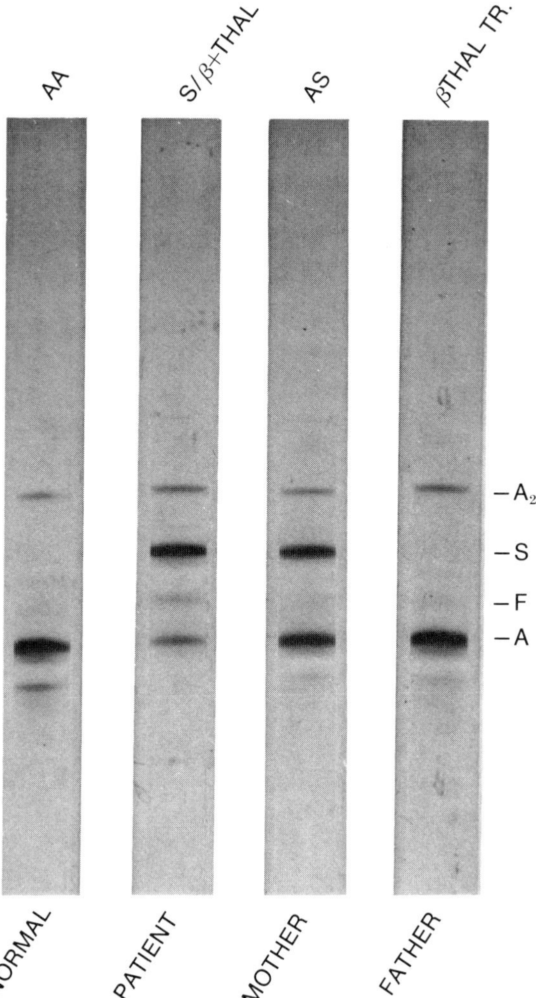

Figure 7–10. Hemoglobin electrophoresis of patient with sickle/β^+ thalassemia and his parents. The mother has sickle trait (AS) and the father has β-thalassemia trait. Note that both the patient and his father have elevated Hb A_2. In addition, the patient has elevated Hb F. The presence of Hb A in the patient's hemolysate indicates that he has S/β^+ thal rather than S/β^0 thal. Hemolysates were analyzed by electrofocusing on polyacrylamide gels.

years) with sickle/β thalassemia than in homozygous sicklers. The hypochromia and microcytosis of the erythrocytes of patients with sickle/β thalassemia is usually established by the age of one year. Hemoglobin electrophoresis provides important independent evidence. If the proportion of Hb A_2 is remarkably increased, e.g., 6 per cent, the diagnosis of sickle/β thalassemia is suggested. Of course, the presence of 10 to 30 per cent hemoglobin A in a patient who has not been transfused, together with Hb S, strongly suggests the presence of S/β^+ thalassemia (Fig. 7–10). The differential between SS and S/β^0 thalassemia is more difficult, since the elevation in hemoglobin A_2 may not be accurately measured, and in either disorder, the sum of Hb S and Hb F accounts for nearly all the hemoglobin. Sometimes family studies are used to establish the diagnosis (Fig. 7–10). The diagnosis of S/β thalassemia can also be made by measuring the biosynthesis of α and β subunits in blood reticulocytes. In S/β thalassemia the β^S/α ratio is 0.5, while it is 1.0 in SS disease. Alpha thalassemia in association with sickle cell anemia is uncommon; the abnormal red cell indices suggest the diagnosis.

Sickle cell thalassemia varies in its severity and outlook; the degree of anemia may be as marked as in sickle cell anemia, or the hemoglobin concentration may be nearly normal. As shown in Table 7–2, S/β^0 thalassemia tends to be more severe than S/β^+ thalassemia. Ocular and bony manifestations may be present, and splenic sequestration crises have been described.

Sickle Cell/Hb D Disease

Sickle cell/Hb D disease is usually due to the presence of Hb S and Hb D-Punjab (in which the glutamic acid residue at β^{121} is replaced by glutamine). The combination of sickle and D-Punjab hemoglobins has been encountered in a number of patients of African origin who have had occasional crises and moderate hemolytic anemia. The electrophoretic pattern of SD disease at alkaline pH is identical with that of SS disease. Hemoglobins S and D-Punjab can be separated by electrophoresis at pH 6.2 in citrate agar. In this acid medium, Hb D migrates like hemoglobin A and is distinct from Hb S.

At least nine hemoglobins with the electrophoretic properties of Hb D (or S) have been found in association with Hb S (McCurdy et al., 1974) (Table 7–4). Of these, only two—Hb D-Punjab and Hb Lepore—each in association with Hb S, have given rise to symptomatic sickle cell disease. Another 12 variants have the same electrophoretic mobility as Hb S but have not thus far been found in association with sickling. The definitive diagnosis of each of these hemoglobins with the electrophoretic properties of Hb D can be made only with detailed structural analysis, since they migrate similarly (like Hb D-Punjab or A, unlike Hb S) on citrate-agar electrophoresis.

Inheritance of Hb S with Other Hemoglobin Variants

Hemoglobin Lepore/S (or Pylos/S) is manifest by the presence of a sickle cell disease of moderate severity, with a thalassemia-like blood picture. The proportion of the nonsickling hemoglobin is lower than in the other β variants.

Hemoglobin S/O-Arab has been described in a number of patients who were previously thought to have Hb SC disease (Milner et al., 1970). Hemoglobin S/O-Arab is generally somewhat more severe than Hb SC disease. A presumptive diagnosis of Hb S/O-Arab disease can be made from the electrophoretic properties at alkaline and acid (pH 6.2) pH: at alkaline pH, Hb O-Arab migrates like Hb C and at pH 6.2 like Hb S (rather than C).

Recently, a patient was found to be doubly heterozygous for hemoglobin S and hemoglobin C-Harlem (Moo-Penn et al., 1975). The hemoglobin electrophoretic patterns resembled that of SC or S/O-Arab. In this disorder, all the β chains have the β6 Glu → Val substitutions and half of the β chains have an additional substitution: β73 Asp → Asn. The patient suffered numerous crises as a child and became less symptomatic as she approached adulthood. The clinical manifestations of hemoglobin S/C-Harlem disease resemble those of SS disease.

The combination of structural α-chain abnormalities with heterozygosity for Hb S has not resulted in sickle cell disease. These combinations can generally be recognized by the appearance of multiple major components ($\alpha_2^A\beta_2^A$, $\alpha_2^X\beta_2^A$,$\alpha_2^X\beta_2^S$, $\alpha_2^A\beta_2^S$) as well as two minor components ($\alpha_2^A\delta_2 \cdot \alpha_2^X\delta_2$) on electrophoresis. Depending upon the charge of the α-chain variant, three or four major bands may be visualized on electrophoresis in alkaline media. (See Figure 6–2.)

Since sickle cell trait is itself asymptomatic, it is perhaps not surprising that amelioration of sickling by the presence of a structural variant has not generally been recognized. However, Hb Memphis ($\alpha_2{}^{23\ \mathrm{Gln}}\ \beta_2^S$) has been observed in association with homozygosity for Hb S. These patients have very mild symptoms of sickling (Kraus et al., 1966; Cooper et al., 1973). In vitro, impaired gelling of Hb S has been demonstrated in the presence of Hb Korle-Bu ($\alpha_2^A\beta_2^{73\ \mathrm{Asn}}$) and Hb F. As might be expected, gelling of Hb S in vitro is favored by the presence of variants which are associated with sickle cell disease—hemoglobins C, D-Punjab, and O-Arab (see Table 7–1).

HEMOGLOBIN S/HPFH

As explained in Chapter 5, the gene for hereditary persistence of fetal hemoglobin (HPFH) is encountered in approximately 0.1 per cent of blacks (Motulsky, 1973). Thus, it is not surprising that occasional individuals have been encountered who are doubly heterozygous for Hb S and HPFH (Bradley et al., 1961). Affected individuals have about 70 per cent Hb S, 20 to 30 per cent Hb F, low Hb A_2, and no Hb A. Peripheral blood counts are usually normal with no evidence of anemia or hemolysis. Red cells are normochromic and normocytic. The peripheral blood film reveals target cells but no fixed sickle forms. Although the sickle preparation and sickle solubility tests are positive, there is rarely clinical evidence of sickling. The mild expression of S/HPFH is due to the fact that the fetal hemoglobin is evenly distributed, thereby protecting all red cells from sickling. This can be demonstrated by differential staining of red cells by acid elution (Kleihauer-Betke stain) or by the use of fluorescently labeled anti-Hb F antibody (Stamatoyannopoulos et al., 1975).

In the great majority of cases the HPFH gene is either allelic or very closely linked to the β-chain structural chain. However, a much less common type of HPFH can be transmitted in cis to the β-chain structural gene (Martinez and Colombo, 1974; Huisman et al., 1975; Stamatoyannopoulos et al., 1975; Friedman and Schwartz, 1976) (see Chapter 5). Stamatoyannopoulos et al. (1975) have reported a patient with homozygous sickle cell disease and HPFH. The increased level of Hb F (20 per cent) and its nearly uniform distribution among red cells probably explain the patient's benign clinical course. This diagnosis should be considered in other patients with mild SS disease and elevated levels of fetal hemoglobin.

Chapter 8

UNSTABLE HEMOGLOBIN VARIANTS—CONGENITAL HEINZ BODY HEMOLYTIC ANEMIA

INTRODUCTION

As mentioned in Chapter 6, most human hemoglobin variants are not associated with detectable clinical manifestations. Many are discovered by chance or during the screening of large populations. However, a growing number of variants are known to have an enhanced propensity to denature, and the denatured hemoglobin precipitates in the red cell. As a result, the abnormal hemoglobin tends to aggregate within the red cell, forming an amorphous mass which has the morphological appearance of a Heinz body. These patients have a disorder of varying clinical severity which is generally called congenital Heinz body hemolytic anemia (CHBA).

In 1952 Cathie described a child with congenital nonspherocytic hemolytic anemia. At 10 months of age the patient had anemia, jaundice, splenomegaly, and pigmenturia. Splenectomy, performed six months later, resulted in no significant clinical improvement. Subsequently, large Heinz bodies were demonstrated in the patient's red cells. Following this report, a number of similar cases have been encountered throughout the world. In most of these cases, a defect in hemoglobin structure and function was suggested by the demonstration of a copious precipitate upon heating the patient's hemolysate (for details, see below). Nearly all these patients have been shown to have a hemoglobin variant. Cathie's patient was found to have Hb

Text continued on page 286.

TABLE 8–1. *Unstable Hemoglobin Variants*

Name	Structure	Helical Site	Inclusion Bodies	Heat Labile	Dark Urine	Hb g/100 ml	Reticulocytes (%)	Per Cent Abnormal Hb	Oxygen Affinity	Comments
I. β-Chain Variants										
Leiden	$\alpha_2\beta_2{}^{6 \text{ or } 7\ Glu \to 0}$	A3 or A4	?			11-13	3-6	30	Decreased	Mild; one residue deletion
Sögn	$\alpha_2\beta_2{}^{14\ Leu \to Arg}$	A11				12-13	0.4	30		No clinical abnormality
Saki	$\alpha_2\beta_2{}^{14\ Leu \to Pro}$	A11								
Belfast	$\alpha_2\beta_2{}^{15\ Trp \to Arg}$	A12	+			11-13	4	28	Slightly increased	
Lyon	$\alpha_2\beta_2{}^{17,18\ Lys,Val \to 0}$	A14,15	+			14.5	4	37	Increased	
Freiburg	$\alpha_2\beta_2{}^{23\ Val \to 0}$	B5		+		13	9	30	Increased	Cyanosis; ↑ methemoglobin, one residue deletion
Riverdale-Bronx	$\alpha_2\beta_2{}^{24\ Gly \to Arg}$	B6		+	0	11-12	10	30		
Savannah	$\alpha_2\beta_2{}^{24\ Gly \to Val}$	B6	+	+		4→6*	50	15-30		Severe
Moscva	$\alpha_2\beta_2{}^{24\ Gly \to Asp}$	B6	+	+				17	Slightly decreased	Patient also had leukemia
St. Louis	$\alpha_2\beta_2{}^{28\ Leu \to Gln}$	B10	+			12	10	29	Increased	15% methemoglobin
Genova	$\alpha_2\beta_2{}^{28\ Leu \to Pro}$	B10	+	+	±	8→14*	10-50	10-25	Increased	
Tacoma	$\alpha_2\beta_2{}^{30\ Arg \to Ser}$	B12	0	+	0	13	4		Increased	No clinical abnormality
Perth	$\alpha_2\beta_2{}^{32\ Leu \to Pro}$	B14	+	+	+	8→11*	27	≃38	Normal	
Philly	$\alpha_2\beta_2{}^{35\ Tyr \to Phe}$	C1	+	+	?	12-14	2-8			
Mequon	$\alpha_2\beta_2{}^{42\ Phe \to Tyr}$	C7								Hemolysis during infection
Hammersmith	$\alpha_2\beta_2{}^{42\ Phe \to Ser}$	CD1	+	+	+	6→7*	20-50	30	Decreased	Severe
Louisville	$\alpha_2\beta_2{}^{42\ Phe \to Leu}$	CD1	+	+		11-13	7-9	30-35	Decreased	
Okaloosa	$\alpha_2\beta_2{}^{48\ Leu \to Arg}$	CD7							Decreased	
Duarte	$\alpha_2\beta_2{}^{62\ Ala \to Pro}$	E6	+	+		15	10	~100	Increased	Heterozygous with β thalassemia

Table continued on following page.

TABLE 8–1. *Unstable Hemoglobin Variants*—Continued

Name	Structure	Helical Site	Inclusion Bodies	Heat Labile	Dark Urine	Hb g/100 ml	Reticulocytes (%)	Per Cent Abnormal Hb	Oxygen Affinity	Comments
Zürich	$\alpha_2\beta_2^{63\ His\to Arg}$	E7	+	+	+	11-12	5-6	25	Increased	Mild; drug-sensitive
Toulouse	$\alpha_2\beta_2^{66\ Lys\to Glu}$	E10	0	+	0	12-15	1-4	40	Normal	No clinical
Sydney	$\alpha_2\beta_2^{67\ Val\to Ala}$	E11	+	+	+	12	8	30		
Bristol	$\alpha_2\beta_2^{67\ Val\to Asp}$	E11	+	+		7→7*	37	36	Decreased	Severe hemolysis
Seattle	$\alpha_2\beta_2^{70\ Ala\to Asp}$	E14	+	+	+	9-10	3	40	Decreased	
Christchurch	$\alpha_2\beta_2^{71\ Phe\to Ser}$	E15	+	+						
Shepherds Bush	$\alpha_2\beta_2^{74\ Gly\to Asp}$	E18				12-13	5-8		Increased	Impaired reactivity of Hb with 2,3-DPG
Bushwick	$\alpha_2\beta_2^{74\ Gly\to Val}$	E18					1-2			Mild; drug-sensitive
St. Antoine	$\alpha_2\beta_2^{74,75\ Gly,Leu\to 0}$	E18,19	+	+	0	11	8	25	Normal	
Buenos Aires	$\alpha_2\beta_2^{85\ Phe\to Ser}$	F1	+	0	0	12-14	8-15		Increased	Compensated hemolysis
Tours	$\alpha_2\beta_2^{87\ Thr\to 0}$	F3	+	+	0	13-14*	9	20	Increased	
Boräs	$\alpha_2\beta_2^{88\ Leu\to Arg}$	F4	+	+		8-12*		10		
Santa Ana	$\alpha_2\beta_2^{88\ Leu\to Pro}$	F4	+	+	+	8-13*	6-28	10		Two hemes per molecule
Gun Hill	$\alpha_2\beta_2^{91\text{-}95\to 0}$	F + FG	0	+	0	13.5	4-10	30	Increased	Five residue deletion; two hemes per molecule
Sabine	$\alpha_2\beta_2^{91\ Leu\to Pro}$	F7	+	+		8-10*	35-65	8		Two hemes per molecule
Istanbul	$\alpha_2\beta_2^{92\ His\to Gln}$	F8	+	+		9-13*	4	12-15	Increased	Two hemes per molecule
Köln	$\alpha_2\beta_2^{98\ Val\to Met}$	FG5	+	+	+	11-13	5-16	10	Increased	Commonest of unstable hemoglobins
Nottingham	$\alpha_2\beta_2^{98\ Val\to Gly}$	FG5	+	+	0	6.7	50		Increased	

Rush	$\alpha_2\beta_2^{101\ \text{Glu}\to\text{Gln}}$	G3		+		11-12	3-7	34	Normal	
Casper	$\alpha_2\beta_2^{106\ \text{Leu}\to\text{Pro}}$	G8	+	+		4-7→13*	20-90		Increased	Severe hemolysis
Peterborough	$\alpha_2\beta_2^{111\ \text{Val}\to\text{Phe}}$	G13	0	+		12	3.5		Decreased	Mild
Madrid	$\alpha_2\beta_2^{115\ \text{Ala}\to\text{Pro}}$	G17	+	+	+	9.7	33	23		Severe hemolysis
Khartoum	$\alpha_2\beta_2^{124\ \text{Pro}\to\text{Arg}}$	H2	0	+						Very mild
Wien	$\alpha_2\beta_2^{130\ \text{Tyr}\to\text{Asp}}$	H8	+	+		10*	43			
Leslie	$\alpha_2\beta_2^{131\ \text{Gln}\to 0}$	H9								
Hope	$\alpha_2\beta_2^{136\ \text{Gly}\to\text{Asp}}$	H14							Decreased	
Olmsted	$\alpha_2\beta_2^{141\ \text{Leu}\to\text{Arg}}$	H19				5-6*	3-8			
Cranston	$\alpha_2\beta_2^{144\to 157}$	C terminus	+	0	0	14	6-8	35	Increased	Elongated β chain
II. α-Chain Variants										
Torino	$\alpha_2^{43\ \text{Phe}\to\text{Val}}\ \beta_2$	CE1	+	+	?	8→12*	6-16	8	Decreased	Moderately severe; aggravated by drugs
L-Ferrara	$\alpha_2^{47\ \text{Asp}\to\text{Gly}}\ \beta_2$	CE5					9	14-20	Normal	Mild
Hasharon	$\alpha_2^{47\ \text{Asp}\to\text{His}}\ \beta_2$	CE5	0	±	0	Normal	1-5	14-19	Normal	Mild
Russ	$\alpha_2^{51\ \text{Gly}\to\text{Arg}}\ \beta_2$	CE9								
Ann Arbor	$\alpha_2^{80\ \text{Leu}\to\text{Arg}}\ \beta_2$	F1				12	10	2-12		Mild
Etobicoke	$\alpha_2^{84\ \text{Ser}\to\text{Arg}}\ \beta_2$	F5		+		11-14	1-3	15	Increased	Mild
Setif	$\alpha_2^{94\ \text{Asp}\to\text{Tyr}}\ \beta_2$	G1		+	0			15	Slightly low	
Bibba	$\alpha_2^{136\ \text{Leu}\to\text{Pro}}\ \beta_2$	H19	+	+		6-7.5	6-16	5-11		Severe
III. γ-Chain Variant										
F-Poole	$\alpha_2\gamma_2^{130\ \text{Trp}\to\text{Gly}}$	H8	+	+						Hemolysis in newborn

*After splenectomy.

Bristol ($\alpha_2\beta_2{}^{67\ Val \rightarrow Asp}$) (Steadman et al., 1970). At present about 60 structurally different unstable hemoglobin variants have been reported (Table 8–1). Some, such as Hb Köln, have been encountered repeatedly in unrelated families from widely scattered parts of the world. Thus, CHBA represents an important type of congenital hemolytic disease. In this chapter we will review its pathogenesis at the cellular and molecular levels, its clinical manifestations, and finally its laboratory diagnosis and treatment.

PATHOGENESIS

The understanding of the mechanism underlying the hemolysis in CHBA was considerably enhanced when Grimes and his associates (Grimes and Meisler, 1962; Grimes et al., 1964) showed that hemolysates from these patients, when incubated at 50° C, formed flocculent precipitates. Such precipitation in stroma-free hemoglobin solutions indicated that an abnormality in soluble cell constituents, probably hemoglobin, was responsible for Heinz body formation. Subsequently, it was shown that heat-labile hemoglobin could be synthesized by reticulocytes (Grimes et al., 1964). Hence its presence was not related to some type of aberrant catabolism or denaturation of aged normal hemoglobin. Hb Zürich was the first unstable variant to be analyzed structurally. Muller and Kingma (1961) demonstrated that at β63(E7), histidine was replaced by arginine. The intimate steric relationship between this residue and the heme group was not known at this time (see Chapter 1). Subsequently, many other patients with CHBA and heat-labile hemoglobin were shown to have electrophoretically abnormal hemoglobins. It became apparent that the great majority of patients whose clinical and laboratory findings suggest the diagnosis of CHBA have structurally abnormal hemoglobin variants. In other patients with the clinical findings of CHBA, current methods may not permit the delineation of structural changes in hemoglobin.

A list of the unstable hemoglobin variants appears in Table 8–1.[1] Its is apparent that there are about four times as many β-chain as α-chain variants. The relatively large number of unstable β-chain variants can be best explained by the strong likelihood that there are four α-chain genes but only two β-chain genes (see Chapter 4). Accordingly, a structural mutation of an α-chain gene would result in the synthesis of only 25 per cent of abnormal α chains. There may

[1]The preparation of Table 8–1 was greatly facilitated by information provided by Dr. Dominique Labie, Dr. Titus Huisman, and Professor Hermann Lehmann and by recent comprehensive reviews by White and Dacie (1971) and White (1974).

be a relatively high incidence of unstable α-chain variants which escape clinical recognition because they make up only a small proportion of the total hemoglobin in the red cell and therefore result in less significant hemolysis. Indeed, most of the α-chain variants listed in Table 8–1 are associated with mild clinical manifestations. It is noteworthy that of the 20-odd *stable* hemoglobin variants associated with increased O_2 affinity and familial polycythemia, all but two are β-chain variants (see Chapter 9).

MOLECULAR BASIS OF INSTABILITY

As discussed in Chapters 1 and 2, considerable knowledge has been amassed on the three-dimensional structure of normal human hemoglobin, allowing rather precise structural-functional interpretations. Thus, the properties of a number of human hemoglobin variants have been explained in terms of the stereochemical consequences arising from an amino acid substitution (or deletion) at a specific site in a globulin subunit (Perutz and Lehmann, 1968; Morimoto et al., 1971). The instability of most of the variants listed in Table 8–1 can be attributed to one of the following five mechanisms:

1. Amino Acid Substitution in the Vicinity of the Heme Pocket. The binding of heme to globin involves a very specific stereochemical fit which helps to stabilize the tertiary conformation of the subunit (see Chapter 1). The heme is inserted into a hydrophobic cleft on the surface of the subunit. The porphyrin interacts with certain nonpolar amino acids in the CD, E, F, and FG regions of the subunits. Most of these nonpolar amino acids are invariant residues. Thus, it is not surprising that substitutions of these residues may result in a decrease in the stability of the heme-globin linkage and, secondarily, of the entire subunit. Figure 8–1 shows a three-dimensional diagram of a β chain. Unstable hemoglobin variants in the vicinity of the heme pocket have been marked by arrows. A number of the unstable hemoglobins have substitutions or deletions in the heme pocket. In some, such as hemoglobins Hammersmith, Zürich, Köln (Jacob et al., 1968; Jacob et al., 1968a), and Sabine (Schneider et al., 1969), experimental evidence supports the prediction that heme binding is impaired. Four of these variants (Bristol, Borås, Olmsted, and Shepherds Bush) involve the substitution of a polar for a nonpolar residue. Such substitutions may allow the entrance of water into the normally hydrophobic heme pocket and thereby weaken heme-globin linkage. The consequences of displacement of heme from its normal binding site will be discussed below in further detail.

2. Disruption of Secondary Structure. The primary amino acid sequence of a protein determines how much of it will be ordered into some form of secondary structure such as the α helix or β pleated

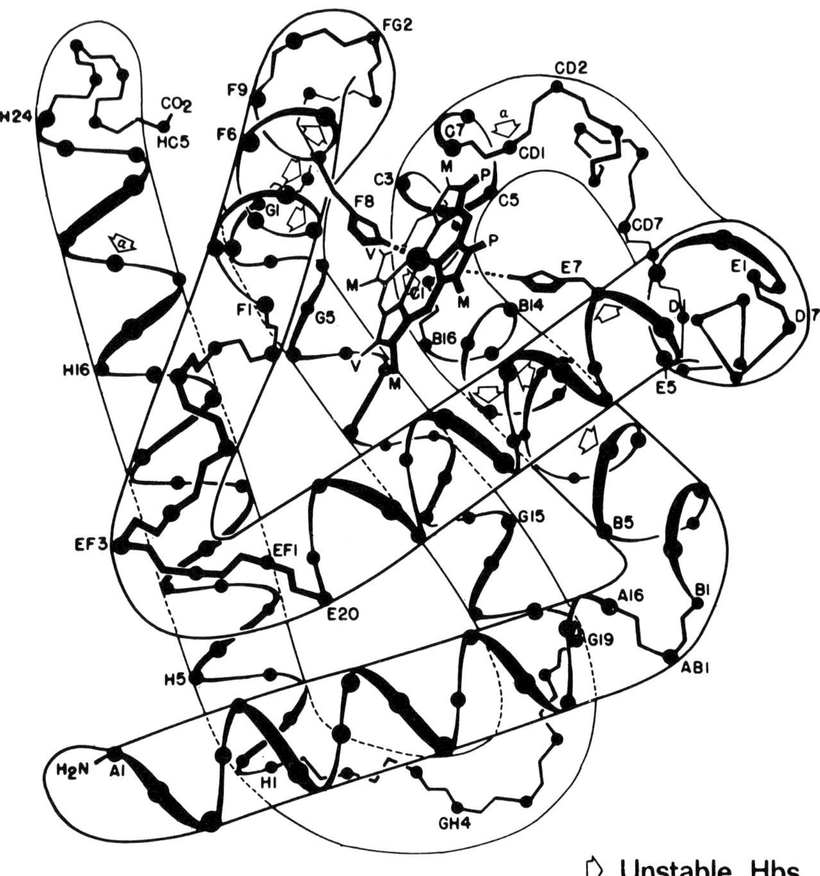

Figure 8–1. Three-dimensional representation of β chain. Arrows indicate sites of substitutions in a number of unstable hemoglobins. Note their proximity to the heme group. (This figure was constructed by Dr. Helen Ranney, using a three-dimensional diagram of myoglobin published by Dickerson, R. E. in Neurath, H. (ed.): The Proteins: Composition, Structure and Function, Vol. II. 2nd ed. New York, Academic Press, 1964, pp. 603–778.)

sheet. As mentioned in Chapter 1, native hemoglobin is about 75 per cent in the form of α helix. The remaining segments of the chains are in random coil. Certain residues have a higher probability of forming an α helix than others. Thus, an analysis of primary structure can give a good prediction of secondary structure (Chou and Fasman, 1974). Certain amino acid substitutions could shift the equilibrium between α helix and random coil in a given segment of the subunit. This would have a marked effect on tertiary structure and the overall stability of the subunit. Proline cannot participate in an α helix except as one of the initial three residues. Eight of the unstable variants are substitutions of proline for leucine. In addition, Hb Duarte and Hb Madrid involve a substitution of proline for alanine. In each case, the substitution involves a residue beyond the third place in the helix. Among the 135 stable hemoglobin variants associated with no clinical manifestations, only one involves a proline substitution at the C-terminal residue of the α chain (Hb Singapore $\alpha^{141\ \mathrm{Arg}\rightarrow\mathrm{Pro}}$). Thus, the disruption of the α helix probably accounts for the instability of the ten variants mentioned above.

3. *Substitution in the Interior of the Subunit.* As mentioned in Chapter 1, the globin subunits are folded in such a way that all the charged amino acids such as lysine, arginine, glutamic acid, and aspartic acid are situated on the surface of the molecule, allowing their ionized groups to be in contact with solvent water. In contrast, the residues oriented toward the interior of the molecule have nonpolar side groups. The interior of the molecule is thus stabilized by hydrophobic interactions. A number of unstable variants involve the substitution of a polar for a nonpolar residue. These include hemoglobins Sögn, Riverdale-Bronx, Bristol, Shepherds Bush, Boräs, Olmsted, Russ, Ann Arbor, and Wien. As mentioned above, four of these (Bristol, Boräs, Shepherds Bush, and Olmsted) are near the heme pocket. Polar for nonpolar substitutions could result in significant alterations in tertiary structure if water is allowed access to the hydrophobic interior of the subunit. In addition, a variant having a neutral amino acid substitution may owe its instability to an alteration of the stereochemical fit of the residue's side group. This is difficult to predict without very precise atomic coordinates. Nevertheless, it is interesting that 17 out of 46 unstable variants (35 per cent) involve the substitution of one noncharged residue for another (including the 6 Leu→Pro substitutions), whereas only 3 out of 110 functionally normal and clinically silent variants encountered to date involve such a substitution (3 per cent). As mentioned in Chapter 1, hemoglobin readily dissociates symmetrically into $\alpha\beta$ dimers: $\alpha_2\beta_2 \rightleftharpoons 2\alpha\beta$. The subunits cleave at the interface between the α_1 and β_2 subunits. In contrast, the bonding between the α_1 and β_1 subunits is considerably stronger. In normal Hb A, the dissociation of the subunits at this interface ($\alpha_1\beta_1 \rightarrow \alpha + \beta$) is observed only under extremes of pH or ionic strength or in solutions which favor disruption of secondary and tertiary structure, such as concentrated urea. A few hemoglobin variants owe their instability to substitutions at the $\alpha_1\beta_1$ interface, which permits the dissociation of the $\alpha\beta$ dimer into monomers and allows hidden sulfhydryl groups to become reactive. Hb Philly is one of the best studied of this type of unstable variant (Rieder et al., 1969).

4. *Amino Acid Deletion(s).* Ten hemoglobin variants have been reported to date to have deletions from one to five residues in

sequence: Leiden, Lyon, Freiburg, Leslie, Coventry, St. Antoine, Tours, Niteroi, Tochigi, and Gun Hill. All of these are unstable variants (Table 8–1). Variants having multiple deletions have only been encountered at or near interhelical corners. Such an alteration in structure can have a marked effect on the overall conformation of the molecule involving intra- and inter-subunit interactions. Distortion of structure is particularly marked in Hb Gun Hill, in which no heme binding to the β chain is possible because of the deletion of five residues in the F–FG region. Despite this, individuals with Hb Gun Hill have relatively mild hemolysis (Bradley and Rieder, 1966; Bradley et al., 1967).

5. *Elongation of Subunit.* A few hemoglobin variants have elongated subunits, owing either to an error in chain termination or to nonhomologous crossover (see Chapter 6). Most of these are present in only small amounts. Hb Cranston is found in association with a compensated hemolytic state (Bunn et al., 1975b). The instability of this variant is probably due to a hydrophobic segment attached to the C-terminal end of the β chain. The stability of the other elongated β chain variant, Hb Tak, has not yet been determined.

Heinz Body Formation

The mechanisms underlying the formation of intracellular inclusions in CHBA have been studied extensively, particularly by Jacob and his associates (1968a, 1968b; Jacob and Winterhalter, 1970a, 1970b), Rachmilewitz (Rachmilewitz and Harari, 1972; Rachmilewitz and White, 1973; Rachmilewitz, 1974), and Winterbourn and Carrell (1972, 1973, 1974). Their experiments were done on selected variants, but the results are likely to be relevant to many of the other unstable hemoglobins. The following phenomena have been demonstrated.

Displacement of the Heme Group in the Abnormal Subunit

The stability of the heme-globin linkage is dependent on the precise stereochemical fit conferred by the surrounding residues in the heme pocket (see Chapter 1). As mentioned above, this fit is perturbed in a number of the unstable variants because of amino acid substitutions or deletions in this region. Furthermore, the oxidation state of the heme iron has an important influence on the stability of the heme-globin linkage. In normal oxyhemoglobin and deoxyhemoglobin, the ferrous heme group remains tightly bound to globin. In contrast, the ferriheme group in methemoglobin has a much lower affinity for globin (Bunn and Jandl, 1968). Jacob and his coworkers (1968b) showed that ferriheme dissociated more readily from methemoglobin Köln than from methemoglobin A. During incubation of hemolysates at 50° C, those containing unstable hemoglobin variants (Köln, Zürich, Hammersmith) showed a rapid decrease in the ratio of absorptions at 540 nm and 280 nm (Jacob and Winterhalter, 1970a, 1970b). These results do not necessarily mean "heme loss." Free hematin is very insoluble at neutral pH and binds avidly and nonspecifically to a number of proteins. It is likely that in many cases the heme group is displaced from its normal position in the subunit during the incubation, and as a result its absorption in the visible spectrum is significantly altered.

Hemichrome Formation

Recent observations by Rachmilewitz and his associates (Rachmilewitz and Harari, 1972; Rachmilewitz and White, 1973; Rachmilewitz, 1974) indicate that hemichromes are a common intermediate in various types of hemoglobin denaturation. They are characterized by a specific absorption in the visible spectrum (Fig. 8–2). The incubation of methemoglobin can lead to hemichromes, particularly under circumstances in which hemoglobin lacks its normal stabilizing interactions. For example, isolated hemoglobin subunits (α or β chains), certain chemically modified hemoglobins, and a number of unstable hemoglobin variants have been shown to form hemichromes readily (Rachmilewitz et al., 1971). Electron paramagnetic (spin) resonance (EPR) has proved a very useful physical measurement in the further characterization of these intermediates (Rachmile-

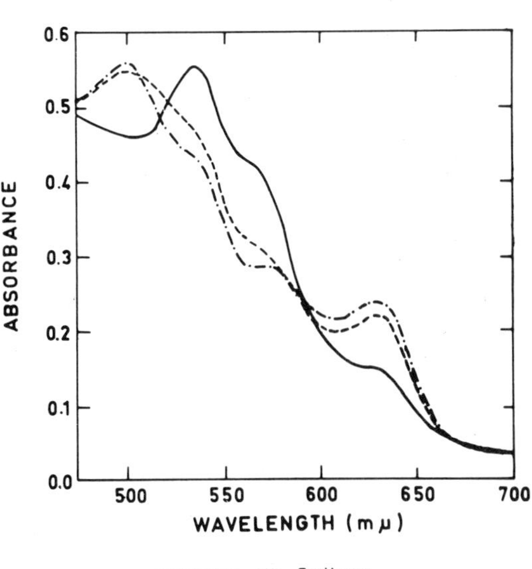

Figure 8–2. Absorption spectra of whole hemolysate and purified hemoglobins from a patient with Hb Freiburg (β23 Val→0), 48 hours after oxidation with ferricyanide (0.05 M phosphate, pH 7.0, 4° C). Purified Hb A (—·—·—·) has an absorption spectrum indicating methemoglobin. Purified Hb Freiburg (———) has an absorption spectrum of a hemichrome. (With permission of Dr. E. A. Rachmilewitz.)

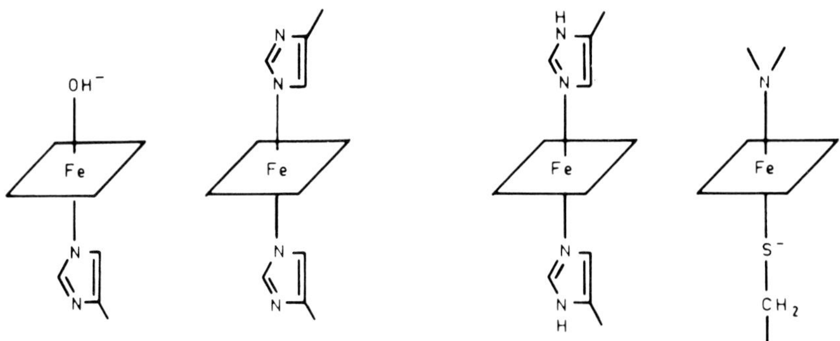

Reversible Hemichromes Irreversible Hemichromes

Figure 8–3. Diagrammatic structure of hemichromes showing proximal histidine below the plane of the porphyrin ring and distal histidine above the plane. (From Rachmilewitz, E. A.: Sem. Hemat. *11*:441, 1974.)

witz et al., 1971). The bonding of the distal (E7) histidine imidazole to the oxidized heme results in the transition from high spin to low spin state having a characteristic EPR signal (Fig. 8–3). This type of hemichrome has been shown to be reversible (hemichrome 1 in Figure 8–5). Upon reduction of the heme iron to the ferrous state, deoxyhemoglobin is formed. Further distortion of the subunit's conformation allows other groups to form an internal ligand with the heme, resulting in the formation of irreversible hemichromes which have distinguishing EPR spectra (hemichrome 2 in Figure 8–5). The formation of irreversible hemichromes is accompanied by precipitation of the hemoglobin.

A number of unstable hemoglobin variants have been shown to form hemichromes, particularly following incubation of the oxidized (methemoglobin) form. These include hemoglobins Köln, β98 Val→Met (Rachmilewitz and Harari, 1972); Louisville (Bucuresti), β42 Phe→Leu (Rachmilewitz, 1974); Freiburg, β23 Val→0 (Rachmilewitz and Harari, 1972); Riverdale-Bronx, β24 Gly→Arg (Rachmilewitz and Harari, 1972); Hammersmith, β42 Phe→Ser (Wajcman et al., 1973b); Seattle, β70 Ala→Asp (Rachmilewitz, 1974); Sydney, β67 Val→Ala (Winterbourn and Carrell, 1974); and Christchurch, β71 Phe→Ser (Winterbourn and Carrell, 1974). It is likely that such hemichromes are formed during the denaturation of other unstable variants. The amino acid substitution apparently causes sufficient disruption in the tertiary structure of the subunit to permit the opposition of the iron atom of the ferriheme group to certain nearby groups of the globin chain. The formation of hemichromes involves a marked reduction in absorption at 540 nm and probably contributes to the decreased ratio of optical density observed for several unstable variants (OD-540/OD-280) (Jacob and Winterhalter, 1970a, 1970b).

Enhanced Reactivity of the β93 Sulfhydryl Groups

Jacob et al. (1968a, 1968b) showed that Hb Köln had an increased rate of reaction with labeled glutathione to form the mixed disulfide. Red cell glutathione has been found to be decreased in a few patients with CHBA (Fairbanks et al., 1969; White and Dacie, 1971; Honig et al., 1973), although normal or elevated in others (Fairbanks et al., 1969; White and Dacie, 1972). The enhanced sulfhydryl reactivity of some of the unstable variants may explain their tendency to become highly labeled with radioactive chromium. White and Dacie (1971) incubated intact CHBA red cells with ^{51}Cr-labeled sodium chromate and then separated the globin peptide chains by column chromatography. The variant β chains (Köln, Hammersmith, and Shepherds Bush) had two- to sixfold higher specific activity than the β^A chains. Jacob and his coworkers (1968a, 1968b) have suggested that in patients with Hb Köln, Heinz bodies may be attached to the inner surface of the red cell membrane by a disulfide bond between hemoglobin and a membrane protein. The inclusions could be released from erythrocyte ghosts by the addition of mercaptoethanol, a reagent capable of reducing disulfide bonds (Jacob et al., 1968a).

Recent studies by Winterbourn and Carrell (1973, 1974) have raised some doubt about the importance of sulfhydryl oxidation in the pathogenesis of CHBA. Experiments on three unstable variants (Köln, Sydney, Christchurch) revealed no blocked cysteines and no protection by reduced glutathione. Although precipitation of the oxy and carboxy forms of these hemoglobins was accompanied by the formation of intermolecular disulfide bonds, there was no evidence that this phenomenon affected the rate of precipitation. Furthermore, these authors examined red cells containing inclusions of Hb Christchurch and failed to demonstrate the presence of any covalent linkage (such as disulfide bonds) between globin and membrane protein. They concluded that the adherence of the Heinz body to the inner surface of the red cell membrane is due to hydrophobic bonding (Winterbourn and Carrell, 1973).

The two phenomena—dissociation of heme and enhanced sulfhydryl reactivity—may be linked according to the following scheme:

$$\begin{array}{ccccc}
\text{Globin—Fe}^{3+}\text{heme} & \underset{K_1}{\rightleftharpoons} & \text{Globin} & + & \text{Fe}^{3+}\text{heme} \\
| & & | & & \\
\text{SH} & & \text{SH} & & \\
K_2 \downarrow\uparrow +\text{RSH} & & K_4 \downarrow\uparrow +\text{RSH} & & \\
\text{Globin—Fe}^{3+}\text{heme} & \underset{K_3}{\rightleftharpoons} & \text{Globin} & + & \text{Fe}^{3+}\text{heme} \\
| & & | & & \\
\text{SSR} & & \text{SSR} & &
\end{array}$$

The following observations support such a relationship: (1) the dissociation of ferriheme from normal methemoglobin A is enhanced when the β93 sulfhydryl group is blocked by N-ethylmaleimide ($K_3 > K_1$) (Bunn and Jandl, 1968); (2) hemoglobin lacking heme groups on the β chains ($\alpha_2\beta_2^0$) has markedly enhanced sulfhydryl reactivity ($K_4 > K_2$) (Jacob and Winterhalter, 1970a; and (3) in several of the unstable variants both of these reactions are favored. From these considerations it is not surprising that the rate of denaturation of the unstable hemoglobins can be enhanced by sulfhydryl blockade (Jacob et al., 1968, 1968a) and that it can be reduced by the addition of a heme ligand such as cyanide (Jacob and Winterhalter, 1970a; Rieder, 1970) which stabilizes the heme-globin linkage (Bunn and Jandl, 1968) (see Figure 8–4). Rieder (1970) has shown that cyanide also inhibits the denaturation of normal hemoglobin.

The unstable hemoglobins have properties very similar to the artificial Hb $\alpha_2\beta_2^0$ (Jacob and Winterhalter, 1970a). As mentioned above, both have enhanced sulfhydryl reactivity. Both form a flocculent precipitate when incubated at 50° C. This denaturation is inhibited by the addition of ligands such as cyanide or hemin. Both $\alpha_2\beta_2^0$ and many of the unstable variants have an increased degree of dissocia-

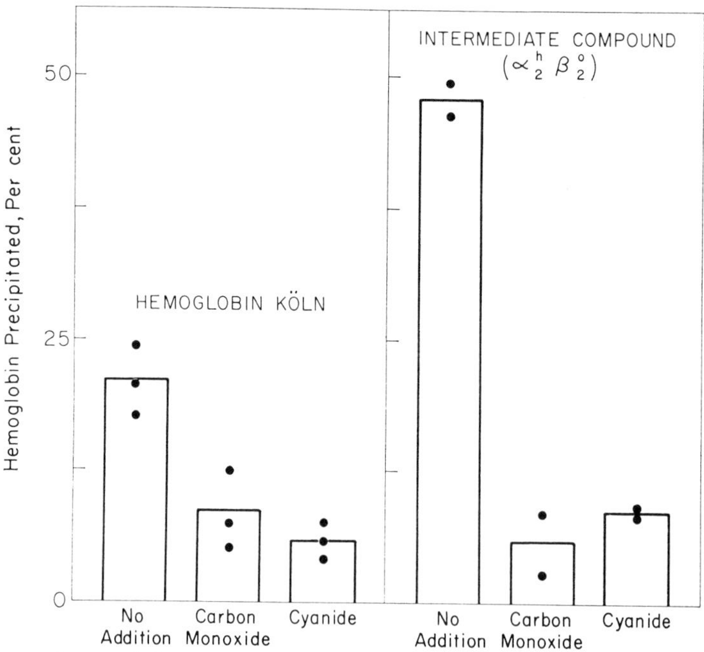

Figure 8–4. Inhibition of heat precipitation of hemoglobin Köln (left) and $\alpha_2^{heme}\beta_2^0$ (right) by cyanide or carbon monoxide. Both heme proteins copiously precipitate when heated at 50° C for 2 hours unless the heme ligands, cyanide or carbon monoxide, are present. (From Jacob, H. S., and Winterhalter, K. H.: J. Clin. Invest. *49*:2008, 1970a.)

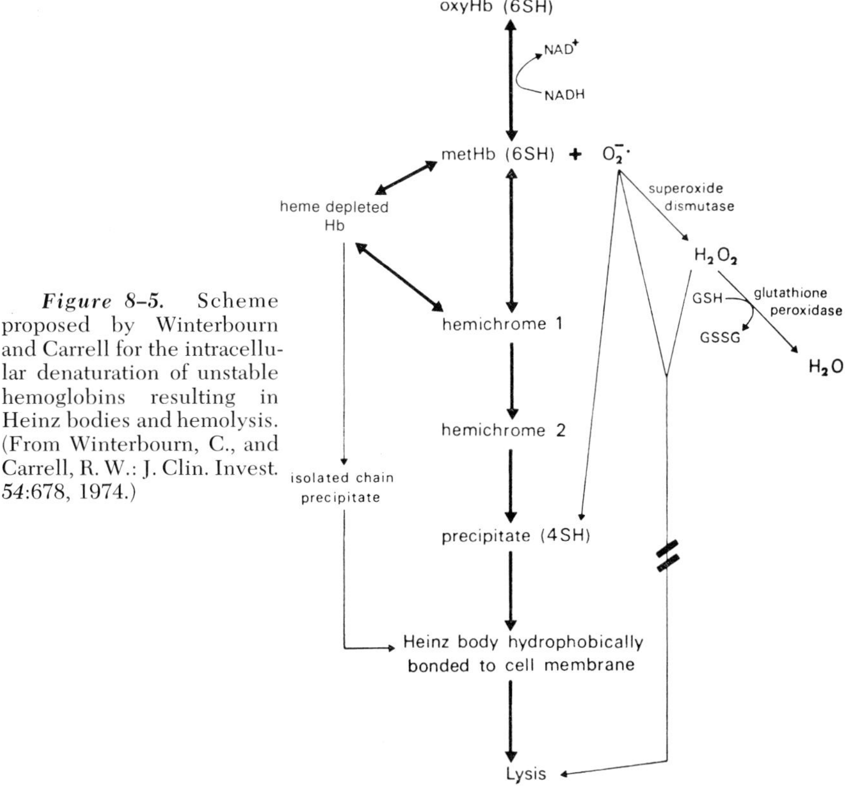

Figure 8–5. Scheme proposed by Winterbourn and Carrell for the intracellular denaturation of unstable hemoglobins resulting in Heinz bodies and hemolysis. (From Winterbourn, C., and Carrell, R. W.: J. Clin. Invest. *54*:678, 1974.)

tion from tetramer to dimer: $\alpha_2\beta_2 \rightarrow 2\alpha\beta$ (Winterhalter, 1972; Waks et al., 1973).

During the circulation of the CHBA red cell in vivo or the incubation of the hemolysate in vitro, the three-dimensional structure of the hemoglobin variant is altered sufficiently so that its solubility decreases and it forms a precipitate. It seems unnecessary to postulate (Rachmilewitz and Harari, 1972; Rachmilewitz, 1974) that the hemoglobin tetramer dissociates into individual subunits prior to the precipitation of the abnormal chain. Winterbourn and Carrell (1972) have performed amino acid analyses and peptide mapping of precipitates of several variants, including Christchurch, Sydney, Köln, and Hammersmith, and have demonstrated the presence of equal amounts of α and β chains. Furthermore, some α chain polymerized with β chain by means of disulfide bond formation. The precipitates of hemoglobins Christchurch and Sydney contained a full complement of heme, whereas Hb Köln appeared to be depleted of half the heme. Thus, the precipitation of most unstable variants probably involves the entire molecule rather than selective heme loss with subsequent aggregation of the denatured globin subunits (Jacob et al., 1968a, 1968b).

The scheme proposed by Winterbourn and Carrell (1974) for the denaturation of unstable hemoglobins is depicted in Figure 8–5. Oxyhemoglobin is converted to methemoglobin. The release of superoxide anion (O_2^-) or its product, H_2O_2, may result in oxidant damage to globin thiols and to the membrane. As yet there is no experimental evidence on this point. Because of its structural abnormality, the unstable methemoglobin is converted first to a reversible hemichrome intermediate and then to an irreversible hemichrome (hemichrome 2). Precipitation of this latter species may be hastened by the formation of disulfide bonds between globin subunits.

MECHANISM OF HEMOLYSIS IN CHBA

There is both morphological (Rifkind, 1965; Schnitzer et al., 1971) and experimental (Jacob et al., 1968a) evidence that in CHBA, Heinz bodies become adherent to the inner surface of the red cell membrane. As mentioned above, this attachment is probably due to hydrophobic rather than covalent interactions (Winterbourn and Carrell, 1973; Chan and Desforges, 1974). The membrane-bound inclusions cause crater-like indentations on the surface of the cell (Schnitzer et al., 1971). Red cells containing Heinz bodies have been shown to have decreased pliability and filterability (Jandl et al., 1961; Miller et al., 1971). It is not surprising that they have difficulty negotiating the microcirculation. Rifkind (1965) has presented convincing morphological evidence that Heinz body red cells get hung up in transit between the cords and sinuses of the spleen. The membrane-bound Heinz body may be ensnared during this passage. The remainder of the red cell then reseals its membrane after it has been relieved of this excess baggage. These considerations help to explain why the number of Heinz bodies increases markedly after patients with CHBA have undergone splenectomy.

The metabolism of CHBA red cells has been studied by a number of investigators. In general, specific enzyme activities have either been normal or increased in keeping with a young population of red cells. In some cases, glucose consumption is increased in conjunction with decreased levels of ATP (Miller et al., 1971; White and Dacie, 1971). Indeed, one case of CHBA (Schneider et al., 1969) was initially reported as a defect in red cell metabolism (Mills et al., 1968). Red cell 2,3-DPG is usually found to be normal. The enhanced potassium efflux (Jacob et al., 1968a; Miller et al., 1971) found in erythrocytes from certain patients with CHBA has been attributed to the adherence of Heinz bodies to the inner surface of the red cell membrane. However, this increased potassium efflux is rather nonspecific and has been reported in a diverse group of hemolytic states, including sickle cell anemia, pyruvate kinase deficiency, hereditary stomatocytosis, and red cells treated with amphotericin B. To the extent that CHBA red cells leak potassium, the energy-dependent Na-K pump is stimulated in order to maintain osmotic equilibrium, thereby increasing the rate of glycolysis and decreasing ATP concentrations. Osmotic fragility is generally normal in CHBA.

The activity of the hexose monophosphate shunt has been increased in some cases of CHBA. Nevertheless, red cell glutathione is more often normal or increased than decreased (White and Dacie, 1971) and does not have an enhanced turnover rate (White and Dacie, 1971) (see above).

Biosynthesis of Unstable Variants

As Table 8–1 shows, the unstable hemoglobin variant usually makes up only a minority of the total hemoglobin. The remainder is Hb A, A_2, and perhaps some F. Furthermore, in some hemolysates of individuals with unstable β-chain variants, a very small amount of free α chains is observed on electrophoresis (Grimes et al., 1964; Sansone and Pik, 1965; Raik et al., 1967; Monn et al., 1968; Rieder and Bradley, 1968; Jacob and Winterhalter, 1970a; Rieder et al., 1975). The presence of free α chains can be explained by either decreased synthesis or enhanced destruction of the unstable β subunit. As the previous discussion on the pathogenesis of CHBA implies, the latter mechanism predominates.

The biosynthesis of a number of unstable variants has been studied. As Table 8–2 shows, the rate of synthesis of normal and variant chains is equal in most cases. Exceptions include hemoglobins Riverdale-Bronx, Boräs, Abraham Lincoln, and Ann Arbor. In all cases, the specific activity of the abnormal β chain greatly exceeded that of β^A because of the selective loss of the unstable variant as CHBA red cells circulate through the RE system (see previous section). It is likely that in red cells containing very unstable variants, a small pool of free α chains exchanges readily with the α chains of the variant. Rieder's (1971) observations on Hb Gun Hill provide a striking illustration of this point. Following incubation of the reticulocyte-rich blood with ^{14}C leucine, hemoglobins A and Gun Hill were separated by electrophoresis. The α chains of the purified hemoglobin A had virtually no radioactivity, while the α chains of Gun Hill were highly labeled. Thus, the newly synthesized α chains appeared to be diluted by a pre-existing pool of unlabeled α chains, thereby lowering α^A radioactivity. The high activity of the α^{GH} chains must have been due to exchange of the partially labeled free α chain pool with the α chains of the unlabeled (but labile) Gun Hill. A similar phenomenon has been noted for hemoglobins Hammersmith (White and

TABLE 8–2. *Synthesis of Globin Chains of Unstable Hemoglobin Variants*

Hb	Per Cent Abnormal Hb	Subunit Specific Activity var/A	Rate of Synthesis of Variant Chain*	Total $\alpha:\beta$ Synthesis	Reference†
Gun Hill β91–95 deleted	32	2.4	120	1.0	Adams et al., 1972†
Köln β98 Val→Met	12	7.4	100	1.2–1.4	White and Brain, 1970; Huehns, 1970†
Hammersmith β42 Phe→Ser	40	1.5	100	1.1	White and Dacie, 1970†
Bristol β67 Val→Asp	36	1.4	98		Steadman et al., 1970†
Riverdale-Bronx β24 Gly→Arg	28	1.4–1.5	56–59	~1.2	Bank et al., 1970, and Zulsky et al., 1970†
Boräs β88 Leu→Arg	10		33		White, 1971†
Shepherds Bush β74 Gly→Asp	25		100		White and Dacie, 1971†
Abraham Lincoln β32 Leu→Pro	18	2.5	50	1.18	Honig et al., 1974
Zürich β63 His→Arg	32		110		Rieder et al., 1965
Leiden β6,7→0	24	1.5	100	1.8	Rieder and James, 1974
Cranston β Elongated chain	30	1.4	100	1.0	Shaeffer et al., in preparation
Bushwick β74 Gly→Val	1–2	20–60	~100	1.0	Rieder et al., 1975
Sabine β91 Leu→Pro	12	~1.5–3	~100		Shaeffer, 1973
Ann Arbor α80 Leu→Arg	2–15	2.5	20	4.0	Adams, 1974

*Expressed as percentage of the rate of synthesis of normal subunit.
†Unless stated otherwise, data have been taken from paper of Honig et al., 1974.

Dacie, 1970), Köln (White and Brain, 1970), Shepherds Bush (White and Dacie, 1971), Riverdale-Bronx (Zalusky et al., 1970), Sabine (Shaeffer, 1973), and Abraham Lincoln (Honig et al., 1974). Because of this exchange of α chains, the ratio of the total radioactivity of the normal and variant hemoglobins is not a reliable indication of the relative synthetic rates. It is curious that despite the marked distortion of primary structure of Hb Gun Hill, which has a deletion of the 5 residue segment at the proximal heme binding site, the rate of translation of $\beta^{\text{Gun Hill}}$ was equal to that of β^{A} (Rieder, 1971). Thus, if heme normally binds to the nascent polypeptide chain, it has no apparent effect on the rate of synthesis. As Table 8–2 shows, in most of the synthesis studies done on reticulocytes containing unstable hemoglobins, total α and β chain production is balanced. However, Hb Leiden is an interesting exception (Rieder and James, 1974). The overall β/α synthetic ratio was found to be 0.47 to 0.63 in peripheral blood and 0.82 in marrow. These values are similar to what has been encountered in individuals with β thalassemia. The mechanism for this imbalance in subunit synthesis is not known.

CLINICAL MANIFESTATIONS

Inheritance

Congenital Heinz body hemolytic anemia exhibits an autosomal dominant pattern of inheritance. Thus, affected individuals are heterozygotes. Because the spleen selectively removes the Heinz bodies, the unstable hemoglobin makes up only a minority (10 to 30 per cent) of the total. As expected in the heterozygous state, the remainder is predominantly normal hemoglobin A. An interesting exception is the recent report of Hb Duarte (Beutler et al., 1974b). This unstable β-chain variant was inherited in conjunction with β thalassemia. Accordingly, the production of normal β^{A} chains was markedly suppressed and, therefore, most of the patient's hemoglobin was Duarte. Fortunately, the variant was only mildly unstable, so that the individual survived into adulthood with a well compensated hemolytic state. Because of the low gene frequency for unstable variants, homozygosity would be very rare (except in offspring of consanguineous marriages) and most often incompatible with life. Such genetic considerations also apply to erythrocytosis accompanying hemoglobin variants with abnormally high oxygen affinity. A sizable minority of cases of CHBA appear to have arisen because of a spontaneous mutation, both parents being unaffected. Viewed another way, of the 20 instances of apparent spontaneous mutations among hemoglobin variants reported up until 1973, 17 involved patients with CHBA (Table 8–3). This is not surprising, since most

TABLE 8–3. Apparent Spontaneous Mutations Among Hemoglobin Variants

HEMOGLOBIN	STRUCTURE	CLINICAL STATUS	BLOOD ANTIGENS TESTED	RNA BASE CHANGE
Hammersmith*	$\alpha_2\beta_2^{42\ \text{Phe}\to\text{Ser}}$	Hemolysis	No	U → C
Köln†	$\alpha_2\beta_2^{98\ \text{Val}\to\text{Met}}$	Hemolysis	Yes (36)	G → A
Santa Ana†	$\alpha_2\beta_2^{88\ \text{Leu}\to\text{Pro}}$	Hemolysis	No	U → C
Olmsted	$\alpha_2\beta_2^{141\ \text{Leu}\to\text{Arg}}$	Hemolysis	No	U → G
Freiburg	$\alpha_2\beta_2^{23\ \text{Val}\to 0}$	Hemolysis	No	
Sabine	$\alpha_2\beta_2^{91\ \text{Leu}\to\text{Pro}}$	Hemolysis	Yes	U → C
Savannah	$\alpha_2\beta_2^{24\ \text{Gly}\to\text{Val}}$	Hemolysis	No	G → U
Toulouse	$\alpha_2\beta_2^{66\ \text{Lys}\to\text{Glu}}$	Hemolysis	No	A → G
Bristol	$\alpha_2\beta_2^{67\ \text{Val}\to\text{Asp}}$	Hemolysis	No	U → A
Bryn Mawr	$\alpha_2\beta_2^{85\ \text{Phe}\to\text{Ser}}$	Hemolysis	No	U → C
Casper†	$\alpha_2\beta_2^{106\ \text{Leu}\to\text{Pro}}$	Hemolysis	Yes	U → C
M-Saskatoon†	$\alpha_2\beta_2^{63\ \text{His}\to\text{Tyr}}$	Cyanosis	Yes	C → U
M-Hyde Park	$\alpha_2\beta_2^{92\ \text{His}\to\text{Tyr}}$	Cyanosis	Yes	C → U
M-Boston	$\alpha_2\beta_2^{58\ \text{His}\to\text{Tyr}}$	Cyanosis	No	C → U
Bethesda	$\alpha_2\beta_2^{145\ \text{Tyr}\to\text{His}}$	Erythrocytosis	Yes	U → C
Abraham Lincoln	$\alpha_2\beta_2^{32\ \text{Leu}\to\text{Pro}}$	Hemolysis	Yes	U → C

*Three instances.
†Two instances.

cases are sufficiently severe that medical attention and evaluation are sought. In contrast, the chances are very remote of finding an asymptomatic individual with a hemoglobin variant due to a spontaneous mutation. Furthermore, the reproductive potential of patients with severe CHBA may be decreased.

PRESENTATION

Congenital Heinz body hemolytic anemia varies widely in clinical severity (Table 8–1). The variability depends primarily on the structural differences among the unstable variants. A given variant tends to produce similar clinical sequelae in affected individuals whether they are within the same family or are unrelated. Thus far, Hb Köln has been the most frequently encountered unstable variant. At least seven unrelated kindred or sporadic cases from various parts of the world have been reported to have Hb Köln. These patients all have a moderate hemolytic state that is well compensated, particularly following splenectomy.

Patients with severe CHBA may present with anemia in early childhood.[2] These include hemoglobins Bristol and Hammersmith. These β-chain variants emerge at approximately 6 months of age when the transition from γ to β chain production is complete. More commonly, patients present at different ages with unexplained hemolytic anemia. In many cases patients come to a physician's attention during an "aplastic" crisis, in which erythropoiesis has been temporarily suppressed by either infection or folic acid deficiency. Like other patients with chronic hemolysis, individuals with CHBA have an increased tendency to develop pigmented gallstones.

In some patients hemolysis may be aggravated by viral or bacterial infections or following the exposure to an oxidant agent such as sulfonamides. Hb Zürich has been encountered in three unrelated families (Frick et al., 1962; Rieder et al., 1965; Dickerman et al., 1973a). Affected individuals have normal hematocrits and absent or minimal hemolysis unless they are exposed to an oxidant stress. A few days of treatment with a sulfa drug can result in a hemolytic crisis with a 50 per cent drop in hematocrit, the emergence of Heinz bodies, and marked hyperbilirubinemia. The anemia remits promptly upon withdrawal of the drug. Those affected family members who have not been exposed to oxidant drugs have no history of hemolysis. Sulfonamides have also been found to exacerbate hemolysis in individuals with hemoglobins Torino (Beretta et al., 1968; Prato et al., 1970), Shepherds Bush (White et al., 1970), and Peterborough (King et al., 1972). Oxidant drugs do not affect hemolysis in patients with Hb Köln (Miller et al., 1971).

A significant proportion of patients with CHBA give a history of passing dark urine. In the absence of liver disease, patients with hemolytic anemia do not have bilirubinuria. Indeed, an outmoded term for hemolytic anemia is "acholuric jaundice." Furthermore, patients with CHBA do not have enough intravascular hemolysis to produce hemoglobinuria. It turns out that the pigmenturia in such patients with CHBA is probably due to dipyrrolmethenes of the mesobilifuscin group (Schmid et al., 1959). The structure of this pigment

---

[2]An unstable γ-chain variant (Hb F-Poole, $\alpha_2{}^G\gamma_2{}^{130\ Trp\rightarrow Gly}$) has been reported to cause hemolytic disease in the newborn (Lee-Potter et al., 1975). The hemolysis disappeared when Hb F switched to Hb A in the first few months of life.

is not yet definitely established. Pigmenturia is an inconsistent finding in CHBA. As shown in Table 8–1, pigmenturia is not well correlated with the severity of hemolysis. Dipyrroluria has also been encountered in β thalassemia (major) (Kreimer-Birnbaum et al., 1966a, b), another disorder associated with Heinz body production (see Chapter 5). It is likely that the urinary pigment is a reflection of aberrant heme catabolism, perhaps via a pathway that bypasses heme oxygenase, an enzyme responsible for the physiological catabolism of heme (Tenhunen et al., 1968). Goldstein et al. (1968) have found that experimentally induced Heinz bodies are also broken down aberrantly with decreased conversion of heme to bilirubin and the formation of a urinary pigment having properties indicative of dipyrroles. It may be that during the auto-oxidation of the unstable hemoglobin in vivo, sufficient superoxide anion or peroxide is generated that heme (or its porphyrin) is oxidized in a nonspecific, nonenzymatic fashion leading to these abnormal products.

A number of the unstable hemoglobin variants are unassociated with any clinical manifestations and have been discovered fortuitously or during surveys of large populations. The frequency of finding these mild unstable variants is increasing because of the development of more sensitive and specific methods for detection (see below).

Physical Findings

The physical findings of patients with CHBA are variable and depend primarily upon the severity of the disease. Those with moderate or severe hemolysis have jaundice and splenomegaly. Some patients may have hypersplenism with significant thrombocytopenia (Hutchison et al., 1964; Pederson et al., 1973). Severe hypersplenic hemolysis has been observed in newborns with Hb Hasharon (Tatsis et al., 1972). A few patients with CHBA may be mildly cyanotic, owing either to the presence of methemoglobinemia (as encountered in Hb Freiburg) (Jones et al., 1966) or to decreased oxygen affinity leading to deoxygenation of the peripheral blood (Hb Hammersmith). Some patients with CHBA have been reported to have leg ulcers (Jackson et al., 1973; White, 1974).

LABORATORY DIAGNOSIS OF CHBA

General Parameters of Hemolysis

Patients with CHBA, like those with other types of chronic hemolysis, will have reticulocytosis accompanied by increased

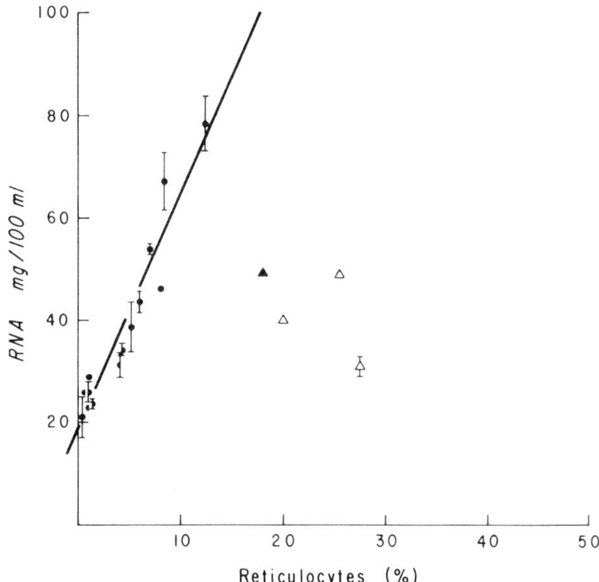

Figure 8–6. The relationship between reticulocytes estimated by supravital stain (abscissa) and by measurement of RNA (ordinate). Normal reticulocytes (●) have a linear relationship between these two measurements. Patients with an unstable hemoglobin variant (Hb Casper) have a falsely high reticulocyte count both prior to (△) and following (▲) splenectomy. (From Koler, R. T., et al.: Amer. J. Med. 55:549, 1973.)

serum bilirubin and decreased haptoglobin. However, the extent of hemolysis is often difficult to evaluate in patients having an unstable hemoglobin. Because the precipitated variant takes up supravital stains, Heinz body–containing cells may be mistaken for reticulocytes. Thus, the estimate of reticulocytes by ordinary methods may be falsely high. As Figure 8–6 shows, measurement of red cell RNA will give a truer indication of reticulocyte number (Koler et al., 1973). In like manner, measurements of red cell life span by tagging red cells with ^{51}Cr are very difficult to interpret. There is no correlation between ^{51}Cr red cell survival and degree of hemolysis in CHBA (Bentley and Lewis, 1974). As mentioned above, ^{51}Cr will bind preferentially to the variant hemoglobin, compared to Hb A (White and Dacie, 1972). Secondly, the isotope appears to elute more readily from the abnormal hemoglobin (Pederson et al., 1973). Finally, as we have discussed, precipitates containing the unstable variant are selectively pitted from red cells during in vivo circulation. These factors make the rate of disappearance of ^{51}Cr radioactivity greatly exceed the rate of red cell destruction. The use of radioactive amino acid precursor (Honig et al., 1973) (Fig. 8–7) or DF^{32}P labeling (Bentley and Lewis, 1974; Hutchinson et al., 1974) will give a more reliable indication of red cell survival.

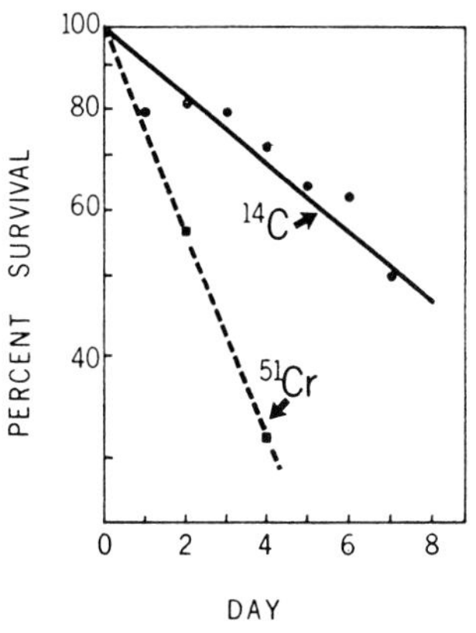

Figure 8–7. Red cell survival of a patient with an unstable hemoglobin variant (Hb Abraham Lincoln) measured by ^{14}C-amino acid labeling of reticulocytes and ^{51}Cr labeling of whole blood. (From Honig, G., et al.: J. Clin. Invest. 52:1748, 1974.)

Red Cell Morphology

Congenital Heinz body anemia red cells may appear entirely normal on a Wright's stained blood film. Often, however, the cells are hypochromic (low MCHC) despite having a normal mean corpuscular volume. This may be a reflection of the pitting function of the spleen. The red cells often show more variation in size and shape than normal, and prominent basophilic stippling may be seen (Fig. 8–8). In some patients the red cells appear as if a bite had been taken from the margin. Again, this may be a morphological sequela of splenic pitting.

The demonstration of Heinz bodies requires the use of a supravital stain such as crystal violet or new methylene blue. Their presence is highly variable. In the most mild forms of CHBA, it may be necessary to incubate red cells for long time periods, either in the presence of an oxidant such as acetylphenylhydrazine or in the absence of substrate (glucose), before Heinz bodies can be demonstrated. It is important to have normal controls for comparison, since numbers of Heinz bodies may be elicited in normal red cells by these maneuvers. Heinz bodies are more readily demonstrable in patients with severe CHBA. In all cases they are much more abundant following splenectomy. They appear as irregular blue-purple inclusions, 0.5 to 2.0μ, often solitary and adjacent to the inner surface of the red cell membrane (Fig. 8–8). In contrast, inclusions generated by the oxidant dye tend to be smaller and multiple. Recent evidence indicates that in CHBA, these bodies are not irreversibly bound to the membrane (Winterbourn and Carrell, 1973). Heinz bodies are not specific for CHBA. They can also be seen in the red cells of patients with some forms of α or β thalassemia and in the red cells of patients exposed to an oxidant stress, particularly those deficient in an enzyme involved in the pentose-phosphate pathway (HMP shunt) or in the synthesis of glutathione.

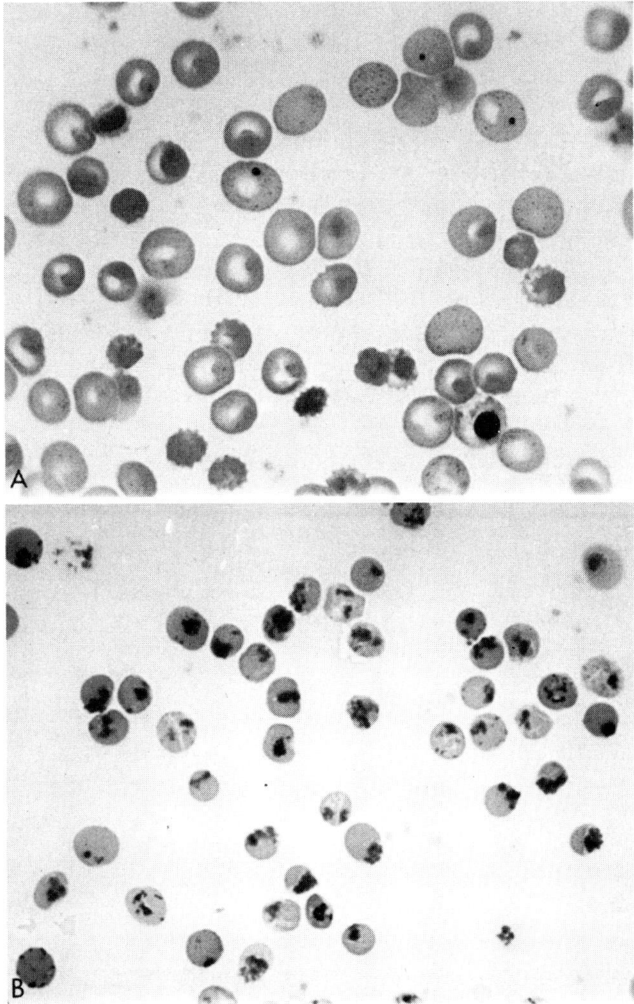

Figure 8–8. *A*, Photomicrograph of peripheral blood from a patient with an unstable hemoglobin variant (Hb Abraham Lincoln). Note basophilic stippling, Howell-Jolly bodies, and normoblast. *B*, Following incubation of blood for 30 minutes with new methylene blue. Most red cells contain large Heinz bodies. (From Honig, G., et al.: J. Clin. Invest. 52:1748, 1974.)

Hemoglobin Denaturation

The diagnosis of CHBA can often be established by the demonstration of denatured hemoglobin in the hemolysate. In most cases the hemoglobin variant will form a flocculent precipitate when a 1 per cent solution of the hemolysate is incubated in a neutral phosphate buffer at 50° C for 1 to 2 hours (Grimes and Meisler, 1962; Grimes et al., 1964). In the preparation of the hemolysate, the stroma should not be removed with organic solvents (White, 1974). The sensitivity of the test may be enhanced by the use of TRIS buffer (Schneiderman et al., 1970), although we have been unable to notice any advantage in this method for the unstable variants which we have tested. Carrell and Kay (1972) showed that incubation of hemolysates in 17 per cent isopropanol at 37° C provides enhanced sensitivity. This test is easy to perform and should be available in clinical laboratories for routine screening. The addition of the sulfhydryl reagent *p*-mercuribenzoate to the hemolysate can result in the precipitation of the abnormal subunit (Rieder et al., 1969; Huisman et al., 1971a; Honig et al., 1973). Those unstable variants which have an increased tendency to dissociate into subunits can be readily attacked by sulfhydryl reagents. This approach has been used to prepare unstable hemoglobin subunits that cannot be separated by conventional means (Huisman et al., 1971a; Honig et al., 1973). In view of the tendency of unstable hemoglobins to denature under a variety of experimental conditions, it is not surprising that the Sickledex Test may give a false-positive result in CHBA (Fairbanks and Pettit, 1972).

Hemoglobin Electrophoresis

The diagnosis of CHBA is confirmed if an abnormal band is demonstrated on hemoglobin electrophoresis. However, only about 45 per cent of the unstable variants have substitutions (or deletions) which involve an alteration in charge. Thus, many of these abnormal hemoglobins are very difficult to separate by ordinary electrophoretic techniques. It may be necessary to try electrophoresis in different media and several pH's before an optimal separation can be achieved. If hemes are lost or displaced from the abnormal subunit, one or more bands (or a smear) migrating less rapidly toward the anode than the intact hemoglobin (i.e., a more positive net charge) may appear. The anomalous electrophoretic behavior of a number of the unstable variants may be related to heme depletion of the abnormal subunits. Another type of electrophoretic heterogeneity was demonstrated in studies on Hb Rush (Adams et al., 1974). Analysis of the hemolysate on cellulose acetate at pH 8.6 revealed two bands migrating cathodally to Hb A. Re-electrophoresis of the middle band produced a pattern similar to that of the whole hemolysate, suggesting that this component was the hybrid tetramer $\alpha_2\beta^A\beta^{Rush}$, and upon re-electrophoresis it dissociated and recombined to form the two parent tetramers.

Hb A_2 may be increased somewhat in patients with CHBA

(White and Dacie, 1972; Honig et al., 1973). This is probably a reflection of the fact that the variant hemoglobin is selectively removed from the red cell as discussed previously, leaving a higher ratio of Hb A_2 to total hemoglobin (Rieder et al., 1965). Similar to other types of chronic hemolysis, Hb F levels may be modestly elevated in CHBA. In some unstable variants, free α chains can be demonstrated on electrophoresis, since the unstable β chains may be selectively precipitated (see previous section on biosynthesis).

If an unstable variant is difficult to separate electrophoretically, it will also be difficult to purify by standard preparative procedures such as column chromatography. For this reason, it may be necessary to take advantage of the relative insolubility or enhanced denaturation of the variant in order to purify it and study its properties. This has been done by *p*-mercuribenzoate precipitation (see above) or isopropanol precipitation (deWeinstein et al., 1973).

Oxygen Equilibria

The unstable hemoglobins tend to have abnormal oxygen affinity. Whole blood oxygen saturation curves have been determined for about half the various unstable variants (Table 8–1). Of these, the oxygen affinity is normal in 20 per cent, decreased in 30 per cent, and increased in 50 per cent. The lattermost finding is not surprising, since the tertiary structure of the variant subunit may be so altered that it cannot form a stable t structure. If the oxygen affinity of the variant hemoglobin differs significantly from that of Hb A, the whole blood oxygen saturation curve will be biphasic (Fig. 8–9).

As Bellingham and Huehns (1968) have pointed out, oxygen affinity may be an important determinant of red cell mass in patients with CHBA. The hemoglobin of individuals with Hb Köln exhibits significantly increased oxygen affinity and, as a consequence, impaired release of oxygen during capillary circulation. The resultant tissue hypoxia stimulates erythropoiesis, presumably via regulation by erythropoietin. As a result, individuals with Hb Köln have minimal anemia, despite a significant amount of hemolysis. One patient actually developed an increase in oxygen affinity and erythrocytosis following splenectomy (Egan and Fairbanks, 1973). Thus, oxygen delivery may not have been improved by the operation (Desforges, 1973). Woodson et al. (1974) have studied oxygen transport in two individuals with Hb Köln. These patients had normal oxygen consumption, hemoglobin concentration, and cardiac output. From the Fick equation discussed in Chapter 3, it follows that A-V oxygen extraction must also be normal. However, because of the increase in red cell oxygen affinity, oxygen delivery could only be achieved at the expense of a significant reduction in mixed venous PO_2. This was

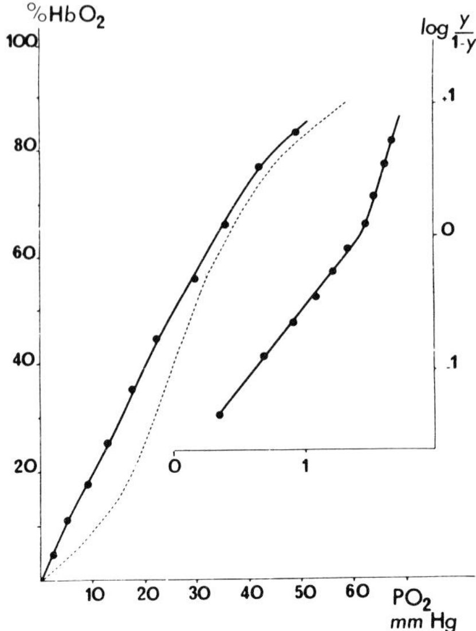

Figure 8–9. Oxygen dissociation curve of blood of a patient with Hb Tours. (Dotted line indicates normal curve.) The Hill plot shown in an inset on the right shows a biphasic curve. The left-hand portion of the curve shows increased oxygen affinity due to the presence of the hemoglobin variant. The right-hand portion of the curve reflects oxygenation of Hb A in the patient's red cells. (From Wajcman, H., et al.: Biochim. Biophys. Acta *295*:495, 1973a.)

documented by direct measurement. The marked increase in urinary erythropoietin in one patient and evidence for redistribution of blood flow to vital organs indicated that these individuals were on the verge of hypoxia.

In contrast, patients with Hb Hammersmith have decreased O_2 affinity (Wajcman et al., 1973b) and severe anemia. Those with Hb Seattle also have a "shift to the right" (Stamatoyannopoulos et al., 1969b), although much less hemolysis than the Hammersmith patients. Because oxygen unloading is enhanced, there is less stimulation to erythropoiesis. The red cell mass of these individuals is thus set at a subnormal level appropriate for their hemoglobin function (Stamatoyannopoulos et al., 1969). This relationship appears to be a general phenomenon among patients with CHBA. As Figure 8–10 shows, those individuals who have unstable variants with increased oxygen affinity tend to have normal or near normal hemoglobin values while those with decreased oxygen affinity may have significant anemia.

It is often difficult to study the functional properties of unstable hemoglobins in detail. During the process of separation from normal Hb A the variant may become irreversibly denatured. Some unstable variants such as Hb Köln (Wajcman et al., 1971; Pederson et al., 1973; Sharma et al., 1974), Hb Savannah (Huisman et al., 1971a), Hb Bibba (Smith et al., 1970), and Hb Istanbul (Aksoy et al., 1972) have an increased tendency to dissociate into dimers. This process appears to be related to the displacement or loss of heme from the β chains. The initial measurements of the oxygen equilibria of purified

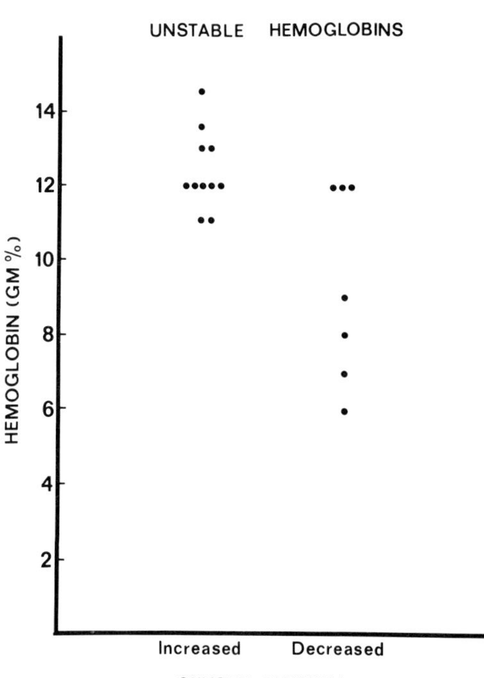

Figure 8–10. Comparison of hemoglobin levels in CHBA patients having increased and decreased oxygen affinity.

Hb Köln by Wajcman et al. (1971) showed it to have high oxygen affinity, low heme-heme interaction, and decreased reactivity with 2,3-DPG. In contrast, DeFuria and Miller (1972) showed that in the presence of added hemin, hemoglobin Köln had a higher degree of heme-heme interaction and normal 2,3-DPG reactivity. Sharma et al. (1974) measured the kinetics of binding of carbon monoxide to Hb Köln and found that in the absence of added hemin, the reaction was fast and monophasic, indicating that deoxy Köln was largely in the R structure. Following the addition of hemin, a biphasic curve was obtained, with the slow component resembling Hb A. These results indicate that the addition of hemin permits Hb Köln to assume the T ("deoxy") conformation and help to explain the conflicting observations on oxygen equilibria noted above.

Besides Hb Köln, two other unstable hemoglobins have been shown to have impaired interaction with 2,3-DPG (May and Huehns, 1972a; Nagel et al., 1973). Hb Leiden ($\alpha_2\beta_2^{6 \text{ or } 7\ \text{Glu}\rightarrow 0}$) (Nagel et al., 1973) probably has weak binding to 2,3-DPG because the deletion increases the distance between the two N termini of the β chains (see Chapter 1). The mechanism for the diminished response of Hb Shepherds Bush ($\alpha_2\beta^{74\ \text{Gly}\rightarrow\text{Asp}}$) to 2,3-DPG is less clear (May and Huehns, 1972a).

TREATMENT

Most individuals with CHBA do not require treatment. Those with severe hemolysis derive benefit from general supportive measures such as folic acid and prompt attention to infections. Oxidant drugs should be avoided. Transfusions are indicated only rarely such as during an aplastic crisis in which erythropoiesis has been suppressed.

As discussed in the section on pathogenesis, the spleen has been shown to sequester CHBA red cells. During the circulation through the spleen Heinz bodies may be "pitted" from the cell, leaving the remainder of the red cell intact. Other cells do not escape from the splenic cords and are destroyed in situ. From these considerations, splenectomy seems to be a reasonable approach in selected cases. In a recent review of the literature, Koler et al. (1973) concluded that splenectomy may be beneficial in severely affected patients. As Figure 8–11 shows, some patients have achieved a significant increase in hemoglobin following splenectomy. Others with equally severe hemolysis have not benefited. It is difficult to predict preoperatively which patients will respond. Measurements of ^{51}Cr red cell survival and splenic uptake are very difficult to interpret (see above). The decision on whether a patient with CHBA should undergo splenectomy may sometimes be resolved by ascertaining whether other patients with the same variant were benefited (see Koler et al., 1973,

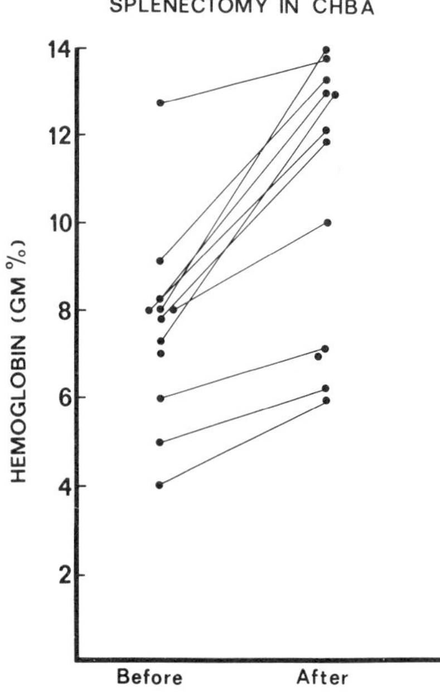

Figure 8–11. Effect of splenectomy on hemoglobin levels in patients with CHBA.

and Figure 8–11). As mentioned earlier, one patient with Hb Köln actually developed polycythemia following splenectomy (Egan and Fairbanks, 1973), probably as a result of the increased oxygen affinity of this variant (see above). It is difficult to appraise the significance of CHBA in the reported deaths of two patients, presumed to have Hb Duarte, following splenectomy, since many relevant details of the hematological status of the individuals either pre- or postoperatively are not known (Beutler et al., 1974b). Splenectomy should not be performed on young children (<6 years of age), since they are at increased risk of developing septicemia following surgery. One 6-year-old child with Hb Hammersmith died of pneumococcal septicemia four years after undergoing a splenectomy (White, 1974).

Chapter 9

HEMOGLOBINOPATHY DUE TO ABNORMAL OXYGEN BINDING*

In 1966, Charache, Weatherall, and Clegg described an individual with unexplained erythrocytosis in association with a hemoglobin variant. Their patient was an 81-year-old man who presented with mild angina pectoris that developed late in life. He had no other significant clinical problems. By chance, he was initially seen in the hematology clinic at Johns Hopkins Hospital (Charache, 1974b). In this setting, Dr. Charache discovered that he had a hemoglobin of 19.9 g/100 ml and an abnormal hemoglobin band on electrophoresis. In an attempt to relate these two findings, Dr. Charache and Dr. Andre Helleghers determined an oxygen dissociation curve on the patient's blood and found that it was significantly displaced to the left. This observation suggested the intriguing possibility that the patient's erythrocytosis might be a secondary compensation to a primary defect in oxygen unloading. A thorough family study revealed 15 other members with both erythrocytosis and the electrophoretically abnormal hemoglobin. Charache then purified the hemoglobin variant and confirmed that it had a marked increase in oxygen affinity. Clegg and Weatherall established that hemoglobin Chesapeake is an α-chain variant with a substitution of leucine for arginine at position 93 (Clegg et al., 1966). This series of observations opened up a new chapter in the developing story of hemoglobin.

Nineteen other variants with increased oxygen affinity have been encountered thus far in individuals with secondary erythrocy-

*This subject has recently been discussed in two excellent reviews (Charache, 1974a; Nagel and Bookchin, 1974b).

TABLE 9–1. *Hemoglobin Variants Associated With Familial Erythrocytosis*

Variant	Structure	Area Affected	Severity	Bohr Effect	Max. Hb. Conc. (g/100 ml)	Reference
Chesapeake	α92 (FG4) Arg→Leu	$\alpha_1\beta_2$	3+	Normal	19.9	Charache et al., 1966
J-Cape Town	α92 (FG4) Arg→Gln	$\alpha_1\beta_2$	+	Normal	16.6	Lines and McIntosh, 1967
Olympia	β20 (B2) Val→Met	$\alpha_1\beta_2$	3+		20.7	Stamatoyannopoulos et al., 1973
Rahere	β82 (EF6) Lys→Thr		2+	Normal	20.0	Lorkin et al., 1975
Creteil	β89 (F5) Ser→Asn					Gavel et al., 1974
Malmö	β97 (FG4) His→Gln	$\alpha_1\beta_2$	3+	Normal	21.3	Fairbanks et al., 1971
Wood	β97 (FG4) His→Leu	$\alpha_1\beta_2$				Taketa et al., 1976
Yakima	β99 (G1) Asp→His	$\alpha_1\beta_2$	3+	Normal	22.9	Jones et al., 1967
Kempsey	β99 (G1) Asp→Asn	$\alpha_1\beta_2$	3+	↓	21.3	Reed et al., 1968
Ypsilanti	β99 (G1) Asp→Tyr	$\alpha_1\beta_2$	2+		22.0	Glynn et al., 1968
Brigham	β100 (G2) Pro→Leu	$\alpha_1\beta_2$	2+	Normal	20.0	Lokich et al., 1973
Heathrow	β103 (G5) Phe→Leu	Heme	3+	Normal	21.0	White et al., 1973
San Diego	β109 (G11) Val→Met	$\alpha_1\beta_2$	2+		18.1	Nute et al., 1974b
Little Rock	β143 (H21) His→Gln	$\beta\beta$	3+	Normal	23.0	Perutz, 1973
Syracuse	β143 (H21) His→Pro	$\beta\beta$	3+	↓	23.8	Jensen et al., 1975
Andrew-Minneapolis	β144 (HC1) Lys→Asn	$\beta\beta$			19.8	Zak et al., 1974
Rainier	β145 (HC2) Tyr→Cys	$\beta\beta$	3+	↓	21.0	Adamson et al., 1969
Bethesda	β145 (HC2) Tyr→His	$\beta\beta$	3+	↓	20.5	Hayashi et al., 1971
Osler (Fort Gordon)	β145 (HC2) Tyr→Asp	$\beta\beta$	3+	↓	22.0	Charache et al., 1975a; Kleckner et al., 1975; Jacon et al., 1975
Hiroshima	β146 (HC3) His→Asp	$\beta\beta$	2+	↓	17.4	Hamilton et al., 1969

tosis (Table 9–1). These variants generally have amino acid substitutions at sites crucial to hemoglobin function. Indeed, the understanding of structural-functional relationships of human hemoglobin is sufficiently advanced that, in most cases, the abnormal oxygen binding of the variant can be readily explained by its specific structural alteration (see below). In addition, a number of other variants are known to have increased oxygen affinity, though they are not associated with secondary erythrocytosis. These variants, shown in Table 9–2, generally do not have such marked increases in oxygen affinity as those listed in Table 9–1. Among the 120-odd variants unassociated with any relevant clinical manifestations, there are probably additional hemoglobins with abnormal functional properties. Until recently, oxygen affinity measurements were not generally included in studies on new hemoglobin variants.

About 30 per cent of the 50-odd unstable hemoglobin variants have significantly increased oxygen affinity (see Table 8–1). In fact, some of these mutant hemoglobins have higher oxygen affinity than those listed in Table 9–1. However, the predominant clinical manifestations are due to accelerated red cell destruction. The oxygen affinity of unstable hemoglobins appears to be an important determinant of the degree to which the patient's hemolysis is compensated: those patients with CHBA due to a variant with high affinity tend to have higher hemoglobin levels than those with normal or decreased oxygen affinity (see Bellingham and Huehns, 1968, and Chapter 8).

MOLECULAR PATHOGENESIS

The functional behavior of normal hemoglobin depends on a transition in its three-dimensional conformation which accompanies the addition and removal of oxygen. This process is discussed in detail in Chapter 1. As formulated in the allosteric model of Monod,

TABLE 9–2. *Hemoglobin Variants Having Increased Oxygen Affinity Without Erythrocytosis*

Variant	Structure	Area Affected	Bohr Effect	References
G-Norfolk	α85 (F6) Asp→Asn		Normal	Cohen-Solal et al., 1975
Denmark Hill	α95 (G2) Pro→Ala	$\alpha_1\beta_2$	↓	Wiltshire et al., 1972
Rampa	α95 (G2) Pro→Ser	$\alpha_1\beta_2$		DeJong et al., 1971
G-Georgia	α95 (G2) Pro→Leu	$\alpha_1\beta_2$	↓	
Hirose	β37 (C3) Trp→Ser	$\alpha_1\beta_2$		
Abruzzo	β143 (H21) His→Arg	$\beta\beta$		

Wyman, and Changeux (MWC) (1965), the hemoglobin tetramer exists in equilibrium between two quaternary conformations: R and T. When normal hemoglobin is fully deoxygenated, it is about 99.99 per cent in the T or "tense" structure. In this state, hemoglobin has a relatively low affinity for oxygen and other heme ligands and a relatively high affinity for allosteric effectors such as Bohr protons and 2,3-DPG. Conversely, normal oxyhemoglobin exists almost exclusively in the R or "relaxed" conformation. In this state it has a relatively high affinity for heme ligands such as oxygen and a low affinity for Bohr protons and 2,3-DPG. The transition between these two conformers involves a considerable free energy change, reflected as cooperativity between subunits or "heme-heme interaction" (Chapter 2). The change from the T to the R conformation involves a rather well-defined series of structural changes including the rupture of the salt bonds that stabilize the T conformation and the rotation of the β chains relative to the α chains. A considerable amount of intramolecular "movement" during this conformational isomerization occurs at the $\alpha_1\beta_2$ interface.

A structural alteration which affects the equilibrium between the R and T states would be expected to have a marked effect on hemoglobin function. Thus, if a specific amino acid substitution decreases the stability of the T structure, the transition to the R state will occur at an earlier stage in ligation, and the hemoglobin will have increased oxygen affinity and decreased heme-heme interaction. This has been demonstrated for a number of chemically modified hemoglobins as well as many of the high-affinity mutants. Hemoglobin Kempsey is a particularly well studied example (Reed et al., 1968; Ogata et al., 1972; Lindstrom et al., 1973; Bunn et al., 1974b; Perutz et al., 1974a). It is a β-chain variant in which β99-aspartic acid has been substituted by asparagine. In deoxyhemoglobin A this aspartic acid residue normally forms an important hydrogen bond with α42-tyrosine at the $\alpha_1\beta_2$ interface (Fig. 9–1). Upon oxygenation, the two subunits shift in a dovetail fashion, so that the β99-α42 hydrogen bond is broken and another one forms between α94-aspartic acid and β102-asparagine (Perutz, 1972). In hemoglobin Kempsey, the substitution at β99 prevents the formation of the former hydrogen bond, and lessens the stability of the "deoxy" or T structure. Thus, when hemoglobin Kempsey is fully deoxygenated it remains partly in the R state. (The equilibrium constant L in the MWC model is drastically reduced.) This has been verified experimentally in a variety of ways. There are a number of physical and chemical properties which distinguish normal oxy- and deoxyhemoglobin. In fact, these can be considered to be properties which distinguish the R and T conformations. In many respects, deoxygenated hemoglobin Kempsey bears more resemblance to oxyhemoglobin A than to deoxyhemoglobin A. These include kinetics of ligand binding, sulf-

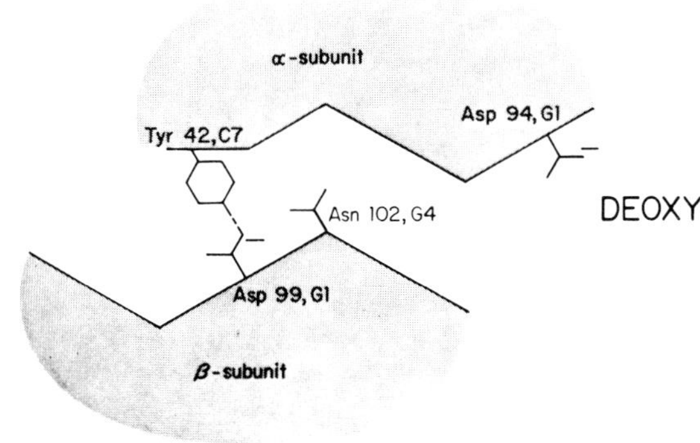

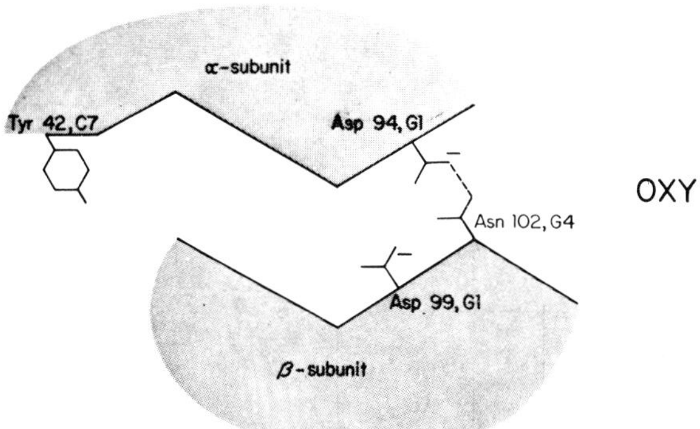

Figure 9–1. Changes at a portion of the $\alpha_2\beta_2$ interface upon oxygenation. The area of contact shifts in a dovetail fashion. Deoxyhemoglobin is stabilized by a hydrogen bond between α42 Tyr and β99 Asp. This bond cannot form in Hb Kempsey (β99 Asp→Asn). Likewise, oxyhemoglobin is stabilized by a bond between α94 Asp and β102 Asn. This bond cannot form in Hb Kansas (β102 Asn→Thr), Hb Beth Israel (β102 Asn→Thr), and Hb Titusville (α94 Asp→Asn). (From Perutz, M. F.: New Scient. Sci. J., June, 1971.)

hydryl reactivity, extent of dissociation into αβ dimers, and binding to haptoglobin (Bunn et al., 1974b). In addition, physical probes such as nuclear magnetic resonance spectroscopy (Lindstrom et al., 1973) and circular dichroism (Perutz et al., 1974a, b) support the conclusion that deoxygenated Hb Kempsey is partially in the R conformation.

Most of the high-affinity variants thus far encountered have substitutions at either of two regions that are crucial to hemoglobin function (see Tables 9–1 and 9–2):

1. The $\alpha_1\beta_2$ interface.
2. The C-terminal end of the β chain.

As discussed in Chapter 2, the C-terminal portions of the α and β chains contribute greatly to the overall stability of the "deoxy" or T conformation (Perutz, 1970a,b). The penultimate tyrosine of both chains (α140, β145) is anchored in a cleft between the F and H helices. In the α chain, the C-terminal arginine is involved in two salt bonds: the guanido group is linked to an aspartate (residue 126) of the α chain and the carboxyl group may be linked to the N-terminal amino group of the other α chain. The C-terminal end of the β chain plays an equally important role. The C-terminal histidine (β146) forms two salt bonds: its carboxyl group is linked to the ϵ amino group of α40-lysine, while its imidazole group forms an intrasubunit bond with the carboxyl of β94-aspartate. In addition, β143-histidine is an important binding site for 2,3-DPG. All these interactions are oxygen-linked. The bonds break upon oxygenation and the molecule then assumes the relaxed (R) conformation. It is not surprising that variants having substitutions at the C-terminal portion of the β chain can have abnormal functional properties, including high oxygen affinity, decreased heme-heme interaction, decreased Bohr effect, and impaired interaction with 2,3-DPG. These will be discussed in more detail in the next section.

PROPERTIES OF THE HIGH-AFFINITY VARIANTS

Oxygen Equilibrium

By definition, this group of hemoglobin variants is associated with a shift to the left of the whole blood oxygen dissociation curve. Under physiologic conditions of pH (7.4) and temperature (37° C), normal red cells in plasma have a P_{50} of 26 mm Hg. That is, at an oxygen tension of 26 mm Hg, hemoglobin in these cells will be half saturated. Increased oxygen affinity is associated with low P_{50}.

In patients with erythrocytosis due to abnormal hemoglobins, whole blood P_{50} values have ranged from 12 mm Hg (hemoglobin Yakima, Novy et al., 1967) to 18 mm Hg (hemoglobin Brigham, Lokich et al., 1973). Figure 9–2 shows a whole blood oxygen dissociation curve from a girl with hemoglobin Bethesda. The red cell organic phosphates were within normal limits. Therefore, the marked shift to the left in the oxygen binding curves indicates the presence of functionally abnormal hemoglobin. From a Hill plot of the data shown in Figure 9–2, it is apparent that the patient has a biphasic curve (Fig. 9–3). The lower portion of the curve is due to the presence of hemoglobin Bethesda. An inflection point is seen at about 50 per cent saturation. The slope of the Hill plot at this point is low, as is the case for a mixture of any two hemoglobins of widely different oxygen affinities. This particular "n" value is *not* a reflection of heme-heme interaction, contrary to some statements in the literature. The upper portion of the patient's curve in Figure 9–3 approaches the normal curve asymptotically and reflects the oxygen-

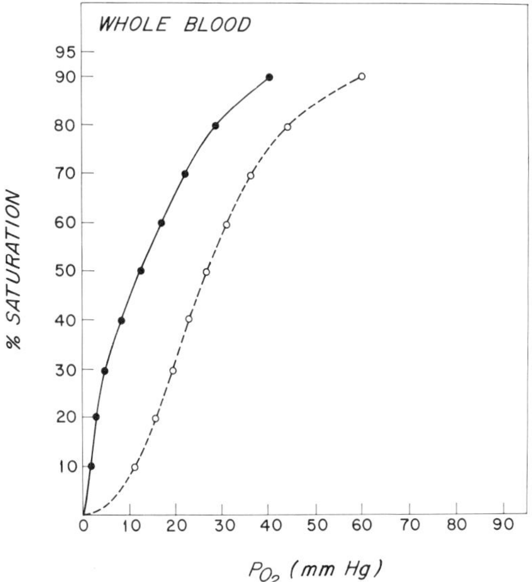

Figure 9–2. Oxygen binding curves of a normal individual ○----○ (P_{50} = 26.5 mm Hg) and of a patient with Hb Bethesda ●——● (P_{50} = 12.8 mm Hg). (Courtesy of Dr. M. B. Laver.)

ation of normal hemoglobin A which coexists in the red cells with an equal amount of hemoglobin Bethesda.

Although the whole blood oxygen dissociation curve provides information which is physiologically relevant, it does not give precise information on the functional properties of the variant hemoglobin. The whole blood curve is determined by the relative oxygen affinities and proportions of the normal and abnormal hemoglobins, as well as by intracellular factors such as organic phosphates, pH, and

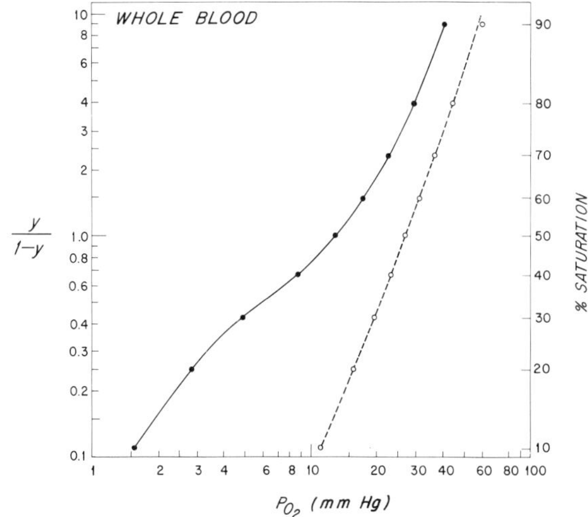

Figure 9–3. Hill plots of data shown in Figure 9–2. Normal (○– – – –○); patient (●——●). Note biphasic curve. (Courtesy of Dr. M. B. Laver.)

TABLE 9–3. Comparison of Functional Properties of High-Affinity Variants Studied under Identical Conditions

HEMOGLOBIN VARIANT	PHOSPHATE-FREE HEMOLYSATE		PURIFIED HEMOGLOBIN			
	% Abnormal	*P_{50}* (mm Hg)*	*P_{50}* (mm Hg)*	*n**	*Bohr Effect***	*$P_{50}DPG/P_{50}$†*
Chesapeake	30		0.55	1.4		
Kempsey	45	1.2	0.23	1.1	−0.22	1.6
Bethesda	50	1.3	0.18	1.1	−0.21	1.6
Brigham	50	2.7	#			
Hiroshima	50		0.90	2.2		
Syracuse	45	1.5	0.33	1.1	−0.24	1.4
A (Normal)	0	4.0	3.4	2.8	−0.55	2.4
α^A Chains			0.45	1.0		
β^A Chains			0.24	1.0		

*0.05 M bis-TRIS buffer (0.1 M Cl^-), pH 7.2, 20° C; hemoglobin concentration = 0.1 mM tetramer.

**$\Delta \log P_{50}/\Delta pH$.

†P_{50} (1 mM 2,3-DPG)/P_{50} (no. 2,3-DPG).

#Hemoglobin Brigham cannot be separated from Hb A by conventional techniques.

carbon dioxide tension. These latter variables are eliminated if measurements are made on a phosphate-free hemolysate. A fuller investigation of the variant requires its isolation by some preparative technique such as column chromatography prior to the measurement of its functional properties. It is difficult to compare the 20-odd high-affinity variants because they have been studied in a number of laboratories by a variety of techniques and under different experimental conditions. In Table 9–3 we show a comparison of the oxygen equilibria of the variants which have been studied in our laboratory. Some of these mutant hemoglobins have oxygen binding properties approaching those of isolated subunits of hemoglobin A. Generally those variants having the highest oxygen affinity have the lowest heme-heme interaction. This abnormality reflects a perturbation in the equilibrium between conformational isomers. These hemoglobins flip from T to R at a relatively early stage in ligation. The reduction in the overall energy of interaction between subunits results in a low n value (see Chapter 2). If the R $\rightleftharpoons$ T equilibrium can be shifted back toward T, then the energy of subunit interaction will be enhanced and Hill's n will increase. For example, the subunit cooperativity of several of the high-affinity variants can be significantly increased by the addition of organic phosphates such as 2,3-DPG and inositol hexaphosphate (Olson and Gibson, 1972; Bunn et al., 1974b) (Fig. 9–4).

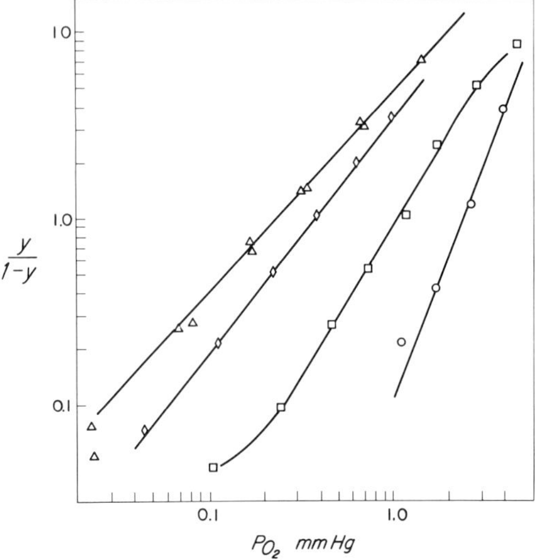

Figure 9–4. Oxygen equilibria of hemoglobin Kempsey and hemoglobin A (isolated from the same column). Hemoglobin (0.4 mM heme) in 0.05 M bis-TRIS buffer, pH 7.2, 0.1 M Cl^-, 20° C.

	P_{50} mm Hg	n
△ Kempsey	0.23	1.1
◇ Kempsey + 1 mM 2,3-DPG	0.37	1.3
□ Kempsey + 1 mM inositol hexaphosphate	1.1	1.7
○ A	2.4	2.6

(From Bunn, H. F., et al.: J. Biol. Chem. *249*:7402, 1974.)

Bohr Effect

Many of the high-affinity hemoglobins have a decreased alkaline Bohr effect (Tables 9–1 and 9–3). In the first place, those variants having substitutions at the C-terminal end of the β chain may have a decreased value because of failure to form the important salt bond (in deoxyhemoglobin) between the imidazole of β146-histidine and the carboxyl group of β94-aspartic acid. This interaction contributes about 50 per cent to the normal alkaline Bohr effect. In hemoglobin Hiroshima, the substitution of aspartic acid for histidine at β146 prevents the formation of this salt bond. The Bohr effect of Hb Hiroshima is half normal. On the other hand, certain variants have a reduced Bohr effect, even though their structural alterations are not at or near one of the residues which are known to contribute Bohr protons. For example, hemoglobin Kempsey (in the absence of organic phosphates) cannot assume a fully T structure upon deoxygenation and thus does not liberate a full complement of Bohr protons upon oxygenation.

INTERACTION WITH 2,3-DPG

Red cell 2,3-DPG has been measured in about half of these variants and has been consistently normal. However, several of these variants have been shown to have a diminished interaction with 2,3-DPG. Two variants, hemoglobins Little Rock and Syracuse, have amino acid substitutions at β143-histidine, one of the residues responsible for the binding of 2,3-DPG to deoxyhemoglobin. Hemoglobin Little Rock ($a_2\beta_2^{143\ \mathrm{His}\rightarrow\mathrm{Gln}}$) is of particular interest, since it has near normal heme-heme interaction and Bohr effect (Bromberg et al., 1973). Its high oxygen affinity may be due to *enhanced* stability of the R structure (Perutz, 1973). Bare et al. (1974) have done careful and extensive oxygen binding studies on hemoglobin Little Rock in the absence and presence of varying concentrations of 2,3-DPG. They have found that deoxyhemoglobin Little Rock binds 2,3-DPG somewhat more weakly than deoxyhemoglobin A. However, the binding of oxyhemoglobin Little Rock with 2,3-DPG is even weaker than that of oxyhemoglobin A with 2,3-DPG, so the overall effect of 2,3-DPG on the oxygenation of hemoglobin Little Rock is normal or even increased. In contrast, hemoglobin Syracuse ($\alpha_2\beta_2^{143\ \mathrm{His}\rightarrow\mathrm{Pro}}$) has decreased 2,3-DPG reactivity, as measured by oxygen affinities (Jensen et al., 1975). The oxygen binding experiments on hemoglobin Syracuse are difficult to interpret in terms of 2,3-DPG interaction with a hemoglobin lacking β143-histidine, because the proline substitution probably disrupts the H helix at position 143 and greatly weakens the overall stability of the T structure.

Beta 82-lysine is another residue involved in the binding of hemoglobin 2,3-DPG (see Figure 1–10). Two variants have recently been encountered which have amino acid substitutions at this site: Hb Rahere ($\alpha_2\beta_2^{82\ \mathrm{Lys}\rightarrow\mathrm{Thr}}$) Lorkin et al., 1975) and Hb Providence ($\alpha_2\beta_2^{82\ \mathrm{Lys}\rightarrow\mathrm{Asn,\ Asp}}$)* (Charache et al., 1975d). Both hemoglobins have nearly normal oxygen affinity in the absence of organic phosphates, but have very little change in P_{50} upon the addition of 2,3-DPG. As a result, heterozygotes have increased whole blood oxygen affinity. The individual with Hb Rahere had a marked increase in hemoglobin (20 g/100 ml) yet his red cell mass was not significantly elevated.

KINETICS OF LIGAND BINDING

Measurement of the rate of binding of oxygen or other ligands to hemoglobin provides information beyond that obtained from equilibrium determinations. In particular, kinetic data have provided insights into the conformational transition that occurs on ligand bind-

*Asparagine is partially deamidated to aspartic acid as a post-translational modification.

ing and into the differential reactivity of the α and β subunits. Gibson and his colleagues have developed very sophisticated methods for studying these fast reactions and have applied them not only to normal human hemoglobin A but to chemically modified hemoglobin and some of the functionally abnormal variants. Those studied in detail at this time include hemoglobins Chesapeake (Nagel et al., 1967; Gibson and Nagel, 1974), Rainier (Amiconi et al., 1972; Salhany, 1972), Hiroshima (Olson et al., 1972), Bethesda (Olson and Gibson, 1972), Kempsey (Bunn et al., 1974b), and Syracuse (McDonald and Gibson, unpublished observations). In general, these variants when fully liganded behave like hemoglobin A. The reaction

$$Hb(O_2)_4 \xrightarrow{k_4} Hb(O_2)_3 + O_2$$

is very similar among these hemoglobins. (The value of k_4 is somewhat low for hemoglobin Hiroshima [Olson et al., 1972] and Syracuse [McDonald and Gibson, unpublished observations] but normal for the others.) Thus, these variants when fully liganded appear to assume a normal R conformation. When deoxygenated, these variants tend to have a rapid and monophasic reaction with heme ligands (such as carbon monoxide), indicating that the deoxygenated hemoglobin exists at least partially in the R state. In contrast, deoxyhemoglobin A has a slow and biphasic reaction with heme ligands, indicating the transition from T to R during heme ligation. In some variants such as Hiroshima (Olson et al., 1972), the abnormal subunit shows particularly fast ligand binding, suggesting that the amino acid substitution has drastically altered the tertiary conformation of the subunit and has exaggerated the asymmetry between α and β chain reactivity for heme ligands. Other variants such as hemoglobin Kempsey do not show such asymmetry between subunits (Bunn et al., 1974b).

X-Ray Crystallography

The precise delineation of the high-affinity variants in three-dimensional space should provide the most direct information on structural-functional relationships. The structure of normal and variant hemoglobins can be compared by difference Fourier analysis. From such information, electron-density maps can be constructed which indicate specific sites where the two molecules differ. Since the three-dimensional structure of deoxyhuman hemoglobin A has been solved at high resolution (2.4 Å), difference Fourier analyses can be obtained by examining crystals prepared from deoxygenated variants. At this time no comparable structural information on the oxygenated forms of these variants is available. X-ray studies have been done on the following high-affinity variants: J-Capetown and Chesapeake (Greer, 1971c), Yakima (Pulsinelli, 1973), Rainier (Greer and Perutz, 1971), Hiroshima (Perutz et al., 1971), Kempsey (Perutz et al., 1974a), and San Diego (Anderson, 1974). In general, difference Fourier analyses of these variants in the deoxy state show marked differences from hemoglobin A that extend beyond the site of amino acid substitution and indicate alterations in both the tertiary structure of the subunit and, in some cases, the quaternary structure of the tetramer. Hemoglobin Chesapeake appears to be an exception. Its deoxy structure appears to differ very little from that of hemoglobin A. In contrast, electron-density maps of the oxy structure at low resolution show marked differences. On occasion, the x-ray studies have provided very specific information. The difference Fourier analysis of deoxyhemoglobin Rainier showed a disulfide bridge between cysteine introduced by mutation at β145 and the cysteine at β93 (Greer and Perutz, 1971). These results indicated that the original structural analysis of hemoglobin Rainier was incorrect. Likewise, x-ray crystallography identified the amino acid substitution of hemoglobin Hiroshima as β146 (Perutz et al., 1971) rather than β143, as was first reported.

Physical Studies

Nuclear magnetic resonance (NMR) and electron paramagnetic resonance (EPR) have proved to be useful conformational probes not only of functionally normal hemoglobin but especially of the high-affinity variants (Davis et al., 1971; Ho and Lindstrom, 1972; Lindstrom et al., 1972b). Since the primary structural alteration in each of these variants is known, a comparison of its NMR spectrum with that of normal hemoglobin under identical conditions permits an assignment of certain peaks to specific structural loci. For example, NMR spectra of hyperfine shifted proton resonance have demonstrated that the environments around the α- and β-chain heme groups are structurally different. From the change in spectra upon partial saturation with ligand, the differential binding to α and β hemes can be demonstrated. This approach was used to show that the β chains of hemoglobin Kempsey have a higher affinity for carbon monoxide than the α chains (Lindstrom et al., 1973). From ring current shift resonances of the carboxy derivatives, assignments can be made to certain residues adjacent to the hemes. Recently, specific NMR signals have also been attributed to certain protons involved in hydrogen bonds at the subunit interfaces. These assignments have been largely based on comparisons with certain high-affinity variants which have amino acid substitutions at these sites (Fung and Ho, 1975).

Synthetic molecules that have paramagnetic resonance (spin labels) have been used to probe the conformation of normal and variant hemoglobins. Spin labels have been employed in several ways: (a) 2,3-DPG analogues (Ogata et al., 1972; Ogata and McConnell, 1972); (b) sulfhydryl reagents (Baldassare et al., 1970); and (c) the heme ligand, nitric oxide (Salhany et al., 1975). Both the binding of organic phosphates to hemoglobin and the environment around the reactive $\beta 93$ sulfhydryl group appear to be strongly dependent upon quaternary structure. Therefore, these measurements can provide a means of monitoring the transition from the T to R structure during ligation of the hemes. Such information on both normal and high-affinity hemoglobins has been useful in testing models of allosteric behavior.

SUBUNIT DISSOCIATION

As discussed in Chapter 2, fully liganded hemoglobin* in solution dissociates readily into dimers:

$$\alpha_2\beta_2 \rightleftharpoons 2\alpha\beta$$

There is ample evidence that the molecule splits at the $\alpha_1\beta_2$ interface. Extremes of pH or denaturing solvent conditions are required to cleave the molecule at the $\alpha_1\beta_1$ interface. In contrast to liganded hemoglobins, deoxyhemoglobin dissociates much less readily into dimers. This difference is due primarily to the inter-subunit salt bonds which stabilize the T structure (Perutz, 1970a and b). As mentioned above and in Table 9–1, many of the high-affinity variants have substitutions at the $\alpha_1\beta_2$ interface. Such structural alterations might be expected to affect the dissociation of the tetramer into dimers. There is convincing evidence that hemoglobins Bethesda (Olson and Gibson, 1972), Kempsey (Bunn et al., 1974b), and Chesapeake (Nagel and Gibson, 1972), when fully deoxygenated, dissociate more readily into dimers than does deoxyhemoglobin A. These observations are in accord with other evidence that neither deoxy Bethesda nor deoxy Kempsey can form a stable T quaternary structure. Furthermore, hemoglobin Chesapeake in the liganded state has *decreased* subunit dissociation (Bunn, 1970), indicating that its R structure is relatively more stable than that of hemoglobin A.

The energy of interaction between hemoglobin subunits in the oxy and deoxy states can be linked thermodynamically to the cooperative binding of ligand to hemes (Briehl, 1964; Noble, 1969; Ackers and Halvorson, 1974). As Figure 9–5 indicates, the oxygen affinity of a mutant or chemically modified hemoglobin will be affected if the

*Oxyhemoglobin, carboxyhemoglobin, cyanmethemoglobin.

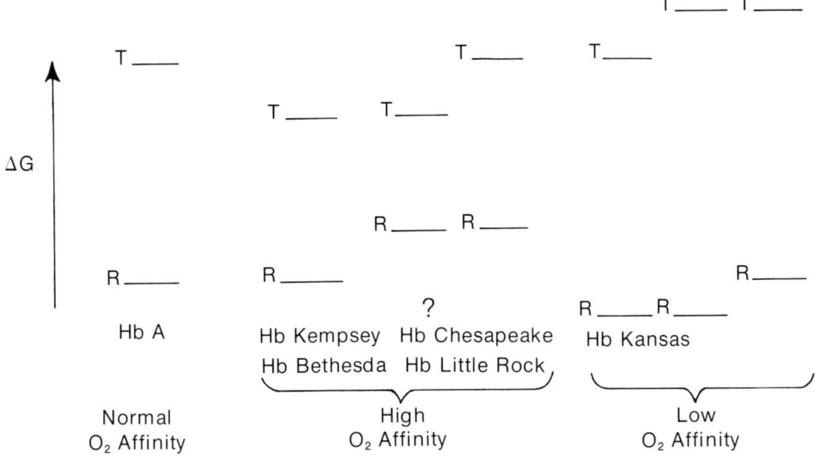

Figure 9–5. Comparison of subunit bonding energies (ΔG) of normal and variant hemoglobins in the oxy (R) and deoxy (T) conformations.

relative stabilities of the R and T structure differ significantly from those of native hemoglobin A. Variants having a relatively unstable T structure like Bethesda and Kempsey will have high oxygen affinity. Similarly, enhanced stability of the R state should also result in high oxygen affinity. Perutz has suggested that the presence of an additional hydrogen bond in oxyhemoglobin Little Rock may be the basis for its high oxygen affinity (Perutz, 1973). If so, this variant in its liganded state should have decreased dissociation into dimers. As mentioned above, this appears to be true for hemoglobin Chesapeake. Greer (1971c) has presented crystallographic evidence that the conformation of oxyhemoglobin Chesapeake differs markedly from that of oxyhemoglobin A, whereas the deoxygenated hemoglobins have very similar three-dimensional structures. However, there are both kinetic (Nagel et al., 1967; Gibson and Nagel, 1974) and NMR data (Ho and Lindstrom, 1972) indicating that deoxy Chesapeake differs significantly from deoxy A. It is likely that both the T and the R forms of this variant have abnormal conformation and subunit interaction. Such a situation is depicted in Figure 9–5.

PHYSIOLOGICAL ASPECTS

In normal man, the oxygen dissociation curve is appropriately poised to permit efficient loading and unloading of oxygen during rest and exercise. Chapter 3 discusses the pathophysiological consequences of significant displacements of the oxygen binding curve. Most commonly, a “shift to the left” or “shift to the right” can be explained by intracellular factors such as alterations in pH and red cell 2,3-DPG or modification of the heme groups, as in carbon monoxide poisoning or methemoglobinemia. In many instances the change in oxygen affinity constitutes an adaptation to some form of environmental stress such as hypoxia. In contrast, individuals with hemoglobin variants of high oxygen affinity exhibit a *primary* displacement of the whole blood oxygen dissociation curve and respond to this molecular lesion with appropriate physiological adjustments. According to the Fick equation cited in Chapter 3, oxygen delivery to tissues (VO_2) is a function of three independent variables:

$$VO_2 = 0.139 \cdot Q \cdot Hb \cdot (S_aO_2 - S_{\bar{v}}O_2)$$

The primary shift to the left in the oxygen dissociation curve results in a marked decrease in oxygen extraction per gram of hemoglobin ($S_aO_2 - S_{\bar{v}}O_2$). Consequently, tissue oxygenation can be maintained by two adjustments: increase in circulating hemoglobin concentration (Hb) or increase in blood flow (Q).

The primary form of compensation appears to be erythrocytosis. An individual with a stable high-affinity variant (normal red cell life span) will have an increase in red cell mass roughly proportional to the "shift to the left" of the whole blood oxygen dissociation curve. This response appears to be mediated through erythropoietin. Adamson et al. (1968, 1969, 1972) have studied individuals with hemoglobins Rainier, Yakima, and Bethesda. The urinary erythropoietin

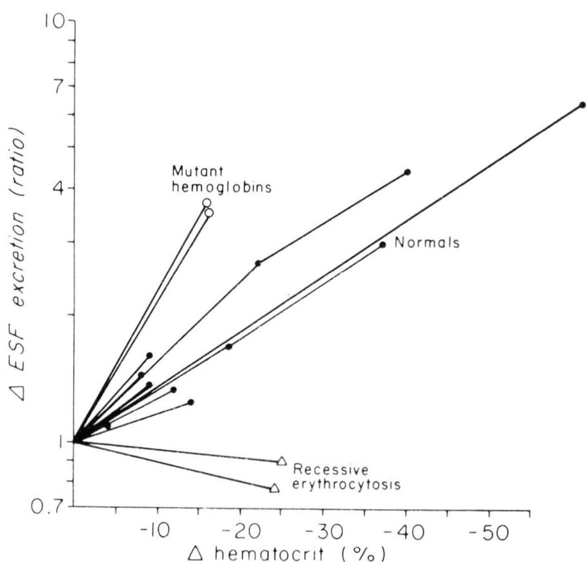

Figure 9–6. Effect of phlebotomy on erythropoietin (ESF) excretion in normal volunteers (●), individuals with high-affinity hemoglobin variants (○), and individuals with autosomal recessive erythrocytosis (△) (see Table 9–4). (From Adamson, J. W., et al.: Blood *41*:641, 1973.)

(ESF) of these polycythemic subjects was normal. However, when these individuals were bled down to a "normal" red cell mass, urinary ESF increased markedly (Fig. 9–6). Similar results have been reported in a patient with hemoglobin Little Rock (Bromberg et al., 1971). These observations attest to the significant hypoxia that these individuals will develop if they are robbed of an important mode of compensation.

Individuals with high-affinity variants have normal arterial oxygen tension. The fact that they develop enhanced erythropoietin production indicates that the sensor for this hormonal regulation must be located in the postarterial region of the renal vasculature (Adamson, 1975).

It is more difficult to assess alterations in blood flow of individuals with high-affinity variants. Total cardiac output and oxygen consumption were found to be normal in a patient with hemoglobin Yakima, whereas the calculated mixed venous oxygen tension was somewhat decreased (Novy et al., 1967). A patient with hemoglobin Little Rock also had a normal resting cardiac output and oxygen consumption but slightly decreased mixed venous oxygen tension (Bromberg et al., 1971). The $P_{\bar{v}}O_2$ dropped more than anticipated when the patient underwent graded exercise. Individuals with hemoglobins Heathrow (White et al., 1973) and Syracuse (Oski, unpublished observations) have been found to have somewhat elevated resting cardiac outputs. The latter patient showed a marked increase in cardiac output during graded exercise. After this patient had been bled down to a normal red cell mass, these measurements became even more abnormal. Changes in total cardiac output do not reflect adjustments in blood flow to specific organs. Individuals with high-affinity variants may have appropriate alterations in regional circulation in order to preserve adequate oxygenation of vital tissues. Recently, a patient with hemoglobin Malmö was shown to have myocardial blood flow that was greater than normal (Gau et al., 1974).

In Chapter 3, a case is made for the importance of red cell 2,3-DPG in the adaptation to hypoxia. However, the high-affinity variants represent one type of hypoxia in which this adaptation does not occur. Red cell 2,3-DPG has been measured in about half the different high-affinity variants and has been consistently normal. It is possible that erythrocytosis provides adequate compensation; however, individuals with this disorder should theoretically derive some benefit from increased red cell 2,3-DPG. An extreme example is depicted in Figure 9–7: these red cells contain half normal hemoglobin A. The remainder of the hemoglobin has very high oxygen affinity and fails to form stable mixed hybrid tetramers with normal hemoglobin (e.g., $\alpha_2\beta^A\beta^X$). Such a lack of interaction has been demonstrated for hemoglobins Bethesda (Bunn et al., 1972a) and Kempsey (Bunn et al., 1974b), two variants which are unable to form a

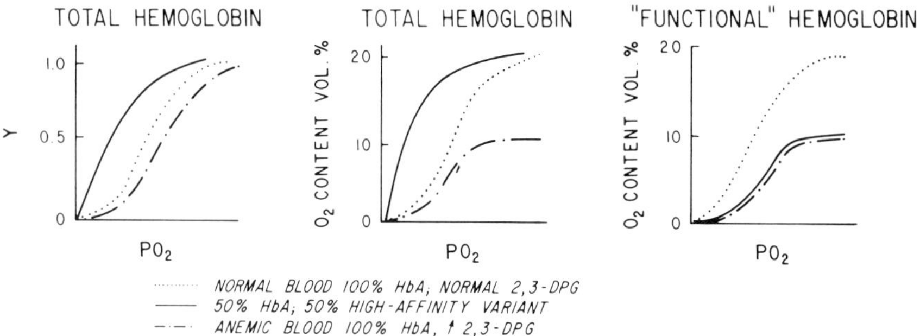

Figure 9–7. Oxygen binding curves of a normal individual (·····), a patient with anemia and increased red cell 2,3-DPG (—·—·—), and a patient with a high affinity variant (———).

stable T structure. In red cells containing such a mixture, the two hemoglobins are oxygenated independently. Furthermore, the high O_2 affinity hemoglobin remains almost fully saturated in all parts of the circulation. Therefore, the abnormal hemoglobin lacks any physiological function and might as well be albumin or some other space-occupying colloid. If so, the individual has a functioning hemoglobin level that is half the total. Such an "anemic" patient should benefit from the interaction of 2,3-DPG on the normal functioning hemoglobin. Actually, in such individuals, red cell 2,3-DPG should be expressed as moles per mole of hemoglobin A, since under physiologic conditions the abnormal hemoglobin remains in the R conformation and fails to interact strongly with 2,3-DPG. Furthermore, several of these variants have impaired interaction with 2,3-DPG (Bunn et al., 1972a, 1974b; Jensen et al., 1975). Viewed in this way, the individual with a high-affinity variant has elevated red cell 2,3-DPG, similar to other patients with anemia!

CLINICAL MANIFESTATIONS

Genetics

Like other structurally abnormal hemoglobins, the high-affinity variants follow an autosomal dominant pattern of inheritance. All affected individuals are heterozygotes; their red cells contain at least as much normal hemoglobin A as the abnormal variant. In most instances the homozygous state would be incompatible with life. A positive family history is very helpful in evaluating a patient for the presence of a high-affinity hemoglobin. However, spontaneous mutations undoubtedly exist. We have seen a girl with hemoglobin Bethesda whose parents were both normal (Bunn et al., 1972a).

Clinical Presentation

The great majority of affected individuals are entirely asymptomatic. Physical examination is unremarkable except for the occasional presence of ruddy complexion. Most commonly, erythrocytosis is detected on a routine blood count. The increase in packed cell volume and red cell mass is generally not severe. Accordingly, affected individuals do not usually have symptoms due to hyperviscosity of the blood. Some individuals with hemoglobin Malmö may be an exception. One patient reliably reported subjective improvement following phlebotomy (Gau et al., 1974). This patient had severe cardiac dysfunction with a history of myocardial infarction, angina, dyspnea, and decreased exercise tolerance. Interestingly, coronary angiography revealed patent vessels except an isolated narrow segment in a branch of the right posterior descending artery. As mentioned in the beginning of this chapter, the first patient in whom this disorder was established had mild angina. However, a survey of the 100-odd individuals that have been reported to date does not indicate a high incidence of myocardial ischemia or any other form of tissue hypoxia.

Some have speculated that in a pregnant woman with a high-affinity variant, the transplacental transport of oxygen may be impaired. In both humans and nearly all other mammals which have been tested, the oxygen affinity of fetal blood is significantly higher than that of maternal blood. The physiological importance of this phenomenon is not well established. There are several instances in which the oxygen binding curve of the mother was shifted to the left of that of the fetus because of an abnormal hemoglobin; these pregnancies were perfectly uneventful and the babies were healthy. An increased incidence of fetal mortality has been reported in a family with hemoglobin Yakima (Jones et al., 1967), but the significance of this is not clear.

Diagnosis

Affected individuals come to the attention of physicians because of unexplained erythrocytosis. Hemoglobin values vary considerably with a mean of about 20 g/100 ml. The increase in red cell mass is less marked than that seen in patients with polycythemia vera. The white count and platelet count are normal and the peripheral blood smear is unremarkable. During the initial evaluation a number of diagnostic possibilities must be ruled out. Table 9–4 is one approach to classifying various types of erythrocytosis. If appropriate clinical and laboratory information does not suggest one of the more common etiologies, the possibility remains that the patient's erythrocytosis is

TABLE 9–4. Differential Diagnosis of Erythrocytosis

- I. Autonomous erythroid proliferation (↓ ESF); polycythemia vera
- II. Secondary erythroid proliferation
  - A. Autonomous or inappropriate increase in ESF
    1. Neoplasm
    2. Renal lesions
    3. Familial erythrocytosis (autosomal recessive inheritance)
  - B. Secondary increase in ESF
    1. Hypoxemia (↓ arterial PO_2)
       - a. High altitude
       - b. Alveolar hypoventilation
       - c. Pulmonary disease
       - d. Cardiac R→L shunt
    2. Abnormal hemoglobin function (normal arterial PO_2)
       - a. High-affinity variants (autosomal dominant inheritance)
       - b. Congenital methemoglobinemia
       - c. Carboxyhemoglobin (smokers)

due to the presence of a functionally abnormal hemoglobin. The likelihood is considerably strengthened if other blood relatives also have unexplained erythrocytosis. However, not all familial erythrocytosis is due to the presence of a functionally abnormal hemoglobin variant. Adamson (1975) has recently reviewed this subject. There is a very rare entity in which familial erythrocytosis is due to a defect in the humoral regulation of red cell mass (Adamson et al., 1973). Unlike the high-affinity variants, this disorder has an autosomal recessive pattern of inheritance.

If hemoglobin electrophoresis reveals the presence of an abnormal band, the diagnosis is virtually established. However, the failure to demonstrate any electrophoretic abnormality by no means rules out the diagnosis. As Table 9–5 shows, only about half the high-affinity variants that have been reported to date can be separated from hemoglobin A by routine electrophoresis on cellulose acetate or starch gel at pH 8.6. Some variants can be detected if other types of electrophoresis are employed, such as agar gel (pH 6.0) or gel electrofocusing. There remains a group that appear to be electrophoretically silent. These include hemoglobins Olympia, Heathrow, Brigham, and Creteil. Certain tricks can be employed to "separate the unseparable." Garel and his colleagues (1974) have taken advantage of the fact that high-affinity mutants may have an altered reactivity to sulfhydryl reagents. This selective chemical modification permits the hemoglobin variant to be separated on the basis of the surface charge.[1] Variants with reduced Bohr effect will have less of a change in isoelectric point upon deoxygenation than has hemoglobin A. Figure 9–8 shows how this approach was used to enhance the

---

[1]Rieder et al. (1969) have utilized differential sulfhydryl reactivity to isolate hemoglobin Philly, an unstable variant with a neutral substitution.

TABLE 9–5. *Electrophoretic Properties of High-Affinity Hemoglobin Variants**

Hemoglobin Variant	Electrophoretic Separation from Hb A			Reference
	Starch Gel (pH 8.6)	*Agar Gel (pH 6.0)*	*Gel Electrofocusing*	
Chesapeake (α92 Arg→Leu)	Yes	Yes	Yes	
J-Cape Town (α92 Arg→Gln)	Yes			
Yakima (β99 Asp→His)	Yes			
Kempsey (β99 Asp→Asn)	Yes		Yes	
Ypsilanti (β99 Asp→Tyr)	Yes			
Hiroshima (β146 His→Asp)	Yes	Yes	Yes	
Andrew-Minneapolis (β144 Lys→Asn)	Yes		Yes	
Abruzzo (β143 His→Arg)	Yes			
Rainier (β145 Tyr→Cys)	No	Yes		
Bethesda (β145 Tyr→His)	No	Yes	No	
Little Rock (β143 His→Gln)	No	Yes	Yes	
Malmö (β97 His→Gln)	No	No	Yes	Jeppson and Berglund, 1972
Wood (β97 His→Leu)	No		Yes	Taketa et al., 1975
Syracuse (β143 His→Pro)	No	No	Yes	Jensen et al., 1975
San Diego (B109 Val→Met)	No	No	Yes	Monte et al., 1976
Creteil (β89 Ser→Asn)	No	No	Yes	Monte et al., 1976
Olympia (β20 Val→Met)	No	No	No	
Brigham (β100 Pro→Leu)	No	No	No	
Heathrow (β103 Phe→Leu)	No	No	No	

*Taken from Jensen et al., 1975.

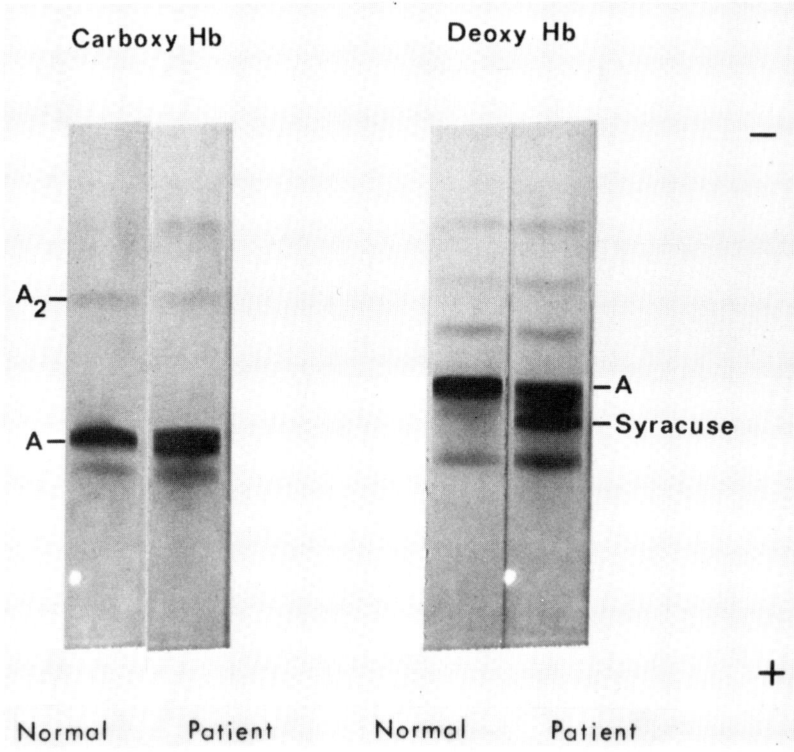

Figure 9–8. Comparison of gel electrofocusing patterns of normal hemolysate and hemolysate of a patient with hemoglobin Syracuse. *Left,* Hemoglobin treated with CO. *Right,* Deoxygenated hemoglobin. The improved separation of Hb Syracuse from Hb A following deoxygenation is a reflection of the fact that Hb Syracuse has a decreased Bohr effect (see text). (From Jensen, M., et al.: J. Clin. Invest. 55:469, 1975.)

electrophoretic separation of hemoglobin Syracuse from hemoglobin A (Jensen et al., 1975).

Since high-affinity hemoglobins may not be detectable by electrophoresis, measurement of oxygen affinity is required to establish the diagnosis. The relative merits of measurements on whole blood versus phosphate-free hemolysate are discussed in a previous section. If the patient's erythrocytosis is due to a hemoglobin variant, there will be a marked and reproducible "shift to the left" of the oxygen dissociation curve. It is advisable to measure red cell 2,3-DPG to rule out the possibility that the increase in whole blood oxygen affinity is due to an abnormality in red cell metabolism, leading to deficiency of 2,3-DPG. Such a finding would be quite unexpected, since most red cell enzymopathies are associated with nonspherocytic hemolytic anemia. This uncertainty is obviated if oxygen affinity is measured on hemolysate stripped of organic phosphates.

Treatment

Once the diagnosis is established, all affected family members should be reassured that they have a benign condition. The great majority of individuals require no treatment at all. However, it is prudent to perform follow-up blood counts at regular intervals. A minority of patients may develop a hematocrit high enough that the viscosity of the blood poses a potential threat. As mentioned earlier, occasional patients have derived subjective benefit from phlebotomy. However, this treatment should be used sparingly, since the increased cell mass is an important mode of compensation. Some affected individuals have been "treated" with radiomimetic drugs such as phosphorus-32 or phenylalanine mustard because they were thought to have polycythemia vera. As Charache (1974a) has pointed out, the avoidance of such inappropriate therapy is one of the important reasons to establish a diagnosis in these patients.

VARIANTS HAVING LOW OXYGEN AFFINITY

The six stable hemoglobin variants that have been found to have abnormally low oxygen affinity are listed in Table 9–6. In addition, a number of the unstable variants and some of the M hemoglobins have been found to have decreased oxygen affinity (see Chapters 8 and 10).

Hemoglobin Kansas is of particular interest, since it has the most abnormal functional properties. In 1961, Reissman, Ruth, and Nomura studied a mother and son with unexplained cyanosis. The subjects were otherwise asymptomatic and had normal hemoglobin levels without any evidence of hemolysis. The cyanosis was explained by an oxygen saturation of only 60 per cent in samples of arterial blood, despite a P_aO_2 of 100 mm Hg. Upon breathing 100 per cent O_2, the oxygen saturation increased by about 35 per cent. These results indicated a marked decrease in whole blood oxygen affinity. At first glance, it is surprising that the red cell mass is "set" at a normal level, in view of such abnormal oxygenation of hemoglobin. However, the amount of oxygen unloaded during the circulation through capillaries is probably within normal limits. Despite the reduced oxygen content of the arterial blood, the shape of the curve permits adequate oxygen release. However, it seems likely that individuals with hemoglobin Kansas would have a limited tolerance to strenuous muscular exercise, which depends upon a marked increase in oxygen unloading.

The structure-function relationships of hemoglobin Kansas have been studied in considerable detail. Bonaventura and Riggs (1968) showed that the structural abnormality was a substitution of threo-

TABLE 9–6. *Stable Hemoglobin Variants Having Decreased Oxygen Affinity*

Variant	Structure	Area Affected	Bohr Effect	Comment	Reference
Titusville	α94 (G1) Asp→Asn	$\alpha_1\beta_2$	Low		Schneider et al., 1975
Providence	β82 (EF6) Leu→Asn,Asp		Low		Charache et al., 1975
Agenogi	β90 (F6) Glu→Lys				Imai et al., 1970
Kansas	β102 (G4) Asn→Thr	$\alpha_1\beta_2$	Normal	Familial cyanosis	Reissman et al., 1961 Bonaventura and Riggs, 1968
Beth Israel	β102 (G4) Asn→Ser	$\alpha_1\beta_2$	Normal	Cyanosis	Nagel et al., 1976
Yoshizuka	β108 (G10) Asn→Asp	$\alpha_1\beta_2$			Imamura et al., 1969

nine for asparagine at β102. Like many of the high-affinity variants, this site is at the $\alpha_1\beta_2$ interface. Indeed, as shown in Figure 9–1, when normal hemoglobin A is oxygenated, β102 Asn forms a hydrogen bond with α94 Asp. Such a bond is not possible in oxyhemoglobin Kansas. Therefore, it is interesting to note that oxyhemoglobin Kansas dissociates more readily into $\alpha\beta$ dimers than does oxyhemoglobin A (Bonaventura and Riggs, 1968). Its low oxygen affinity appears to be due in part to a relatively unstable R structure. In hemoglobin Kansas, the transition from the T to the R structure occurs relatively late in heme ligation. Indeed, in the presence of organic phosphates such as 2,3-DPG and inositol hexaphosphate, fully liganded hemoglobin Kansas has the NMR characteristics of the T structure (Ogawa et al., 1972). Difference Fourier analyses of crystals of deoxyhemoglobin Kansas indicate widespread abnormalities in the T structure (Greer, 1971a). Furthermore, isolated β chains of Kansas subunits also have relatively low oxygen affinity (Riggs and Gibson, 1973). The interpretation of these results is complicated by the fact that these preparations of β subunits showed a considerable amount of kinetic heterogeneity that is unexplained.

Recently, Nagel et al. (1976) have reported a patient with cyanosis due to Hb Beth Israel (β102 Asn $\rightarrow$ Ser). This variant has an amino acid substitution at the same site as Hb Kansas. The functional properties of the two variants are very similar. Hb Beth Israel probably arose as a spontaneous mutation, since neither parent is cyanotic.

Hb Titusville (α94 Asp $\rightarrow$ Asn) (Schneider et al., 1975) appears to have an oxygen affinity nearly as low as that of Hb Kansas and Hb Beth Israel. The amino acid substitution prevents the formation of the bond between α94 and β102 which normally stabilizes oxyhemoglobin (Figure 9–1). As a result, Hb Titusville resembles Hb Kansas in having enhanced dissociation of tetramer into dimers. The proposita had no apparent clinical or hematological abnormalities.

Hemoglobins Yoshizuka (Imamura et al., 1969) and Agenogi (Imai et al., 1970) also have decreased O_2 affinity, although less marked than Hbs Kansas, Beth Israel, or Titusville. Some affected family members have slightly decreased hemoglobin levels. It may be that this "anemia" is the opposite of the polycythemia found in association with high-affinity variants; the enhanced oxygen release provided by the right-shifted curve would reduce the erythropoietin-mediated stimulus to erythropoiesis. Such a mechanism has been offered to explain the anemia in patients with hemoglobin Seattle (Stamatoyannopoulos et al., 1969b), an unstable variant. However, this situation is more complex, since the shortened red cell survival in these individuals also contributes to the reduction in their red cell mass.

Chapter 10

M HEMOGLOBINS, METHEMOGLOBINEMIA, AND CARBOXYHEMOGLOBINEMIA

THE M HEMOGLOBINS

In 1948, a young physician, H. Hörlein, and a medical student, G. Weber, described a family in which certain members had congenital cyanosis. The abnormality was transmitted as an autosomal dominant trait through four generations. The affected individuals had a "lavender-blue" appearance while their blood appeared brown. Hemolysates had absorption spectra which were similar but not identical to that of methemoglobin. Hörlein and Weber proved that the abnormality lay with the globin and not with the heme by forming hybrids of patient's globin with normal heme and patient's heme with normal globin. Only the former produced the spectral changes present in the native hemolysate. These results provided the first convincing evidence of a familial hemoglobinopathy, antedating by one year Itano and Pauling's discovery of the abnormal electrophoretic behavior of Hb S.

In 1955, Singer designated this type of hemoglobin variant as Hb M. Subsequently other examples of Hb M were discovered (Kiese et al., 1956; Gerald et al., 1957; Pisciotta et al., 1959) and were found to have abnormal electrophoretic (Gerald, 1958) as well as spectral properties.

The existence of familial cyanosis having an autosomal dominant inheritance pattern has been recognized in Japan since 1800 (Shibata et al., 1967a). This disorder, called "Kochikuro" (black mouth), was restricted to the prefecture of Iwate in the northeast corner of Honshu. In the 1950's there were about 70 affected individuals residing in this region who had blood "as black as Japanese soy sauce."

The structural analysis of the M hemoglobins was first completed by Gerald and Efron (1961). They identified three variants: M-Boston ($\alpha^{58\ \mathrm{His} \to \mathrm{Tyr}}\beta_2$), M-Saskatoon ($\alpha_2\beta_2^{63\ \mathrm{His} \to \mathrm{Tyr}}$), and M-Milwaukee-1 ($\alpha_2\beta_2{}^{67\ \mathrm{Val\to Glu}}$). Subsequently, the family described by Hörlein and Weber (1948) was shown to have Hb M-Saskatoon. The Japanese with "Kochikuro" were found to have a fourth variant, Hb M-Iwate ($\alpha_2{}^{87\ \mathrm{His\to Tyr}}\beta_2$) (Shibata et al., 1964). In 1966, Heller et al. described a fifth M hemoglobin: Hyde Park ($\alpha_2\beta_2{}^{92\ \mathrm{His\to Tyr}}$). No other new M hemoglobins have been discovered in subsequent years. The unstable variant Hb St. Louis almost qualifies as an M hemoglobin. The substitution of glutamine for leucine at $\beta 28$ causes the heme iron in the abnormal subunits to become completely oxidized to methemoglobin (Cohen-Solal et al., 1975). In addition, another unstable variant, Hb Freiburg ($\alpha_2\beta_2{}^{23\ \mathrm{Val\to 0}}$), has an enhanced tendency toward auto-oxidation (Jones et al., 1966). However, these two hemoglobins lack the clinical, electrophoretic, and spectral properties shared by the five M hemoglobins.

Because individuals affected with one of the M hemoglobins have a distinctive physical appearance they have been discovered

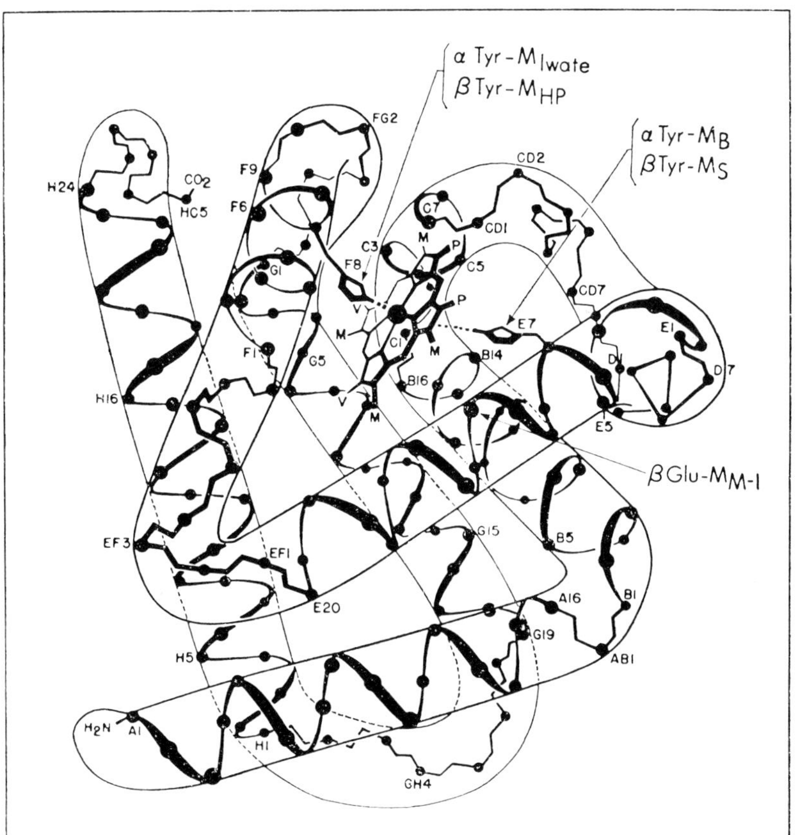

Figure 10–1. Three-dimensional model of hemoglobin subunit modified from Dickerson (1963) showing substituted sites in the M hemoglobins. (From Ranney, H. M., et al.: Proc. First Inter-Am. Symp. on Hemoglobins, 1971.) $M_{HP} = M_{\mathrm{Hyde\ Park}}$; $M_{M\text{-}1} = M_{\mathrm{Milwaukee\text{-}1}}$; $M_B = M_{\mathrm{Boston}}$; $M_S = M_{\mathrm{Saskatoon}}$.

quite readily in far-flung parts of the globe. For example, Hb M-Saskatoon has been found in Germany, Canada, Britain, the United States, France, Denmark, Norway, Poland, Italy, South Africa, and Japan (Vella et al., 1974). The various exotic names that have been applied to the M hemoglobins (Table 6–2) provide further testimony to the worldwide distribution of these variants. Understandably, Hb M has only rarely been recognized in blacks (Heller et al., 1966).

As discussed in detail in Chapter 1, the iron atom of the heme group is normally linked to the imidazole group of the proximal (F8) histidine of the α and β chains. Another histidine residue at position E7 is situated on the opposite side, near the sixth coordination position of the heme iron, where oxygen normally binds. Its imidazole group does not form a bond with heme iron unless hemichrome is engendered during hemoglobin denaturation (see Chapter 8). As shown in Figure 10–1, four of the five M hemoglobins involve a substitution of a tyrosine for either the proximal (F8) or distal (E7) histidine in the α or β chain. Gerald and Efron (1961) postulated that the phenolic group of the tyrosine residues are able to form a covalent link with the heme iron, thus stabilizing the atom in the oxidized (Fe^{+++}) form.

Structure-Function Relationships

Studies on chemically modified hemoglobins have provided important insights into how the protein functions. Among the most thoroughly investigated are the valence hybrids in which the heme iron of either the α or the β chain has been selectively oxidized and then stabilized by the addition of a heme ligand such as cyanide. For example, in $\alpha_2^{CNMet}\beta_2$, the α-chain hemes are frozen in the oxidized state and only the β chains are able to bind oxygen. These valence hybrids may be suitable analogues of partially oxygenated intermediates such as $Hb(O_2)_2$ which have been so difficult to study. Comparable attention has been devoted to the functional properties of the M hemoglobins which are naturally occurring valence hybrids.

Oxygen Equilibria

Because of the close homology between the structure of the α and β chains, one might expect that mutants having a substitution (His→Tyr) at the proximal heme binding site (F8) would have functional properties similar to each other, yet different from those having the substitution at the distal heme binding site (E7). In fact, the experimental results are totally contrary to this expectation. The oxygen equilibria of the M hemoglobins depend primarily upon which subunit is affected, rather than whether the substitution is at the

TABLE 10–1. Properties of M Hemoglobins

	M-Boston	M-Iwate	M-Saskatoon	M-Hyde Park	M-Milwaukee-1
Structure	$\alpha_2{}^{58\ \mathrm{His}\rightarrow\mathrm{Tyr}}\beta_2$	$\alpha_2{}^{87\ \mathrm{His}\rightarrow\mathrm{Tyr}}\beta_2$	$\alpha_2\beta_2{}^{63\ \mathrm{His}\rightarrow\mathrm{Tyr}}$	$\alpha_2\beta_2{}^{92\ \mathrm{His}\rightarrow\mathrm{Tyr}}$	$\alpha_2\beta_2{}^{67\ \mathrm{Val}\rightarrow\mathrm{Glu}}$
Helical residue	E7	F8	E7	F8	E11
O_2 affinity at P_{50}	Low	Low	Normal	Normal	Low
Bohr effect	Low	Low	Present	Present	Present
Hill's *n*	1.2	1.1	1.2	1.3	1.1–1.3
Quaternary Structure					
Deoxygenated	T*	T*		T*	T*
Oxygenated	T**	T**		R**	R**
Rate of reduction of Fe^{+++} in abn chains†	↓↓	↓↓	↓		↓
Rate of binding of Fe^{+++} in abn chains with cyanide	↓↓	↓↓	↓	↓	
Rate of heat denaturation	↓		↑	↑	Normal

*Determined from x-ray data.

**Assumed but unproved (see text).

†Rate of reduction of Fe^{+++} in abnormal chains with dithionite in presence of CO.

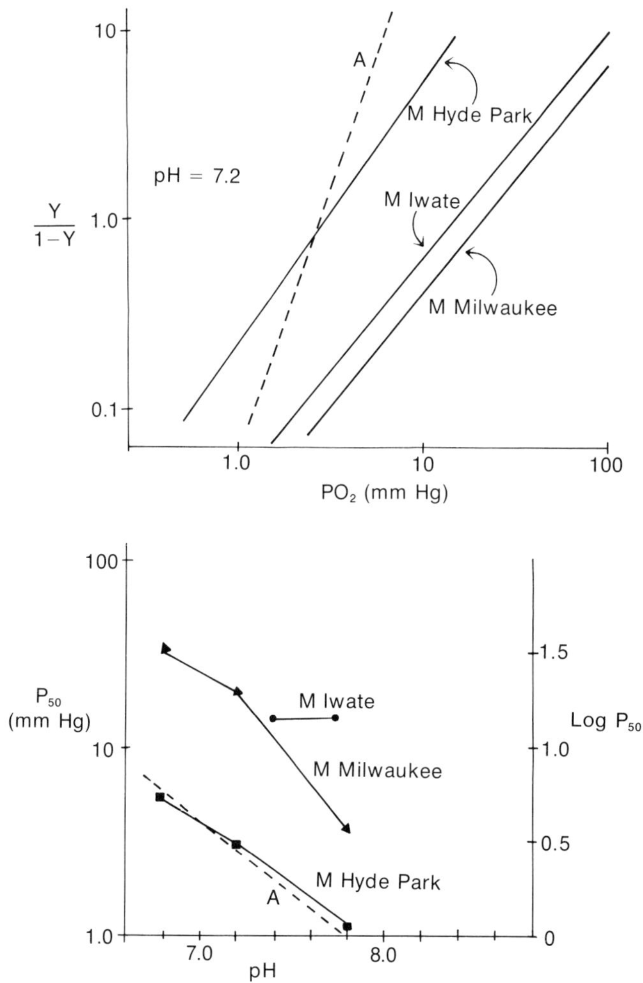

Figure 10–2. Oxygen equilibria of M hemoglobins.

Top Panel, Hill plots of Hbs M Hyde Park (β92 Tyr), M Iwate (α87 Tyr), and M Milwaukee (β67 Glu). Note that all the M hemoglobins have decreased subunit cooperativity as shown by slopes of Hill plots ($n = 1.1$–1.3). In contrast Hb A (– – –) has n of 2.9 (0.1 M PO_4, pH 7.2, 10° C).

Bottom Panel, Relationship of P_{50} to pH. Note that Hb M Hyde Park (■) and Hb M Milwaukee (▲) appear to have a normal Bohr effect (Δ log P_{50}/Δ pH). However, since the M hemoglobins bind only two oxygen molecules, the total number of protons released upon oxygenation of Hb A is 4 (Δ log P_{50}/Δ pH). Thus, the alkaline Bohr effect of Hbs M Hyde Park and M Milwaukee is about half normal. It is nearly absent in Hb M Iwate (●).

(This figure was constructed from the data of Ranney, H. M., et al.: Biochem. Biophys. Res. Commun. *33*:1004, 1968b, and Udem, L., et al.: J. Mol. Biol. *48*:489, 1970.)

proximal or distal histidine. The α-chain M hemoglobins (Boston and Iwate), in which only the β chains react with oxygen, have low oxygen affinity and nearly absent Bohr effect (Kikuchi et al., 1964; Suzuki et al., 1965). In contrast, the β-chain variants (Saskatoon and Hyde Park), which carry O_2 only on the α chains, have nearly normal P_{50} and a substantial Bohr effect. (Suzuki et al., 1966; Ranney et al., 1968b.) Representative oxygen binding curves are shown in Figure 10–2. Hemoglobin M-Milwaukee-1 differs from the other two β variants in having low oxygen affinity (Udem et al., 1970) (Table 10–1).

Hill plots of oxygen binding curves of the M hemoglobins reveal n values ranging from 1.1 to 1.3. Since only two of the subunits can bind oxygen, the maximal value of n is 2.0, rather than 4.0 as for Hb A. Even so, the M hemoglobins have markedly reduced subunit cooperativity compared to Hb A.

Whole blood oxygen binding curves of individuals with M hemoglobin tend to be markedly right-shifted, particularly if the variant has low oxygen affinity or if red cell 2,3-DPG is markedly elevated (Byckova et al., 1971). Because of low subunit cooperativity, the M hemoglobin is less saturated at high oxygen tensions compared to Hb A. These factors increase the amount of deoxyhemoglobin in arterial blood and may contribute to the individual's cyanosis.

X-Ray Crystallography

Analysis of the three-dimensional structure of the M hemoglobins by x-ray crystallography has proved useful in explaining their puzzling functional properties. Thus far four of the variants have been examined: M-Hyde Park (Greer, 1971b), M-Iwate (Greer, 1971b), M-Milwaukee-1 (Perutz et al., 1972), and M-Boston (Pulsinelli et al., 1973).

When deoxygenated, both Hb M-Hyde Park (βF8 Tyr) and Hb M-Iwate (αF8 Tyr) are isomorphous with deoxy Hb A. This means that the abnormal oxidized subunit assumes the t tertiary conformation. Hb M-Iwate remains in the T quaternary conformation, even after it is fully oxidized. It is likely that the oxygenated form of Hb M-Iwate ($\alpha_2^M\beta_2^{O_2}$) would also remain in the T structure. The stable T structure of Hb M-Iwate and the failure to switch to the R structure upon oxygen binding explains the low oxygen affinity and absent Bohr effect of this hemoglobin variant. There is some uncertainty about the interaction of the heme group with the tyrosine at F8 or with histidine at E7, since the analysis of Hb M-Iwate was done at relatively low resolution (5.5 Å).

Hb M-Hyde Park differs from Hb M-Iwate in its ability to assume an R conformation when fully oxidized. In view of its Bohr effect, Hb M-Hyde Park probably switches from the T to the R conformation upon full oxygenation. The x-ray data indicated a loss of about 20 to 30 per cent of the β-chain heme groups. This observation helps to explain the relative instability of Hb M-Hyde Park (Hayashi et al., 1968b). Because of heme loss, the resolution in the vicinity of the β hemes of Hb M-Hyde Park was reduced and therefore the position of the tyrosine at βF8 remains uncertain. However, from the position of the heme group relative to E7-histidine, F8-tyrosine probably does not act as an internal ligand stabilizing the Fe^{+++} atom. On the other hand, the x-ray data on Hb M-Iwate do indicate that such a linkage occurs as predicted by Gerald and Efron (1961). There are kinetic data which support the structural evidence for a difference between Hb M-Hyde Park and Hb M-Iwate in the stability of the internal ligand at F8. For example, both Hb M-Iwate and the other α variant, Hb M-Boston, have a much slower rate of reduction of the abnormal subunit's heme Fe^{+++} than have M-Hyde Park and the other two β-chain M hemoglobins (Shibata et al., 1961; Hayashi et al., 1968a). Secondly, the α-chain M hemoglobins have a very slow rate of reaction with cyanide in keeping with the presence of a strong internal ligand (Hayashi et al., 1967) (see Table 10–1).

The x-ray analysis of Hb M-Boston (αE7 Tyr) produced quite surprising results (Pulsinelli et al., 1973). Deoxygenated Hb M-Boston was isomorphous with deoxyhemoglobin A. The α heme Fe^{+++} was bonded to the phenolate group of E7-tyrosine! The iron atom is displaced to the distal side of the porphyrin ring and is no longer bonded to the proximal (F8) histidine. Thus the Fe^{+++} heme of the abnormal subunit is five-coordinated. These relationships are shown diagrammatically in Figure 10–3. It is likely that Hb M-Boston remains in the T conformation even after it is oxygenated. Pulsinelli et al. (1973) found that the x-ray diffraction pattern of the deoxy crystals

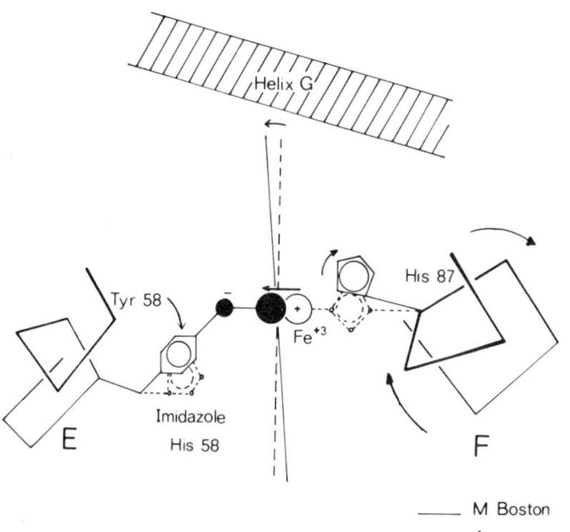

Figure 10–3. Schematic diagram of the abnormal β chain of Hb M Boston showing the relationship of the iron atom to the plane of the porphyrin ring (shown as straight and dotted lines) and the substituted tyrosine at α58 (E7) forming a bond with the iron atom. (From Pulsinelli, P. D., et al.: Proc. Natl. Acad. Sci. USA *70*:3870, 1973.)

was preserved even after exposure to air. Failure to undergo a switch to the R conformation would explain the low oxygen affinity and absent Bohr effect of Hb M-Boston. When Hb M-Boston is chemically reduced to $\alpha_2^{++}\beta_2^{++}$, it has normal heme-heme interaction and near normal Bohr effect (Nishikura et al., 1975). It is likely that the reduced iron (Fe^{++}) binds to the proximal (F8) histidine, since the phenolate group has a relatively weak affinity for Fe^{++}. If so, the iron atom would have to go through the porphyrin ring and come out the other side!

When deoxygenated, Hb M-Milwaukee-1 (βE11 Glu) had a quaternary (T) structure like that of deoxyhemoglobin A (Perutz et al., 1972). The carboxyl group of the substituted glutamic acid at β67 was shown to be coordinated with the heme iron at the sixth position. In contrast, when fully oxidized, Hb M-Milwaukee-1 assumed an R quaternary structure isomorphous with that of oxyhemoglobin A. Thus, the abnormal β chains of Hb M-Milwaukee-1 can form either the t or the r tertiary structure, dependent upon the state of the normal α chain. This conclusion gained strong independent support from optical data (Perutz et al., 1972) showing a shift in the red absorption spectrum contributed by the abnormal β chains when the normal α chains reacted with carbon monoxide. In addition, NMR data of Lindstrom et al. (1972a) indicate that such a change in quaternary conformation occurs when deoxyhemoglobin M-Milwaukee is treated with carbon monoxide. The fact that Hb M-Milwaukee-1 has a substantial Bohr effect is also consistent with this conclusion.

Clinical Manifestations

Patients have obvious cyanosis but are otherwise totally asymptomatic. A family history will often elicit a dominant inheritance pattern. However, in a number of affected individuals, the M hemoglobin has apparently arisen as a spontaneous mutation (Josephson et al., 1962; Farmer et al., 1964; Becroft et al., 1968; Stavem et al., 1972; Kohne et al., 1975). If the individual's cyanosis was apparent at birth, an α-chain M hemoglobin is likely. The β-chain M hemoglobins do not present clinically until the γ chain has been replaced by β chains at about six months of age.

The blood has a chocolate brown appearance and does not "pink up" when equilibrated with room air. Routine hematological parameters are usually within normal limits. Some but not all individuals with the β-chain M hemoglobins (Hyde Park and Saskatoon) have a mild compensated hemolytic state (Josephson et al., 1962; Hobolth, 1965a, b; Shibata et al., 1967b; Heller, 1969; Stavem et al., 1972), reflecting the fact that these two hemoglobin variants are slightly unstable (Hayashi et al., 1968a). The fact that x-ray crystallography of Hb

M-Hyde Park revealed a partial loss of hemes from the β chains supports this contention. One individual with Hb M-Saskatoon had a significant decrease in hemoglobin following the ingestion of an oxidant drug (Stavem et al., 1972).

Diagnosis

The presumptive diagnosis of M hemoglobin is made from absorption spectra of hemolysate and hemoglobin electrophoresis.

Spectral abnormalities of the M hemoglobins are best seen if all the hemoglobin is oxidized to the Fe^{+++} state with ferricyanide. As Figure 10–4 shows, the absorption spectrum of each of the M hemoglobins differs slightly from the others and can be readily distin-

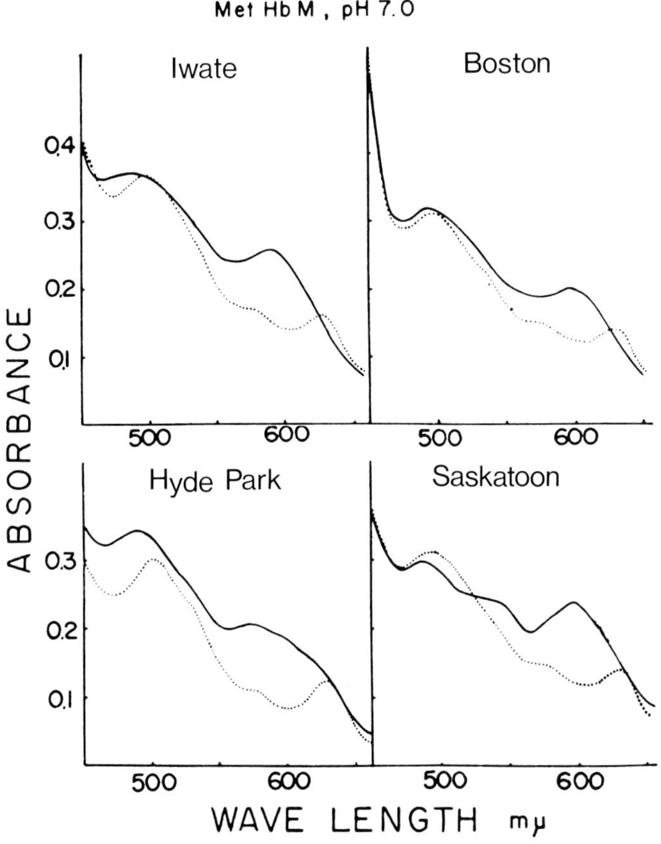

Figure 10–4. Absorption spectra of purified M hemoglobins after they had been fully oxidized with ferricyanide. The absorption spectrum of normal methemoglobin A is shown by the dotted line. (From Shibata, S., et al.: Bull. Yamaguchi Med. Sch. *14*:141, 1967a.)

guished from that of normal methemoglobin. However, it is not possible to identify any of the M hemoglobins on the basis of absorption spectra, since the results are affected by differences in the composition of the buffer and the purity of the sample. Shibata et al. (1967a) have published a very thorough treatment of the spectroscopy of the M hemoglobins. Hayashi et al. (1966) have shown that EPR spectroscopy provides a more specific identification of several of the M hemoglobins.

ELECTROPHORESIS. The M hemoglobins can also be demonstrated by electrophoresis under appropriate conditions. Routine electrophoresis of the oxygenated hemolysate at pH 8.6 usually fails to separate the normal and abnormal hemoglobins. However, electrophoresis on agar gel at pH 7.1 will generally reveal a brown band (Hb M) running slightly on the anodal side of a red band (Hb A). A much sharper pattern can be obtained with gel electrofocusing (Fig. 10–5). A wider separation of M and A hemoglobins is achieved if the hemolysate is oxidized with ferricyanide (Gerald, 1958). Methemoglobin A has a much higher isoelectric point (more positive surface charge) than methemoglobin M, since the Fe^{+++} atoms of the abnormal subunits are neutralized by an internal ligand.

The *differential diagnosis* rests between hemoglobin M and congenital methemoglobinemia (diaphorase I deficiency). The former has a dominant inheritance pattern while the latter has a recessive pattern. The two disorders can be readily distinguished by a spectral analysis of the hemolysate and hemoglobin electrophoresis. Diaphorase I deficiency is discussed below.

Once the presumptive diagnosis of Hb M is made, it is necessary to identify the structural abnormality. The M hemoglobins can be purified by chromatography on Biorex-70. In Dr. Ranney's laboratory the hemolysate is applied to a column equilibrated with sodium phosphate buffer (0.130 M Na^+, pH 6.42) at room temperature. The red Hb A elutes faster than the brown Hbs M, which remain at the top of the column. It is convenient to split the column, once the separation has been achieved, and then elute the purified components. Usually the α-chain M hemoglobins make up 15 to 30 per cent of the total while the β-chain variants make up 40 to 50 per cent (see Figure 6–4). The structural abnormality can be identified from peptide maps of tryptic digests of the abnormal subunit. Specific stains for histidine and tyrosine are very useful in interpreting the fingerprints.

Treatment

No specific treatment of these individuals is either indicated or possible. It is important that the patient be thoroughly informed of the benign nature of the disorder. The primary reason for establish-

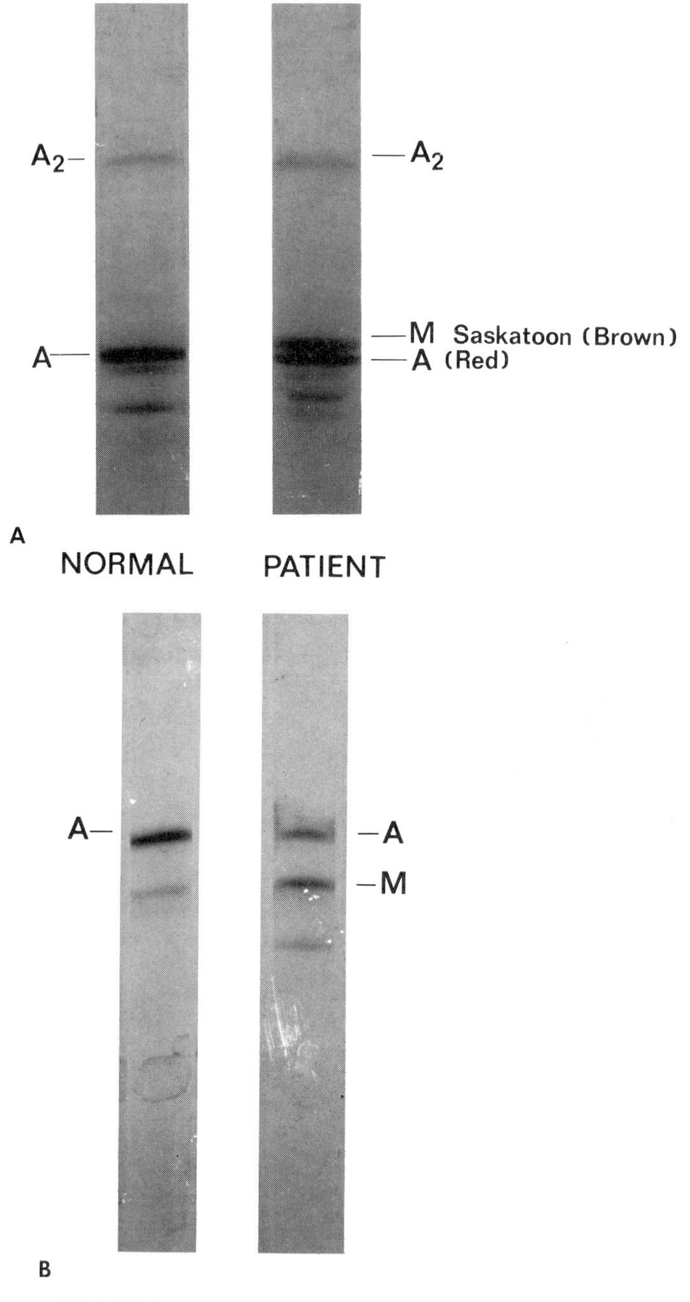

Figure 10–5. Gel electrofocusing patterns obtained on hemolysate of patient with Hb M Saskatoon. *A*, Pattern obtained on oxygenated specimens showing separation of red Hb A band and brown Hb M Saskatoon band. *B*, Pattern obtained after ferricyanide, showing wider separation of Hbs A and M Saskatoon. (The structural analysis of Hb M Saskatoon was done by Dr. Thomas Bradley.)

ing the diagnosis is to provide adequate reassurance and prevent iatrogenic misadventures that might arise under the mistaken impression that the patient has a cardiac or pulmonary disorder. One member of the original family described by Hörlein and Weber was barred from military service during the Franco-Prussian war. Individuals with M hemoglobins have undergone cardiac catheterization (Overly et al., 1967) and even exploratory surgery (Bookchin and Nagel, 1974) because of presumed heart disease. One woman in labor was refused anesthesia because "she was already cyanotic" (Vella et al., 1974). A patient believing she had heart disease declined to have abdominal surgery (Baltzan and Sugarman, 1950). Another unfortunate subject was confined to a bed and chair existence because his solicitous family felt he had a life-threatening illness (Lehmann and Huntsman, 1974).

METHEMOGLOBINEMIA

The oxidation of the iron in normal hemoglobin from Fe^{++} to Fe^{+++} results in the formation of methemoglobin. Ferriheme is incapable of binding oxygen or carbon monoxide. If methemoglobin exceeds 1.5 g/100 ml (10 per cent of the total hemoglobin), affected individuals will have clinically obvious cyanosis. The color of the skin is indistinguishable from the much commoner cyanosis due to the failure of oxygen saturation that may occur in pulmonary and cardiac disorders. Methemoglobinemia occurs in metabolically abnormal red cells with diaphorase I deficiency or in metabolically normal cells exposed to oxidant stress.

Congenital methemoglobinemia is due either to deficiency in diaphorase I (NADH-dependent methemoglobin reductase) or, less commonly, to the presence of one of the M hemoglobins (see below). Diaphorase I deficiency is inherited in an autosomal recessive pattern. This enzyme is a flavoprotein having properties similar to those of liver microsomal cytochrome b_5 reductase. The erythrocyte and hepatic enzymes have long segments of identical primary structure (Hultquist et al., 1974; Douglas and Hultquist, 1976). It would be of interest to determine whether patients with deficiency of erythrocyte diaphorase I have any abnormality in hepatic microsomal function.

Individuals with diaphorase I deficiency have life-long cyanosis of variable degree but no associated symptoms or physical findings. Some may have mild polycythemia. Untreated individuals usually have 15 to 30 per cent methemoglobin. The α- and β-chain hemes are oxidized to approximately equal extent (Fig. 10–6). Methemoglobin levels increase in the older population of red cells (Keitt et al., 1966) because the activity of the abnormal enzyme declines markedly with red cell age (Feig et al., 1972; Schwartz et al., 1972). There

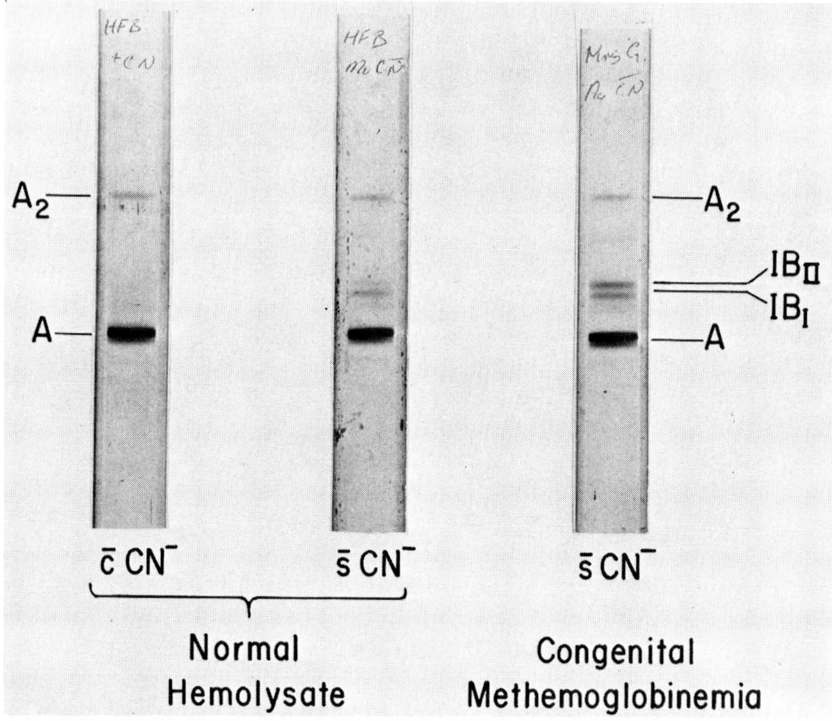

Figure 10–6. Gel electrofocusing pattern of hemolysate of a patient with congenital methemoglobinemia (diaphorase I deficiency). IB_I and IB_{II} are half-oxidized hemoglobins ($\alpha_2^+\beta_2$ and $\alpha_2\beta_2^+$, respectively). This specimen contained 10 per cent methemoglobin. Note that the intermediate bands are much fainter in the normal hemolysate. If cyanide was added to the hemolysate prior to application, no intermediate bands were detectable in either the normal hemolysate (left) or the diaphorase-I deficient hemolysate (not shown). (From Bunn, H. F.: Ann. N.Y. Acad. Sci. *209*:345, 1973.)

appears to be considerable polymorphism in the variant enzymes from different families as shown by differences in electrophoretic mobility and kinetic parameters. In these ways, diaphorase I deficiency resembles glucose-6-phosphate dehydrogenase deficiency. The oral administration of methylene blue (100 to 300 mg/day) or ascorbic acid (300 to 500 mg/day) will result in a marked reduction in the level of methemoglobin. The purpose of such treatment is primarily cosmetic.

Acquired methemoglobinemia is generally due to exposure to an agent capable of oxidizing heme iron to the ferric state. Compounds which can cause clinically significant methemoglobinemia include nitrites, nitrates, aniline derivatives, and certain oxidant drugs such as sulfonamides, vitamin K analogues, Pyridium, antimalarials, and certain anesthetics and analgesics. As might be expected, individuals heterozygous for diaphorase I deficiency (NADH-dependent methemoglobin reductase) are much more likely than normals to develop clinically apparent methemoglobinemia following exposure to an oxidant stress (Cohen et al., 1968).

The extent of methemoglobinemia depends not only on the dose of the toxic agent but also on the susceptibility of the exposed individual. At a methemoglobin level of about 35 per cent, the affected individual becomes symptomatic, experiencing headache, weakness, and breathlessness. Levels in excess of 70 per cent are incompatible with life.

The toxicity of methemoglobinemia can be readily explained in terms of our current understanding of hemoglobin function, as outlined in Chapter 2. The fact that a certain proportion of hemes is no longer able to bind oxygen is not a serious physiological handicap per se. Thirty per cent methemoglobinemia is much more deleterious than a 30 per cent decrement in red cell mass, because the oxidized hemes have a profound effect on the remaining functional hemes in the hemoglobin tetramer. The conformation of methemoglobin (as well as of carboxyhemoglobin and cyanmethemoglobin) is very close to that of oxyhemoglobin. Thus, a partially oxidized hemoglobin tetramer has the same tertiary and quaternary structure as a molecule which is comparably oxygenated. In each case, the affinity of the remaining hemes for oxygen is increased. For this reason, methemoglobinemia (as well as carbon monoxide) causes a "shift to the left" of the oxyhemoglobin dissociation curve and, consequently, impaired unloading of oxygen to tissues.

Severe toxic methemoglobinemia is treated by the intravenous administration of methylene blue (2 mg/Kg). Usually, within an hour, the methemoglobin level is reduced by at least 50 per cent.

CARBOXYHEMOGLOBINEMIA

Carbon monoxide (CO) has an effect on hemoglobin function similar to that of heme oxidation. Patients having increased levels of carboxyhemoglobin have a normal or "cherry red" color rather than cyanosis. This gas has received belated recognition as an important and widespread industrial pollutant and toxin. CO may be engendered from the combustion of any organic material but, most commonly, that of hydrocarbons, such as petroleum and tobacco tar. In addition, one mole of CO is formed endogenously in the breakdown of heme into bile pigment. Accordingly, individuals with significant hemolysis or ineffective erythropoiesis have a measurably increased amount of circulating carboxyhemoglobin.

Like oxygen, CO is a ligand which binds reversibly to hemoglobin when heme iron is in the reduced (ferrous) state. The toxicity of CO is due to its very high affinity for heme, approximately 210 times that of oxygen. Following an acute exposure, CO remains so tightly bound to hemoglobin that about four hours are required for an individual with normal ventilation to expel half of it. Because of its slow disappearance time, a toxic level of carboxyhemoglobin may accumulate from continued exposure to a relatively low dose of CO. CO also binds to other heme proteins, such as cytochrome P-450. Whether this contributes significantly to the toxicity of CO is not yet known.

As expected, the clinical manifestations of CO intoxication are directly related to the duration and extent of exposure. Impaired visual and time discrimination have been documented in individuals with carboxyhemoglogin levels of 5 per cent (Coburn, 1970). Above approximately 20 per cent carboxyhemoglobin, more overt and subjective symptoms develop, such as headache, weakness, and so forth (Coburn, 1970). At levels of 40 to 60 per cent, unconsciousness is followed by death. Like methemoglobinemia, the toxic effect of CO is primarily due to increased oxygen affinity of the blood.

The mechanism by which CO shifts the oxyhemoglobin dissociation curve to the left is identical to that of methemoglobin (see above). However, a given per cent carboxyhemoglobin appears to be more deleterious than a comparable level of methemoglobin. This may be because of a more even distribution of CO among red cells of all ages.

The treatment of carbon monoxide intoxication is directed primarily at removing the source of toxic exposure and facilitating the expulsion of gas by the lungs. Thus, it is very important to maintain adequate ventilation. If the patient is transferred from room air to 100 per cent oxygen, the disappearance half time for CO is reduced from four hours to one hour. Other therapeutic approaches, such as hyperbaric oxygen or exchange transfusion, may have theoretical merit but are not readily available.

REFERENCES

Abramson, R. K., Rucknagel, D. L., Shreffler, D. C., et al.: Homozygous Hb J Tongariki: evidence for only one alpha chain structural locus in Melanesians. Science *169*:194, 1970.

Ackers, G. K., and Halvorson, H. R.: Linkage between oxygenation and subunit dissociation in human hemoglobin. Proc. Natl. Acad. Sci. USA *71*:4312, 1974.

Adair, G. S.: The osmotic pressure of haemoglobin in the absence of salts. Proc. Roy. Soc. London *109A*:292, 1925.

Adams, J. G., III: Hemoglobin Ann Arbor: Disturbance in the coordinated biosynthesis of globin chains? Ann. NY Acad. Sci. *241*:232, 1974.

Adams, J. G., III, Winter, W. P., Rucknagel, D. L., et al.: Biosynthesis of hemoglobin Ann Arbor: Evidence for catabolic and feedback regulation. Science *176*:1427, 1972.

Adams, J. G., III, Winter, W. P., Tausk, K., et al.: Hemoglobin Rush (β101[G3] Glutamine): A new unstable hemoglobin causing mild hemolytic anemia. Blood *43*:261, 1974.

Adamson, J. W.: Familial polycythemia. Semin. Hematol. *12*:383, 1975.

Adamson, J. W., and Finch, C. A.: Erythropoietin and the polycythemias. Ann. NY Acad. Sci. *149*:560, 1968.

Adamson, J. W., and Finch, C. A.: Hemoglobin function, oxygen affinity and erythropoietin. Ann. Rev. Physiol. *37*:351, 1975.

Adamson, J. W., and Stamatoyannopoulos, G.: Activation of hemoglobin C synthesis in sheep marrow culture. Science *180*:130, 1973.

Adamson, J. W., Parer, J. T., and Stamatoyannopoulos, G.: Erythrocytosis associated with hemoglobin Rainier: oxygen equilibria and marrow regulation. J. Clin. Invest. *48*:1376, 1969.

Adamson, J. W., Hayashi, A., Stamatoyannopoulos, G. and Burger, W. F.: Erythrocyte function and marrow regulation in hemoglobin Bethesda (β145 Histidine). J. Clin. Invest. *51*:2883, 1972.

Adamson, J. W., Stamatoyannopoulos, G., Kontras, S., et al.: Recessive familial erythrocytosis: aspects of marrow regulation in two families. Blood *41*:641, 1973.

Adamson, S. D., Herbert, E., and Godchaux, W.: Factors affecting the rate of protein synthesis in lysate systems from reticulocytes. Arch. Biochem. Biophys. *125*:671, 1968.

Adamson, S. D., Herbert, E., and Kemp S.: Effects of hemin and other porphyrins on protein synthesis in a reticulocyte lysate cell-free system. J. Mol. Biol. *42*:247, 1969.

Adamson, S. D., Howard, G. A., and Herbert, E.: The ribosome cycle in a reconstituted cell-free system from reticulocytes. Cold Spring Harbor Symp. Quant. Biol. *37*:547, 1969.

Adamson, S. D., Yau, P. M., Herbert, E., et al.: Involvement of hemin, a stimulatory fraction from ribosomes and a protein synthesis inhibitor in the regulation of hemoglobin synthesis. J. Mol. Biol. *63*:247, 1972.

Agostoni, A., Berfasconi, C., Gerli, G. C., et al.: Oxygen affinity and electrolyte distribution of human blood: changes induced by propranolol. Science *182*:300, 1973.

Agostoni, A., Lotto, A., Stabilini, R., et al.: Hemoglobin oxygen affinity in patients with low-output heart failure and cardiogenic shock after acute myocardial infarction. Eur. J. Cardiol. *3*:53, 1975.

Akerblöm, O., De Verdier, C. H., Garby, L., et al.: Restoration of defective oxygen-transport function of stored red blood cells by addition of inosine. Scand. J. Clin. Lab. Invest. *21*:245, 1968.

Aksoy, M.: The hemoglobin E syndromes. II. Sickle-cell–hemoglobin E disease. Blood *15*:610, 1960.

Aksoy, M.: The first observation of homozygous hemoglobin S–alpha thalassemia disease and two types of sickle cell thalassemia disease: (a) Sickle cell–alpha thalassemia disease; (b) sickle cell–beta thalassemia disease. Blood *22*:757, 1963.

Aksoy, M.: Thalassemia intermedia: a genetic study in 11 patients. J. Med. Genet. *7*:47, 1970.

Aksoy, M., and Erdem, S.: Some problems of hemoglobin patterns in different thalassemic syndromes showing the heterogeneity of beta-thalassemia genes. Ann. NY Acad. Sci. *165*:13, 1969.

Aksoy, M., Erdem, S., Efremov, G. D., et al.: Hemoglobin Istanbul: Substitution of glutamine for histidine in a proximal histidine (F8[92]β). J. Clin. Invest. *51*:2380, 1972.

Alavi, A., Bond, J. P., Kuhl, D. E., et al.: Scan detection of bone marrow infarcts in sickle cell disorders. J. Nucl. Med. *15*:1003, 1974.

Alberti, K. G. M., Emerson, P. M., Darley, J. H., et al.: 2,3-Diphosphoglycerate and tissue oxygenation in uncontrolled diabetes. Lancet *2*:391, 1972.

Alexanian, R., and Nadell, J.: Oxymetholone treatment for sickle cell anemia. Blood *45*:769, 1975.

Ali, M. A., and Brain, M. C.: Ethanol inhibition of haemoglobin synthesis: in vitro evidence for a haem correctable defect in normal subjects and in alcoholics. Br. J. Haematol. *28*:311, 1974.

Alkjaersig, N., Fletcher, A., Joist, H., and Chaplin, H.: Hemostatic alterations accompanying sickle cell pain crises. J. Lab. Clin. Med. *88*:440, 1976.

Allen, D. W., and Wyman, J.: Equilibre de l'hémoglobine de drepanocytose avec l'oxygène. Rev. Hématol. *9*:155, 1954.

Allen, D. W., Schroeder, W. A., and Balog, J.: Observations on the chromatographic heterogeneity of normal adult and fetal human hemoglobin: A study of the effects of crystallization and chromatography on the heterogeneity and isoleucine content. J. Am. Soc. *80*:1628, 1958.

Allison, A. C.: Protection afforded by sickle cell trait against subtertian malarial infection. Br. Med. J. *1*:290, 1954.

Allison, A. C.: Observations on the sickling phenomenon and on the distribution of different haemoglobin types in erythrocyte populations. Clin. Sci. *15*:497, 1956.

Allison, A. C.: Malaria in carriers of the sickle-cell trait and in newborn children. Exp. Parasitol. *6*:418, 1957a.

Allison, A. C.: Properties of sickle-cell haemoglobin. Biochem. J. *65*:212, 1957b.

Allison, A. C., and Cecil, R.: The thiol groups of normal adult human haemoglobin. Biochem. J. *69*:27, 1958.

Alter, B. P., Rappeport, J. M., Huisman, T. H. J., et al.: Fetal erythropoiesis following bone marrow transplantation. Blood *46*:1054, 1975, and Blood *48*:843, 1976.

Alter, B. P., Friedman, S., Hobbins, J. C., et al.: Prenatal diagnosis of sickle-cell anemia and alpha G-Philadelphia. N. Engl. J. Med. *294*:1040, 1976a.

Alter, B. P., Sherman, A. S., Hobbins, J. C., et al.: Prenatal diagnosis of hemoglobinopathies: Experience in 17 cases. Clin. Res. *24*:293A, 1976b, and N. Engl. J. Med., *295*:1437, 1976.

Amiconi, G., Winterhalter, K. H., Antonini, E., et al.: Functional properties of hemoglobin Rainier. FEBS Lett., *21*:341, 1972.

Anderson, N. L.: Hemoglobin San Diego (β109[G11] Val→Met): crystal structure of the deoxy form. J. Clin. Invest. *53*:329, 1974.

Anderson, N. L., Perutz, M. F., and Stamatoyannopoulos, G.: Site of amino acid substitution in hemoglobin Seattle ($\alpha_2{}^A\beta_2{}^{70\ Asp}$). Nature [New Biol.] *243*:274, 1973.

Anderson, W. F., and Gilbert, J.: tRNA-dependent translational control of *in vitro* hemoglobin synthesis. Biochem. Biophys. Res. Commun. *36*:456, 1969.

Anderson, W. F., Steggles, A., Wilson, G., et al.: Cell-free transcription of human bone marrow chromatin. Ann. NY Acad. Sci. *241*:262, 1974.

Anfinsen, C. B.: Principles that govern the folding of protein chains. Science *181*:223, 1973.

Antonini, E., Wyman, J., Zito, R., et al.: Studies on carboxypeptidase digests of human hemoglobin. J. Biol. Chem., *236*:PC60, 1961.

Antonini, E., Wyman, J., Moretti, R., et al.: The interaction of bromthymol blue with hemoglobin and its effect on oxygen equilibrium. Biochim. Biophys. Acta *71*:124, 1963.

Antonovych, T. T.: Ultrastructural changes in glomeruli of patients with sickle cell disease and nephrotic syndrome. In Abstracts, Fifth Annual Meeting, Washington, D.C. The American Society of Nephrology, 1971, p. 3.

Armaly, M. F.: Ocular manifestations in sickle cell disease. Arch. Intern. Med. *133*:670, 1974.

Arnone, A.: X-ray diffraction study of binding of 2,3-diphosphoglycerate to human deoxyhaemoglobin. Nature *237*:146, 1972.

Arnone, A.: X-ray studies of the interaction of CO_2 with human deoxyhaemoglobin. Nature *247*:143, 1974.

Arnone, A., and Perutz, M. F.: Structure of inositol hexaphosphate—human deoxyhaemoglobin complex. Nature *249*:34, 1974.

Arturson, G., Garby, L., Robert, M., et al.: Oxygen affinity of whole blood *in vivo* and under standard conditions in subjects with diabetes mellitus. Scand. J. Clin. Lab. Invest. *34*:19, 1974a.

Arturson, G., Garby, L., Wranne, B., et al.: Effect of 2,3-diphosphoglycerate on the oxygen affinity and on the proton- and carbamino-linked oxygen affinity of hemoglobin in human whole blood. Acta Physiol. Scand. *92*:332, 1974b.

Asakura, T., Agarwal, P. L., Relman, D. A., et al.: Mechanical instability of the oxyform of sickle haemoglobin. Nature *244*:437, 1973.

Asakura, T., Ohnishi, T., Friedman, S., et al.: Abnormal precipitation of oxyhemoglobin S by mechanical shaking. Proc. Natl. Acad. Sci. USA *71*:1594, 1974.

Askari, A., and Rao, S. N.: Regulation of AMP deaminase by 2,3-diphosphoglyceric acid: a possible mechanism for the control of adenine nucleotide metabolism in human erythrocytes. Biochim. Biophys. Acta *151*:198, 1968.

Astrup, P.: Oxygen dissociation curves in some diseases. Försvarsmedicin *5*:199, 1969.

Astrup, P.: Red cell pH and oxygen affinity of hemoglobin. N. Engl. J. Med. *283*:202, 1970.

Astrup, P., and Rørth, M.: Oxygen affinity of hemoglobin and red cell 2,3-diphosphoglycerate in hepatic cirrhosis. Scand. J. Clin. Lab. Invest. *31*:311, 1973.

Astrup, P., Engel, K., Severinghaus, J. W., et al.: The influence of temperature and pH on the dissociation curve of oxyhemoglobin of human blood. Scand. J. Clin. Lab. Invest. *17*:515, 1965.

Astrup, P., Rørth, M., and Thorshauge, C.: Dependency on acid-base status of oxyhemoglobin dissociation and 2,3-diphosphoglycerate level in human erythrocytes. II. In vivo studies. Scand. J. Clin. Lab. Invest. *26*:47, 1970.

Attah, E. B., and Ekere, M. C.: Death patterns in sickle cell anemia. JAMA *233*:889, 1975.

Atwater, J., Schwartz, I. R., Erslev, A. J., et al.: Sickling of erythrocytes in a patient with thalassemia-hemoglobin I disease. N. Engl. J. Med. *263*:1215, 1960.

Axel, R., Cedar, H., and Felsenfeld, G.: Synthesis of globin ribonucleic acid from duck-reticulocyte chromatin *in vitro*. Proc. Natl. Acad. Sci. USA *70*:2029, 1973.

Axel, R., Cedar, H., and Felsenfeld, G.: The structure of the globin genes in chromatin. Biochemistry *14*:2489, 1975.

Azevêdo, E.: Historical note on inheritance of sickle cell anemia. Am. J. Hum. Genet. *25*:457, 1973.

Badr, F. M., Lorkin, P. A., and Lehmann, H.: Haemoglobin P-Nilotic containing a β-δ chain. Nature [New Biol.] *242*:107, 1973.

Baglioni, C.: Chemical studies on haemoglobin D. Biochim. Biophys. Acta *59*:437, 1962a.

Baglioni, C.: The fusion of two peptide chains in hemoglobin Lepore and its interpretation as a genetic deletion. Proc. Natl. Acad. Sci. USA *48*:1880, 1962b.

Baglioni, C.: Correlations between genetics and chemistry of human hemoglobins. In Taylor, H. J. (ed.): Molecular Genetics, Part I. New York, Academic Press, 1963, pp. 405–475.

Baglioni, C., and Campana, T.: Alpha chain and globin intermediates in the formation of rabbit hemoglobin. Eur. J. Biochem. *2*:480, 1967.

Baglioni, C., Colombo, B., and Jacobs-Lorena, M.: Chain termination: a test for a possible explanation of thalassemia. Ann. NY Acad. Sci. *165*:212, 1969.

Baine, R. M., Rucknagel, D. L., Dublin, P. A., et al.: Trimodality in the proportion of hemoglobin G Philadelphia in heterozygotes: evidence for heterogeneity in the number of human alpha chain loci. Proc. Natl. Acad. Sci. USA *73*:3633, 1976.

Baker, R., Powers, D., and Haywood, L. J.: Restoration of the deformability of "irreversibly" sickled cells by procaine hydrochloride. Biochem. Biophys. Res. Commun. *59*:548, 1974.

Baldassare, J. J., Charache, S., Jones, R. T., and Ho, C.: Electron paramagnetic resonance studies of spin-labeled hemoglobins. II. Roles of subunit interactions and of intermediate structures in the cooperative oxygenation of hemoglobin and the results on hemoglobin Yakima, hemoglobin J Cape Town and carboxypeptidases A– and B–treated hemoglobin A. Biochemistry *9*:4707, 1970.

Ball, G. V., and Sorenson, L. B.: The pathogenesis of hyperuricemia and gout in sickle cell anemia. Arthritis Rheum. *13*:846, 1970.

Baltzman, D. M., and Sugarman, H.: Hereditary cyanosis. Can. Med. Assoc. J. *62*:348, 1950.

Bank, A., and Marks, P. A.: Excess alpha chain synthesis relative to beta chain synthesis in thalassemia major and minor. Nature *212*:1158, 1966a.

Bank, A., and Marks, P. A.: Protein synthesis in a cell-free human reticulocyte system: ribosome function in thalassemia, J. Clin. Invest. *45*:330, 1966b.

Bank, A., Braverman, S., O'Donnell, J. V., and Marks, P. A.: Absolute rates of globin chain synthesis in thalassemia. Blood *31*:226, 1968.

Bank, A., O'Donnell, J. V., and Braverman, A. D.: Globin chain synthesis in heterozygotes for beta chain mutations. J. Lab. Clin. Med. *76*:616, 1970.

Bank, A., Mears, G., Weiss, R., et al.: Preferential binding of β^S globin chains associated with stroma in sickle cell disorder. J. Clin. Invest. *54*:805, 1974.

Bannerman, R. M.: Abnormalities of heme and pyrrole metabolism in thalassemia. Ann. NY Acad. Sci. *119*:503, 1964.

Bannerman, R. M., Grinstein, M., and Moore, C. V.: Haemoglobin synthesis in thalassemia; *in vitro* studies. Br. J. Haematol. 5:102, 1959.

Bannerman, R. M., Callender, S. T., Hardisty, R. M., et al.: Iron absorption in thalassemia. Br. J. Haematol. *10*:490, 1964.

Barcroft, J.: The respiratory function of the blood. Part II. Haemoglobin. London, Cambridge University Press, 1928.

Bard, H.: Études préliminaire de la synthèse des hémoglobines foetales et adultes chez le prémature. Union Medicale du Canada *100*:1097, 1971.

Bard, H.: Postnatal fetal and adult hemoglobin synthesis in D1 trisomy syndrome. Blood *40*:523, 1972.

Bard, H.: Postnatal, fetal and adult hemoglobin synthesis in early preterm newborn infants. J. Clin. Invest. 52:1789, 1973.

Bard, H.: The postnatal decline of hemoglobin F synthesis in normal full-term infants. J. Clin. Invest. *55*:395, 1975.

Bard, H., Makowski, E. L., Meschia, G., et al.: The relative rates of synthesis of hemoglobin A and F in immature red cells of newborn infants. Pediatrics *45*:766, 1970.

Bare, G. H., Alben, J., Bromberg, P. A., et al.: Hemoglobin Little Rock (β143 [H21] His→Gln). Effects of an amino acid substitution at the 2,3-diphosphoglycerate binding site. J. Biol. Chem. *249*:773, 1974.

Bargellesi, A., Pontremoli, S., and Conconi, F.: Absence of beta-globin synthesis and excess of alpha-globin synthesis in homozygous beta-thalassemia. Eur. J. Biochem. *1*:73, 1967.

Bargellesi, A., Pontremoli, S., Menini, C., et al.: Excess of alpha globin synthesis in homozygous beta-thalassemia and its removal from the red blood cell cytoplasm. Eur. J. Biochem. *3*:364, 1968.

Barnes, P. M., Hendrickse, R. G., and Watson-Williams, E. J.: Low-molecular-weight dextran in treatment of bone-pain crises in sickle cell disease: a double-blind trial. Lancet *2*:1271, 1965.

Barreras, L., Diggs, L. W., and Bell, A.: Erythrocyte morphology in patients with sickle cell anemia and pulmonary emboli. JAMA *203*:569, 1968.

Barrett, T., Maryanka, D., Hamlyn, P. H., et al.: Nonhistone proteins control gene expression in reconstituted chromatin. Proc. Natl. Acad. Sci. USA *71*:5057, 1974.

Barrett-Connor, E.: Cholelithiasis in sickle cell anemia. Am. J. Med. *45*:889, 1968.

Barrett-Connor, E.: Bacterial infection and sickle cell anemia. Medicine (Baltimore) *50*:97, 1971.

Barrett-Connor, E.: Anemia and infection. Am. J. Med. *52*:242, 1972.

Barrett-Connor, E.: Pneumonia and pulmonary infarction in sickle cell anemia. JAMA *224*:997, 1973.

Barry, M., Flynn, D. M., Letsky, E. A., et al.: Long-term chelation therapy in thalassemia major: effect on liver iron concentration, liver histology and clinical progress. Br. Med. J. *2*:16, 1974.

Bartels, H., and Harms, H.: Sauerstoffdissoziationskurven des Blutes von Säugetieren. Pfluegers Arch. *268*:334, 1959.

Bartels, H., Betke, K., Hilpert, P., et al.: Die sogenannte Standard-O_2-dissoziationskurve des gesunden erwachsenen Menschen. Pfluegers Arch. *272*:372, 1961.

Basch, R. A.: Hemoglobin synthesis in short term cultures of human fetal hematopoietic tissues. Blood *39*:530, 1972.

Basu, A. K., and Woodruff, A. W.: Effect of pyrexia on sicklaemic states. Lancet *ii*:1088, 1963.

Battaglia, F. C., McGaughey, H., Makowski, E. L., and Meschia, G.: Postnatal changes in oxygen affinity of sheep red cells: a dual role of 2,3-diphosphoglyceric acid. Am. J. Physiol. *219*:217, 1970.

Bauer, C.: Antagonistic influence of CO_2 and 2,3-diphosphoglycerate on the Bohr effect of human haemoglobin. Life Sci. *8*:1041, 1969.

Bauer, C., and Rathschlag-Schaefer, A.-M.: The influence of aldosterone and cortisol on oxygen affinity and cation concentration of the blood. Respir. Physiol. *5*:360, 1968.

Bauer, C., and Schroeder, E.: Carbamino compounds of haemoglobin in human adult and foetal blood. J. Physiol. (London) *227*:457, 1972.

Bauer, C., Ludwig, I., and Ludwig, M.: Different effects of 2,3-diphosphoglycerate and adenosine triphosphate on the oxygen affinity of adult and foetal human haemoglobin. Life Sci. *7*:1339, 1968.

Bauer, C., Henry, Y., and Banerjee, R.: Binding of 2,3-diphosphoglycerate to haemoglobin valency hybrids. Nature [New Biol.] *242*:208, 1973.

Baur, E. W., and Motulsky, A. G.: Hemoglobin Tacoma—a β chain variant associated with increased Hb A_2. Humangenetik *1*:621, 1965.

Beard, M. E. J., Necheles, T. F., and Allen, D. M.: Clinical experience with intensive transfusion therapy in Cooley's anemia. Ann. NY Acad. Sci. *165*:415, 1969.

Beaven, G. H., Stevens, B. L., Dance, H., and White, J. C.: Occurrence of haemoglobin H in leukaemia. Nature *199*:1297, 1963.

Beaven, G. H., Hornabrook, R. W., Fox, R. H., et al.: Occurrence of heterozygotes and homozygotes for the alpha chain haemoglobin variant Hb J (Tongariki) in New Guinea. Nature (London) *235*:46, 1972.

Beck, W. S. (ed.): Hematology. 2nd ed. Boston, MIT Press, 1976.

Becroft, D. M. O., Douglas, R., Carrell, R. W., and Lehmann, H.: Haemoglobin M Hyde Park: A hereditary methaemoglobinaemia in a Caucasian child. NZ Med. J. *68*:72, 1968.

Beet, E. A.: The genetics of the sickle cell trait in a Bantu tribe. Ann. Eugen. *14*:279, 1949.

Bellingham, A. J., and Huehns, E. R.: Compensation in haemolytic anaemias caused by abnormal haemoglobins. Nature *218*:924, 1968.

Bellingham, A. J., Detter, J. C., and Lenfant, C.: The role of hemoglobin affinity for oxygen and red-cell 2,3-diphosphoglycerate in the management of diabetic ketoacidosis. Trans. Assoc. Am. Physicians *83*:113, 1970.

Bellingham, A. J., Detter, J. C., and Lenfant, C.: Regulatory mechanisms of hemoglobin oxygen affinity in acidosis and alkalosis. J. Clin. Invest. *50*:700, 1971.

Beltrami, C. A., Bearzi, I., and Fabris, G.: Storage cells of spleen and bone marrow in thalassemia: an ultrastructural study. Blood *41*:901, 1973.

Benesch, R. E., and Benesch, R.: The influence of oxygenation on the reactivity of the —SH groups of hemoglobin. Biochemistry *1*:735, 1962.

Benesch, R., and Benesch, R. E.: The effect of organic phosphates from the human erythrocyte on the allosteric properties of hemoglobin. Biochem. Biophys. Res. Commun. *26*:162, 1967.

Benesch, R. E., Ranney, H. M., Benesch, R., et al.: The chemistry of the Bohr effect. II. Some properties of hemoglobin H. J. Biol. Chem. *236*:2926, 1961.

Benesch, R. E., Benesch, R., and Williamson, M. E.: The influence of reversible oxygen binding on the interaction between hemoglobin subunits. Proc. Natl. Acad. Sci. USA *48*:2071, 1962.

Benesch, R., Benesch, R. E., and Enoki, Y.: The interaction of hemoglobin and its subunits with 2,3-diphosphoglycerate. Proc. Natl. Acad. Sci. USA *61*:1102, 1968a.

Benesch, R., Benesch, R. E., and Yu, C. I.: Reciprocal binding of oxygen and diphosphoglycerate by human hemoglobin. Proc. Natl. Acad. Sci. USA *59*:526, 1968b.

Benesch, R. E., Benesch, R., and Yu, C. I.: The oxygenation of hemoglobin in the presence of diphosphoglycerate. Effect of temperature, pH, ionic strength and hemoglobin concentration. Biochemistry *8*:2567, 1969.

Benesch, R. E., Benesch, R., Renthal, R. D., and Maeda, N.: Affinity labeling of the polyphosphate binding site of hemoglobin. Biochemistry *11*:3526, 1972.

Benesch, R., Benesch, R. E., and Yung, S.: Chemical modifications that inhibit gelation of sickle hemoglobin. Proc. Natl. Acad. Sci. USA *71*:1504, 1974.

Benesch, R. E., Yung, S., Benesch, R., et al.: α-Chain contacts in the polymerisation of sickle haemoglobin. Nature *260*:219, 1976.

Bennett, M. A., Heslop, R. W., and Meynell, M. J.. Massive haematuria associated with sickle-cell trait. Br. Med. J. *1*:677, 1967.

Bentley, S. A., Lewis, S. M., and White, J. M.: Red cell survival studies in patients with unstable hemoglobin disorders. Br. J. Haematol. *26*:85, 1974.

Benz, E. J., Jr., and Forget, B. G.: Defect in messenger RNA for human hemoglobin synthesis in beta thalassemia. J. Clin. Invest. *50*:2755, 1971.

Benz, E. J., Jr., and Forget, B. G.: The biosynthesis of hemoglobin. Semin. Hematol. *11*:463, 1974.

Benz, E. J., Jr., and Forget, B. G.: The molecular genetics of the thalassemia syndromes. *In* Brown, E. B. (ed.): Progress in Hematology. New York, Grune & Stratton, Vol IX, p. 107, 1975.

Benz, E. J., Jr., Swerdlow, P. S., and Forget, B. G.: Globin messenger RNA in Hb H disease. Blood *42*:825, 1973.

Benz, E. J., Jr., Housman, D., Pritchard, J., and Forget, B. G.: Non-functioning globin messenger RNA for Lepore globin chains in Hb Lepore-β°-thalassemia. Clin. Res. *23*:269A, 1975a.

Benz, E. J., Jr., Swerdlow, P. S., and Forget, B. G.: Absence of functional messenger RNA activity for beta globin chain synthesis in β^0-thalassemia. Blood *45*:1, 1975b.

Beresford, C. H., Clegg, J. B., and Weatherall, D. J.: Haemoglobin Ocho Rios (β52 (D3) aspartic acid→alanine): A new β chain variant of haemoglobin A found in combination with haemoglobin S. J. Med. Genet. *9*:151, 1972.

Beretta, A., Prato, V., Gallo, E., and Lehmann, H.: Haemoglobin Torino – α43 (CD1) phenylalanine→valine. Nature *217*:1016, 1968.

Berger, H., Jänig, G.-R., Gerber, G., et al.:Interaction of haemoglobin with ions. Interactions among magnesium, adenosine 5′-triphosphate, 2,3-disphosphoglycerate and oxygenated and deoxygenated human haemoglobin under simulated intracellular conditions. Eur. J. Biochem. *38*:553, 1973.

Berman, M., Benesch, R., and Benesch, R. E.: The removal of organic phosphates from hemoglobin. Arch. Biochem. Biophys. *145*:236, 1971.

Bernal, J. D., and Crowfoot, D.: X-ray photographs of crystalline pepsin. Nature *133*: 794, 1934.

Bernini, L., Colucci, C. F., deMichele, D., et al.: A possible case of alpha-beta thalassemia. Acta Genet. Stat. Med. *12*:202, 1962.

Berns, A., Jansen, P., and Bloemendal, H.: The separation of α- and β-rabbit globin mRNA by polyacrylamide gel electrophoresis. FEBS Lett. *47*:343, 1974.

Berns, A., Salden, M., Bogdanovsky, D., et al.: Non-specific stimulation of cell-free protein synthesis by a dialyzable factor isolated from reticulocyte initiation factors (iRNA). Proc. Natl. Acad. Sci. USA *72*:714, 1975.

Bernstein, J., and Whitten, C. F.: A histologic appraisal of the kidney in sickle cell anemia. Arch. Pathol. *70*:407, 1960.

Bernstein, R. E.: Alterations in metabolic energetics and cation transport during aging of red cells. J. Clin. Invest. *38*:1572, 1959.

Bertles, J. F., and Döbler, J.: Reversible and irreversible sickling: A distinction by electron microscopy. Blood *33*:884, 1969.

Bertles, J. F., and Milner, P. F. A.: Irreversibly sickled erythrocytes: a consequence of the heterogeneous distribution of hemoglobin types in sickle cell anemia. J. Clin. Invest. *47*:1731, 1968.

Bertles, J. F., Rabinowitz, R., and Döbler, J.: Hemoglobin interaction: modification of solid phase composition in the sickling phenomenon. Science *169*:375, 1970.

Bester, A. J., Kennedy, D. S., and Heywood, S. M.: Two classes of translational control RNA; their role in the regulation of protein synthesis. Proc. Natl. Acad. Sci. USA *72*: 1523, 1975.

Beutler, E.: The effect of methemoglobin formation in sickle cell disease. J. Clin. Invest. *40*:1856, 1961.

Beutler, E.: 2,3-diphosphoglycerate affects enzymes of glucose metabolism in red blood cells. Nature [New Biol.] *232*:20, 1971.

Beutler, E., and Wood, L. A.: The in vivo regeneration of red cell 2,3-diphosphoglyceric acid after transfusion of stored blood. J. Lab. Clin. Med. *74*:300, 1969.

Beutler, E., Johnson, C., Powars, D., and West, C.: Prevalence of glucose-6-phosphate dehydrogenase deficiency in sickle cell disease. N. Engl. J. Med. *290*:826, 1974a.

Beutler, E., Lang, A., and Lehmann, H.: Hemoglobin Duarte ($\alpha_2\beta_2{}^{62}$ [E6] Ala→Pro): A new unstable hemoglobin with increased oxygen affinity. Blood *43*:527, 1974b.

Beuzard, Y., Courvalin, J. C., Cohen-Solal, M., et al.: Structural studies on hemoglobin St. Etienne (β92 [F8] His→Gln): a new abnormal hemoglobin with loss of β proximal histidine and absence of heme on the β chain. FEBS Lett. *27*:76, 1972.

Beuzard, Y., Rodvien, R., and London, I.: Effect of hemin on the synthesis of hemoglobin and other proteins in mammalian cells. Proc. Natl. Acad. Sci. USA *70*:1022, 1973.

Beychok, S., Tyuma, I., Benesch, R. E., and Benesch, R.: Optically active absorption bands of hemoglobin and its subunits. J. Biol. Chem. *242*:2460, 1967.

Bhoyroo, S. I., and Storrs, C. N.: Adult and fetal haemoglobin haemolytic disease of the newborn. Arch. Dis. Child. *46*:570, 1971.

Bilinski, R. T., Kandel, G. L., and Rabiner, S. F.: Epsilon aminocaproic acid therapy of hematuria due to heterozygous sickle cell diseases. J. Urol. *102*:93, 1969.

Bird, G. W. G., and Lehmann, H.: Haemoglobin D in India. Br. Med. J. *1*:514, 1956.

Bishop, J. O., and Jones, K. W.: Chromosomal localization of human haemoglobin structural genes. Nature *240*:149, 1972.

Bishop, J. O., and Rosbash, M.: Reiteration frequency of duck haemoglobin genes. Nature [New Biol.] *241*:204, 1973.

Bishop, J. O., Pemberton, R., and Baglioni, C.: Reiteration frequency of haemoglobin genes in the duck. Nature [New Biol.], *235*:231, 1972.

Blendis, L. M., Modell, C. B., Bowdler, A. J., and Williams, R.: Some effects of splenectomy in thalassaemia major. Br. J. Haematol. *28*:77, 1974.

Blobel, G.: Protein tightly bound to globin mRNA. Biochem. Biophys. Res. Commun. *47*:88, 1972.

Blobel, G.: A protein of molecular weight 78,000 bound to the polyadenylate region of eukaryotic messenger RNA's. Proc. Natl. Acad. Sci. USA *70*:924, 1973.

Blum, N., and Schapira, G.: Régulation de la synthèse de l'hémoglobine par addition de α hémoglobine libre. C. R. Acad. Sci. [D.] *264*:1211, 1967.

Blum, N., Maleknia, N., Schapira, G., et al.: α hémoglobine libre et biosynthèse de l'hémoglobine. Biochim. Biophys. Acta *179*:448, 1969.

Blum, N., Maleknia, M., Schapira, G., et al.: α- et β-globines libres et biosynthèse de l'hémoglobine. Biochim. Biophys. Acta *199*:236, 1970.

Blum, M., Kneip, B., and Schapira, G.: Influence d'origine specifique des chaines α d'hémoglobine sur la biosynthèse de l'hémoglobine de lapin. Biochimie *54*:1121, 1972.

Blunt, M. H., and Evans, J. V.: Changes in the concentration of potassium in the erythrocyte and in haemoglobin type in Merino sheep under a severe anaemic stress. Nature *200*:1215, 1963.

Bogdanovsky, D., Hermann, W., and Schapira, G.: Presence of a new RNA species among the initiation protein factors active in eukaryotes translation. Biochem. Biophys. Res. Commun. *54*:25, 1973.

Boggs, D. R., Hyde, F., and Srodes C.: An unusual pattern of neutrophil kinetics in sickle cell anemia. Blood *41*:59, 1973.

Bohr, C.: Theoretische Behandlung der quantitativen Verhältnis bei der Sauerstoffaufnahme des Hämoglobins. Zbl. Physiol. *17*:682, 1904.

Bohr, C., Hasselbalch, K., and Krogh, A.: Ueber einen in biologischer Beziehung wichtigen Einfluss, den die Kohlensäurespannung des Blutes auf dessen Sauerstoffbindung übt. Skand. Arch. Physiol. *16*:402, 1904.

Bonanou-Tzedaki, S. A., Pragnell, I. B., and Arnstein, H. R. V.: Presence of haemoglobin messenger RNA in the postribosomal supernatant of rabbit reticulocytes and conditions necessary for its translation. FEBS Lett. *26*:77, 1972.

Bonaventura, J., and Riggs, A.: Hemoglobin Kansas, a human hemoglobin with a neutral amino acid substitution and an abnormal oxygen equilibrium. J. Biol. Chem. *243*: 980, 1968.

Bookchin, R. M., and Gallop, P. M.: Structure of hemoglobin A_{Ic}: Nature of the N-terminal β chain blocking group. Biochem. Biophys. Res. Commun. *32*:86, 1968.

Bookchin, R. M., and Nagel, R. L.: Ligand-induced conformational dependence of hemoglobin in sickling interactions. J. Mol. Biol. *60*:263, 1971.

Bookchin, R. M., and Nagel, R. L.: Conformational requirements for the polymerization of hemoglobin S: Studies of mixed liganded hybrids. J. Mol. Biol. *76*:233, 1973a.

Bookchin, R., and Nagel, R. L.: Molecular interactions of sickling hemoglobins. In Abramson, H., Bertles, J. F., and Wethers, D. L. (eds.): Sickle Cell Disease. St. Louis, The C. V. Mosby Co., 1973b, p. 140.

Bookchin, R. M., Nagel, R. L., and Ranney, H. M.: Structure and properties of hemoglobin C-Harlem, a human hemoglobin variant with amino acid substitutions in 2 residues of the β-polypeptide chain. J. Biol. Chem. *242*:248, 1967.

Bookchin, R. M., Nagel, R. L., and Ranney, H. M.: The effect of $\beta^{73\ Asn}$ on the interactions of sickling hemoglobins. Biochim. Biophys. Acta *221*:373, 1970.

Bookchin, R. M., Nagel, R. L., and Balazs, T.: Role of hybrid tetramers in gelation of deoxy Hb mixtures containing hemoglobin S. Blood *44*:942 (Abst.), 1974.

Bookchin, R. M., Nagel, R. L., and Balazs, T.: Role of hybrid tetramer formation in gelation of haemoglobin S. Nature *256*:667, 1975.

Boyer, S. H., Rucknagel, D. L., Weatherall, D. J., et al.: Further evidence for linkage between the β and δ loci governing human hemoglobin and the population dynamics of linked genes. Am. J. Hum. Genet. *15*:438, 1963.

Boyer, S. H., Hathaway, P., Pascasio, F., et al.: Differences in the amino acid sequences of tryptic peptides from three sheep hemoglobin β chains. J. Biol. Chem. *242*:2211, 1967.

Boyer, S. H., Smith, K. D., Noyes, A. N., and Mullen, M. A.: Immunological characterization of rabbit hemoglobin α- and β-chain–synthesizing polysomes. J. Biol. Chem. *249*:7210, 1974.

Boyer, S. H., Belding, T. K., Margolet, L., and Noyes, A. N.: Fetal hemoglobin restriction to a few erythrocytes (F cells) in normal human adults. Science *188*:361, 1975.

Bradley, T. B., and Rieder, R. F.: Hemoglobin Gun Hill: a β chain abnormality associated with a hemolytic state. Blood *28*:975, 1966.

Bradley, T. B., Brawner, J. N., and Conley, C. L.: Further observations on an inherited anomaly characterized by persistence of fetal hemoglobin. Bull. Johns Hopkins Hosp. *108*:242, 1961.

Bradley, T. B., Wohl, R. C., and Rieder, R. F.: Hemoglobin Gun Hill: Deletion of five amino acid residues and impaired heme-globin binding. Science *157*:1581, 1967.

Bradley, T. B., Wohl, R. C., Murphy, S. B., et al.: Properties of hemoglobin Bryn Mawr, $\beta^{85\ Phe \longrightarrow Ser}$, a new spontaneous mutation producing an unstable hemoglobin with high oxygen affinity. Blood *40*:947, 1972.

Bradley, T. B., Wohl, R. C., and Smith, G. J.: Elongation of the α-globin chain in a Black family: interaction with Hb G-Philadelphia. Clin. Res. *23*:131A, 1975.

Bratu, V., Lorkin, P. A., Lehmann, H., and Predescu, C.: Haemoglobin Buchuresti, β42 (CD1) Phe→Leu, a cause of unstable haemoglobin haemolytic anaemia. Biochim. Biophys. Acta *251*:1, 1971.

Braunitzer, G.: Vergleichende Untersuchungen zur Primärstruktur der Proteinkomponente einiger Hämoglobine. Z. Physiol. Chemie *312*:72, 1958.

Braverman, A. S., and Bank, A.: Changing rates of globin chain synthesis during erythroid cell maturation in thalassemia. J. Mol. Biol. *42*:57, 1969.

Braverman, A. S., McCurdy, P. R., Manos, O., et al.: Homozygous beta-thalassemia in American blacks: the problem of mild thalassemia. J. Lab. Clin. Med. *81*:857, 1973.

Brawerman, G.: Alterations in the size of the poly (A) segment in newly synthesized messenger RNA of mouse sarcoma 180 ascites cells. Mol. Biol. Rep. *1*:7, 1973.

Brenna, O., Luzzana, M., Pace, M., et al.: The interaction between hemoglobin and its "oxygen-linked" ligands. In Brewer, G. J. (ed.): Hemoglobin and Red Cell Structure and Function. New York, Plenum Press, 1972, p. 19. Adv. Exp. Med. Biol., Vol. 28.

Brewer, G. J.: Erythrocyte metabolism and function: hexokinase inhibition by 2,3-diphosphoglycerate and interaction with ATP and Mg^{2+}. Biochim. Biophys. Acta *192*:157, 1969.

Brewer, G. J.: Clinical implications of variation in erythrocyte oxygen affinity: A, Blood storage, and B, Arteriosclerosis. In Rørth, M., and Astrup, P. (eds.): Oxygen Affinity of Hemoglobin and Red Cell Acid-Base Status. New York, Academic Press, 1972, p. 629.

Brewer, G. J., and Oelshlegel, F. J., Jr.: Antisickling effects of zinc. Biochem. Biophys. Res. Commun. *58*:854, 1974.

Brewer, G. J., Oelshlegel, F. J., Jr., and Eaton, J. A.: Biochemical, physiological and genetic factors in the regulation of mammalian erythrocyte metabolism and DPG levels. In Rørth, M., and Astrup, P. (eds.): Oxygen Affinity of Hemoglobin and Red Cell Acid-Base Status. New York, Academic Press, 1972, p. 539.

Briehl, R. W.: Relations between aggregation and oxygen equilibrium in human and lamprey haemoglobin. In Goodwin, T. W., Harris, J. I., and Hartley, B. S. (eds.): Structure and Activity of Enzymes. New York, Academic Press, 1964, p. 171.

Briehl, R. W., and Ewert, S.: Effects of pH, 2,3-diphosphoglycerate and salts on gelation of sickle cell deoxyhemoglobin. J. Mol. Biol. *80*:445, 1973.

Briehl, R. W., and Ewert, S. M.: Gelation of sickle cell hemoglobin. II. Methemoglobin. J. Mol. Biol. *89*:759, 1974.

Briehl, R. W., and Salhany, J. M.: R-T conformational switch in nitrosyl hemoglobin S as judged by gelation. Fed. Proc. *34*:654, (Abst. 2471) 1975.

Brimhall, B., Jones, R. T., Baur, E. W., and Motulsky, A. G.: Structural characterization of hemoglobin Tacoma. Biochemistry *8*:2125, 1969.

Brittain, H. P., de la Torre, A., and Willey, E. N.: A case of sickle cell disease with an abscess arising in an infarct of the liver. Ann. Intern. Med. *65*:560, 1966.

Brittenham, G., Lozoff, B., and Narasimhan, S.: Sickle cell disease among the Veddoid groups of South India. In Hechter, J. I., Schechter, A. N., Eaton, W. A., et al. (eds.): Proceedings of First National Symposium on Sickle Cell Disease. Washington, D.C. DHEW Pub. No. 75–723 (NIH), Bethesda, Md., 1974, p. 257.

Brody, J. I., Goldsmith, M. H., Park, S. K., et al.: Symptomatic crises of sickle cell anemia treated by limited exchange transfusion. Ann. Intern. Med. *72*:327, 1970.

Bromberg, P. A.: Pulmonary aspects of sickle cell disease. Arch. Intern. Med. *133*:652, 1974.

Bromberg, P. A., and Jensen, W. N.: Arterial oxygen unsaturation in sickle cell disease. Am. Rev. Respir. Dis. *96*:400, 1967a.

Bromberg, P. A., and Jensen, W. N.: Blood oxygen dissociation curves in sickle cell disease. J. Lab. Clin. Med. *70*:480, 1967b.

Bromberg, P. A., Padilla, F., Guy, J. T., and Balcerzak, S. P.: Effect of a new hemoglobin (Hb Little Rock) on the physiology of oxygen delivery. J. Lab. Clin. Med. *78*:837, 1971.

Bromberg, P. A., Alben, T. O., Bare, G. H., et al.: High oxygen affinity variant of haemoglobin Little Rock with unique properties. Nature [New Biol.] *243*:177, 1973.

Bromberg, Y. M., Abrahamov, A., and Salzberger, M.: The effect of maternal anoxaemia on the foetal haemoglobin of the newborn. J. Obstet. Gynaecol. Br. Commonw. *63*: 875, 1956.

Brook, C. G. D., Thompson, E. N., Marshall, W. C., et al.: Growth in children with thalassemia major and effect of two different transfusion regimens. Arch. Dis. Child. *44*:612, 1969.

Brown, M. J., Weatherall, D. J., Clegg, J. B., et al.: Benign sickle cell anaemia. Br. J. Haematol. *22*:635, 1972.

Brunori, M., Noble, R. W., Antonini, E., and Wyman, J.: The reactions of the isolated α and β chains of human hemoglobin with oxygen and carbon monoxide. J. Biol. Chem. *241*:5238, 1966.

Bruns, G. P., and London, I. M.: The effect of hemin on the synthesis of globin. Biochem. Biophys. Res. Commun. *18*:236, 1965.

Bucci, E., and Fronticelli, C.: A new method for the preparation of α and β subunits of human hemoglobin. J. Biol. Chem. *240*:PC551, 1964.

Buckalew, V. M., and Someren, A.: Renal manifestations of sickle cell disease. Arch. Intern. Med. *133*:660, 1974.

Bunn, H. F.: Dissociation of haemoglobin Chesapeake into subunits. Nature *227*:839, 1970.

Bunn, H. F.: Differences in the interaction of 2,3-diphosphoglycerate with certain mammalian hemoglobins. Science *172*:1049, 1971.

Bunn, H. F.: The interaction of sickle hemoglobin with DPG, CO_2 and with other hemoglobins: formation of asymmetrical hybrids. In Brewer, G. J. (ed.): Hemoglobin and Red Cell Structure and Function. New York, Plenum Press, 1972, p. 41. (Adv. Exp. Med. Biol., Vol. 28.)

Bunn, H. F.: The use of gel electrofocusing in the study of human hemoglobins. Ann. N. Y. Acad. Sci. *209*:345, 1973.

Bunn, H. F., and Briehl, R. W.: The interaction of 2,3-diphosphoglycerate with various human hemoglobins. J. Clin. Invest. *49*:1088, 1970.

Bunn, H. F., and Jandl, J. H.: Exchange of heme among hemoglobins and between hemoglobin and albumin. J. Biol. Chem. *243*:465, 1968.

Bunn, H. F., and Kitchen, H.: Hemoglobin function in the horse: the role of 2,3-diphosphoglycerate in modifying the oxygen affinity of maternal and fetal blood. Blood *42*:471, 1973.

Bunn, H. F., and McDonough, M.: Asymmetrical hemoglobin hybrids. An approach to the study of subunit interactions. Biochemistry *13*:988, 1974.

Bunn, H. F., Esham, W. T., and Bull, R. W.: The renal handling of hemoglobin. I. Glomerular filtration. J. Exp. Med. *129*:909, 1969a.

Bunn, H. F., May, M. H., Kocholaty, W., and Shields, C. E.: Hemoglobin function in stored blood. J. Clin. Invest. *48*:311, 1969b.

Bunn, H. F., Ransil, B. J., and Chao, A.: The interaction between erythrocyte organic phosphates, magnesium ion and hemoglobin. J. Biol. Chem. *246*:5273, 1971.

Bunn, H. F., Bradley, T. B., Davis, W. E., et al.: Structural and functional studies on hemoglobin Bethesda ($\alpha_2\beta_2{}^{145\ His}$), a variant associated with compensatory erythrocytosis. J. Clin. Invest. *51*:2299, 1972a.

Bunn, H. F., Meriwether, W. D., Balcerzak, S. P., and Rucknagel, D. L.: Oxygen equilibrium of hemoglobin E. J. Clin. Invest. *51*:2984, 1972b.

Bunn, H. F., Seal, U. S., and Scott, A. F.: The role of 2,3-diphosphoglycerate in mediating hemoglobin function of mammalian red cells. Ann. NY Acad. Sci. *241*:498, 1974a.

Bunn, H. F., Wohl, R. C., Bradley, T. B., et al.: Functional properties of hemoglobin Kempsey. J. Biol. Chem. *249*:7402, 1974b.

Bunn, H. F., Haney, D. N., Gabbay, K. H., and Gallop, P.: Further identification of the nature and linkage of the carbohydrate in hemoglobin A_{Ic}. Biochem. Biophys. Res. Commun. *67*:103, 1975a.

Bunn, H. F., Schmidt, G. J., Haney, D. N., et al.: Hemoglobin Cranston, an unstable variant having an elongated β chain due to nonhomologous crossover between two normal β chain genes. Proc. Natl. Acad. Sci. USA *72*:3609, 1975b.

Bunn, H. F., Haney, D. N., Kamin, S., et al.: Biosynthesis of human hemoglobin A_{Ic}. Slow glycosylation of hemoglobin *in vivo.* J. Clin. Invest. *57*:1652, 1976.

Burka, E. R., and Marks, P. A.: Ribosomes active in protein synthesis in human reticulocytes: a defect in thalassemia major. Nature *199*:706, 1963.

Burkert, L. B., Sharma, V. S., Pisciotta, A. V., et al.: Hemoglobin Mequon β41 (C7) Phenylalanine→Tyrosine. Clin. Res. *22*:176 (Abst.), 1974.

Burr, H., and Lingrel, J. B.: Poly A sequences at the 3′ termini of rabbit globin mRNA's. Nature [New Biol.] *233*:41, 1971.

Byckova, V., Wajcman, H., Labie, D., et al.: Hemoglobin M Saskatoon: further data on biophysics and oxygen equilibrium. Biochim. Biophys. Acta *243*:117, 1971.

Caldwell, P. R. B., Fritts, H. W., and Cournand, A.: Oxyhemoglobin dissociation curve in liver disease. J. Appl. Physiol. *20*:316, 1965.

Caldwell, P. R. B., Nagel, R. L., and Jaffé, E. R.: The effect of oxygen, carbon dioxide, pH and cyanate on the binding of 2,3-diphosphoglycerate to human hemoglobin. Biochem. Biophys. Res. Commun. *44*:1504, 1971.

Campbell, J. H., and Cummins, S. D.: Priapism in sickle cell anemia. J. Urol. *66*:697, 1951.

Cann, A., Gambino, R., Banks, J., et al.: Polyadenylate sequences and biologic activity of human globin messenger ribonucleic acid. J. Biol. Chem. *249*:7536, 1974.

Capp, G. L., Rigas, D. A., and Jones, R. T.: Hemoglobin Portland 1: a new human hemoglobin unique in structure. Science *157*:65, 1967.

Capp, G. L., Rigas, D. A., and Jones, R. T.: Evidence for a new haemoglobin chain (ζ-chain). Nature *228*:278, 1970.

Card, R., and Brain, M.: The "anemia" of childhood. N. Engl. J. Med. *288*:388, 1973.

Carrell, R. W., and Kay, R.: A simple method for the detection of unstable hemoglobins. Br. J. Haematol. *23*:615, 1972.

Carrell, R. W., and Owen, M. C.: A new approach to haemoglobin variant identification. Haemoglobin Christchurch β71 (E15) Phenylalanine→Serine. Biochim. Biophys. Acta *236*:507, 1971.

Carrell, R. W., Lehmann, H., and Hutchison, H. E.: Haemoglobin Köln (β98 Valine→Methionine): an unstable protein causing inclusion-body anaemia. Nature *210*:915, 1966.

Carrell, R. W., Lehmann, H., Lorkin, P. A., et al.: Haemoglobin Sydney: β67 (E11) Valine→Alanine: An emerging pattern of unstable haemoglobins. Nature *215*:626, 1967.

Cassel, J., Kogure, K., Busto, R., et al.: The effect on cerebral energy metabolites of the cyanate produced shift of the oxygen saturation curve. In Bicher, H. I., and Bruley, D. F. (eds.): Oxygen Transport to Tissue. New York, Plenum Press, 1973, p. 319. (Adv. Exp. Med. Biol., Vol. 37A.)

Castle, W. B., and Jandl, J. H.: Blood viscosity and blood volumes: opposing influences upon oxygen transport in polycythemia. Semin. Hematol. *3*:193, 1966.

Cathie, I. A. B.: Apparent idiopathic Heinz body anemia. Great Ormond St. J. *3*:43, 1952.

Cerami, A., and Manning, J. M.: Potassium cyanate as an inhibitor of the sickling of erythrocytes *in vitro*. Proc. Natl. Acad. Sci. USA *68*:1180, 1971.

Chalevelakis, G., Clegg, J. B., and Weatherall, D. J.: Imbalanced globin chain synthesis in heterozygous β-thalassemic bone marrow. Proc. Natl. Acad. Sci. USA *72*:3853, 1975.

Chan, E., and Desforges, J.: Role of disulfide bonds in Heinz body attachment to membranes. Blood *44*:921, 1974.

Chance, B., Cohen, P., and Jobsis, F.: Intracellular oxidation reduction states in vivo. Science *137*:499, 1962.

Chang, H., Hobbins, J. C., Cividalli, G., et al.: In utero diagnosis of hemoglobinopathies. Hemoglobin synthesis in fetal red cells. N. Engl. J. Med. *290*:1067, 1974.

Chang, H., Modell, C. B., Alter, B. P., et al.: Expression of the β-thalassemia gene in the first trimester fetus. Proc. Natl. Acad. Sci. USA *72*:3633, 1975.

Chanutin, A., and Curnish, R. R.: Effect of organic and inorganic phosphates on the oxygen equilibrium of human erythrocytes. Arch. Biochem. Biophys. *121*:96, 1967.

Chanutin, A., and Hermann, E.: The interaction of organic and inorganic phosphates with hemoglobin. Arch. Biochem. Biophys. *131*:180, 1969.

Charache, S.: Haemoglobins with altered oxygen affinity. Clin. Haematol. *3*:357, 1974a.

Charache, S.: A manifestation of abnormal hemoglobins of man: altered oxygen affinity. Hemoglobin Chesapeake: from the clinic to the laboratory and back again. Ann. NY Acad. Sci. *241*:449, 1974b.

Charache, S.: The treatment of sickle cell anemia. Arch. Intern. Med. *133*:698, 1974c.

Charache, S., and Conley, C. L.: Rate of sickling of red cells during deoxygenation of blood from persons with various sickling disorders. Blood *24*:25, 1964.

Charache, S., and Conley, C. L.: Factors leading to vascular occlusion in sickle cell anemia. In Brewer, G. J. (ed.): Erythrocyte Structure and Function. (Third International Conference on Red Cell Metabolism and Function, University of Michigan, 1974–1975.) A. R. Liss, 1975, p. 243.

Charache, S., and Page, D. L.: Infarction of bone marrow in the sickle cell disorders. Ann. Intern. Med. *67*:1195, 1967.

Charache, S., and Weatherall, D. J.: Fast hemoglobin in lead poisoning. Blood *28*:377, 1966.

Charache, S., Weatherall, D. J., and Clegg, J. B.: Polycythemia associated with a hemoglobinopathy. J. Clin. Invest. *45*:813, 1966.

Charache, S., Conley, C. L., Waugh, D. F., et al.: Pathogenesis of hemolytic anemia in homozygous hemoglobin C disease. J. Clin. Invest. *46*:1795, 1967.

Charache, S., Mondzac, A. M., and Gessner, U.: Hemoglobin Hasharon ($\alpha_2^{47\ \mathrm{His}}$ [CD5] β_2): a hemoglobin found in low concentration. J. Clin. Invest. *48*:834, 1969.

Charache, S., Grisolia, S., Fiedler, A. J., and Hellegers, A.: Effect of 2,3-diphosphoglycerate on oxygen affinity of blood in sickle cell anemia. J. Clin. Invest. *49*:806, 1970.
Charache, S., Brimhall, B., and Milner, P.: Hemoglobin Okaloosa (β48(CD7) Leucine→Arginine): An unstable variant with low oxygen affinity. J. Clin. Invest. *52*:2858, 1973.
Charache, S., Brimhall, B., and Jones, R. T.: Polycythemia produced by hemoglobin Osler (β145 [HC2] Tyr→Asp). Johns Hopkins Med. J. *136*:132, 1975a.
Charache, S., Clegg, J. B., Weatherall, D. J., and Conley, C. L.: Unbalanced globin synthesis in hereditary persistence of fetal hemoglobin. Clin. Res. *23*:587A, 1975b.
Charache, S., Duffy, T. R., Jander, N., et al.: Toxic-therapeutic ratio of sodium cyanate. Arch. Intern. Med. *135*:1043, 1975c.
Charache, S., McCurdy, P., and Fox, J.: Hemoglobin Providence (Hb Prov), a fetal-like hemoglobin. Blood *46*:1030, 1975d.
Chernoff, A. I.: The human hemoglobins in health and disease. N. Engl. J. Med. *253*: 365, 1955.
Chernoff, A. I.: Studies of hemoglobin E. I. The clinical, hematologic and genetic characteristics of the hemoglobin E syndromes. J. Lab. Clin. Med. *47*:455, 1956.
Chernoff, A. I.: The hemoglobin D syndromes. Blood *13*:116, 1958.
Chernoff, A. I.: The amino acid composition of hemoglobin. I. An improved method for separating the peptide chains of human hemoglobin. J. Chromatogr. *6*:252, 1961.
Chernoff, A. I.: A method for the quantitative determination of HgB A_2. Ann. NY Acad. Sci. *119*:557, 1964.
Chernoff, A. I., and Singer, K.: Studies on abnormal hemoglobins. IV. Persistence of fetal hemoglobin in the erythrocytes of normal children. Pediatrics *9*:469, 1952.
Chien, S., Usami, S., and Bertles, J. F.: Abnormal rheology of oxygenated blood in sickle cell anemia. J. Clin. Invest. *49*:623, 1970.
Chillar, R. K., Slawsky, P., and Desforges, J. F.: Red cell 2,3-diphosphoglycerate and adenosine triphosphate in patients with shock. Br. J. Haematol. *21*:183, 1971.
Chiodi, H.: Comparative study of blood gas transport in high altitude and sea level Camelidae and goats. Respir. Physiol. *11*:84, 1971.
Chiu, J. F., Tsai, Y. H., Sakuma, K., et al.: Regulation of *in vitro* mRNA transcription by a fraction of chromosomal proteins. J. Biol. Chem. *250*:9431, 1975.
Chou, P. Y., and Fasman, G. D.: Prediction of protein conformation. Biochemistry *13*: 222, 1974.
Chuang, A. H., Waterman, M. R., Yamaoka, K., et al.: Effect of pH, carbamylation and other hemoglobins on deoxyhemoglobin S aggregation inside intact erythrocytes as detected by proton relaxation rate measurements. Arch. Biochem. Biophys. *167*:145, 1975.
Cimadevilla, J. M., and Hardesty, B.: Evidence for a non-hemin regulated translational repressor in Friend leukemia virus–transformed murine proerythroblasts. Biochem. Biophys. Res. Commun. *63*:931, 1975.
Cimadevilla, J. M., Kramer, G., Pinphanichakarn, P., et al.: Inhibition of peptide chain initiation by a nonhemin-regulated translational repressor from Friend leukemia cells. Arch. Biochem. Biophys. *171*:145, 1975.
Cividalli, G., Nathan, D. G., Kan, Y. W., et al.: Relation of beta to gamma synthesis during the first trimester: An approach to prenatal diagnosis of thalassemia. Pediatr. Res. *8*:553, 1974a.
Cividalli, G., Nathan, D. G., and Lodish, H. F.: Translational control of hemoglobin synthesis in thalassemic bone marrow. J. Clin. Invest. *53*:955, 1974b.
Clark, M. R., and Shohet, S. B.: Hybrid erythrocytes for membrane studies in sickle cell disease. Blood *47*:121, 1976.
Clegg, J. B., and Weatherall, D. J.: Hemoglobin synthesis in α-thalassemia (haemoglobin H disease). Nature *215*:1241, 1967.
Clegg, J. B., and Weatherall, D. J.: Hemoglobin synthesis during erythroid maturation in β-thalassemia. Nature [New Biol.] *240*:190, 1972.
Clegg, J. B., Naughton, M. A., and Weatherall, D. J.: Abnormal human hemoglobins. Separation and characterization of the α and β chains by chromatography, and the determination of two new variants Hb Chesapeake and Hb J (Bangkok). J. Mol. Biol. *19*:91, 1966.
Clegg, J. B., Weatherall, D. J., Na-Nakorn, S., et al.: Haemoglobin synthesis in beta thalassemia. Nature *220*:664, 1968.

Clegg, J. B., Weatherall, D. J., and Eunson, C. E.: The distribution of nascent globin chains on human reticulocyte polysomes. Biochim. Biophys. Acta *247*:109, 1971a.

Clegg, J. B., Weatherall, D. J., and Milner, P. F.: Haemoglobin Constant Spring—a chain-termination mutant? Nature *234*:337, 1971b.

Clegg, J. B., Weatherall, D. J., Contopolou-Griva, I., et al.: Haemoglobin Icaria, a new chain-termination mutant which causes α-thalassaemia. Nature *251*:245, 1974a.

Clegg, J. B., Weatherall, D. J., Smith, D. H., et al.: Hb Kenya: a clue to the genetic control of human foetal haemoglobin synthesis. Br. J. Haematol. *28*:141, 1974b.

Coburn, R. F. (ed.): Biological effects of carbon monoxide. Ann. NY Acad. Sci. *174*:all, 1970.

Coburn, R. F., Ploegmakers, F., Gondrie, P., and Abboud, R.: Myocardial myoglobin oxygen tension. Am. J. Physiol. *224*:870, 1973.

Cohen-Solal, M., Thillet, J., Gaillardon, J., et al.: Functional properties of hemoglobin Saint Etienne, a variant carrying heme only on α chains. Rev. Eur. Etud. Clin. Biol. *17*:988, 1972.

Cohen-Solal, M., Seligmann, M., Thillet, J., and Rosa, J.: Haemoglobin Saint Louis β28 (B10) leucine→glutamine. A new unstable haemoglobin only present in a ferri form. FEBS Lett. *33*:37, 1973.

Cohen-Solal, M., Manesse, B., Thillet, J., and Rosa, J.: Haemoglobin G-Norfolk α85(F6) Asp→Asn. Structural characterization by sequenator analysis and functional properties of a new variant with high oxygen affinity. FEBS Lett. *50*:163, 1975.

Cohen-Solal, M., Blouquit, Y., Garel, M. C., et al.: Haemoglobin Lyon (β17–18 [A14–15] Lys→Val→0). Determination by sequenator analysis. Biochim. Biophys. Acta *351*:306, 1974.

Collett, L. C., and O'Gower, A. K.: Molluscan hemoglobins with unusual temperature-dependent characteristics. Comp. Biochem. Physiol. *41A*:843, 1972.

Colombo, B., Kim, B., Perez Atencio, R., et al.: The pattern of fetal haeomoglobin disappearance after birth. Br. J. Haematol. *32*:79, 1976.

Colvard, M. C., and Longmuir, I. S.: The effects of pacing on oxygen hemoglobin dissociation and oxygen carrying capacity in patients suspected of coronary artery disease. Am. Heart J. *85*:662, 1973.

Comroe, J. H., Jr.: Physiology of Respiration. Chicago, Year Book Medical Publishers, 1965.

Comroe, J. H., Jr., Forster, R. E., DuBois, A. B., et al.: The Lung. Clinical Physiology and Pulmonary Function Tests. 2nd ed. Chicago, Year Book Medical Publishers, 1962.

Conconi, F., and Del Senno, L.: The molecular defect of Ferrara β-thalassemia. Ann. NY Acad. Sci. *232*:54, 1974.

Conconi, F., Bargellesi, A., Del Senno, L., et al.: Globin chain synthesis in Sicilian thalassaemic subjects. Br. J. Haematol. *19*:469, 1970.

Conconi, F., Rowley, P. T., Del Senno, L., et al.: Induction of β-globin synthesis in the β-thalassaemia of Ferrara. Nature [New Biol.] *238*:83, 1972.

Conconi, F., Del Senno, L., Ferrarese, P., et al.: Appearance of β globin synthesis in erythroid cells of Ferrara β^0-thalassaemic patients following blood transfusion. Nature *254*:256, 1975.

Condon, P. I., and Serjeant, G. R.: Ocular findings in homozygous sickle cell anemia in Jamaica. Am. J. Ophthalmol. *73*:533, 1972a.

Condon, P. I., and Serjeant, G. R.: Ocular findings in hemoglobin sickle cell disease in Jamaica. Am. J. Ophthalmol. *74*:921, 1972b.

Conkie, D., Affara, N., Harrison, P. R., et al.: In situ localization of globin messenger RNA formation. II. After treatment of Friend virus–transformed mouse cells with dimethyl sulfoxide. J. Cell. Biol. *63*:414, 1974.

Conkie, D., Kleiman, L., Harrison, P. R., and Paul, J.: Increase in the accumulation of globin mRNA in immature erythroblasts in response to erythropoietin *in vivo* or *in vitro*. Exp. Cell Res. *93*:315, 1975.

Conley, C. L., Weatherall, D. J., Richardson, S. N., et al.: Hereditary persistence of fetal hemoglobin: A study of 79 affected persons in 15 Negro families in Baltimore. Blood *21*:261, 1963.

Constantoulakis, M., Economidou, J., Karagiorga, M., et al.: Combined long term treatment of hemosiderosis with desferrioxamine and DTPA in homozygous β-thalassemia. Ann. NY Acad. Sci. *232*:193, 1974.

Cooper, H. A., and Hoagland, H. C.: Fetal hemoglobin. Mayo Clin. Proc. *47*:402, 1972.

Cooper, M. R., Kraus, A. P., Felts, J. H., et al.: A third case of hemoglobin Memphis/sickle cell disease: whole blood viscosity used as a screening test. Am. J. Med. *55*: 535, 1973.

Cooperative Urea Trials Group: Clinical trials of therapy for sickle cell vaso-occlusive crises. JAMA *228*:1120, 1974.

Cottam, G. L., Valentine, K. M., Yamaoka, K., and Waterman, M. R.: The gelatin of deoxyhemoglobin S in erythrocytes as detected by transverse water proton relaxation measurements. Arch. Biochem. Biophys. *162*:487, 1974.

Craddock, P. R. Hunt, F. A., and Rozenberg, M. C.: The effective use of oxymetholone in the therapy of thalassaemia with anaemia. Med. J. Aust. *2*:199, 1972.

Crookston, J. H., Farquharson, H. A., Beale, D., et al.: Hemoglobin Etobicoke: α84 (F5) serine replaced by arginine. Can. J. Biochem. *47*:143, 1969.

Crystal, R. G., Shafritz, D., Prichard, P., et al.: Initial dipeptide formation in hemoglobin biosynthesis. Proc. Natl. Acad. Sci. USA *68*:1810, 1971.

Crystal, R. G., Nienhuis, A. W., Elson, N. A., et al.: Initiation of globin synthesis: preparation and use of reticulocyte ribosomes retaining initiation region messenger ribonucleic acid fragments. J. Biol. Chem. *247*:5357, 1972.

Crystal, R. G., Elson, N. A., Nienhuis, A. W., et al.: Initiation of globin synthesis in β-thalassemia. N. Engl. J. Med. *288*:1091, 1973.

Czernik, A. J., Psychoyos, S., and Cash, W. D.: Failure of thyroid hormones to enhance the activity of diphosphoglycerate mutase. Endocrinology *96*:508, 1974.

Dacie, J. V., Shinton, N. K., Gaffney, P. J., et al.: Haemoglobin Hammersmith (β42 [CD1] Phe$\rightarrow$Ser). Nature (London) *216*:663, 1967.

Darnell, J. E., Jolinek, W. R., and Molloy, G. R.: Biogenesis of mRNA: genetic regulation in mammalian cells. Science *181*:1215, 1973.

Davis, D. G., Lindstrom, T. R., Mock, N. H., et al.: Nuclear magnetic resonance studies of hemoglobins. VI. Heme proton spectra of human deoxyhemoglobins and their relevance to the nature of cooperative oxygenation of hemoglobin. J. Mol. Biol. *60*:101, 1971.

Dawson, R. B.: Hemoglobin function: effects of salts and glutathione. Vox Sang. *22*:26, 1972.

Dawson, R. B., and Ellis, T. J.: The hemoglobin function of blood stored at 4° C in ACD and CPD with adenine and inosine. Transfusion *10*:113, 1970.

Dawson, R. B., and Kocholaty, W. F.: Hemoglobin function during blood storage. XV. Effects of metabolic additives inosine and methylene blue on P_{50} and 2,3-DPG. In Brewer, G. J. (ed.): Hemoglobin and Red Cell Structure and Function. New York, Plenum Press, 1972, p. 495. (Adv. Exp. Med. Biol., Vol. 28.)

Dawson, R. B., Jr., Kocholaty, W. F., and Gray, J. L.: Hemoglobin function and 2,3-DPG levels of blood stored at 4° C in ACD and CPD: pH effect. Transfusion *10*:279, 1970.

Dayhoff, M. O.: Computer analysis of protein evolution. Sci. Am. *221*:86, 1969.

Dayhoff, M. O.: Atlas of Protein Sequence and Structure. Vol. 5. Washington, D.C., National Biomedical Research Foundation, 1972.

DeBruin, S. H., and Janssen, L. H. M.: Comparison of the oxygen and proton binding behavior of human hemoglobin A and A_2. Biochim. Biophys. Acta *295*:490, 1973.

DeFuria, F. G., and Miller, D. R.: Oxygen affinity in hemoglobin Köln disease. Blood *39*:398, 1972.

DeFuria, F. G., Miller, D. R., Cerami, A., and Manning, J. M.: The effects of cyanate in vitro on red blood cell metabolism and function in sickle cell anemia. J. Clin. Invest. *51*:566, 1972.

DeFuria, F. G., Miller, D. R., and Canale, V. C.: Red blood cell metabolism and function in transfused β-thalassemia. Ann. NY Acad. Sci. *232*:323, 1974.

Deisseroth, A., Velez, R., and Nienhuis, A. W.: Hemoglobin synthesis in somatic cell hybrids: independent segregation of the human alpha- and beta-globin genes. Science *191*:1262, 1976.

DeJong, W. W. W.: Structure of the δ-chain of chimpanzee haemoglobin A_2. Nature [New Biol.] *234*:176, 1971.

DeJong, W. W. W., Went, L. N., and Bernini, L. F.: Haemoglobin Leiden: Deletion of β6 or 7 glutamic acid. Nature *220*:788, 1968.

DeJong, W. W. W., Bernini, L. F., and Khan, P. M.: Haemoglobin Rampa: α95 Pro$\rightarrow$Ser. Biochim. Biophys. Acta *236*:197, 1971.

DeJong, W. W. W., Khan, P. M., and Bernini, L. F.: Hemoglobin Koya Dora: High frequency of a chain termination mutant. Am. J. Hum. Genet. *27*:81, 1975.

Delivoria-Papadopoulos, M. D., Monow, G., and Oski, F. A.: Exchange transfusion in the newborn infant with fresh and "old" blood. The role of storage on 2,3-diphosphoglycerate, hemoglobin-oxygen affinity and oxygen release. J. Pediatr. *79*:898, 1971a.

Delivoria-Papadopoulos, M., Roncevic, N. P., and Oski, F. A.: Postnatal changes in oxygen transport of term, premature and sick infants. The role of red cell 2,3-diphosphoglycerate and adult hemoglobin. Pediatr. Res. *5*:235, 1971b.

Delivoria-Papadopoulos, M., Martens, R. J., Oski, F. A., et al.: Effect of oxygen-hemoglobin affinity on oxygen consumption and cardiac output of newborn piglets following exchange transfusion. Pediatr. Res. *6*:342, 1972.

Desforges, J. F.: Unstable oxygen delivery. N. Engl. J. Med. *288*:965, 1973.

DeSimone, J., Kleve, L., Longley, M. A., and Shaeffer, J.: Rapid turnover of newly-synthesized β^S chains in reticulocytes from individuals with sickle cell trait. Biochem. Biophys. Res. Commun. *57*:248, 1974a.

DeSimone, J., Kleve, L., Longley, M. A., et al.: Unbalanced globin chain synthesis in reticulocytes of sickle cell trait individuals. Biochem. Biophys. Res. Commun. *59*:564, 1974b.

deVerdier, C. H., and Garby, L.: Glucose metabolism in normal erythrocytes: II. Factors influencing the hexokinase step. Scand. J. Haematol. *2*:305, 1965.

deVerdier, C. H., and Garby, L.: Low binding of 2,3-diphosphoglycerate to haemoglobin F: a contribution to the knowledge of the binding site and an explanation for the high oxygen affinity of foetal blood. Scand. J. Clin. Lab. Invest. *23*:149, 1969.

de Weinstein, B. I., White, J. M., Wiltshire, B. G., and Lehmann, H.: A new unstable haemoglobin: Hb Buenos Aires, β85 (F1) Phe→Ser. Acta Haematol. *50*:357, 1973.

Dhindsa, D. S., Hoversland, A. S., and Templeton, J. W.: Postnatal changes in oxygen affinity and concentrations of 2,3-diphosphoglycerate in dog blood. Biol. Neonate *20*:226, 1972.

Diamond, H. S., Meisel, A., Sharon, E., et al.: Hyperuricosuria and increased tubular secretion of urate in sickle cell anemia. Am. J. Med. *59*:796, 1976.

Diamond, M. P., Cotgrove, I., and Parker, A.: Case of intrauterine death due to α-thalassemia. Br. Med. J. *2*:278, 1965.

Dickerman, J. D., Holtzman, N. A., and Zinkham, W. H.: Hemoglobin Zürich. A third family presenting with hemolytic reactions to sulfonamides. Am. J. Med. *55*:638, 1973a.

Dickerman, J. D., Ostrea, E. M., and Zinkham, W. H.: In vivo aging of transfused erythrocytes and 2,3-diphosphoglycerate levels. Blood *42*:9, 1973b.

Dickerson, R. E.: X-ray analysis and protein structure. In Neurath, H. (ed.): The Proteins: Composition, Structure and Function. Vol. II. 2nd ed. New York, Academic Press, 1963, p. 603.

Diederich, D., Gill, P., and Larsen, W.: The irreversibly sickled erythrocyte: response to *in vitro* carbamylation. In Hercules, J. I., Schechter, A. N., Eaton, W. A., et al. (eds.): Proceedings of First National Symposium on Sickle Cell Disease, Washington, D.C. DHEW Pub. No. 75–723 (NIH), Bethesda, Md., 1974, p. 53.

Diggs, L. W.: Pulmonary lesions in sickle cell anemia. Blood *34*:734, 1969.

Diggs, L. W.: Anatomic lesions in sickle cell disease. *In* Abramson, H., Bertles, J. F., and Wethers, D. L. (eds.): Sickle Cell Disease: Diagnosis, Management, Education and Research. St. Louis, The C. V. Mosby Co., 1973, p. 189.

Diggs, L. W., and Bell, A.: Intraerythrocytic hemoglobin crystals in sickle cell-hemoglobin C disease. Blood *25*:218, 1965.

Dinman, B. D., Eaton, J. W., and Brewer, G. J.: Effects of carbon monoxide on DPG concentrations in the erythrocyte. Ann. NY Acad. Sci. *174*:246, 1970.

Dische, Z.: The pentose phosphate metabolism in red cells. In Bishop, C., and Surgenor, D. M. (eds.): The Red Blood Cell: A Comprehensive Treatise. New York, Academic Press, 1964, p. 189.

Donahue, R. P., Bias, W. B., Renwick, J. H., and McKusick, V. A.: Probable assignment of the Duffy blood group locus to chromosome 1 in man. Proc. Natl. Acad. Sci. USA *61*:949, 1968.

Dos-Santos, W. D., and Lehmann, H.: Acetazolamide in sickle-cell anaemia. Br. Med. J. *2*:139, 1959.

Douglas, R. H., and Hultquist, D. E.: Evidence that two forms of bovine erythrocyte cytochrome b_5 are identical to segments of microsomal cytochrome b_5. Proc. Natl. Acad. Sci. USA, in press, 1976.

Dow, L., Terada, M., Natta, C., et al.: Globin synthesis of intact cells and activity of isolated mRNA in β-thalassemia. Nature [New Biol.] *243*:114, 1973.

Drabkin, D. L.: Aspects of the oxygenation and oxidation functions. In Roughton, F. J. W., and Kendrew, J. C. (eds.): Haemoglobin (Barcroft Symposium). New York, Interscience, 1949, p. 35.

Dreyfus, J. C., Labie, D., Vibert, M., et al.: An attempt at demonstrating the existence of a nonsense mutation in β-thalassemia. Eur. J. Biochem. *27*:291, 1972.

Dubochet, J., Morel, C., Lebleu, B., and Herzberg, M.: Structure of globin mRNA and mRNA-protein particles. Eur. J. Biochem. *36*:465, 1973.

Duhm, J.: Effects of 2,3-diphosphoglycerate and other organic phosphate compounds on oxygen affinity and intracellular pH of human erythrocytes. Pfluegers Arch. *326*:341, 1971.

Duhm, J., and Gerlach, E.: On the mechanisms of the hypoxia-induced increase of 2,3-diphosphoglycerate in erythrocytes. Pfluegers Arch. *326*:254, 1971.

Duhm, J., Deuticke, B., and Gerlach, E.: Beeinflusst Trijodthyronin den 2,3-Diphosphoglycerat-Gehalt von Erythrocyten? Naturwissenschaften *56*:329, 1969.

Eaton, J. W., and Brewer, G. J.: The relationship between red cell 2,3-diphosphoglycerate and levels of hemoglobin in the human. Proc. Natl. Acad. Sci. USA *61*:756, 1968.

Eaton, J. W., Brewer, G. J., and Grover, R. F.: Role of red cell 2,3-diphosphoglycerate in the adaptation of man to altitude. J. Lab. Clin. Med. *73*:603, 1969.

Eaton, J. W., Skelton, T. D., Swofford, H. S., et al.: Elevated erythrocyte calcium in sickle cell disease. Nature *246*:105, 1973.

Eaton, J. W., Skelton, T. D., and Berger, E.: Survival at extreme altitude: Protective effect of increased hemoglobin-oxygen affinity. Science *183*:743, 1974.

Eaton, J. W., White, J. G., Jacob, H. S., et al.: Ca^{2+}-induced maintenance of sickling in Hb SS erythrocytes. Blood *46*:1051, 1975.

Economidou, J., Constantoulakis, M., Augoustaki, O., et al.: Frequency of antibodies to various antigenic determinants in polytransfused patients with homozygous thalassemia in Greece. Vox Sang. *20*:252, 1971.

Eddison, G. G., Briehl, R. W., and Ranney, H. M.: Oxygen equilibria of hemoglobin A_2 and hemoglobin Lepore. J. Clin. Invest. *43*:2323, 1964.

Edelstein, S. J., Telford, J. N., and Crepeaw, R. H.: Structure of fibers of sickle cell hemoglobin. Proc. Natl. Acad. Sci. USA *70*:1104, 1973.

Edsall, J. T.: Blood and hemoglobin: the evolution of knowledge of functional adaptation in a biochemical system. Part I. The adaptation of chemical structure to function in hemoglobin. J. Hist. Biol. *5*:205, 1972.

Edwards, M. J., and Rigas, D. A.: Electrolyte-labile increase of oxygen affinity during in vivo aging of hemoglobin. J. Clin. Invest. *46*:1579, 1967.

Edwards, M. J., Koler, R. D., Rigas, D. A., and Pitcairn, D. M.: The effect of in vivo aging of normal human erythrocytes and erythrocyte macromolecules upon oxyhemoglobin dissociation. J. Clin. Invest. *40*:636, 1961.

Edwards, M. J., Novy, M. J., Walters, C.-L., et al.: Improved oxygen release: an adaptation of mature red cells to hypoxia. J. Clin. Invest. *47*:1851, 1968.

Edwards, M. J., Canon, B., Albertson, J., and Bigley, R. H.: Mean red cell age, a determinant of blood oxygen affinity. Nature *230*:583, 1971.

Efremov, G. D., Huisman, T. H. J., Smith, L. L., et al.: Haemoglobin Richmond, a human hemoglobin which forms asymmetric hybrids with other hemoglobins. J. Biol. Chem. *244*:6105, 1969.

Egan, E. L., and Fairbanks, V. F.: Postsplenectomy erythrocytosis in hemoglobin Köln disease. N. Engl. J. Med. *288*:929, 1973.

Elbaum, D., Nagel, R. L., Bookchin, R. M., et al.: Effect of alkylureas on the polymerization of hemoglobin S. Proc. Natl. Acad. Sci. USA *71*:4718, 1974.

Eliot, R. S., and Bratt, G.: The paradox of myocardial ischemia and necrosis in young women with normal coronary angiograms. Am. J. Cardiol. *23*:633, 1969.

Eliot, R. S., Salhany, J., and Mizukami, H.: Angina and infarction occurring with patent coronary arteries and decreased rate of oxygen release. Adv. Cardiol. *5*:106, 1970.

Engelhard, D., Cividalli, G., and Rachmilewitz, E. A.: Splenectomy in homozygous beta thalassaemia: a retrospective study of 30 pateints. Br. J. Haematol. *31*:391, 1975.

England, J. M., and Fraser, P. M.: Differentiation of iron deficiency from thalassaemia trait by routine blood-count. Lancet *1*:449, 1973.

Engle, M. A.: Cardiac involvement in Cooley's anemia. Ann. NY Acad. Sci. *119*:694, 1964.

Englehardt, J. F.: Doctoral Dissertation, Göttingen, Germany, 1825.

Eraklis, A. J., Kevy, S. V., Diamond, L. K., et al.: Hazard of overwhelming infection after splenectomy in childhood. N. Engl. J. Med. *276*:1225, 1967.

Erlandson, M. E., Walden, B., Stern, G., et al.: Studies on congenital hemolytic syndrome: IV. Gastrointestinal absorption of iron. Blood *19*:359, 1962.

Ernst, V., and Arnstein, H. R. V.: Synthesis of α and β globin directed by messenger ribonucleoprotein from rabbit reticulocytes. Biochim. Biophys. Acta *378*:251, 1975.

Esan, G. J. F., Morgan, F. J., O'Donnell, J. V. et al.: Diminished synthesis of an alpha chain mutant, hemoglobin I (α16 Lys→Glu). J. Clin. Invest. *49*:2218, 1970.

Fairbanks, V. F., and Pettit, R. M.: Sickledex test in unstable hemoglobin disorders. JAMA *220*:128, 1972.

Fairbanks, V. F., Opfell, R. W., and Burgert, E. O.: Three families with unstable hemoglobinopathies (Köln, Olmsted and Santa Ana) causing hemolytic anemia with inclusion bodies and pigmenturia. Am. J. Med. *46*:344, 1969.

Fairbanks, V. F., Maldanado, J. E., Charache, S., et al.: Familial erythrocytosis due to electrophoretically undetectable hemoglobin with impaired oxygen dissociation (Hemoglobin Malmö, $\alpha_2\beta_2^{97Gln}$). Mayo Clin. Proc. *46*:721, 1971.

Farmer, M. B., Lehmann, H., and Raine, D. N.: Two unrelated patients with congenital cyanosis due to haemoglobinopathy M. Lancet *II*:786, 1964.

Favre, A., Morel, C., and Scherrer, K.: The secondary structure and poly(A) content of globin messenger RNA as a pure RNA and in polyribosome-derived ribonucleoprotein complexes. Eur. J. Biochem. *57*:147, 1975.

Feig, S. A., Nathan, D. G., Gerald, P. S., et al.: Congenital methemoglobinemia: the result of age dependent decay of methemoglobin reductase. Blood *39*:407, 1972.

Felicetti, L., Colombo, B., and Baglioni, C.: Assembly of hemoglobin. Biochim. Biophys. Acta *129*:380, 1966.

Ferguson, J. K. W., and Roughton, F. J. W.: The chemical relationships with physiological importance of carbamino compounds of CO_2 with haemoglobin. J. Physiol. (London) *83*:87, 1934.

Fermi, G.: Three-dimensional Fourier synthesis of human deoxyhaemoglobin at 2.5-Å resolution: refinement of the atomic model. J. Mol. Biol. *97*:237, 1975.

Fernandez, L. A., and Erslev, A. J.: Oxygen affinity and compensated hemolysis in hereditary spherocytosis. J. Lab. Clin. Med. *80*:780, 1972.

Fessas, P.: Inclusions of hemoglobin in erythroblasts and erythrocytes of thalassemia. Blood *21*:21, 1963.

Fessas, P.: Forms of thalassemia. In Jonxis, J. H. P. (ed.): Abnormal Hemoglobins in Africa. Oxford, Blackwell Scientific Publications, 1965, p. 71.

Fessas, P., and Loukopoulos, D.: Alpha-chain of human hemoglòbin: occurrence *in vivo*. Science *143*:590, 1964.

Fessas, P., and Stamatoyannopoulos, G.: Absence of hemoglobin A_2 in an adult. Nature *195*:1215, 1962.

Fessas, P., and Stamatoyannopoulos, G.: Hereditary persistence of fetal hemoglobin in Greece. A study and a comparison. Blood *24*:223, 1964.

Fessas, P., and Yataganas, X.: Intraerythroblastic instability of hemoglobin β_4 (Hgb H). Blood *31*:323, 1968.

Fessas, P., Loukopoulos, D., and Kaltsoya, A.: Peptide analysis of the inclusions of erythroid cells in β-thalassemia. Biochim. Biophys. Acta *124*:430, 1966.

Finch, C. A., Deubelbeiss, K., Cook, J. D., et al.: Ferrokinetics in man. Medicine (Baltimore) *49*:17, 1970.

Finch, J. T., Perutz, M. F., Bertles, J. F., and Döbler, J.: Structure of sickled erythrocytes and of sickle-cell hemoglobin fibers. Proc. Natl. Acad. Sci. USA *70*:718, 1973.

Finne, P. H., and Halvorsen, S.: Regulation of erythropoiesis in the fetus and newborn. Arch. Dis. Child. *47*:683, 1972.

Finney, R. A., Jr., and Hatch, F. E., Jr.: Effect of a carbonic anhydrase inhibitor (dichlorphenamide) on sickle cell anemia. Am. J. Med. Sci. *250*:154, 1965.

Fischer, H., and Orth, H.: Die Chemie des Pyrrols, Pyrrolfarbstoffe. II. Erste hälfte. Leipzig Akadem. Verlagsgesellschaft, 1937, p. 372.

Fischer, H., and Zeile, K.: Synthese des Hämatoporphyrins, Protoporphyrins und Hämins. Justus Liebig's Annalen der Chemie *468*:98, 1929.

Fischer, S., Nagel, R., Bookchin, R., et al.: The binding of hemoglobin to membranes of normal and sickled erythrocytes. Biochim. Biophys. Acta *375*:422, 1975.

Fitch, W. M.: A comparison between evolutionary substitutions and variants in human hemoglobins. Ann. NY Acad. Sci. *241*:439, 1974.

Flatz, G., Kinderlerer, J. L., Kilmartin, J. V., et al.: Haemoglobin Tak: a variant with additional residues at the end of the β-chains. Lancet *1*:732, 1971.

Flenley, D. C., Fairweather, L. J., Cooke, N. J., and Kerby, B. J.: Changes in haemoglobin binding curve and oxygen transport in chronic hypoxia lung disease. Br. Med. J. *1*:602, 1975.

Flye, M. W., and Silver, D.: The role of surgery in sickle cell disease. Surg. Gynecol. Obstet. *137*:115, 1973.

Forget, B. G.: The molecular basis of thalassemia. CRC Crit. Rev. Biochem. *2*:311, 1974.

Forget, B. G., and Nathan, D. G.: Molecular pathology of the thalassemias. Adv. Intern. Med. *21*:97, 1975.

Forget, B. G., Baltimore, D., Benz, E. J., Jr., et al.: Globin messenger RNA in the thalassemia syndromes. Ann. NY Acad. Sci. *232*:76, 1974a.

Forget, B. G., Marotta, C. A., Weissman, S. M., et al.: Nucleotide sequences of human globin messenger RNA. Ann NY Acad. Sci. *241*:290, 1974b.

Forget, B. G., Benz, E. J., Jr., Skoultchi, A., et al.: Absence of messenger RNA for beta globin chain in β^0-thalassemia. Nature *247*:379, 1974c.

Forget, B. G., Housman, D., Benz, E. J., Jr., et al.: Synthesis of DNA complementary to separated human alpha and beta globin messenger RNA's. Proc. Natl. Acad. Sci. USA *72*:984, 1975a.

Forget, B. G., Marotta, C. A., Weissman, S. M., et al.: Nucleotide sequences of the 3′-terminal untranslated region of messenger RNA for human beta globin chain. Proc. Natl. Acad. Sci. USA *72*:3614, 1975b.

Forget, B. G., Glass, J., and Housman, D.: Erythroid cell differentiation. In Neth, R., and Moloney, W. C. (eds.): Modern Trends in Human Leukemia II. Munich, Lehmanns Verlag, in press, 1976a.

Forget, B. G., Hillman, D. G., Lazarus, H., et al.: Absence of messenger RNA and gene DNA for β-globin chains in hereditary persistence of fetal hemoglobin. Cell *7*:323, 1976b.

Forget, B. G., Hillman, D. G., Cohen-Solal, M., et al.: Beta globin messenger RNA in $beta^0$ thalassemia. Blood *48*:998A, 1976c.

Fraser, I. D.: Adult and foetal haemoglobin in Rh haemolytic disease. Br. J. Haematol. *23*:269, 1972.

Frazer, G. R., Kitsos, C., Motulsky, A. G., et al.: Thalassemias, abnormal hemoglobins, and glucose-6-phosphate dehydrogenase deficiency in the Arta area of Greece: diagnostic and genetic aspects of complete village studies. Ann NY Acad. Sci. *119*:415, 1964.

Freedman, M. L., and Karpatkin, S.: Short communication: elevated platelet count and megathrombocyte number in sickle cell anemia. Blood *46*:579, 1975.

Freedman, M. L., Geraghty, M., and Rosman, J.: Hemin control of globin synthesis: isolation of a hemin reversible translational repressor from human mature erythrocytes. J. Biol. Chem. *249*:7290, 1974.

Frick, P. G., Hitzig, W. H., and Betke, K.: Hemoglobin Zürich. A new hemoglobin anomaly associated with acute hemolytic episodes with inclusion bodies after sulfonamide therapy. Blood *20*:261, 1962.

Friedman, E. A., Sreepada Rao, T. K., Sprung, C. L., et al.: Uremia in sickle-cell anemia treated by maintenance hemodialysis. N. Engl. J. Med. *291*:431, 1974.

Friedman, S., and Schwartz, E.: Hereditary persistence of foetal haemoglobin with β-chain synthesis in cis position ($^{G}\gamma$-β^+-HPFH) in a Negro family. Nature *259*:138, 1976.

Friedman, S., Oski, F. A., and Schwartz, E.: Bone marrow and peripheral blood globin synthesis in an American Black family with beta thalassemia. Blood *39*:785, 1972.

Friedman, S., Hamilton, R. W., and Schwartz, E.: β-thalassemia in the American Negro. J. Clin. Invest. *52*:1453, 1973.

Friedman, S., Özsoylu, S., Luddy, R., et al.: Heterozygous beta thalassaemia of unusual severity. Br. J. Haematol. *32*:65, 1976a.

Friedman, S., Schwartz, E., Ahern, E., et al.: Variations in globin chain synthesis in hereditary persistence of fetal haemoglobin. Br. J. Haematol. *32*:357, 1976b.

Friend, C., Scher, W., Holland, J. G., and Sato, T.: Hemoglobin synthesis in murine virus-induced leukemic cells in vitro. Stimulation of erythroid differentiation by dimethyl sulfoxide. Proc. Natl. Acad. Sci. USA *68*:378, 1971.

Frischer, H., and Bowman, J.: Hemoglobin E, an oxidatively unstable mutation. J. Lab. Clin. Med. *85*:531, 1975.

Fuhr, J. E., and Gengozian, N.: Coordination of heme and globin synthesis in primate reticulocytes. Biochim. Biophys. Acta *320*:53, 1973.

Fuhr, J. E., and Overton, M.: Translational control of globin synthesis by low molecular weight RNA. Biochem. Biophys. Res. Commun. *63*:742, 1975.

Fuhr, J. E., Natta, C., Marks, P. A., and Bank, A.: Protein synthesis in cell-free systems from reticulocytes of thalassemic patients. Nature *224*:1305, 1969.

Fung, L. W., and Ho., C.: A proton nuclear magnetic resonance study of the quaternary structure of human hemoglobins in water. Biochemistry *14*:2526, 1975.

Gaburro, D., Volpato, S., and Vigi, V.: Diagnosis of beta thalassemia in the newborn by means of hemoglobin synthesis. Acta Pediatr. Scand. *59*:523, 1970.

Gabuzda, T. G., Nathan, D. G., and Gardner, F. H.: The turnover of hemoglobins A, F, and A_2 in the peripheral blood of three patients with thalassemia. J. Clin. Invest. *42*:1678, 1963.

Gabuzda, T. G., Nathan, D. G., and Gardner, F. H.: The metabolism of the individual $C.^{14}$ Labelled hemoglobin in patients with H-thalassemia; with observations on radiochromate binding to the hemoglobins during red cell survival. J. Clin. Invest. *44*:315, 1965.

Gacon, G., Wajcman, H., and Labie, D.: Hemoglobin E: Its oxygen affinity in relation with the ionic environment. FEBS Lett. *41*:147, 1974.

Gahlenbeck, H., and Bartels, H.: Veränderung der Sauerstoffbindungskurven des Blutes bei Hyperthyreosen und nach Gabe von Trijodthyronin bei Gesunden und bei Ratten. Klin. Wochenschr. *46*:547, 1968.

Gahlenbeck, H., Rathschlag-Schaefer and Bartels, H.: Triiodothyronine induced changes of oxygen affinity of blood. Respir. Physiol. *6*:16, 1968.

Gallagher, P. J.: 2,3-Diphosphoglycerate in acute asthma. J. Clin. Pathol. *24*:518, 1971.

Gambino, R., Kacian, D., O'Donnel, J., et al.: A limited number of globin genes in human DNA. Proc. Natl. Acad. Sci USA *71*:3966, 1974.

Gander, E. S., Stewart, A. G., Morel, C. M., et al.: Isolation and characterization of ribosome-free cytoplasmic messenger ribonucleoprotein complexes from avian erythroblasts. Eur. J. Biochem. *38*:443, 1973.

Garby, L., and deVerdier, C. H.: Affinity of human hemoglobin A to 2,3-diphosphoglycerate. Effect of hemoglobin concentration and of pH. Scand. J. Clin. Lab. Invest. *27*:345, 1971.

Garby, L., Robert, M., and Zaar, B.: Proton and carbamino linked oxygen affinity of normal human blood. Acta Physiol. Scand. *84*:482, 1972.

Garel, M. C., Cohen-Solal, M., Bluoquit, Y., et al.: A method for isolation of abnormal haemoglobins with high oxygen affinity due to a frozen quaternary R-structure: Application to Hb Creteil $\alpha_2{}^A\beta_2$ (F5) 89 Asn. FEBS Lett. *43*:93, 1974.

Garner, M. H., Bogardt, R. A., and Gurd, F. R. N.: Determination of the pK values of the α amino groups of human hemoglobin. J. Biol. Chem. *250*:4398, 1975.

Garrick, L. M., Dembure, P. P., and Garrick, M. D.: Interaction between the synthesis of α and β globin. Eur. J. Biochem. *58*:339, 1975.

Garrick, M. D., Reichlin, M., Mattioli, M., and Manning, R.: The anemia-induced reversible switch from hemoglobin A to hemoglobin C in Caprine ruminants: immunochemical evidence that both hemoglobins are found in the same cell. Dev. Biol. *30*:1, 1973.

Gau, G. T., Fairbanks, V. F., Maldonado, J. E., et al.: Cardiac dysfunction in a patient with hemoglobin Malmö treated with repeated transfusions. Clin. Res. *22*:276A, 1974.

Gerald, P. S.: The electrophoretic and spectroscopic characterization of Hgb M. Blood *13*:936, 1958.

Gerald, P. S., and Diamond, L. K.: The diagnosis of thalassemia trait by starch block electrophoresis of the hemoglobin. Blood *13*:61, 1958.
Gerald, P. S., and Efron, M. L.: Chemical studies of several varieties of Hb M. Proc. Natl. Acad. Sci. USA *47*:1758, 1961.
Gerald, P. S., Cook, C. D., and Diamond, L. K.: Hemoglobin M. Science *126*:300, 1957.
Gerber, G., Berger, H., Jänig, G.-R., and Rapoport, S.: Interaction of haemoglobin with ions. Quantitative description of the state of magnesium adenosine 5′-triphosphate, 2,3-disphosphoglycerate and human hemoglobin under simulated intracellular conditions. Eur. J. Biochem. *38*:563, 1973.
Gianni, A. M., Giglioni, B., Ottolenghi, S., et al.: Globin α-chain synthesis directed by "supernatant" 10S RNA from rabbit reticulocytes. Nature [New Biol.] *240*:183, 1972.
Gibson, Q. H., and Nagel, R. L.: Allosteric transition and ligand binding in hemoglobin Chesapeake. J. Biol. Chem. *249*:7255, 1974.
Gibson, Q. H., and Parkhurst, L. J.: Kinetic evidence for a tetrameric functional unit in hemoglobin. J. Biol. Chem. *243*:5521, 1968.
Gilbert, J. M., and Anderson, W. F.: Cell-free hemoglobin synthesis. II. Characteristics of the transfer ribonucleic acid-dependent assay system. J. Biol. Chem. *245*:2342, 1970.
Gilbert, J. M., Thornton, A. G., Nienhuis, A., et al.: Cell-free hemoglobin synthesis in beta thalassemia. Proc. Natl. Acad. Sci. USA *67*:1854, 1970.
Gill, F., and Schwartz, E.: Free α globin pool in human bone marrow. J. Clin. Invest. *52*:3057, 1973.
Gill, F., Atwater, J., and Schwartz, E.: Hemoglobin Lepore trait: Globin synthesis in bone marrow and peripheral blood. Science *178*:623, 1972.
Gillette, P. N., Lu, Y. S., and Peterson, C. M.: The pharmacology of cyanate with a summary of its initial usage in sickle cell disease. Progr. Hematol. *8*:181, 1973.
Gilmour, R. S., and Paul, J.: Tissue-specific transcription of the globin gene in isolated chromatin. Proc. Natl. Acad. Sci. USA *70*:3440, 1973.
Gilmour, R. S., Harrison, P. R., Windass, J. D., et al.: Globin messenger RNA synthesis and processing during haemoglobin induction in Friend cells. I. Evidence for transcriptional control in clone. Cell Differ. *3*:9, 1974.
Glader, B. E., Lux, S. E., Muller, A., et al.: Cation water and ATP content of irrerversibly sickled RBC's (ISC's) *in vivo*. Clin. Res. *24*:309, 1976.
Glass, J., Lavidor, L. M., and Robinson, S. H.: Studies of murine erythroid cell development. Synthesis of heme and hemoglobin. J. Cell Biol. *65*:298, 1975.
Glynn, K. P., Penner, J. A., Smith, J. R., et al.: Familial erythrocytosis: description of three families, one with Hemoglobin Ypsilanti. Ann. Intern. Med. *69*:769, 1968.
Goldberg, A.: Lead poisoning and haem biosynthesis. Br. J. Haematol. *23*:521, 1972.
Goldberg, M. A., Bunn, H. F., and Harkness, D. R.: The use of centrifugation in studying the interaction of sickle and non-sickle hemoglobins. Clin. Res. *23*:581A, 1975.
Goldberg, M. F.: Treatment of proliferative sickle retinopathy. Trans. Am. Acad. Ophthalmol. Otolaryngol. *75*:532, 1971.
Goldstein, G. W., Hammaker, L., and Schmid, R.: The catabolism of Heinz bodies: An experimental model demonstrating conversion to non-bilirubin catabolites. Blood *31*:388, 1968.
Gordon, P. A., Breeze, G. R., Mann, J. R., et al.: Coagulation fibrinolysis in sickle cell disease. J. Clin. Pathol. *27*:485, 1974.
Gordon-Smith, E. C., Dacie, J. V., Blecher, T. E., et al.: Haemoglobin Nottingham β FG5 (98) Val→Gly: A new unstable haemoglobin producing severe haemolysis. Proc. Roy. Soc. Med. *66*:507, 1973.
Gorshein, D., Oski, F. A., and Delivoria-Papadopoulos, M.: Effect of androgens on the red cell 2,3-diphosphoglycerate hemoglobin oxygen affinity and red cell mass in mammals. Proc. Soc. Exp. Biol. Med. *147*:616, 1974.
Gorski, J., Morrison, M. R., Merkel, C. G., and Lingrel, J. B.: Size heterogeneity of polyadenylate sequences in mouse globin messenger RNA. J. Mol. Biol. *86*:363, 1974.
Gorski, J., Morrison, M. R., Merkel, C. G., and Lingrel, J. B.: Poly (A) size class distribution in globin mRNAs as a function of time. Nature *253*:749, 1975.
Gould, H. J., and Hamlyn, P. H.: The molecular weight of rabbit globin messenger RNA's. FEBS Lett. *30*:301, 1973.
Grace, D. A., and Winter, C. C.: Priapism: an appraisal of management of twenty-three patients. J. Urol. *99*:301, 1968.

Granick, S., and Kappas, A.: Steroid induction of porphyrin synthesis in liver cell culture. I. Structural basis and possible physiological role in the control of heme formation. J. Biol. Chem. *242*:4587, 1967.

Grayzel, A. I., Hörchner, P., and London, I. M.: The stimulation of globin synthesis by heme. Proc. Natl. Acad. Sci. USA *55*:650, 1966.

Grayzel, A., Fuhr, J. E., and London, I. M.: The effects of inhibitors of protein synthesis on the synthesis of heme in rabbit reticulocytes. Biochem. Biophys. Res. Commun. *28*:705, 1967.

Graziano, J. H., Grady, R. W., and Cerami, A.: The identification of 2,3-dihydroxybenzoic acid as a potentially useful iron-chelating drug. J. Pharmacol. Exp. Ther. *190*:570, 1974.

Graziano, J. H., Miller, D. R., Grady, R. W., et al.: Inhibition of membrane peroxidation in thalassaemic erythrocytes by 2,3-dihydroxybenzoic acid. Br. J. Haematol. *32*:351, 1976.

Green, D. W., Ingram, V. M., and Perutz, M. F.: The structure of haemoglobin. IV. Sign determination by the isomorphous replacement method. Proc. Roy. Soc. London A *225*:287, 1954.

Green, T. W., Conley, C. L., and Berthrong, M.: The liver in sickle cell anemias. Bull. Johns Hopkins Hosp. *92*:99, 1953.

Greenberg, M. S., and Kass, E. H.: Studies on the destruction of red blood cells. XIII. Observation on the role of pH in the pathogenesis and treatment of painful crisis in sickle cell disease. Arch. Intern. Med. *101*:355, 1958.

Greer, J.: Three-dimensional structure of abnormal human haemoglobins Kansas and Richmond. J. Mol. Biol. *59*:99, 1971a.

Greer, J.: Three-dimensional structure of abnormal human haemoglobins M Hyde Park and M Iwate. J. Mol. Biol. *59* 107, 1971b.

Greer, J.: Three-dimensional structure of abnormal human haemoglobins Chesapeake and J-Capetown. J. Mol. Biol. *62*:241, 1971c.

Greer, J., and Perutz, M. F.: Three-dimensional structure and haemoglobin Rainier. Nature [New Biol.] *230*:261, 1971.

Griggs, R. C., and Harris, J. W.: Biophysics of the variants of sickle cell disease. Arch. Intern. Med. *97*:315, 1956.

Grimes, A. J., and Meisler, A.: Possible cause of Heinz bodies in congenital Heinz-body anaemia. Nature *194*:190, 1962.

Grimes, A. J., Meisler, A., and Dacie, J. V.: Congenital Heinz-body anaemia: Further evidence on the cause of Heinz-body production in red cells. Br. J. Haematol. *10*:281, 1964.

Gross, G. J., and Hardman, H. F.: Alteration in oxyhemoglobin equilibrium (P-50) and myocardial oxygen consumption (mVO_2) by nitroglycerin (GTN). J. Pharmacol. Exp. Ther. *193*:346, 1975.

Gross, M.: Control of globin synthesis by hemin. Regulation by hemin of the formation and inactivation of a translational repressor of globin synthesis in rabbit reticulocytes lysates. Biochim. Biophys. Acta *340*:484, 1974.

Gross, M., and Rabinovitz, M.: Control of globin synthesis by hemin: factors influencing formation of an inhibitor of globin chain initiation in reticulocyte lysates. Biochim. Biophys. Acta *287*:340, 1972a.

Gross, M., and Rabinovitz, M.: Control of globin synthesis in cell-free preparations of reticulocytes by formation of a translational repressor that is inactivated by hemin. Proc. Natl. Acad. Sci. USA *69*:1565, 1972b.

Gross, M., and Rabinovitz, M.: Partial purification of a translational repressor mediating hemin control of globin synthesis and implication of results on the site of inhibition. Biochem. Biophys. Res. Commun. *50*:832, 1973.

Gross, R. T., Kriss, J. P., and Spaet, T. H.: The hematopoietic and goitrogenic effects of cobaltous chloride in patients with sickle cell anemia. Pediatrics *15*:284, 1955.

Grossbard, E., Terada, M., Dow, L. W., and Bank, A.: Decreased α globin messenger RNA activity associated with polyribosomes in α thalassemia. Nature [New Biol.] *241*:209, 1973.

Guest, G. M., and Rapoport, S.: Role of acid soluble phosphorous compounds in red blood cells in experimental rickets, renal insufficiency, pyloric obstruction, gastroenteritis, ammonium chloride acidosis and diabetes acidosis. Am. J. Dis. Child. *58*:1072, 1939.

Guidotti, G.: Thalassemia. In "Conference on Hemoglobin," Arden House, Columbia University, New York, 1962.

Gullbring, B., and Ström, G.: Changes in oxygen carrying function of human hemoglobin during storage in cold acid-citrate-dextrose solution. Acta Med. Scand. *155*:413, 1956.

Gunn, R. B., Silvers, D. N., and Rosse, W. F.: Potassium permeability in β-thalassemia minor red blood cells. J. Clin. Invest. *51*:1043, 1972.

Guy, J. T., Bromberg, P. A., Metz, E. N., et al.: Oxygen delivery following transfusion of stored blood. I. Normal rats. J. Appl. Physiol. *37*:60, 1974.

Haber, J. E., and Koshland, D. E.: The effect of 2,3-diphosphoglyceric acid on the changes in ββ interactions in hemoglobin during oxygenation. J. Biol. Chem. *246*:7790, 1971.

Hahn, E. V., and Gillespie, E. B.: Sickle cell anemia. Arch. Intern. Med. *39*:233, 1927.

Haidas, S., Labie, D., and Kaplan, J. C.: 2,3-Diphosphoglycerate content and oxygen affinity as a function of red cell age in normal individuals. Blood *38*:463, 1971.

Hakim, J., Boucherot, J., Troube, H., et al.: Red cell 2,3-diphosphoglycerate and adenosine triphosphate levels in patients with polycythemia vera. Rev. Eur. Etud. Clin. Biol. *17*:99, 1972.

Halbrecht, I., Isaacs, W. A., Lehmann, H., and Ben-Porat, F.: Hemoglobin Hasharon (α47 aspartic acid-histidine). Isr. J. Med. Sci. *3*:827, 1967.

Hall-Craggs, M., Marsden, P. D., Raper, A. B., et al.: Homozygous sickle-cell anaemia arising from two different haemoglobins S. Interaction of haemoglobins S and Stanleyville-II. Br. Med. J. *2*:87, 1964.

Ham, T. H., and Castle, W. B.: Relation of increased hypotonic fragility and of erythrostasis to the mechanism of hemolysis in certain anemias. Trans. Assn. Am. Physicians *55*:127, 1940.

Hamasaki, N., and Rose, Z. B.: The binding of phosphorylated red cell metabolites to human hemoglobin A. J. Biol. Chem. *249*:7896, 1974.

Hamasaki, N., Minakami, S., and Aono, K.: 2,3-Diphosphoglycerate content of human arterial and venous blood. Nature [New Biol.] *229*:215, 1971.

Hamilton, H. G., Iuchi, I., Miyaji, T., et al.: Hemoglobin Hiroshima (β^{143} Histidine→ Aspartic acid): a newly identified fast moving beta chain variant associated with increased oxygen affinity and compensatory erythremia. J. Clin. Invest. *48*:525, 1969.

Hamilton, R. W., Schwartz, E., Atwater, J., et al.: Acquired hemoglobin H disease. N. Engl. J. Med. *285*:1217, 1971.

Hamlyn, P. H., and Gould, H. J.: Isolation and identification of separated messenger RNAs for rabbit α and β globin. J. Mol. Biol. *94*:101, 1975.

Hammes, G. G., and Wu, C. W.: Regulation of enzyme activity. Science *172*:1205, 1971.

Harkness, D. R., and Roth, S.: Purification and properties of 2,3-diphosphoglyceric acid phosphatase from human erythrocytes. Biochem Biophys. Res. Commun. *34*:849, 1969.

Harkness, D. R., and Roth, S.: Clinical evaluation of cyanate in sickle cell anemia. Progr. Hematol. *9*:157, 1975.

Harkness, D. R., Ponce, J., and Grayson, V.: A comparative study on the phosphoglyceric acid cycle in mammalian erythrocytes. Comp. Biochem. Physiol. *28*:129, 1969.

Harkness, D. R., Ponce, J., and Roth, S.: Kinetic studies of the inhibition of glycolytic kinases of human erythrocytes by 2,3-diphosphoglyceric acid. Biochim. Biophys. Acta *250*:63, 1971.

Harris, J. W.: Studies on the destruction of red blood cells. VIII. Molecular orientation in sickle cell hemoglobin solution. Proc. Soc. Exp. Biol. Med. *75*:197, 1950.

Harris, J. W., and Bensusan, H. B.: The kinetics of the sol-gel transformation of deoxyhemoglobin S by continuous monitoring of viscosity. J. Lab. Clin. Med. *86*:564, 1975.

Harris, J. W., and Kellermeyer, R. W.: The Red Cell. Cambridge, Mass., Harvard University Press, 1970, p. 170.

Harris, J. W., Brewster, H. H., Ham, T. H., and Castle W. B.: Studies on the destruction of red blood cells. The biophysics and biology of sickle cell disease. Arch. Intern. Med. 97:145, 1956.

Harrison, P. R., Hell, A., Birnie, G. D., and Paul, J.: Evidence for single copies of globin genes in the mouse genome. Nature *239*:219, 1972.

Harrison, P. R., Conkie, D., Paul, J., et al.: Localization of cellular globin messenger RNA by in situ hybridization to complementary DNA. FEBS Lett. *32*:109, 1973.

Harrison, P. R., Conkie, D., Affara, N., and Paul, J.: In situ localization of globin messenger RNA formation. I. During mouse fetal liver development. J. Cell. Biol. *63*:402, 1974a.

Harrison, P. R., Gilmour, R. S., Affara, N. A., et al.: Globin messenger RNA synthesis and processing during haemoglobin induction in Friend cells. II. Evidence for post-transcriptional control in clone 707. Cell Differ. *3*:23, 1974b.

Hartz, W. H., and Schwartz, S. O.: Hemoglobin C disease, report of four cases. Blood *10*:235, 1955.

Hasen, H. B., and Raines, S. L.: Priapism associated with sickle cell disease. J. Urol. *88*:71, 1962.

Hathorn, M., and Lewis, R. A.: Inhibition of sickling by phenothiazines. Effect on red cell survival. Br. J. Haematol. *12*:195, 1966.

Haurowitz, F.: Zur Chemie des Blutfarbstoffes. 8 Mitteilung. Hoppe-Seyler's Z. Physiol. Chem. *173*:118, 1928.

Haurowitz, F.: Das Gleichgewicht zwischen Hämoglobin und Sauerstoff. Hoppe-Seyler's Z. Physiol. Chem. *254*:266, 1938.

Haut, M. J., Cowan, D. H., and Harris, J. W.: Platelet function and survival in sickle cell disease. J. Lab. Clin. Med. *82*:44, 1973.

Hayashi, A., Shimizu, A., Yamamura, Y., and Watari, H.: Hemoglobins M: Identification of Iwate, Boston and Saskatoon variants. Science *152*:207, 1966.

Hayashi, A., Shimizu, A., Suzuki, T., and Yamamura, Y.: The properties of hemoglobin M. Reactivity of methemoglobin M to cyanide, azide and fluoride. Biochim. Biophys. Acta *140*:251, 1967.

Hayashi, A., Suzuki, T., Shimizu, A., et al.: Properties of hemoglobin M. Unequivalent nature of the α and β subunits in the hemoglobin molecule. Biochim. Biophys. Acta *168*:262, 1968a.

Hayashi, A., Suzuki, T., Shimizu, A., et al.: Some observations on the physicochemical properties of hemoglobin $M_{Hyde\ Park}$. Arch. Biochem. Biophys. *125*:895, 1968b.

Hayashi, A., Stamatoyannopoulos, G., Yoshida, A., et al.: Haemoglobin Rainier: β145 (HC2) Tyrosine→Cysteine and Haemoglobin Bethesda: β145 (HC2) Tyrosine→Histidine. Nature [New Biol.] *230*:264, 1971.

Hecht, F., Motulsky, A. G., Lemire, R. J., and Shepard, T. E.: Predominance of hemoglobin Gower 1 in early human embryonic development. Science *152*:91, 1966.

Hecht, F., Jones, R. T., and Koler, R. D.: Newborn infants with Hb Portland 1; an indicator of α-chain deficiency. Ann. Hum. Genet. *31*:215, 1967.

Hedlund, B. E., and Lovrien, R.: Thermodynamics of 2,3-diphosphoglycerate association with human oxy- and deoxyhemoglobin. Biochem. Biophys. Res. Commun. *61*:859, 1974.

Heilmeyer, L.: Spectrophotometry in Medicine. Translated by A. Jordan and T. L. Tippell. Glasgow, Maclehose, 1943, 280 pp.

Heilmeyer, L.: Disturbances in Heme Synthesis. Springfield, Illinois, Charles C Thomas, 1966.

Heinemann, H. O., and Cheung, M. W.: Renal concentrating mechanism in sickle cell anemia. J. Lab. Clin. Med. *49*:923, 1957.

Heinrich, H. C., Gabbe, E. E., Oppitz, K. H., et al.: Absorption of inorganic and food iron in children with heterozygous and homozygous β-thalassemia. Z. Kinderheilkd. *115*:1, 1973.

Heller, P.: Hemoglobin M—An early chapter in the saga of molecular pathology. Ann. Intern. Med. *70*:1038, 1969.

Heller, P.: Does the sickle cell trait have pathogenic significance? In Hercules, J. I., Schechter, A. N., Eaton, W. A., et al. (eds.): Proceedings of First National Symposium on Sickle Cell Disease, Washington, D.C. DHEW Pub. No. 75–723, (NIH), Bethesda, Md., 1974, p. 293.

Heller, P., and Yakulis, V.: The distribution of hemoglobin A_2. Ann. NY Acad. Sci. *165*:54, 1969.

Heller, P., Henderson, W., and Yakulis, V.: Autosomal inactivation in the sickle-cell trait. Lancet 2:197, 1963a.

Heller, P., Yakulis, V., Epstein, R., and Friedland, S.: Variation in the amount of hemoglobin S in a patient with sickle cell trait and megaloblastic anemia. Blood *21*:479, 1963b.

Heller, P., Coleman, R. D., and Yakulis, V. J.: Structural studies of haemoglobin M-Hyde Park. Proceedings of the XI Congress of the International Society of Hematology, Sydney, 1966, pp. 427–434.

Hemmingsen, E. A.: Enhanced transport of oxygen by hemoglobin and myoglobin. In Proceedings of International Symposium on the Cardiovascular and Respiratory Effects of Hypoxia, Kingston, Ontario, 1965. New York, Hafner Publishing Co., 1966, pp. 41–54.

Henry, Y., and Cassoly, R.: Chain non-equivalence in nitric oxide binding to hemoglobin. Biochem. Biophys. Res. Commun. *51*:659, 1973.

Hensley, P., Edelstein, S. J., Wharton, D. C., et al.: Conformation and spin state in methemoglobin. J. Biol. Chem. *250*:952, 1975.

Hercules, J. I., Schechter, A. N., Eaton, W. A., et al. (eds.): Proceedings of First National Symposium on Sickle Cell Disease, Washington, D.C. DHEW Pub. No. 75–723 (NIH), Bethesda, Md., 1974.

Herrick, J. B.: Peculiar elongated and sickle-shaped red blood corpuscles in a case of severe anemia. Arch. Intern. Med. *6*:517, 1910.

Hershko, A., Razin, A., and Mager, J.: Regulation of the synthesis of 5-phosphoribosyl-I-pyrophosphate in intact red blood cell and in cell free preparations. Biochim. Biophys. Acta *184*:64, 1969.

Heywood, J. D., Karon, M., and Weissman, S.: Amino acids: incorporation into alpha- and beta-chains of hemoglobin by normal and thalassemic reticulocytes. Science *146*:530, 1964.

Heywood, J. D., Karon, M., and Weissman, S.: Asymmetrical incorporation of amino acids into the alpha- and beta-chains of hemoglobin synthesized in thalassemic reticulocytes. J. Lab. Clin. Med. *66*:476, 1965.

Heywood, S. M., Kennedy, D. S., and Bester, A. J.: Separation of specific initiation factors involved in the translation of myosin and myoglobin messenger RNAs and the isolation of a new RNA involved in translation. Proc. Natl. Acad. Sci. USA *71*:2428, 1974.

Hilkovitz, G.: Sickle cell disease: New method of treatment. Preliminary report. Br. Med. J. *2*:266, 1957.

Hill, A. V.: The possible effects of the aggregation of the molecules of haemoglobin on its dissociation current. J. Physiol. *40*:iv-vii, 1910.

Hill, R. J., and Craig, L. C.: Countercurrent distribution studies with adult human hemoglobin. J. Am. Chem. Soc. *81*:2272, 1959.

Hill, R. L., Swenson, R. T., and Schwartz, H. C.: The chemical and genetic relationships between hemoglobins S and $G_{San\ Jose}$. Blood *19*:573, 1962.

Hines, J. D., and Cowan, D. H.: Studies on the pathogenesis of alcohol-induced sideroblastic bone-marrow abnormalities. N. Engl. J. Med. *283*:441, 1970.

Hines, J. D., and Grasso, J. A.: The sideroblastic anemias. Semin. Hematol. *7*:86, 1970.

Hjelm, M.: The content of 2,3-diphosphoglycerate and some other phosphocompounds in human erythrocytes from healthy adults and subjects with different types of anaemia. Försvarsmedicin *5*:219, 1969.

Hjelm, M., and Wadman, B.: Erythrocyte-DPG and creatine in polycythemia. N. Engl. J. Med. *287*:45, 1972.

Ho, C., and Lindstrom, T. R.: Functional non-equivalence of α and β hemes in human hemoglobins. Adv. Exp. Med. Biol. *28*:65, 1972.

Hobbins, J. C., and Mahoney, M. J.: In utero diagnosis of hemoglobinopathies. I. Technique for obtaining fetal blood. N. Engl. J. Med. *290*:1065, 1974.

Hobbins, J. C., and Mahoney, M. J.: Fetal blood drawing. Lancet *2*:107, 1975.

Hobolth, N.: Haemoglobin $M_{Århus}$. I. Clinical family study. Acta Paediatr. Scand. *54*:357, 1965a.

Hobolth, N.: Haemoglobin $M_{Århus}$. II. Studies on a new haemoglobin which causes congenital methaemoglobinaemia. Acta Paediatr. Scand. *54*:357, 1965b.

Hofrichter, J., Hendricker, D., and Eaton, W. A.: Structure of hemoglobin S fibers: optical determination of the molecular orientation in sickled erythrocytes. Proc. Natl. Acad. Sci. USA *70*:3604, 1973.

Hofrichter, J., Ross, P. D., and Eaton, W. A.: Supersaturation in sickle cell hemoglobin globin S gelatin: a new approach to understanding sickle cell disease. Proc. Natl. Acad. Sci. USA *71*:4864, 1974.

Hofrichter, J., Ross, P. D., and Eaton, W. A.: Supersaturation in sickle cell hemoglobin solutions. Proc. Natl. Acad. Sci. U.S.A. *73*:3035, 1976.

Hollan, S. R., Szelenyi, J. G., Brimhall, B., et al.: Multiple alpha chain loci for human haemoglobins: Hb J-Buda and Hb G-Pest. Nature *235*:47, 1972.

Hollenberg, M. D., Kalback, M. M., and Kazazian, H. H., Jr.: Adult hemoglobin synthesis by reticulocytes from the human fetus at midtrimester. Science *174*:698, 1971.

Hollender, A., Lorkin, P. A., Lehmann, H., and Svensson, B.: New unstable haemoglobin Borås, β88 (F4) Leucine→Arginine. Nature (London) *222*:953, 1969.

Holmquist, W. R., and Schroeder, W. A.: A new N-terminal blocking group involving a Schiff base in hemoglobin A_{Ic}. Biochemistry *5*:2489, 1966.

Holsinger, J. W., Salhany, J. M., and Eliot, R. S.: Physiologic observations on the effect of impaired blood oxygen release on the myocardium. Adv. Cardiol. *9*:81, 1973.

Honig, G. R.: Inhibition of synthesis of fetal haemoglobin by an isoleucine analogue. J. Clin. Invest. *46*:1778, 1967.

Honig, G. R., Rowan, B., and Mason, R.: Unequal synthesis of complementary globin chains of human fetal hemoglobin by the effect of L-O-methyl threonine. J. Biol. Chem. *244*:2027, 1969.

Honig, G. R., Green, D., Shamsuddin, M., et al.: Hemoglobin Abraham Lincoln, β32 (B14) leucine→proline, an unstable variant producing severe hemolytic disease. J. Clin. Invest. *52*:1746, 1973.

Honig, G. R., Mason, R. G., Vida, L. N., and Shamsuddin, M.: Synthesis of Hemoglobin Abraham Lincoln (β32 Leu→Pro). Blood *43*:657, 1974.

Hoppe-Seyler, F.: Ueber die chemischen und optischen Eigenschaften des Blutfarbstoffs. Virchow's Arch. Pathol. Anat. *29*:233, 1864.

Hörlein, H., and Weber, G.: Über chronische familiäre Methämoglobinämie und eine neue Modifikation des Methämoglobins. Dtsch. Med. Wochenschr. *73*:476, 1948.

Hosoi, T.: Studies on hemoglobin F within a single erythrocyte by fluorescent antibody technique. Exp. Cell Res. *37*:680, 1965.

Housman, D., Jacobs-Lorena, M., et al.: Initiation of hemoglobin synthesis by methionyl-tRNA. Nature *227*:913, 1970.

Housman, D., Forget, B. G., Skoutchi, A., and Benz, E. J., Jr.: Quantitative deficiency of chain specific globin mRNA in the thalassemia syndromes. Proc. Natl. Acad. Sci. USA *70*:1809, 1973.

Housman, D., Skoultchi, A., Forget, B. G., et al.: Use of globin cDNA as a hybridization probe for globin mRNA. Ann. NY Acad. Sci. *241*:280, 1974.

Howard, G., Adamson, S., and Herbert, E.: Studies on cessation of protein synthesis in a reticulocyte lysate cell free system. Biochim. Biophys. Acta *213*:237, 1970.

Huehns, E. R.: The unstable hemoglobins. Bull. Soc. Chim. Biol. *52*:1131, 1970.

Huehns, E. R., and Farooqui, A. M.: Oxygen dissociation properties of human embryonic red cells. Nature *254*:335, 1975.

Huehns, E. R., and Shooter, E. M.: The properties and reactions of hemoblogin F and their bearing on the dissociation equilibrium of hemoglobin. Biochem. J. *101*:852, 1966.

Huehns, E. R., Flynn, F. V., Butler, E. A., and Beaven, G. H.: Two new haemoglobin variants in a very young human embryo. Nature *189*:496, 1961.

Huehns, E. R., Dance, N., Beaven, G. H., et al.: Human embryonic hemoglobins. Cold Spring Harbor Symp. Quant. Biol. *21*:327, 1964.

Huehns, E. R., Dance, N., Beaven, G. H., et al.: Human embryonic haemoglobins. Nature (London) *201*:1095, 1969.

Huehns, E. R., Hecht, F., Yoshida, A., et al.: Hemoglobin Seattle ($\alpha_2{}^A\beta_2{}^{76}$): An unstable hemoglobin causing chronic hemolytic anemia. Blood *36*:209, 1970.

Huestis, W. H., and Raftery, M. A.: ^{31}P-NMR studies of the release of diphosphoglyceric acid on carbon monoxide binding to hemoglobin. Biochem. Biophys. Res. Commun. *49*:428, 1972.

Huestis, W. H., and Raftery, M. A.: Characterization of intermediate states in the ligation of hemoglobin. Biochemistry *12*:2531, 1973.

Huez, G., Marbaix, G., Hubert, E., et al.: Role of the polyadenylate segment in the translation of globin messenger RNA in Xenopus oocytes. Proc. Natl. Acad. Sci. USA *71*:3143, 1974.

Hugh-Jones, K., Lehmann, H., and McAlister, J. M.: Some experiences in managing sickle-cell anaemia in children and young adults, using alkalis and magnesium. Br. Med. J. *2*:226, 1964.

Huisman, T. H. J.: Chromatographic separation of hemoglobins A_2 and C. The quantities of hemoglobin A_2 in patients with AC trait, CC disease and C–β-thalassemia. Clin. Chim. Acta *40*:159, 1972.

Huisman, T. H. J., and Meyering, C. A.: Studies on the heterogeneity of hemoglobin. I. The heterogeneity of different human hemoglobin types in carboxymethylcellulose and in Amberlite IRC-50 chromatography: Qualitatative aspects. Clin. Chim. Acta *5*:103, 1960.

Huisman, T. H. J., Martis, E. A., and Dozy, A. M.: Chromatography of hemoglobin types on carboxymethylcellulose. J. Lab. Clin. Med. *52*:312, 1958a.
Huisman, T. H. J., Van Vliet, G., and Sebens, T.: Sheep hemoglobins. Nature *182*:171, 1958b.
Huisman, T. H. J., Boyd, E. M., Kitchens, J., et al.: Oxygen equilibria and biochemical changes of whole blood stored in different preservation media. Transfusion *9*:180, 1969.
Huisman, T. H. J., Schroeder, W. A., et al.: Nature of fetal hemoglobin in the Greek type of hereditary persistence of fetal hemoglobin, with and without concurrent β-thalassemia. J. Clin. Invest. *49*:1035, 1970.
Huisman, T. H. J., Brown, A. K., Efremov, G. D., et al.: Hemoglobin Savannah (B6[24] β-glycine→valine): an unstable variant causing anemia with inclusion bodies. J. Clin. Invest. *50*:650, 1971a.
Huisman, T. H. J., Schroeder, W. A., and Charache, S.: Hereditary persistence of fetal hemoglobin: heterogeneity of fetal hemoglobin in homozygotes and in conjunction with β-thalassemia. N. Engl. J. Med. *285*:711, 1971b.
Huisman, T. H. J., Schroeder, W. A., et al.: Evidence for four nonallelic structural genes for the γ chain of human fetal hemoglobin. Biochem. Genet. *7*:131, 1972a.
Huisman, T. H. J., Wrightstone, R. N., Wilson, J. B., et al.: Hemoglobin Kenya, the product of fusion of γ and β polypeptide chains. Arch. Biochem. Biophys. *153*:850, 1972b.
Huisman, T. H. J., Wilson, J. B., Gravely, M., et al.: Hemoglobin Grady: the first example of a variant with elongated chains due to an insertion of residues. Proc. Natl. Acad. Sci. USA *71*:3270, 1974.
Huisman, T. H. J., Miller, A., and Schroeder, W. A.: $A^{G}\gamma$ type of hereditary persistence of fetal hemoglobin with β chain production *in cis*. Am. J. Hum. Genet. *27*:765, 1975.
Hultquist, D. E., Dean, R. T., and Douglas, R. H.: Homogeneous cytochrome b_5 from human erythrocytes. Biochem. Biophys. Res. Commun. *60*:28, 1974.
Humpeler, E., and Amor, H.: Sex differences in the oxygen affinity of hemoglobin. Pfluegers Arch. *343*:151, 1973.
Humpeler, E., Amor, H., and Braunsteiner, H.: Unterschedliche Sauerstoffaffinität des Hämoglobins bei Anämien verschiedener Åtiologie. Blut *29*:382, 1974.
Humphries, S., Doel, M., and Williamson, R.: The translation of mouse globin mRNA from which the polyadenylic acid sequence has been removed in a reinitiation protein synthesis system. Biochem. Biophys. Res. Commun. *58*:927, 1974.
Hunt, J. T., and Ingram, V. M.: Abnormal human haemoglobins. IV. The chemical difference between normal human haemoglobin and haemoglobin C. Biochim. Biophys. Acta *42*:409, 1960.
Hunt, R. T., Hunter, A. J., and Munro, A. J.: Control of hemoglobin synthesis: Distribution of ribosomes on the mRNA for α and β chains. J. Mol. Biol. *36*:31, 1968a.
Hunt, R. T., Munro, A. J., and Hunter, A. R.: Control of haemoglobin synthesis: A difference in the size of polysomes making α and β chains. Nature *220*:481, 1968b.
Hunt, R. T., Hunter, A. R., and Munro, A. J.: Control of hemoglobin synthesis: Rate of translation of the messenger RNA for the α and β chains. J. Mol. Biol. *43*:123, 1969.
Hunt, T.: The control of globin synthesis in rabbit reticulocytes. Ann. NY Acad. Sci. *241*:223, 1974.
Hunt, T., Vanderhoff, G., and London, I.: Control of globin synthesis: the role of heme. J. Mol. Biol. *66*:471, 1972.
Huntsman, R. G., and Lehmann, H.: The hemoglobinopathies. In Stanbury, J. B., et al. (eds.): Metabolic Basis of Inherited Diseases. New York, McGraw-Hill Book Co., 3rd ed. 1972, pp. 297–369.
Hurt, G. A., and Chanutin, A.: Organic phosphate compounds of erythrocytes from individuals with uremia. J. Lab. Clin. Med. *64*:675, 1964.
Hurt, G. A., and Chanutin, A.: Organic phosphate compounds of erythrocytes from individuals with cirrhosis of the liver. Proc. Soc. Exp. Biol. Med. *118*:167, 1965.
Hutchison, H. E., Pinkerton, P. H., Waters, P., et al.: Hereditary Heinz body anaemia, thrombocytopenia and haemoglobinopathy (Hb Köln) in a Glasgow family. Br. Med. J. *2*:1099, 1964.
Idelson, L. I., Didkowsky, N. A., Casey, R., et al.: New unstable haemoglobin (Hb Moscva, β24(B4)Gly→Asp) found in the USSR. Nature *249*:768, 1974.
Imai, K., and Tyuma, I.: Thermodynamical analysis of oxygen equilibrium of stripped hemoglobin. Biochem. Biophys. Res. Commun. *51*:52, 1973.

Imai, K., Morimoto, H., Kotan, M., et al.: Studies on the function of abnormal hemoglobins. II. Oxygen equilibrium of abnormal hemoglobins: Shimonosecki, Ube II, Hikari, Gifu and Agenogi. Biochim. Biophys. Acta *200*:197, 1970.

Imaizumi, T., Digglemann, H., and Scherrer, K.: Demonstration of globin messenger sequences in giant nuclear precursors of messenger RNA of avian erythroblasts. Proc. Natl. Acad. Sci. USA *70*:1122, 1973.

Imamura, T., Fujita, S., and Ohta, Y.: Hemoglobin Yoshizuka (G10[108] β asparagine→aspartic acid): A new variant with a reduced oxygen affinity from a Japanese family. J. Clin. Invest. *48*:2341, 1969.

Ingram, V. M.: Sulphhydryl groups in haemoglobins. Biochem. J. *59*:653, 1955.

Ingram, V. M.: A specific chemical difference between the globins of normal human and sickle cell anaemia haemoglobin. Nature *178*:792, 1956.

Ingram, V. M.: Abnormal human haemoglobins. II. The chemical difference between normal and sickle cell haemoglobins. Biochim. Biophys. Acta *36*:402, 1959.

Ingram, V. M.: A molecular model for thalassemia. Ann. NY Acad. Sci. *119*:485, 1964.

Ingram, V. M., and Stretton, A. O. W.: Human hemoglobin A_2: chemistry, genetics and evolution. Nature *190*:1079, 1961.

Isaacs, W. A., and Hayhoe, F. G. J.: Steroid hormones in sickle-cell disease. Nature *215*:1139, 1967.

Itano, H. A.: A third abnormal hemoglobin associated with hereditary hemolytic anemia. Proc. Natl. Acad. Sci. USA *37*:775, 1951.

Itano, H. A.: The synthesis and structure of normal and abnormal hemoglobins. In Jonxis, J. H. P. (ed.): Abnormal Haemoglobins in Africa. Oxford, Blackwell Scientific Publications, 1965, p. 3.

Itano, H. A., and Neel, J. V.: A new inherited abnormality of human hemoglobin. Proc. Natl. Acad. Sci. USA *36*:613, 1950.

Jackson, J. F., Odom, J. L., and Bell, W. N.: Amelioration of sickle cell disease by persistent fetal hemoglobin. JAMA *177*:867, 1961.

Jackson, J. M., Yates, A., and Huehns, E. R.: Haemoglobin Perth: β32 (B14) leu→pro, an unstable haemoglobin causing haemolysis. Br. J. Haematol. *25*:607, 1973.

Jackson, R., and Hunter, T.: Role of methionine in the initiation of haemoglobin synthesis. Nature *227*:672, 1970.

Jacob, H. S., and Amsden, T.: Acute hemolytic anemia with rigid red cells in hypophosphatemia. N. Engl. J. Med. *285*:1446, 1971.

Jacob, H. S., and Winterhalter, K. H.: The role of hemoglobin heme loss in Heinz body formation: Studies with a partially heme-deficient hemoglobin and with genetically unstable hemoglobin. J. Clin. Invest. *49*:2008, 1970a.

Jacob, H. S., and Winterhalter, K. H.: Unstable hemoglobins: The role of heme loss in Heinz body formation. Proc. Natl. Acad. Sci. USA *65*:697, 1970b.

Jacob, H. S., Brain, M. C., and Dacie, J. V.: Altered sulfhydryl reactivity of hemoglobins and red blood cell membranes in congenital Heinz body hemolytic anemia. J. Clin. Invest. *47*:2664, 1968a.

Jacob, H. S., Brain, M. C., Dacie, J. V., et al.: Abnormal haem binding and globin SH group blockade in unstable haemoglobins. Nature *218*:1214, 1968b.

Jacobs-Lorena, M., and Baglioni, C.: Messenger RNA for globin in the postribosomal supernatant of rabbit reticulocytes. Proc. Natl. Acad. Sci. USA *69*:1425, 1972.

Jacobs-Lorena, M., and Baglioni, C.: Synthesis of rabbit globin by reticulocyte postribosomal supernatant and heterologous ribosomes. Eur. J. Biochem. *35*:559, 1973.

Jacon, G., Wajcman, H., and Labie, D.: Structural and functional study of Hb Nancy, β145 (HC2) Tyr→Asp. A high oxygen affinity hemoglobin. FEBS Lett. *56*:39, 1975.

Jandl, J. H., and Greenberg, M. S.: Bone marrow failure due to relative nutritional deficiency in Cooley's hemolytic anemia. N. Engl. J. Med. *280*:461, 1959.

Jandl, J. H., Simmons, R. L., and Castle, W. B.: Red cell filtration and the pathogenesis of certain hemolytic anemias. Blood *18*:133, 1961.

Jenkins, M. E., Scott, R. B., and Baird, R. L.: Studies in sickle cell anemia. XVI. Sudden death during sickle cell anemia crises in young children. J. Pediatr. *56*:30, 1960.

Jensen, M., Bunn, H. F., Halikas, G., et al.: Effect of cyanate and 2,3-diphosphoglycerate on sickling. J. Clin. Invest. *52*:2542, 1973a.

Jensen, M., Nathan, D., and Bunn, H. F.: The reaction of cyanate with the α and β subunits of hemoglobin: Effects of oxygenation, phosphates and carbon dioxide. J. Biol. Chem. *248*:8057, 1973b.

Jensen, M., Shohet, S. B., and Nathan, D. G.: The role of red cell energy metabolism in the generation of irreversibly sickled cells in vitro. Blood *42*:835, 1973c.

Jensen, M., Oski, F. A., Nathan, D. G., and Bunn, H. F.: Hemoglobin Syracuse (α_2 $\beta_2{}^{143\,[H21]\,His \rightarrow Pro}$). A new high-affinity variant detected by special electrophoretic methods. J. Clin. Invest. *55*:469, 1975.

Jensen, W. N., Schofield, R. A., and Agner, R.: Clinical and necropsy findings in hemoglobin C disease. Blood *12*:74, 1957.

Jensen, W. N., Ricknagel, D. L., and Taylor, W. J.: In vivo study of the sickle cell phenomenon. J. Lab. Clin. Med. *56*:854, 1960.

Jensen, W. N., Bromberg, P. A., and Barefield, K.: Membrane deformation: A cause of the irreversibly sickled cell (ISC). Clin. Res. *17*:464, 1969.

Jeppson, J. O., and Berglund, S.: Thin layer isoelectric focusing and its application to haemoglobin Malmö. Clin. Chim. Acta *40*:153, 1972.

Johnston, F. E., Hertzog, K. P., and Malina, R. M.: Longitudinal growth in thalassemia major. Am. J. Dis. Child. *112*:396, 1966.

Johnston, R. B.: Increased susceptibility to infection in sickle cell disease: Review of its occurrence and possible causes. South. Med. J. *67*:1342, 1974.

Johnston, R. B., Newman, S. L., and Struth, A. G.: An abnormality of the alternate pathway of complement activation in sickle-cell disease. N. Engl. J. Med. *288*:803, 1973.

Jones, R. L., Peterson, C. M., Graziano, J. R., et al.: 2,3-Dihydroxybenzoic acid and iron overload. Blood *46*:1027(Abst.), 1975.

Jones, R. T.: Structural studies of aminoethylated hemoglobins by automatic peptide chromatography. Cold Spring Harbor Symp. Quant. Biol. *29*:297, 1964.

Jones, R. T., and Schroeder, W. A.: Chemical characterization and subunit hybridization of human hemoglobin H and associated compounds. Biochemistry *2*:1357, 1963.

Jones, R. T., Brimhall, B., Huisman, T. H. J., et al.: Hemoglobin Freiburg: Abnormal hemoglobin due to deletion of a single amino acid residue. Science *154*:1024, 1966.

Jones, R. T., Osgood, E. E., Brimhall, B., and Koler, R. D.: Hemoglobin Yakima. I. Clinical and biochemical studies. J. Clin. Invest. *46*:1840, 1967.

Jones, S. R., Binder, R. A., and Donowho, E. M.: Sudden death in sickle-cell trait. N. Engl. J. Med. *282*:323, 1970.

Jope, H. M., and O'Brien, J. R. P.: Crystallization and solubility studies on human adult and foetal haemoglobins. In Roughton, F. J. W., and Kendrew, J. C. (eds.): Haemoglobin (Barcroft Symposium). New York, Interscience, 1949, p. 269.

Josephs, R., Jarosch, H. S., and Edelstein, S. J.: Polymorphism of sickle cell hemoglobin fibers. J. Mol. Biol. *102*:409, 1976.

Josephson, A. M., Masri, M. S., Singer, L., et al.: Starch block electrophoretic studies of human hemoglobin solutions. II. Results in cord blood, thalassemia and other hematologic disorders: comparison with Tiselius electrophoresis. Blood *13*:543, 1958.

Josephson, A. M., Weinstein, H. G., Yakulis, B. S., et al.: A new variant of hemoglobin M disease: Hemoglobin $M_{Chicago}$. J. Lab. Clin. Med. *59*:918, 1962.

Jurkiewicz, M. J., Pearson, H. A., and Furlow, L. T.: Reconstruction of the maxilla in thalassemia. Ann. NY Acad. Sci. *165*:437, 1969.

Kabat, D.: The switch from fetal to adult hemoglobin in humans: evidence suggesting a role for γ-β gene linkage. Ann. NY Acad. Sci. *241*:119, 1974.

Kacian, D. L., Spiegelman, S., Bank, A., et al.: *In vitro* synthesis of DNA components of human genes for globins. Nature [New Biol.] *235*:167, 1972.

Kacian, D. L., Gambino, R., Dow, L. W., et al.: Decreased globin messenger RNA in thalassemia detected by molecular hybridization. Proc. Natl. Acad. Sci. USA *70*:1886, 1973.

Kaempfer, R.: Identification and RNA-binding properties of an initiation factor capable of relieving translational inhibition induced by heme deprivation or double stranded RNA. Biochem. Biophys. Res. Commun. *61*:591, 1974.

Kaempfer, R., and Kaufman, J.: Translational control of hemoglobin synthesis by an initiation factor required for recycling of ribosomes and their binding to messenger RNA. Proc. Natl. Acad. Sci. USA *69*:3317, 1972.

Kamuzora, H., and Lehmann, H.: A new haemoglobin variant—Haemoglobin J Birmingham, α120 (H3) Ala→Glu. Ann. Clin. Biochem. *11*:53, 1974.

Kamuzora, H., and Lehmann, H.: Human embryonic haemoglobins including a comparison by homology of the human ζ and α chains. Nature *256*:511, 1975.

Kamuzora, H., Jones, R. T., and Lehmann, H.: The ζ chain, an α-like chain of human embryonic haemoglobin. FEBS Lett. *46*:195, 1974.

Kan, Y. W., and Golbus, M. S.: Prenatal diagnosis of hereditary hemoglobin disorders: current developments. Pediatr. Res. *10*:367(Abstr. 397), 1976.

Kan, Y. W., and Nathan, D. G.: Mild thalassemia: the result of interaction of alpha and beta thalassemia genes. J. Clin. Invest. *49*:635, 1970.

Kan, Y. W., Allen, A., and Lowenstein, L.: Hydrops fetalis with alpha thalassemia. N. Engl. J. Med. *276*:18, 1967.

Kan, Y. W., Schwartz, E., and Nathan, D. G.: Globin chain synthesis in the alpha thalassemia syndromes. J. Clin. Invest. *47*:2515, 1968.

Kan, Y. W., Dozy, A. M., Alter, B. P., et al.: Detection of the sickle gene in the human fetus. Potential for intrauterine diagnosis of sickle cell anemia. N. Engl. J. Med. *287*:1, 1972a.

Kan, Y. W., Forget, B. G., and Nathan, D. G.: Gamma-beta thalassemia: a cause of hemolytic disease of newborns. N. Engl. J. Med. *286*:129, 1972b.

Kan, Y. W., Nathan, D. G., and Lodish, H. F.: Equal synthesis of α- and β-globin chains in erythroid precursors in heterozygous β-thalassemia. J. Clin. Invest. *51*:1906, 1972c.

Kan, Y. W., Todd, D., and Dozy, A. M.: Hemoglobin Constant Spring: possibly unstable mRNA and evidence for 2 locus theory for α chain production. Clin. Res. *20*:471, 1972d.

Kan, Y. W., Bellevue, R., Rieder, R., et al.: Prenatal diagnosis of α thalassemia. Clin. Res. *22*:374A, 1974a.

Kan, Y. W., Nathan, D. G., Cividalli, G., et al.: Concentration of fetal red blood cells from a mixture of maternal and fetal blood by anti-i serum: an aid to prenatal diagnosis of hemoglobinopathies. Blood *43*:411, 1974b.

Kan, Y. W., Todd, D., and Dozy, A. M.: Haemoglobin Constant Spring synthesis in red cell precursors. Br. J. Haematol. *28*:103, 1974c.

Kan, Y. W., Valenti, C., Guidotti, R., et al.: Fetal blood-sampling *in utero*. Lancet *1*:79, 1974d.

Kan, Y. W., Dozy, A. M., Varmus, H. E., et al.: Deletion of α-globin genes in haemoglobin-H disease demonstrates multiple α-globin structural loci. Nature *255*:255, 1975a.

Kan, Y. W., Globus, M. S., Klein, P., et al.: Successful application of prenatal diagnosis in a pregnancy at risk for homozygous β-thalassemia N. Engl. J. Med. *292*:1096, 1975b.

Kan, Y. W., Golbus, M. S., Trecartin, R., et al.: Prenatal diagnosis of homozygous β-thalassaemia. Lancet *2*:790, 1975c.

Kan, Y. W., Holland, J. P., Dozy, A. M., et al.: Deletion of the β-globin structure gene in hereditary persistence of foetal hemoglobin. Nature *258*:162, 1975d.

Kan, Y. W., Holland, J. P., Dozy, A. M., et al.: Demonstration of non-functional β-globin mRNA in homozygous β°-thalassemia. Proc. Natl. Acad. Sci. USA *72*:5140, 1975e.

Kan, Y. W., Golbus, M. S., and Dozy, A. M.: Application of molecular hybridization to prenatal diagnosis of α thalassemia. Clin. Res. *24*:435(Abst.), 1976a.

Kan, Y. W., Golbus, M. S., and Trecartin, R.: Prenatal diagnosis of sickle-cell anemia. N. Engl. J. Med. *294*:1039, 1976b.

Kaplan, E., Zuelzer, W. W., and Neel, J. V.: A new inherited abnormality of hemoglobin and its interaction with sickle cell hemoglobin. Blood *6*:1240, 1951.

Kappas, A., and Granick, S.: Steroid induction of porphyrin synthesis in liver cell culture. II. The effects of heme, uridine diphosphate glucuronic acid and inhibition of protein synthesis on the process. J. Biol. Chem. *243*:346, 1968.

Kappel, W. K., and Hass, L. F.: The isolation and partial characterization of diphosphoglycerate mutase from human erythrocytes. Biochemistry *15*:290, 1975.

Karayalcin, G., Imran, M., and Rosner, F.: Priapism in sickle cell disease: report of five cases. Am. J. Med. Sci. *264*:289, 1972.

Karibian, D., and London, I.: Control of heme synthesis by feedback inhibition. Biochem. Biophys. Res. Commun. *18*:243, 1965.

Kattamis, C., and Lehmann, H.: Duplication of alpha thalassaemia gene in three Greek families with haemoglobin H disease. Lancet *2*:635, 1970.

Kattamis, C., Touliatos, N., Haidas, S., and Matsaniotis, N.: Growth of children with thalassemia: effect of different transfusion regimens. Arch. Dis. Child. *45*:502, 1970.

Kattamis, C., Lagos, P., Metaxotou-Mavromati, A., et al.: Serum iron and unsaturated iron-binding capacity in the β-thalassemia trait: their relation to the levels of haemoglobins A, A_2, and F. J. Med. Genet. *9*:154, 1972.

Kattamis, C., Metaxotou-Mavromati, A., Karamboula, K., et al.: The clinical and haematological findings in children inheriting two types of thalassaemia: high-A_2 type β-thalassaemia, and high-F type of $\delta\beta$-thalassaemia. Br. J. Haematol. *25*:375, 1973.

Kazazian, H. H., Jr., and Freedman, M.: The characterization of separated α and β chain polysomes in rabbit reticulocytes. J. Biol. Chem. *243*:6446, 1968.

Kazazian, H. H., Jr., and Woodhead, A. P.: Hemoglobin A synthesis in the developing fetus. N. Engl. J. Med., *289*:58, 1973.

Kazazian, H. H., Jr., Snyder, P. G., and Cheng, T. C.: Separation of α- and β-globin messenger RNAs by formamide gel electrophoresis. Biochem. Biophys. Res. Commun. *59*:1053, 1974.

Kazazian, H. H., Jr., Ginder, G. D., Snyder, P. G., et al.: Further evidence of a quantitative deficiency of chain-specific globin mRNA in the thalassemia syndromes. Proc. Natl. Acad. Sci. USA *72*:567, 1975.

Kazazian, H. H., Jr., Silverstein, A. M., Snyder, P. G., et al.: Increasing haemoglobin β-chain synthesis in foetal development is associated with a declining γ- to α-mRNA ratio. Nature *260*:67, 1976.

Keberle, H.: The biochemistry of desferrioxamine and its relation to iron metabolism. Ann. NY Acad. Sci. *119*:758, 1964.

Keeling, M. M., Ogden, L. L., Wrightstone, R. N., et al.: Hemoglobin Louisville (β42 [CD1] Phe→Leu): an unstable variant causing mild hemolytic anemia. J. Clin. Invest. *50*:2395, 1971.

Keitel, A. G., Thompson, D., and Itano, H. A.: Hyposthenuria in sickle cell anemia: a reversible renal defect. J. Clin. Invest. *35*:998, 1958.

Keitt, A. S.: Pyruvate kinase deficiency and related disorders of red cell glycolysis. Am. J. Med. *41*:762, 1966.

Keitt, A. S.: Hemolytic anemia with impaired hexokinase activity. J. Clin. Invest. *48*:1997, 1969.

Keitt, A. S.: Reduced nicotinamide adenine dinucleotide-linked analysis of 2,3-diphosphoglyceric acid: spectrophotometric and fluorometric procedures. J. Lab. Clin. Med. *77*:470, 1971.

Keitt, A. S., Smith, T. W., and Jandl, J. H.: Red-cell "pseudo-mosaicism" in congenital methaemoglobinemia. N. Engl. J. Med. *275*:397, 1966.

Keitt, A. S., Hinkes, C., and Block, A. J.: Comparison of factors regulating red cell 2,3-diphosphoglycerate (2,3-DPG) in acute and chronic hypoxemia. J. Lab. Clin. Med. *84*:275, 1974.

Kendall, A. G., Ojwang, P. J., et al.: Hemoglobin Kenya, the product of a γ-β fusion gene: studies of the family. Am. J. Hum. Genet. *25*:548, 1973.

Kendrew, J. C.: The three-dimensional structure of a protein molecule. Sci. Am. *205*:104, 1961.

Kennedy, C. C., Blundell, G., Lorkin, P. A., et al.: Haemoglobin Belfast (β15(A12) Tryptophan→Arginine: A new unstable haemoglobin variant. Br. Med. J. *4*:324, 1974.

Kennedy, D. S., Bester, A. J., and Heywood, S. M.: The regulation of protein synthesis by translational control RNA. Biochem. Biophys. Res. Commun. *61*:415, 1974.

Keys, A., and Snell, A. M.: Respiratory properties of the arterial blood in normal man and in patients with disease of the liver: position of the oxygen dissociation curve. J. Clin. Invest. *17*:59, 1938.

Kiese, M., Kurz, H., and Schneider, C.: Chronische Hämoglobinämie durch pathologischen Blutfarbstoff. Klin. Wochenschr. *34*:957, 1956.

Kiesow, L. A., Bless, J. W., and Shelton, J. B.: Oxygen dissociation in human erythrocytes: its response to hyperbaric environments. Science *179*:1236, 1973.

Kikochi, G., Hayashi, N., and Tamura, A.: Oxygen equilibrium of hemoglobin M_{Iwate}. Biochim. Biophys. Acta *90*:199, 1964.

Killam, K. F.: Convulsant hydrazides. II. Comparison of electrical changes and enzyme inhibition induced by the administration of thiosemicarbazide. J. Pharmacol. Exp. Ther. *119*:263, 1957.

Kilmartin, J. V., and Rossi-Bernardi, L.: Inhibition of CO_2 combination and reduction of the Bohr effect in haemoglobin chemically modified at its α-amino groups. Nature *222*:1243, 1969.

Kilmartin, J. V., and Rossi-Bernardi, L.: The binding of carbon dioxide by horse haemoglobin. Biochem. J. *124*:31, 1971.

Kilmartin, J. V., and Rossi-Bernardi, L.: Interaction of hemoglobin with hydrogen ions, carbon dioxide, and organic phosphates. Physiol. Rev. *53*:836, 1973.

Kilmartin, J. V., Breen, J. J., Roberts, G. C. K., and Ho, C.: Direct measurement of the pK values of an alkaline Bohr group in human hemoglobin. Proc. Natl. Acad. Sci. USA *70*:1246, 1973a.

Kilmartin, J. V., Fogg, J., Luzzana, M., and Rossi-Bernardi, L.: Role of the α-amino groups of the α and β chains of human hemoglobin in oxygen-linked binding of carbon dioxide. J. Biol. Chem. *248*:7039, 1973b.

Kim, H. C., Marks, P. A., Rifkind, R. A., et al.: Isolation and *in vitro* differentiation of human erythroid precursor cells. Blood *47*:767, 1976.

King, M. A. R., Wiltshire, B. G., Lehmann, H., and Morimoto, H.: An unstable haemoglobin with reduced oxygen affinity: Haemoglobin Peterborough, β 111 (C13) valine→phenylalanine, its interaction with normal haemoglobin and with haemoglobin Lepore. Br. J. Haematol. *22*:125, 1972.

Kleckner, H. B., Wilson, J. B., Lindeman, J. G., et al.: Hemoglobin Fort-Gordon or $\alpha_2\beta_2^{145\ Tyr \rightarrow Asp}$, a new high-affinity variant. Biochim. Biophys. Acta *400*(2):343, 1975.

Kleihauer, E. F., Reynolds, C. A., Dozy, A. M., et al.: Hemoglobin Bibba or $\alpha_2^{136\ Pro}\beta_2$, an unstable α chain abnormal hemoglobin. Biochim. Biophys. Acta *154*:220, 1968.

Klinefelter, H. F.: The heart in sickle cell anemia. Am. J. Med. Sci. *203*:34, 1942.

Klion, F. M., Weiner, M. J., and Schaffner, F.: Cholestasis in sickle cell anemia. Am. J. Med. *37*:829, 1964.

Klocke, R. A.: Oxygen transport and 2,3-diphosphoglycerate. Chest *62*:795, 1972.

Knöchel, W., and Tiedemann, H.: Size distribution and cell-free translation of globin-coding HnRNA from avian erythroblasts. Biochim. Biophys. Acta *378*:383, 1975.

Knox-Macauley, H. H. M., Weatherall, D. J., Clegg, J. B., et al.: The clinical and biosynthetic characterization of $\alpha\beta$-thalassemia. Br. J. Haematol. *22*:497, 1972.

Koch, H.-H., and Schröter, W.: Kompensatorische Veränderungen der erythrocytären 2,3-Diphosphoglycerat Konzentration bei Anämien and Polyglobulien. Monatsschr. Kinderheilkd. *121*:392, 1973.

Koenig, R. J., and Cerami, A.: Synthesis of hemoglobin A_{Ic} in normal and diabetic mice: potential model of basement membrane thickening. Proc. Natl. Acad. Sci. USA *72*:3687, 1975.

Koenig, R. J., Peterson, C. M., Jones, R. L., et al.: Correlation of glucose regulation and hemoglobin A_{IC} in diabetes mellitus. N. Engl. J. Med. *295*:417, 1976.

Kohne, E., Grosse, H. P., Versmold, K., et al.: Hb M Erlangen: $\alpha_2\beta_2^{63(E7)\ Tyr}$: Eine neue Mutation mit Hämolyse und Diaphorasemangel. Z. Kinderheilkd. *120*:69, 1975.

Kolatat, T.: Oxygen affinity of hemoglobin E. Siriraj Hosp. Gaz. *16*:205, 1964.

Koler, R. D., and Rigas, D. A.: Genetics of haemoglobin H. Ann. Hum. Genet. *25*:95, 1961.

Koler, R. D., Jones, R. T., Wasi, P., and Pootrakul, S.: Genetics of haemoglobin H and α-thalassaemia. Ann. Hum. Genet. *34*:371, 1971.

Koler, R. D., Jones, R. T., Bigley, R. H., et al.: Hemoglobin Casper β106 (G8) Leu→Pro, a contemporary mutation. Am. J. Med. *55*:549, 1973.

Konotey-Ahulu, F. I. D.: Effect of environment on sickle cell disease in West Africa: Epidemiologic and clinical considerations. In Abramson, H., Bertles, J. F., and Wethers, D. L. (eds.): Sickle Cell Disease: Diagnosis, Management, Education and Research. St. Louis, The C. V. Mosby Co., 1973, p. 20.

Konotey-Ahulu, F. I. D.: The sickle cell diseases. Arch. Intern. Med. *133*:611, 1974.

Konotey-Ahulu, F. I. D., Gallo, E., Lehmann, H., et al.: Haemoglobin Korle-Bu (β^{73} Aspartic acid→Asparagine) showing one of the two amino acids substitutions of haemoglobin C Harlem. J. Med. Genet. *5*:107, 1968.

Konotey-Ahulu, F. I. D., Kinderlerer, J. L., Lehmann, H., et al.: Haemoglobin Osu-Christiansborg: A new β-chain variant of haemoglobin A (β^{52} [D3] Aspartic acid→ Asparagine) in combination with haemoglobin S. J. Med. Genet. *8*:302, 1971.

Körber, E.: Inaugural dissertation: "Uber differenzen Blutfarbstoffes." Dorpat, 1866. Cited by Bischoff, H.: Z. Exp. Med. *48*:472, 1926.

Koshland, D. E., Jr., Némethy, G., and Filmer, D.: Comparison of experimental binding data and theoretical models in proteins containing subunits. Biochemistry *5*:365, 1966.

Kostuk, W. J., Suwa, K., Bernstein, E. F., and Sobel, B. E.: Altered hemoglobin oxygen affinity in patients with acute myocardial infarction. Am. J. Cardiol. *31*:295, 1973.

Koutras, G. A., Hattori, M., Schneider, A. S., et al.: Studies on chromated erythrocytes. Effect of sodium chromate on erythrocyte glutathione reductase. J. Clin. Invest. *43*:323. 1964.

Kramer, G., Cimadevilla, J. M., and Hardesty, B.: Specificity of the protein kinase activity associated with the hemin controlled repressor of rabbit reticulocytes. Proc. Natl. Acad. Sci. USA *73*:3078, 1976.

Krantz, S. B.: Recent contributions to the mechanism of action and clinical relevance of erythropoietin. J. Lab. Clin. Med. *82*:847, 1973.

Kraus, A. P., and Diggs, L. W.: In vitro crystallization of hemoglobin occurring in citrated blood from patients with hemoglobin C. J. Lab. Clin. Med. *47*:700, 1956.

Kraus, L. M., Miyaji, T., Iuchi, I., and Kraus, A. P.: Characterization of $\alpha^{23}GluNH_2$ in hemoglobin Memphis. Hemoglobin Memphis/S, a new variant of molecular disease. Biochemistry *5*:3701, 1966.

Kreimer-Birnbaum, M., Pinkerton, P. H., Bannerman, R. M., et al.: Dipyrrolic urinary pigments in congenital Heinz-body anaemia due to Hb Köln and in thalassaemia. Br. Med. J. *2*:396, 1966a.

Kreimer-Birnbaum, M., Pinkerton, P. H., Bannerman, R. M., et al.: Urinary "dipyrroles"; their occurrence and significance in thalassemia and other disorders. Blood *28*:993, 1966b.

Krogh, A.: The number and distribution of capillaries in muscles with calculation of the oxygen pressure head necessary for supplying the tissue. J. Physiol. (London) *52*:409, 1919.

Kunkel, H. G., and Wallenius, G.: New hemoglobins in normal adult blood. Science *122*:288, 1955.

Kunkel, H. G., Ceppellini, R., Müller-Eberhard, U., et al.: Observations on the minor basic hemoglobin components in the blood of normal individuals and patients with thalassemia. J. Clin. Invest. *36*:1615, 1957.

Küster, W.: Beiträge zur Kenntnis des Bilirubins und Hämins. Hoppe-Seyler's Z. Physiol. Chem. *82*:463, 1912.

Kwan, S., and Brawerman, G.: A particle associated with the polyadenylate segment in mammalian messenger RNA. Proc. Natl. Acad. Sci. USA *69*:3247, 1972.

Laforet, M. T., Butterfield, J. B., and Alpers, J. D.: The biosynthesis of 2,3-diphosphoglycerate by monophosphoglycerate mutase from muscle and erythrocytes. Arch. Biochem. Biophys. *165*:179, 1974.

Lane, C. D., Gregory, C. M., Iyazumi, T., and Scherrer, K.: The use of the Xenopus oocyte to prove the existence of messenger sequences in high molecular weight RNA. Nature [New Biol.] *243*:78, 1973.

Lanyon, W. G., Ottolenghi, S., and Williamson, R.: Human globin gene expression and linkage in bone marrow and fetal liver. Proc. Natl. Acad. Sci. USA *72*:258, 1975.

Lassman, M. N., Genel, M., and Wise, J. K.: Carbohydrate homeostasis and pancreatic islet cell function in thalassemia. Ann. Intern. Med. *80*:65, 1974.

Laux, B., Dennis, D., and White, H. B., III: Human α-chain globin messenger: prediction of a nucleotide sequence. Biochem. Biophys. Res. Commun. *54*:894, 1973.

Laver, M. B., Tung, C., Jackson, E., et al.: Effect of benzoic acid derivatives of O_2 affinity of hemoglobin solutions, intact RBCs in vitro and in vivo. Fed. Proc. *33*:335, 1974.

Lawson, W. H., Jr., and Forster, R. E.: Oxygen tension gradients in peripheral capillary blood. J. Appl. Physiol. *22*:970, 1967.

Lebleu, B., Marbaix, G., Huez, G., et al.: Characterization of the messenger ribonucleoprotein released from reticulocyte polyribosomes by EDTA treatment. Eur. J. Biochem. *19*:264, 1971.

LeCrone, C. N.: Absence of special fetal hemoglobin in beagle dogs. Blood *35*:451, 1970.

Lee, C. K., and Manning, J. M.: Kinetics of carbamylation of the amino groups of sickle cell hemoglobin by cyanate. J. Biol. Chem. *248*:5861, 1973.

Lee-Potter, J. P., Deacon-Smith, R. A., Simpkiss, M. J., et al.: A new cause of haemolytic anaemia in the newborn. A description of an unstable fetal haemoglobin: F Poole, $\alpha_2{}^{G}\gamma_2{}^{130\,Trp \rightarrow Gly}$. J. Clin. Pathol. *28*:317, 1975.
Legon, S., Jackson, R. J., and Hunt, T.: Control of protein synthesis in reticulocytes by haemin. Nature [New Biol.] *24*:150, 1973.
Legon, S., Brayley, A., Hunt, T., and Jackson, R. J.: The effect of cyclic AMP and related compounds on the control of protein synthesis in reticulocyte lysates. Biochem. Biophys. Res. Commun. *56*:745, 1974.
Lehmann, H.: Different types of alpha thalassaemia and significance of haemoglobin Bart's in neonates. Lancet *2*:78, 1970.
Lehmann, H., and Carrell, R. W.: Differences between α and β chain mutants of human hemoglobin and between α and β thalassaemia. Possible duplication of the α-chain gene. Br. Med. J. 4:748, 1968.
Lehmann, H., and Carrell, R. W.: Variations in the structure of human haemoglobin with particular reference to the unstable haemoglobins. Br. Med. Bull. *25*:14, 1969.
Lehmann, H., and Charlesworth, D.: Observations on hemoglobin P (Congo type). Biochem. J. *119*:43, 1970.
Lehmann, H., and Huntsman, R. G.: Man's Haemoglobins. 2nd ed. Philadelphia, J. B. Lippincott Co., 1974.
Lehmann, H., Story, P., and Thien, H.: Hemoglobin E in Burmese. Br. Med. J. *1*:544, 1956.
Lehmann, H., Casey, R., Lang, A., et al.: Haemoglobin Tak: a β-chain elongation. Br. J. Haematol. *31*(Suppl.):119, 1975.
Lenfant, C., and Sullivan, K.: Adaptation to high altitude. N. Engl. J. Med. *284*:1298, 1971.
Lenfant, C., Torrance, J., English, E., et al.: Effect of altitude on oxygen binding by hemoglobin and on organic phosphate levels. J. Clin. Invest. *47*:2652, 1968.
Lenfant, C., Torrance, J. D., and Reynafarje, C.: Shift of the O_2-Hb dissociation curve at altitude: Mechanism and effect. J. Appl. Physiol. *30*:625, 1971.
Lessin, L. S., Jensen, W. N., and Ponder, E.: Molecular mechanism of hemolytic anemia in homozygous hemoglobin C disease. J. Exp. Med. *130*:443, 1969.
Levere, R. D., Lichtman, H. C., and Levine, J.: Effect of iron deficiency anaemia on the metabolism of the heterogenic haemoglobins in sickle cell trait. Nature *202*:499, 1964.
Levin, D. H., Ranu, R. S., Ernst, V., et al.: Association of a cyclic AMP-dependent protein kinase with a purified translational inhibitor isolated from hemin-deficient rabbit reticulocyte lysates. Proc. Natl. Acad. Sci. USA *72*:4849, 1975.
Levin, D. H., Ranu, R. S., Ernst, V., et al.: Regulation of protein synthesis in reticulocyte lysates: phosphorylation of methionyl-tRNAf binding factor by protein kinase activity of translational inhibitor isolated from heme-deficient lysates. Proc. Natl. Acad. Sci. USA *73*:3112, 1976.
Lian, C.-Y., and Harkness, D. R.: The kinetic properties of adenylate deaminase from human erythrocytes. Biochim. Biophys. Acta *341*:27, 1974.
Libnoch, J. A., Taketa, F., Mauk, A. G., et al.: Hemoglobin Wood β97 (FG4) His→Leu. Cause of familial erythrocytosis and drug-induced methemoglobinemia. Blood *46*:1030, 1975.
Lichtman, M. A.: Oxygen binding to hemoglobin in hypoproliferative anemia: adaptation to alkalosis, not hemoglobin deficit. Blood *42*:996, 1973.
Lichtman, M. A., and Miller, D. R.: Erythrocyte glycolysis 2,3-diphosphoglycerate and adenosine triphosphate concentration in uremic subjects: Relationship to extracellular phosphate concentration. J. Lab. Clin. Med. *76*:267, 1970.
Lichtman, M. A., Miller, D. R., Cohen, J., et al.: Reduced red cell glycolysis, 2,3-diphosphoglycerate and adenosine triphosphate concentration and increased hemoglobin-oxygen affinity caused by hypophosphatemia. Ann. Intern. Med. *74*:562, 1971.
Lichtman, M. A., Cohen, J., Young, J. A., et al.: The relationships between arterial oxygen flow rate, oxygen binding by hemoglobin and oxygen utilization after myocardial infarction. J. Clin. Invest. *54*:501, 1974a.
Lichtman, M. A., Murphy, M. S., Byer, B. J., and Freeman, R. B.: Hemoglobin affinity for oxygen in chronic renal disease. The effect of hemodialysis. Blood *43*:417, 1974b.

Lichtman, M. A., Murphy, M. S., Whitbeck, A. A., et al.: Oxygen binding to hemoglobin in subjects with hypoproliferative anaemia, with and without chronic renal disease: role of pH. Br. J. Haematol. *27*:438, 1974c.

Lichtman, M. A., Whitbeck, A. A., and Murphy, M.: Fictitious changes in binding of oxygen to hemoglobin when based on extracellular pH in the presence of certain blood additives like radiographic contrast media. Invest. Radiol. *10*:225, 1975.

Liebman, J., Lucas, R., Moss, A., et al.: Airline travel for children with chronic pulmonary disease. Pediatrics *57*:408, 1976.

Lief, P. D., Sullivan, A., and Goldberg, M.: Physiological contributions of thin and thick loops of Henle to the renal concentrating mechanism. J. Clin. Invest. *48*:52(Abst.), 1969.

Lie-Injo, L. E.: Alpha-chain thalassemia and hydrops fetalis in Malaya: report of five cases. Blood *20*:581, 1962.

Lie-Injo, L. E., and Jo, B. H.: A fast-moving haemoglobin in hydrops fetalis. Nature *185*:698, 1960.

Lie-Injo, L. E., Ganesan, J., Clegg, J. B., and Weatherall, D. J.: The homozygous state for Hb Constant Spring. Blood *43*:251, 1974.

Lim, L., and Canellakis, E. S.: Adenine-rich polymer associated with rabbit reticulocyte messenger RNA. Nature *227*:710, 1970.

Lindsay, J., Meshel, J. C., and Patterson, R. M.: The cardiovascular manifestations of sickle cell disease. Arch. Intern. Med. *133*:643, 1974.

Lindstrom, T. R., and Ho., C.: Functional non-equivalence of α and β hemes in human adult hemoglobin. Proc. Natl. Acad. Sci. USA *69*:1707, 1972.

Lindstrom, T. R., Ho, C., and Pisciotta, A. V.: Nuclear magnetic resonance studies of haemoglobin M Milwaukee. Nature [New Biol.] *237*:263, 1972a.

Lindstrom, T. R., Noren, I. B. E., Charache, S., et al.: Nuclear magnetic resonance studies of hemoglobins. VII. Tertiary structure around ligand binding site in carbonmonoxy-hemoglobin. Biochemistry *11*:1677, 1972b.

Lindstrom, T. R., Baldassare, J. J., Bunn, H. F., and Ho., C.: Nuclear magnetic resonance and spin-label studies of hemoglobin Kempsey. Biochemistry. *12*:4212, 1973.

Lindstrom, T. R., Koenig, S. H., Boussios, T., et al.: Intermolecular interactions of oxygenated sickle hemoglobin molecules in cells and cell-free solutions. Biophys. J. *16*:679, 1976.

Lines, J. G., and McIntosh, R.: Oxygen binding by haemoglobin J-Cape Town ($\alpha_2{}^{92}{}_{\mathrm{Arg}\rightarrow\mathrm{Gln}}$). Nature *215*:297, 1967.

Lingrel, J. B., Lockard, R. E., Jones, R. F., et al.: Biologically active messenger RNA for hemoglobin. Ser. Haematol. *4*:37, 1971.

Lipschitz, D. A., Dugard, J., Simon, M. O., et al.: The site of action of desferrioxamine. Br. J. Haematol. *20*:395, 1971.

Lo, H. H., and Schimmel, P. R.: Interaction of human hemoglobin with adenine nucleotides. J. Biol. Chem. *244*:5084, 1969.

Lodish, H. F.: Alpha and beta globin messenger ribonucleic acid: different amounts and rates of initiation of translation. J. Biol. Chem. *246*:7131, 1971.

Lodish, H. F.: Model for the regulation of mRNA translation applied to haemoglobin synthesis. Nature *251*:385, 1974.

Lodish, H. F., and Jacobsen, M.: Regulation of hemoglobin synthesis: equal rates of translation and termination of α- and β-globin chains. J. Biol. Chem. *247*:3622, 1972.

Logothetis, J., Economidou, J., Constantoulakis, M., et al.: Cephalofacial deformities in thalassemia major (Cooley's anemia). Am. J. Dis. Child. *121*:300, 1971.

Logothetis, J., Loewenson, R. B., Augoustaki, O., et al.: Body growth in Cooley's anemia (homozygous beta-thalassemia) with a correlative study as to other aspects of the illness in 138 cases. Pediatrics *50*:92, 1972.

Lokich, J. J., Maloney, W. C., Bunn, H. F., et al.: Hemoglobin Brigham ($\alpha_2{}^{A}\beta_2{}^{100}{}_{\mathrm{Pro}\rightarrow\mathrm{Leu}}$), hemoglobin variant associated with familial erythrocytosis. J. Clin. Invest. *52*:2060, 1973.

Longmuir, I. S., and Bourke, A.: The measurement of the diffusion of oxygen through respiring tissue. Biochem. J. *76*:225, 1960.

Lorkin, P. A.: Fetal and embryonic haemoglobins. J. Med. Genet. *10*:50, 1973.

Lorkin, P. A., and Lehmann, H.: Fetal and embryonic haemoglobins. J. Med. Genet. *10*:50, 1973.

Lorkin, P. A., Lehmann, H., Fairbanks, V. P., et al.: Two new pathological haemoglobins: Olmsted β141 (H19) Leu→Arg and Malmö β97 (FG4) His→Gln. Biochem. J. *119*:68, 1970.

Lorkin, P. A., Stephens, A. D., Beard, M. E. J., et al.: Haemoglobin Rahere (β82 Lys→Thr): a new high affinity haemoglobin associated with decreased 2,3-diphosphoglycerate binding and relative polycythaemia. Br. Med. J. *4*:200, 1975.

Loukopoulos, D., and Fessas, P.: The distribution of hemoglobin types in thalassemic erythrocytes. J. Clin. Invest. *44*:231, 1965.

Lubin, A., and Desforges, J.: Effect of Heinz bodies on red cell deformability. Blood *39*:658, 1972.

Lubin, B. H., Pena, V., Mentzer, W. C., et al.: Dimethyl adipimidate: a new antisickling agent. Proc. Natl. Acad. Sci. USA *72*:43, 1975.

Lucas, W. M., and Bullock, W.: Hematuria in sickle cell disease. J. Urol. *83*:733, 1960.

Luhby, A. L., and Cooperman, J. M.: Folic acid deficiency in thalassaemia major. Lancet *2*:490, 1961.

Luhby, A. L., Cooperman, J. M., Feldman, R., et al.: Folic acid deficiency as a limiting factor in the anemias of thalassemia major. Blood *18*:786, 1961.

Lukanidin, E. M., Georgieo, G. P., and Williamson, R.: A comparative study of the protein components of nuclear and polysomal messenger ribonucleoprotein. FEBS Lett. *19*:152, 1971.

Lukens, J. N., and Neuman, L. A.: Excretion and distribution of iron during chronic deferoxamine therapy. Blood *38*:614, 1971.

Lumeng, L., and Li, T. K.: Vitamin B_6 metabolism in chronic alcohol abuse. Pyridoxal phosphate levels in plasma and the effects of acetaldehyde on pyridoxal phosphate synthesis and degradation in human erythrocytes. J. Clin. Invest. *53*:693, 1974.

Lundh, B., and Gardner, F. H.: The haematological response to androgens in sickle cell anemia. Scand. J. Haematol. *7*:389, 1970.

Luque, J., Diederich, D., and Grisolia, S.: Binding of 2,3-diphosphoglycerate to oxyhemoglobin. Biochem. Biophys. Res. Commun. *36*:1019, 1969.

Lutcher, C. L., Wilson, J. B., Gravely, M. E., et al.: Hb Leslie, an unstable hemoglobin due to deletion of glutaminyl residue β131 (H9) occurring in association with β^0-thalassemia, Hb C and Hb S. Blood *47*:99, 1976.

Lux, S. E., and John, K. M.: The membrane defect in irreversibly sickled red cells (ISC's). Irreversible deformation of the spectrin-actin lattice. Blood *46*:1052, 1975.

Luzzato, L., Nwachuku-Jarrett, E. S., and Reddy, S.: Increased sickling of parasitized erythrocytes as mechanism of resistance against malaria in sickle-cell trait. Lancet *1*:319, 1970.

Macnaughton, M., Freeman, K. B., and Bishop, J. O.: A precursor to hemoglobin mRNA in nuclei of immature duck red blood cells. Cell *1*:117, 1974.

Magdoff-Fairchild, B., Swerdlow, P. H., and Bertles, J. F.: Intermolecular organization of deoxygenated sickle haemoglobin determined by X-ray diffraction. Nature *239*:217, 1972.

Malfa, R., and Steinhardt, J.: A temperature-dependent latent-period in the aggregation of sickle-cell deoxyhemoglobin. Biochem. Biophys. Res. Commun. *59*:887, 1974.

Mann, J. R., and Stuart, J.: Sodium bicarbonate prophylaxis of sickle cell crisis. Pediatrics *53*:414, 1974.

Mann, J. R., MacNeish, A. S., Bannister, D., et al.: δβ-Thalassemia in a Chinese family. Br. J. Haematol. *23*:393, 1972.

Mansbridge, J. N., Crossley, J. A., Lanyon, W. G., and Williamson, R.: The poly (adenylic acid) sequence of mouse globin messenger RNA. Eur. J. Biochem. *44*:261, 1974.

Marbaix, G., Huez, G., Burny, A., et al.: Absence of polyadenylate segment in globin messenger RNA accelerates its degradation in Xenopus oocytes. Proc. Natl. Acad. Sci. USA *72*:3065, 1975.

Marks, P. A., and Rifkind, R. A.: Protein synthesis; its control in erythropoiesis. Science *175*:955, 1972.

Marotta, C. A., Forget, B. G., Weissman, S. M., et al.: Nucleotide sequences of human globin messenger RNA. Proc. Natl. Acad. Sci. USA *71*:2300, 1974.

Marotta, C. A., Forget, B. G., Cohen-Solal, M., et al.: Nucleotide sequence analysis of coding and noncoding regions of human β-globin mRNA. *In* Cohn, W. E. (ed.): Progress in Nucleic Acid Research and Molecular Biology, New York, Academic Press, Vol. 19, p. 165, 1977.

Maroun, L. E., Driscoll, B. F., and Nardone, R. M.: Possible cytoplasmic precursor of haemoglobin messenger RNA. Nature [New Biol.] *231*:270, 1971.

Marti, H. R.: Normale und Anormale Menschliche Hämoglobine. Berlin, Springer Verlag, 1963, p. 81.

Martinez, G., and Colombo, B.: A new type of hereditary persistence of foetal haemoglobin: is a diffusible factor regulating γ-chain synthesis? Nature *252*:735, 1974.

Masys, D. R., Bromberg, P. A., and Balcerzak, S. P.: Red cells shrink during sickling. Blood *44*:885, 1974.

Mathews, M. B., Pragnell, I., Osborn, M., and Arnstein, H.: Stimulation by reticulocyte initiation factors of protein synthesis in a cell-free system from Krebs II ascites cells. Biochim. Biophys. Acta *287*:113, 1972.

Mathews, M. B., Hunt, T., and Brayley, A.: Specificity of the control of protein synthesis by haemin. Nature [New Biol.] *243*:230, 1973.

Mattii, R., Weinger, R., and Sise, H. S.: Coagulation, fibrinogen survival and fibrin split products in sickle cell disease. Blood *42*:1004 (Abst.), 1973.

Maurer, H. S., Behrman, R. E., and Honig, G. R.: Dependence of the oxygen affinity of blood on the presence of foetal or adult hemoglobin. Nature *227*:388, 1970.

Maurer, H. S., Vida, L. N., and Honig, G. R.: Similarities of the erythocytes in juvenile chronic myelogenic leukemia to fetal erythrocytes. Blood *39*:778, 1972.

Maxwell, C., and Rabinovitz, M.: Evidence for an inhibitor in the control of globin synthesis by hemin in a reticulocyte lysate. Biochem. Biophys. Res. Commun. *35*:79, 1969.

Maxwell, C., Kamper, C., and Rabinovitz, M.: Hemin control of globin synthesis: an assay for the inhibitor formed in the absence of hemin and some characteristics of its formation. J. Mol. Biol. *58*:317, 1971.

May, A., and Huehns, E. R.: The control of oxygen affinity of red cells with Hb Shepherds Bush. Br. J. Haematol. *22*:599, 1972a.

May, A., and Huehns, E. R.: The mechanism of the low oxygen affinity of red cells in sickle cell disease. Haematol. Bluttransfus. *10*:279, 1972b.

McCarthy, G. M., Temperley, I. J., Clegg, J. B., and Weatherall, D. J.: Thalassemia in an Irish family. Ir. J. Med. Sci. (7th Series) *1*:303, 1968.

McCormick, D. B., and Snell, E. E.: Pyridoxal phosphokinases. II. Effects of inhibitors. J. Biol. Chem. *236*:2085, 1961.

McCoy, R. C.: Ultrastructural alterations in the kidney of patients with sickle cell disease and the nephrotic syndrome. Lab. Invest. *21*:85, 1969.

McCurdy, P. R.: Clinical and physiological studies in a Negro with sickle cell hemoglobin D disease. N. Engl. J. Med. *262*:961, 1960.

McCurdy, P. R., Lorkin, P. A., Casey, R., et al.: Hemoglobin S-G (S-D) syndrome. Am. J. Med. *57*:665, 1974.

McCurdy, P. R., Sherman, A. S., Kamuzora, H., et al.: Globin synthesis in subjects doubly heterozygous for hemoglobin G Philadelphia and hemoglobin S or C. J. Lab. Clin. Med. *85*:891, 1975.

McDonald, M. J., Noble, R. W., Sharma, V. S., and Ranney, H. M.: Equilibrium and kinetic studies of hemoglobin I: a functionally silent amino acid substitution at an invariant residue. J. Mol. Biol. *89*:245, 1974.

McKeehan, W. L.: Regulation of hemoglobin synthesis. J. Biol. Chem. *249*:6517, 1974.

Melderis, H., Steinheider, G., and Ostertag, W.: Evidence for a unique kind of α-type globin chains in early mammalian embryos. Nature *250*:774, 1974.

Melli, M., and Pemberton, R. E.: New method of studying the precursor-product relationship betwen high molecular weight RNA and messenger RNA. Nature [New Biol.] *236*:172, 1972.

Mentzer, W. C.: Differentiation of iron deficiency from thalassaemia trait. Lancet *1*:882, 1973.

Merkel, C. G., Kwan, S. P., and Lingrel, J. B.: Size of the polyadenylic acid region of newly synthesized globin messenger ribonucleic acid. J. Biol. Chem. *250*:3725, 1975.

Messer, M. J., and Harris, J. W.: Filtration characteristics of sickle cells: Rates of alteration of filterability after deoxygenation, reoxygenation and correlations with sickling and unsickling. J. Lab. Clin. Med. *76*:537, 1970.

Messer, M. J., Hahn, J. A., and Bradley, T. B.: The kinetics of sickling and unsickling of red cells under physiologic conditions: rheologic and ultrastructural correlations. Presented at Symposium on Molecular and Cellular Aspects of Sickle Cell Disease., December 10, 1975. DHEW Publ. No. (NIH)76-1007.

Metafora, S., Terada, M., Dow, L. W., et al.: Increased efficiency of exogenous messenger RNA translation in a Krebs ascites cell lysate. Proc. Natl. Acad. Sci. USA *69*:1299, 1972.

Miller, D. R., Weed, R. I., Stamatoyannopoulos, G., and Yoshida, A.: Hemoglobin Köln disease occurring as a fresh mutation: Erythrocyte metabolism and survival. Blood *38*:715, 1971.

Miller, L. D., Oski, F. A., Diaco, J. F., et al.: The affinity of hemoglobin for oxygen: its control and in vivo significance. Surgery *68*:187, 1970.

Miller, M. E., Rørth, M., Parving, H. H., et al.: pH effect of erythropoietin response to hypoxia. N. Engl. J. Med. *288*:706, 1973.

Miller, W. W., Delivoria-Papadopoulos, M., Miller, L., and Oski, F. A.: Oxygen releasing factor in hyperthyroidism. JAMA *211*:1824, 1970.

Mills, G. C., Bowman, A. B., and Johnson, J. E.: Effects of triiodothyronine on glutathione and phosphate esters of human erythrocytes. Tex. Rep. Biol. Med. *24*:629, 1966.

Mills, G. C., Levin, W. C., and Alperin, J. B.: Hemolytic anemia associated with low erythrocyte ATP. Blood *32*:15, 1968.

Milner, P. F.: The sickling disorders. Clin. Haematol. *3*:289, 1974.

Milner, P. F., Miller, C., Grey, R., et al.: Hemoglobin O Arab in four Negro families and its interaction with hemoglobin S and hemoglobin C. N. Engl. J. Med. *283*:1417, 1970.

Milner, P. F., Clegg, J. B., and Weatherall, D. J.: Haemoglobin H disease due to a unique haemoglobin variant with an elongated α-chain. Lancet *1*:729, 1971.

Milosz, A., and Settle, W.: A new approach to the treatment of sickle cell anemia. Res. Commun. Chem. Pathol. Pharmacol. *12*:137, 1975.

Minikami, S.: Effect of oxygen tension on glycolysis in erythrocytes. Försvarsmedicin 5:181, 1969.

Minnich, V., Hill, R. J., Khuri, P. D., and Anderson, M. E.: Hemoglobin Hope: A beta chain variant. Blood *25*:830, 1965.

Mitchell, T. R., and Pegrum, G. D.: The oxygen affinity in chronic renal failure. Br. J. Haematol. *21*:463, 1971.

Mizuno, S., Fisher, J., and Rabinovitz, M.: Hemin control of globin synthesis: Action of an inhibitor formed in the absence of hemin on the reticulocyte cell-free system and its reversal by a ribosomal factor. Biochim. Biophys. Acta *272*:638, 1972.

Modell, C. B., and Beck, J.: Long-term desferrioxamine therapy in thalassemia. Ann. NY Acad. Sci. *232*:201, 1974.

Modell, C. B., Latter, A., Steadman, J. H., et al.: Haemoglobin synthesis in β-thalassaemia. Br. J. Haematol. *17*:485, 1969.

Moffat, K.: Gelation of sickle cell hemoglobin: effects of hybrid tetramer formation in hemoglobin mixtures. Science *185*:274, 1974.

Moffat, K., and Gibson, Q. H.: The rates of polymerization and depolymerization of sickle cell hemoglobin. Biochem. Biophys. Res. Commun. *61*:237, 1974.

Molinari, P. F., Chung, S. K., and Snyder, L. M.: Variations of erythrocyte glycolysis following androgens. J. Lab. Clin. Med. *81*:443, 1973.

Monn, E., and Bjark, P.: Hb Sögn (β14 arginine). Haematological and genetical studies. Scand. J. Haematol. *7*:455, 1970.

Monn, E., Gaffney, P. J., Jr., and Lehmann, H.: Haemoglobin Sögn (β14 arginine). A new haemoglobin variant. Scand. J. Haematol. *5*:353, 1968.

Monod, J., Wyman, J., and Changeux, J. P.: On the nature of allosteric transitions: A plausible model. J. Mol. Biol. *12*:88, 1965.

Monte, M., Beuzard, U., and Rosa, J.: Mapping of several abnormal hemoglobins by horizontal polyacrylamide gel isoelectric focusing. Am. J. Clin. Path. *66*:753, 1976.

Monti, M.: Red cell 2,3-diphosphoglycerate in patients with hyperthyroidism before and after treatment. Acta Med. Scand. *196*:263, 1974.

Moo-Penn, W., Bechtel, K., Jue, M. S., et al.: The presence of hemoglobin S and C-Harlem in an individual in the United States. Blood *46*:363, 1975.

Morel, C., Kayibanda, B., and Scherrer, K.: Proteins associated with globin messenger RNA in avian erythroblasts: isolation and comparison with proteins bound to nuclear messenger-like RNA. FEBS Lett. *18*:84, 1971.

Morel, C., Gander, E. S., Herzberg, M., et al.: The duck-globin messenger-ribonucleoprotein complex. Eur. J. Biochem. *36*:455, 1973.

Morell, S. A., Ayers, V. A., Hoffman, P., and Taketa, F.: Reversible changes in the NEM-reactive SH groups of hemoglobin on oxygenation-deoxygenation. Proc. Natl. Acad. Sci. USA *48*:1057, 1962.

Morimoto, H., Lehmann, H., and Perutz, M. F.: Molecular pathology of human haemoglobin: Stereochemical interpretation of abnormal oxygen affinities. Nature *232*:408, 1971.

Morrison, M. R., Merkel, C. G., and Lingrel, J. B.: Size of the poly (A) region in mouse globin messenger RNA. Mol. Biol. Rep. *1*:55, 1973.

Morrison, M. R., Brinkley, S. A., Gorski, J., and Lingrel, J. B.: The separation and identification of α- and β-globin messenger ribonucleic acids. J. Biol. Chem. *249*:5290, 1974.

Moser, K. M., and Shea, J. C. L.: The relationship between pulmonary infarction, cor pulmonale and sickle states. Am. J. Med. *22*:561, 1957.

Mostofi, F. K., and Bruegge, C. F.V.: Lesions in kidneys removed for unilateral hematuria in sickle cell disease. Arch. Pathol. *63*:336, 1957.

Motulsky, A. G.: Frequency of sickling disorders in U.S. Blacks. N. Engl. J. Med. *288*:31, 1973.

Muirhead, H., et al.: Structure and function of haemoglobin. III. A three-dimensional Fourier synthesis of human deoxyhaemoglobin at 5.5 Ångström resolution. J. Mol. Biol. *28*:117, 1967.

Mulhausen, R., Astrup, P., and Kjeldsen, K.: Oxygen affinity of hemoglobin in patients with cardiovascular diseases, anemia, and cirrhosis of the liver. Scand. J. Clin. Lab. Invest. *19*:291, 1967.

Muller, C. J., and Kingma, S.: Haemoglobin Zürich, $\alpha_2{}^A\beta_2{}^{63\ Arg}$. Biochim. Biophys. Acta *50*:595, 1961.

Murayama, M.: Molecular mechanism of red cell "sickling." Science *153*:145, 1966.

Murayama, M., in Nalbandian, R. M. (ed.): Molecular Aspects of Sickle Cell Hemoglobin. Springfield, Illinois, Charles C Thomas, 1971.

Murphy, J. R.: Hemoglobin CC disease: rheological properties of erythrocytes and abnormalities in cell water. J. Clin. Invest. *47*:1483, 1968.

Murphy, J. R.: Sickle cell hemoglobin (Hb AS) in black football players. JAMA *225*:981, 1973.

Murphy, J. R., Wengerd, M., and Kellermeyer, R. W.: Erythrocyte O_2 affinity: influence of cell density and *in vitro* changes in hemoglobin concentration. J. Lab. Clin. Med. *84*:218, 1974.

Nagel, R. L., and Bookchin, R. M.: The effect of 2,3-diphosphoglycerate on gelation of hemoglobin S and its molecular mechanism. Clin. Res. *22*:399A, 1974a.

Nagel, R. L., and Bookchin, R. M.: Human hemoglobin mutants with abnormal oxygen binding. Semin. Hematol. *11*:385, 1974b.

Nagel, R. L., and Gibson, Q. H.: The binding of hemoglobin to haptoglobin in its relation to subunit dissociation of hemoglobin. J. Biol. Chem. *246*:69, 1971.

Nagel, R. L., and Gibson, Q. H.: The hemoglobin-haptoglobin reaction as a probe of hemoglobin conformation. Biochem. Biophys. Res. Commun. *48*:959, 1972.

Nagel, R. L., Rothman, M. C., Bradley, T. B., and Ranney, H. M.: Comparative haptoglobin binding properties of oxyhemoglobin and deoxyhemoglobin. J. Biol. Chem. *240*:PC4543, 1965.

Nagel, R. L., Gibson, Q. H., and Charache, S.: Relation between structure and function in hemoglobin Chesapeake. Biochemistry *6*:2395, 1967.

Nagel, R. L., Ranney, H. M., Bradley, T. B., Jr., et al.: Hemoglobin L Ferrara trait in a Jewish family associated with a hemolytic state in the propositus. Blood *34*:157, 1969.

Nagel, R. L., Lynfield, J., Johnson, J., et al.: Hemoglobin Beth Israel: A mutant causing clinically apparent cyanosis. N. Engl. J. Med. *295*:125, 1976.

Najman, A., Duhamel, G., Andre, R., et al.: Hemolytic anemia due to unstable hemoglobin with deletion. Study of 2 new cases—Hb Tours (Thr β87 deleted) and Hb St. Antoine (Gly→Leu β74, 75 deleted). Nouv. Rev. Fr. Hematol. *13*:803, 1973.

Na-Nakorn, S., and Wasi, P.: Alpha-thalassemia in Northern Thailand. Am. J. Hum. Genet. *22*:645, 1970.

Na-Nakorn, S., Wasi, P., Pornpatkul, M., et al.: Further evidence for a genetic basis of haemoglobin H disease from newborn offspring of patients. Nature *223*:59, 1969.

Nance, W. E., Conneally, M., Kang, K. W., et al.: Genetic linkage analysis of human hemoglobin variants. Am. J. Hum. Genet. *22*:453, 1970.

Nathan, D. G.: Thalassemia. N. Engl. J. Med. *286*:586, 1972.
Nathan, D. G.: Thalassemia: a progress report in applied molecular biology. N. Engl. J. Med. *288*:1122, 1973.
Nathan, D. G., and Alter, B. P.: Antenatal diagnosis of the haemoglobinopathies. Br. J. Haematol. *31*(Suppl.):143, 1975.
Nathan, D. G., and Gunn, R. B.: Thalassemia: the consequences of unbalanced hemoglobin synthesis. Am. J. Med. *41*:815, 1966.
Nathan, D. G., and Oski, F. A. (eds.): Hematology of Infancy and Childhood. Philadelphia, W. B. Saunders Co., 1971.
Nathan, D. G., Stossel, T. B., Gunn, R. B., et al.: Influence of hemoglobin precipitation on erythrocyte metabolism in alpha and beta thalassemia. J. Clin. Invest. *48*:33, 1969.
Nathan, D. G., Lodish, H., Kan, Y. M., and Housman, D.: Beta thalassemia and translation of globin messenger RNA. Proc. Natl. Acad. Sci. USA *68*:2514, 1971.
Natta, C. L., Banks, J., Niazi, G., et al.: Decreased β-globin mRNA activity in bone marrow cells in homozygous and heterozygous β-thalassaemia. Nature [New Biol.] *244*:280, 1973a.
Natta, C. L., Niazi, G., Ford, S., et al.: Balanced globin chain synthesis in hereditary persistence of fetal hemoglobin (HPFH). Blood *42*:991, 1973b.
Necheles, T. F., Allen, D. M., and Finkel, H. E.: Clinical Disorders of Hemoglobin Structure and Synthesis. New York, Appleton-Century-Crofts, 1969a.
Necheles, T. F., Beard, M. E. J., and Allen, D. M.: Myocardial hemosiderosis in hypoxic mice. Ann NY Acad. Sci. *165*:167, 1969b.
Necheles, T. F., Sabbah, R., and Chung, S., et al.: Intensive transfusion therapy in thalassemia major. An eight year follow-up. Ann NY Acad. Sci. *232*:179, 1974.
Neel, J. V.: The clinical detection of the genetic carriers of inherited disease. Medicine (Baltimore) *26*:115, 1947.
Neel, J. V.: The inheritance of sickle cell anemia. Science *110*:64, 1949.
Neel, J. V.: The inheritance of the sickling phenomenon, with particular reference to sickle cell disease. Blood *6*:389, 1951.
Neer, E. J., and Konigsberg, W.: The characterization of modified human hemoglobin. II. Reaction with 1-fluoro-2,4-dinitrobenzene. J. Biol. Chem. *243*:1966, 1968.
Newman, D. R., Pierre, R. V., and Linman, J. W.: Studies on the diagnostic significance of hemoglobin F levels. Mayo Clin. Proc. *48*:199, 1973.
Nienhuis, A. W., and Anderson, W. F.: Isolation and translation of hemoglobin messenger RNA from thalassemia, sickle cell anemia and normal human reticulocytes. J. Clin. Invest. *50*:2458, 1971.
Nienhuis, A. W., and Bunn, H. F.: Hemoglobin switching in sheep and goats: Occurrence of hemoglobins A and C in the same red cell. Science *185*:946, 1974.
Nienhuis, A. W., Laycock, D. G., and Anderson, W. F.: Translation of rabbit haemoglobin messenger RNA by thalassaemic and non-thalassaemic ribosomes. Nature [New Biol.] *231*:205, 1971.
Nienhuis, A. W., Canfield, P. H., and Anderson, W. F.: Hemoglobin messenger RNA from human bone marrow: isolation and translation in homozygous and heterozygous β-thalassemia. J. Clin. Invest. *52*:1735, 1973.
Nienhuis, A. W., Delea, C., Aamodt, R., et al.: Potential role for desferrioxamine and ascorbic acid in the treatment of chronic iron overload. Blood *46*:1026(Abst.), 1975.
Nigen, A. M., Njikam, N., Lee, C. K., and Manning, J. M.: Studies on mechanism of action of cyanate in sickle cell disease. Oxygen affinity and gelling properties of hemoglobin S carbamylated on specific chains. J. Biol. Chem. *249*:6611, 1974.
Nishikura, K., Sugita, Y., Nagai, M., et al.: High cooperativity of haemoglobin M Boston in the completely reduced state. Nature *254*:727, 1975.
Noble, R. W.: Relation between allosteric effects and changes in the energy of bonding between molecular subunits. J. Mol. Biol. *39*:479, 1969.
Novy, M. J., and Parer, J. T.: Absence of high blood oxygen affinity in the fetal cat. Respir. Physiol. *6*:144, 1969.
Novy, M. J., Edwards, M. J., and Metcalfe, J.: Hemoglobin Yakima. II. High blood oxygen affinity associated with compensatory erythrocytosis and normal hemodynamics. J. Clin. Invest. *46*:1848, 1967.
Nudel, U., Lebleu, B., Zchavi-Willner, T., and Revel, M.: Messenger ribonucleoprotein and initiation factors in rabbit-reticulocyte polyribosomes. Eur. J. Biochem. *33*:314, 1973.

Nute, P. E., et al.: Multiple hemoglobin α-chain loci in monkeys, apes, and man. Ann. NY Acad. Sci. *241*:39, 1974a.

Nute, P. E., Stamatoyannopoulos, G., Hermodson, M. A., and Roth, D.: Hemoglobinopathic erythrocytosis due to a new electrophoretically silent variant, Hemoglobin San Diego (β109 (G11) Val→Met). J. Clin. Invest. *53*:320, 1974b.

Nute, P. E., Wood, W. G., Stamatoyannopoulos, G., et al.: The Kenya form of hereditary persistence of fetal haemoglobin: structural studies and evidence for homogeneous distribution of haemoglobin F using fluorescent anti-haemoglobin F antibodies. Br. J. Haematol. *32*:55, 1976.

O'Brien, R. T.: The effect of iron deficiency on the expression of hemoglobin H. Blood *41*:853, 1973.

O'Brien, R. T.: Ascorbic acid enhancement of desferrioxamine-induced urinary iron excretion in thalassemia major. Ann. NY Acad. Sci. *232*:221, 1974.

O'Brien, R. T., and Pearson, H. A.: Splenic function and hematologic changes during the first year of life in sickle cell anemia. In Hercules, J. I., Schechter, A. N., Eaton, W. A., et al. (eds.): Proceedings of First National Symposium on Sickle Cell Disease, Washington, D.C. DHEW Pub. No. 75–723 (NIH), Bethesda, Md., 1974, p. 73.

O'Brien, R. T., Pearson, H. A., and Spencer, R. P.: Transfusion-induced decrease in spleen size in thalassemia major: documentation by radioisotopic scan. J. Pediatr. *81*:105, 1972.

Oelshlegel, F. J., Brewer, G. J., Prasad, A. S., et al.: Effect of zinc on increasing oxygen affinity of sickle and normal red blood cells. Biochem. Biophys. Res. Commun. *53*:560, 1973.

Ogata, R., and McConnell, H. M.: The binding of a spin-labeled triphosphate to hemoglobin. Cold Spring Harbor Symp. Quant. Biol. *36*:325, 1971.

Ogata, R., and McConnell, H. M.: Mechanism of cooperative oxygen binding to hemoglobin. Proc. Natl. Acad. Sci. USA *69*:334, 1972.

Ogata, R. T., McConnell, H. M., and Jones, R. T.: Binding of triphosphate spin labels to hemoglobin Kempsey. Biochem. Biophys. Res. Commun. *47*:157, 1972.

Ogawa, S., Mayer, A., and Shulman, R. G.: High resolution proton magnetic resonance study of the two quaternary states in fully ligated hemoglobin Kansas. Biochem. Biophys. Res. Commun. *49*:1485, 1972.

O'Gorman, P., Allsopp, K. M., Lehmann, H., and Sukumaran, P. K.: Sickle-cell haemoglobin K disease. Br. Med. J. *2*:1381, 1963.

Ohta, Y., Yamaoka, K., Sumida, I., et al.: Two unique structural and synthetic variants, Hb Miyada and homozygous δ-thalassemia, discovered in Japanese. XIII International Congress of Haematology, Munich. Abstracts, Munich, R. F. Lehmanns Verlag, 1970, p. 233.

Ohta, Y., Yamaoka, K., Sumida, I., et al.: Haemoglobin Miyada, a β-δ fusion peptide (anti-Lepore) type discovered in a Japanese family. Nature [New Biol.] *234*:218, 1971.

Olsen, G. D., Gaskill, P., and Kabat, D.: Presence of hemoglobin messenger ribonucleoprotein in a reticulocyte supernatant fraction. Biochim. Biophys. Acta *272*:297, 1972.

Olson, J. S., and Gibson, Q. H.: The functional properties of hemoglobin Bethesda ($\alpha_2\beta_2{}^{145\ His}$). J. Biol. Chem. *247*:3662, 1972.

Olson, J. S., Gibson, Q. H., Nagel, R. L., et al.: The ligand-binding properties of hemoglobin Hiroshima ($\alpha_2\beta_2{}^{146\ Asp}$). J. Biol. Chem. *247*:7485, 1972.

Opalinski, A., and Beutler, E.: Creatine, 2,3-diphosphoglycerate and anemia. N. Engl. J. Med. *285*:483, 1971.

Opfell, R. W., Lorkin, P. A., and Lehmann, H.: Hereditary non-spherocytic haemolytic anaemia with post-splenectomy inclusion bodies and pigmenturia caused by an unstable haemoglobin Santa Ana—β88 (F4) leucine→proline. J. Med. Genet. *5*:292, 1968.

Oski, F. A., and Gottlieb, A. J.: The interrelationships between red blood cell metabolites, hemoglobin and the oxygen-equilibrium curve. Progr. Hematol. *7*:33, 1971.

Oski, F. A., Viner, E. D., Purugganan, H. B., and McElfresh, A. E.: Low molecular weight dextran in sickle cell crisis. JAMA *191*:43, 1965.

Oski, F. A., Call, F. L., and Lessen, L.: Failure of promazine HCl to prevent the painful episodes in sickle cell anemia. J. Pediatr. *73*:265, 1968.

Oski, F. A., Gottlieb, A. J., Delivoria-Papadopoulos, M., and Miller, W. W.: Red-cell 2,3-diphosphoglycerate levels in subjects with chronic hypoxemia. N. Engl. J. Med. *280*:1165, 1969.
Oski, F. A., Gottlieb, A. J., Miller, W. W., et al.: The effects of deoxygenation of adult and fetal hemoglobin on the synthesis of red cell 2,3-diphosphoglycerate and its in vivo consequences. J. Clin. Invest. *49*:400, 1970.
Oski, F. A., Marshall, B. E., Cohen, P. F., et al.: Exercise with anemia. The role of the left-shifted or right-shifted oxygen-hemoglobin equilibrium curve. Ann. Intern. Med. *74*:44, 1971a.
Oski, F. A., Travis, S. F., Miller, L. D., et al.: The in vitro restoration of red cell 2,3-diphosphoglycerate levels in banked blood. Blood *37*:52, 1971b.
Oski, F. A., Miller, L. D., Delivoria-Papadopoulos, M., et al.: Oxygen affinity in red cells: changes induced in vivo by propranolol. Science *175*:1372, 1972.
Oster, J. R., Lee, S. M., Lespier, L. E., et al.: Renal acidification in sickle-cell trait. Arch. Intern. Med. *136*:30, 1976.
Ostertag, W., Melderis, H., Steinheider, G., et al.: Synthesis of mouse haemoglobin and globin mRNA in leukaemic cell cultures. Nature [New Biol.] *239*:231, 1972a.
Ostertag, W., von Ehrenstein, G., and Charache, S.: Duplicated α-chain genes in Hopkins-2 haemoglobin of man and evidence for unequal crossing-over between them. Nature [New Biol.] *237*:90, 1972b.
Ottolenghi, S., Lanyon, W. G., Paul, J., et al.: The severe form of α-thalassaemia is caused by a haemoglobin gene deletion. Nature *251*:389, 1974.
Ottolenghi, S., Lanyon, W. G., Williamson, R., et al.: Human globin gene analysis for a patient with $\beta^0/\delta\beta^0$-thalassemia. Proc. Natl. Acad. Sci. USA *72*:2294, 1975.
Ottolenghi, S., Comi, P., Giglioni, B., et al.: $\delta\beta$-thalassemia is due to a gene deletion. Cell *9*:71, 1976.
Overly, W. L., Rosenberg, A., and Harris, J. W.: Hemoglobin M Reserve: studies on identification and characterization. J. Lab. Clin. Med. *69*:62, 1967.
Özsoylu, S.: Homozygous hemoglobin D-Punjab. Acta Haematol. (Basel) *43*:353, 1970.
Packman, S., Aviv, H., Ross, J., and Leder, P.: A comparison of globin genes in duck reticulocytes and liver cells. Biochem. Biophys. Res. Commun. *49*:813, 1972.
Padilla, F., Bromberg, P. A., and Jensen, W. N.: The sickle-unsickle cycle: a cause of fragmentation leading to permanently deformed cells. Blood *41*:653, 1973.
Pagnier, J., Labie, D., Kaplan, J. C., et al.: Étude biochimique d'un cas d'érythroleucémie. Nouv. Rev. Fr. Hematol. *12*:317, 1972.
Pagnier, J., Wajcman, H., and Labie, D.: Defect in hemoglobin synthesis possibly due to a disturbed association. FEBS Lett. *45*:252, 1974.
Palek, J.: Calcium accumulation during sickling of hemoglobin S (HbSS) red cells. Blood *42*:988, 1973.
Palek, J., Mirčevová, A., and Brabec, V.: 2,3-Diphosphoglycerate metabolism in hereditary spherocytosis. Br. J. Haematol. *17*:59, 1969.
Palek, J., Church, A., and Fairbanks, G.: Trans-membrane movements and distribution of calcium in normal and hemoglobin S erythrocytes. In Leaf, A.,Hoffman, J. F., and Bolis, L. (eds.): Membranes and Diseases. Proceedings of International Conference on Biological Membranes. Craus-sur-Sierre, Switzerland, 1975.
Paniker, N. V., Ben-Bassat, I., and Beutler, E.: Evaluation of sickle hemoglobin and desickling agents by falling ball viscometry. J. Lab. Clin. Med. *80*:282, 1972.
Pardo, V., Strauss, J., Kramer, H., et al.: Nephropathy associated with sickle cell anemia: an autologous immune complex nephritis. Am. J. Med. *59*:650, 1975.
Park, C. M.: Isoelectric focusing and the study of interacting protein systems: ligand binding, phosphate binding and subunit exchange in hemoglobin. Ann NY Acad. Sci. *209*:237, 1973.
Parker, J. C.: Influence of 2,3-diphosphoglycerate metabolism on sodium-potassium permeability in human red blood cells: studies with bisulfite and other redox reagents. J. Clin. Invest. *48*:117, 1969.
Parker, J. P., Beirne, G. J., Desai, J. N., et al.: Androgen-induced increase in red-cell 2,3-diphosphoglycerate. N. Engl. J. Med. *287*:381, 1972.
Pataryas, H. A., and Stamatoyannopoulos, G.: Hemoglobins in human fetuses; evidence for adult hemoglobin production after the 11th gestational week. Blood *39*:688, 1972.
Paul, J., Gilmour, R. S., Affara, N., et al.: The globin gene: structure and expression. Cold Spring Harbor Symp. Quant. Biol. *38*:885, 1973.

Pauling, L., and Corey, R. B.: Atomic coordinates and structure factors for two helical configurations of polypeptide chains. Proc. Natl. Acad. Sci. USA *37*:235, 1951.

Pauling, L., Itano, H. A., Singer, S. J., and Wells, I. C.: Sickle cell anemia: A molecular disease. Science *110*:543, 1949.

Paulsen, E. P.: Hemoglobin A_{Ic} in childhood diabetes. Metabolism *22*:269, 1973.

Pearson, H. A.: Hemoglobin S–thalassemia syndrome in Negro children. Ann. NY Acad. Sci. *165*:83, 1969.

Pearson, H. A.: Progress in early diagnosis of sickle cell disease. Children *18*:222, 1971.

Pearson, H. A.: Sickle cell anemia: Clinical managment during the early years of life. In Abramson, H., Bertles, J. F., and Wethers, D. L. (eds.): Sickle Cell Disease, Diagnosis, Management, Education and Research. St. Louis, The C. V. Mosby Co., 1973, p. 244.

Pearson, H. A.: Routine screening of umbilical cord blood for sickle cell diseases. JAMA *227*:420, 1974.

Pearson, H. A.: O_2 dissociation and RBC 2,3-DPG in thalassemia. Blood *46*:1027, 1975.

Pearson, H. A., and Moore, M. M.: Human hemoglobin gene linkage: report of a family with hemoglobin β_2, hemoglobin S and β-thalassemia, including a probable crossover between thalassemia and the delta loci. Am. J. Hum. Genet. *17*:125, 1965.

Pearson, H. A., and Noyes, W. D.: Failure of phenothiazines in sickle cell anemia. JAMA *199*:33, 1967.

Pearson, H. A., Cornelius, E. A., Schwartz, A. D., et al.: Transfusion-reversible functional asplenia in young children with sickle-cell anemia. N. Engl. J. Med. *283*:334, 1970.

Pearson, H. A., O'Brien, R. T., and McIntosh, S.: Screening for thalassemia trait by electronic measurement of mean corpuscular volume (MCV). N. Engl. J. Med. *288*:351, 1973.

Pederson, P. R., McCurdy, P. R., Wrightstone, R. N., et al.: Hemoglobin Köln in a Black: Pre- and post-splenectomy red cell survival ($DF^{32}P$ and ^{51}Cr) and the pathogenesis of hemoglobin instability. Blood *42*:771, 1973.

Pemberton, R. E., and Baglioni, C.: Duck hemoglobin messenger RNA contains a polynucleotide sequence rich in adenylic acid. J. Mol. Biol. *65*:531, 1972.

Pemberton, R. E., and Baglioni, C.: Newly synthesized polyribosomal RNA of duck erythroid cells. J. Mol. Biol. *81*:255, 1973.

Pembrey, M. E., Weatherall, D. J., and Clegg, J. B.: Maternal synthesis of haemoglobin F in pregnancy. Lancet *1*:1350, 1973.

Pendleton, R. G., Newman, D. J., Sherman, S. S., et al.: Effect of propranolol upon the hemoglobin-oxygen dissociation curve. J. Pharmacol. Exp. Ther. *180*:647, 1972.

Perella, M., Bresciani, D., and Rossi-Bernardi, L.: The binding of CO_2 to human hemoglobin. J. Biol. Chem. *250*:5413, 1975.

Perillie, P. E., and Epstein, F. H.: Sickling phenomenon produced by hypertonic solutions: a possible explanation for the hyposthenuria of sicklemia. J. Clin. Invest. *42*:570, 1963.

Perrine, R. P.: Cholelithiasis in sickle cell anemia in a Caucasian population. Am. J. Med. *54*:327, 1973.

Perutz, M. F.: Stereochemistry of cooperative effects in haemoglobin. Nature *228*:726, 1970a.

Perutz, M. F.: The Bohr effect and combination with organic phosphates. Nature *228*:734, 1970b.

Perutz, M. F.: Sir Lawrence Bragg. N. Scient. Sci. J. July 8, 1971, p. 67.

Perutz, M. F.: Nature of haem-haem interaction. Nature [New Biol.] *237*:495, 1972.

Perutz, M. F.: Stereochemical interpretation of high oxygen affinity of haemoglobin Little Rock ($\alpha_2\beta_2$ 143 His→Glu). Nature [New Biol.] *243*:180, 1973.

Perutz, M. F.: Mechanism of denaturation of haemoglobin by alkali. Nature *247*:341, 1974.

Perutz, M. F., and Lehmann, H.: Molecular pathology of human haemoglobin. Nature *219*:902, 1968.

Perutz, M. F., and Mazzarella, L.: A preliminary X-ray analysis of haemoglobin H. Nature *199*:639, 1963.

Perutz, M. F., and Mitchison, J. M.: State of haemoglobin in sickle cell anaemia. Nature *166*:677, 1950.

Perutz, M. F., Pulsinelli, P., Ten Eyck, L., et al.: Haemoglobin Hiroshima and the mechanism of the alkaline Bohr effect. Nature [New Biol.] *232*:147, 1971.

Perutz, M. F., Pulsinelli, P. D., and Ranney, H. M.: Structure and subunit interaction of haemoglobin M Milwaukee. Nature [New Biol.] *237*:259, 1972.

Perutz, M. F., Ladner, J. E., Simon, S. R., and Ho, C.: Influence of globin structure on the state of the heme. Biochemistry *13*:2163, 1974a.

Perutz, M. F., Fersht, A. R., Simon, S. R., and Roberts, G. C. K.: Influence of globin structure on the state of the heme. II. Allosteric transitions in methemoglobin. Biochemistry *13*:2174, 1974b.

Peters, R. A.: Chemical nature of specific oxygen capacity in haemoglobin. J. Physiol. (London) *44*:131, 1912.

Peterson, C. M., Graziano, J. H., de Ciutiis, A., et al.: Metal metabolism, sickle cell disease and response to cyanate. Blood *44*:945(Abst.), 1974a.

Peterson, C. M., de Ciutiis, A. C., and Cerami, A.: Sodium cyanate and sickle cell disease: efficacy vs. toxicity. In Hercules, J. I., Schechter, A. N., Eaton, W. A., et al. (eds.): Proceedings of First National Symposium on Sickle Cell Disease, Washington, D.C. DHEW Pub. No. 75–723 (NIH), Bethesda, Md., 1974b, pp. 37–38.

Peterson, C. M., Tsairis, P., Ohnishi, A., et al.: Sodium cyanate induced polyneuropathy in patients with sickle cell disease. Ann. Intern. Med. *81*:152, 1974c.

Pietschmann, H., Kolarz, G., and Singer, F.: Zytochemische Untersuchungen bei einer neuen Hämoglobinopathie (Hämoglobin Wien). Wien Klin. Wochenschr. *83*:362, 1971.

Piomelli, S., Danoff, S. J., Becker, M. H., et al.: Prevention of bone malformations and cardiomegaly in Cooley's anemia by early hypertransfusion regimen. Ann. NY Acad. Sci. *165*:427, 1969.

Piomelli, S., Reindorf, C. A., Arzanian, M. T., et al.: Clinical and biochemical interactions of glucose-6-phosphate dehydrogenase deficiency and sickle-cell anemia. N. Engl. J. Med. *287*:213, 1972.

Piomelli, S., Becker, M., Arzanian, M. T., et al.: Early hypertransfusion regimen in patients with Cooley's anemia. Ann. NY Acad. Sci. *232*:186, 1974.

Pisciotta, A. V., Ebbe, S. N., and Hinz, J. E.: Clinical and laboratory features of two variants of methemoglobin M disease. J. Lab. Clin. Med. *54*:73, 1959.

Pitcock, J. A., Muirhead, E. E., Hatch, F. E., et al.: Early renal changes in sickle cell anemia. Arch. Pathol. *90*:403, 1970.

Ponka, P., and Neuwirt, J.: Haem synthesis and iron uptake by reticulocytes. Br. J. Haematol. *28*:1, 1974.

Pootrakul, S., Wasi, P., and Na-Nakorn, S.: Haemoglobin Bart's hydrops foetalis in Thailand. Ann. Hum. Genet. *30*:203, 1967a.

Pootrakul, S., Wasi, P., and Na-Nakorn, S.: Studies on haemoglobin Bart's (Hb-γ^4) in Thailand: the incidence and the mechanism of occurrence in cord blood. Ann. Hum. Genet. *31*:149, 1967b.

Pootrakul, S., Wasi, P., Pornpatkul, M., et al.: Incidence of alpha thalassemia in Bangkok. J. Med. Assn. Thai. *53*:250, 1970.

Pootrakul, S., Wasi, P., and Na-Nakorn, S., et al.: Haematological data in 312 cases of β-thalassaemia trait in Thailand. Br. J. Haematol. *24*:703, 1973.

Pootrakul, S., Pongsamart, S., Prawatmuang, P., et al.: Hb Constant Spring: degradation and Hb synthesis studies. Proceedings of the 16th International Congress of Hematology, Kyoto, Japan, 1976. Excerpta Medica (in press).

Portnoy, B. A., and Herion, J. C.: Neurological manifestations in sickle-cell disease; with a review of the literature and emphasis on the prevalence of hemiplegia. Ann. Inter. Med. *76*:643, 1972.

Powars, D. R.: The natural history of sickle cell disease—the first ten years. Semin. Hematol. *12*:267, 1975.

Power, H. W.: A model of how the sickle-cell gene produces malaria resistance. J. Theor. Biol. *50*:121, 1975.

Pragnell, I. R., and Arnstein, H. R. V.: Interaction of haemoglobin messenger RNA with the small subparticle of reticulocyte ribosomes. FEBS Lett. *9*:331, 1970.

Prankerd, T. A. J.: The spleen and anaemia. Br. Med. J. *2*:517, 1963.

Prato, V., Gallo, E., Ricco, G., et al.: Haemolytic anaemia due to haemoglobin Torino. Br. J. Haematol. *19*:105, 1970.

Preisler, H. D., Housman, D., Scher, W., and Friend, C.: Effects of 5-bromo-2′-deoxyuridine on production of globin messenger RNA in dimethyl sulfoxide–stimulated Friend leukemia cells. Proc. Natl. Acad. Sci. USA *70*:2956, 1973.

Prensky, W., and Holmquist, G.: Chromosomal localization of human haemoglobin structural genes: techniques queried. Nature *241*:44, 1973.

Pribilla, W., Klesse, P., Betke, K., et al.: Hämoglobin-Köln-Krankheit: Familiäre hypochrome hämolytische Anämie mit Hämoglobinanomalie. Klin. Wochenschr. *43*:1049, 1965.

Price, P. M., Conover, J. H., and Hirschhorn, K.: Chromosomal localization of human haemoglobin structural genes. Nature *237*:340, 1972.

Prichard, P. M., Gilbert, J. M., Shafritz, D. A., et al.: Factors for the initiation of haemoglobin synthesis by rabbit reticulocyte ribosomes. Nature *226*:511, 1970.

Prindle, K. M., and McCurdy, P. R.: Red cell life span in hemoglobin C disorders. Clin. Res. *17*:33, 1969.

Pritchard, J. A., Scott, D. E., and Whalley, P.: The effects of maternal sickle cell hemoglobinopathies and sickle cell trait on reproductive performance. Am. J. Obstet. Gynecol. *117*:662, 1971.

Pritchard, J., Hillman, D. G., Glass, J., et al.: Deficiency of β-globin chain messenger RNA (mRNA) in nucleated red cell precursors from heterozygous β-thalassemia (Hetero β-Thal) marrow. Blood *46*:1050, 1975.

Propper, R. D., Shurin, S. B., and Nathan, D. G.: Reassessment of the use of desferrioxamine B in iron overload. N. Engl. J. Med. *294*:1421, 1976.

Proudfoot, N. J., and Brownlee, G. G.: Sequence at the 3′ end of globin mRNA shows homology with immunoglobulin light chain mRNA. Nature *252*:359, 1974.

Proudfoot, N. J., and Brownlee, G. G.: 3′ non-coding region sequences in eukaryotic messenger RNA. Nature *263*:211, 1976a.

Proudfoot, N. J., and Brownlee, G. G.: Nucleotide sequences of globin messenger RNA. Br. Med. Bull. *32*:251, 1976b.

Pugh, R. P., Monical, T. V., and Minnich, V.: Sickle cell anemia with two adult hemoglobins—Hb S and Hb G-Philadelphia/S. Blood *23*:206, 1964.

Pulsinelli, P. D.: Structure of deoxyhaemoglobin Yakima: a high affinity mutant form exhibiting oxy-like $\alpha_1\beta_2$ subunit interactions. J. Mol. Biol. *74*:57, 1973.

Pulsinelli, P. D., Perutz, M. F., and Nagel, R. L.: Structure of Hemoglobin M Boston, a variant with a five coordinated ferric heme. Proc. Natl. Acad. Sci. USA *70*:3870, 1973.

Purcell, Y., and Brozovic, B.: Red cell 2,3-diphosphoglycerate concentration in man decreases with age. Nature *251*:511, 1974.

Purugganan, H. B., and McElfresh, A. E.: Failure of carbonmonoxy sickle-cell haemoglobin to alter the sickle state. Lancet *1*:79, 1964.

Rabinovitz, M., Freedman, M. L., Fisher, J. M., Maxwell, C. R.: Translational control in hemoglobin synthesis. Cold Spring Harbor Symp. Quant. Biol. *34*:567, 1969.

Rachmilewitz, E. A.: Denaturation of the normal and abnormal hemoglobin molecule. Semin. Hematol. *11*:441, 1974.

Rachmilewitz, E. A., and Harari, E.: Intermediate hemichrome formation after oxidation of three unstable hemoglobins (Freiburg, Riverdale-Bronx and Köln). Haematol. Bluttransfus. *10*:241, 1972.

Rachmilewitz, E. A., and Thorell, B.: Hemichromes in single inclusion bodies in red cells of beta thalassemia. Blood *39*:794, 1972.

Rachmilewitz, E. A., and White, J. M.: Haemichrome formation during the *in vitro* oxidation of haemoglobin Köln. Nature [New Biol.] *241*:115, 1973.

Rachmilewitz, E. A., Peisach, J., and Blumberg, W. E.: Studies on the stability of oxyhemoglobin A and its constituent chains and their derivatives. J. Biol. Chem. *246*:3356, 1971.

Rachmilewitz, E. A., Lubin, B. H., and Shohet, S. B.: Lipid membrane peroxidation in β-thalassemia major. Blood *47*:495, 1976.

Raffel, C., Stein, S., and Kaempfer, R.: Role for heme in mammalian protein synthesis: activation of an initiation factor. Proc. Natl. Acad. Sci. USA *71*:4020, 1974.

Rahbar, S.: An abnormal hemoglobin in red cells of diabetics. Clin. Chim. Acta *22*:296, 1968.

Rahbar, S., Blumberg, O., and Ranney, H. M.: Studies of an unusual hemoglobin in patients with diabetes mellitus. Biochem. Biophys. Res. Commun. *36*:838, 1969.

Raich, P. C., Rodriguez, J. M., Desai, J. N., and Shahidi, N. T.: Effect of hemodialysis on erythrocyte 2,3-diphosphoglycerate in patients with uremia. Am. J. Med. Sci. *265*:147, 1973.

Raik, E., Hunter, E. G., and Lindsay, D. A.: Compensated hereditary haemolytic disease resulting from an unstable haemoglobin fraction. Med. J. Aust. *1*:955, 1967.

Ramirez, F., Gambino, R., Maniatis, G. M., et al.: Changes in globin messenger RNA content during erythroid cell differentiation. J. Biol. Chem. *250*:6054, 1975a.
Ramirez, F., Natta, C., O'Donnell, J. V., et al.: Relative numbers of human globin genes assayed with purified α and β complementary human DNA. Proc. Natl. Acad. Sci. USA *72*:1550, 1975b.
Ramirez, F., O'Donnell, J. V., Marks, P. A., et al.: Abnormal or absent βmRNA in β^0 Ferrara and gene deletion in $\delta\beta$ thalassaemia. Nature *263*:471, 1976.
Rampling, M. W., and Sirs, J. A.: The rate of sickling of cells containing sickle-cell haemoglobin. Clin. Sci. Mol. Med. *45*:655, 1973.
Rand, P. W., Norton, J. M., Barker, N. D., et al.: Responses to graded hypoxia at high and low 2,3-diphosphoglycerate concentrations. J. Appl. Physiol. *34*:827, 1973.
Ranney, H. M., Larson, D. L., and McCormack, G. H.: Some clinical, biochemical and genetic observations on hemoglobin C. J. Clin. Invest. *32*:1277, 1953.
Ranney, H. M., Briehl, R. W., and Jacobs, A. S.: Oxygen equilibrium of hemoglobin α^A and of hemoglobin reconstituted from hemoglobins α^A and H. J. Biol. Chem. *240*: 2442, 1965.
Ranney, H. M., Jacobs, A. S., Udem, L., and Zalusky, R.: Hemoglobin Riverdale-Bronx, an unstable hemoglobin resulting from the substitution of arginine for glycine at helical residue B6 of the β polypeptide chain. Biochem. Biophys. Res. Commun. *33*:1004, 1968a.
Ranney, H. M., Nagel, R. L., Heller, P., and Udem, L.: Oxygen equilibrium of hemoglobin M-Hyde Park. Biochim. Biophys. Acta *160*:112, 1968b.
Ranney, H. M., Nagel, R. L., and Udem, L.: Some properties of the M-hemoglobins. In Arends, T., Bemski, G., and Nagel, R. L. (eds.): Proceedings of First Inter-American Symposium on Hemoglobins, Caracas, Venezuela, 1969. Basel, S. Karger, 1971, p. 143.
Raper, A. B., Black, A. J., Huntsman, R. G., and Pollack, M.: Sickling and steroid hormones. Trans. Roy. Soc. Trop. Med. Hyg. *64*:293, 1970.
Rapoport, S., and Luebering, J.: Glycerate-2,3-diphosphatase. J. Biol. Chem. *189*:683, 1951.
Ravin, M. B., Drury, W. L., Keitt, A. S., et al.: Red cell 2,3-diphosphoglycerate in surgical correction of cyanotic congenital heart disease. Anesth. Analg. (Cleveland) *52*:599, 1973.
Redetzki, J. E., Bickers, J. N., and Samuels, M. S.: Homozygous hemoglobin C disease: Clinical review of 15 patients. South. Med. J. *61*:238, 1968.
Reed, C. S., Hampson, R., Gordon, S., et al.: Erythrocytosis secondary to increased oxygen affinity of a mutant hemoglobin, Hemoglobin Kempsey. Blood *31*:623, 1968.
Reed, L. J., and Mollin, D. W.: Synthesis of hemoglobin A_2 in sideroblastic and megaloblastic anemias. Abstracts, XII Congress of the International Society of Hematology, New York, The Society, 1968, p. 63.
Reichert, E. T., and Brown, A. P.: The differentiation and specificity of corresponding proteins and other vital substances in relation to biological classification and organic evolution: The crystallography of hemoglobins. Washington, D.C., Carnegie Institution of Washington Pub. No. 116, 1909.
Reichlin, M., Bucci, E., Antonini, E., et al.: The immunochemical difference between horse oxy- and deoxyhemoglobin. J. Mol. Biol. *9*:785, 1964.
Reynolds, C. A., and Huisman, T. H. J.: Hemoglobin Russ or $\alpha_2{}^{51\ \mathrm{Arg}}\beta_2$. Biochim. Biophys. Acta *130*:541, 1966.
Reynolds, J.: Roentgenological features of sickle cell disease and related hemoglobinopathies. Springfield, Illinois, Charles C Thomas, 1965.
Reynolds, J. D. H.: Painful sickle cell crisis— successful treatment with hyperbaric oxygen therapy. JAMA *216*:1977, 1971.
Rhinesmith, H. S., Schroeder, W. A., and Pauling, L.: A quantitative study of the hydrolysis of human dinitrophenyl (DNP) globin: The number and kind of polypeptide chains in normal adult human hemoglobin. J. Am. Chem. Soc. *79*:4682, 1957.
Rickles, F. R., and O'Leary, D. S.: Role of coagulation system in pathophysiology of sickle cell disease. Arch. Intern. Med. *133*:635, 1974.
Rieder, R. F.: Hemoglobin stability: Observations on the denaturation of normal and abnormal hemoglobins by oxidant dyes, heat and alkali. J. Clin. Invest. *49*:2369, 1970.

Rieder, R. F.: Synthesis of hemoglobin Gun Hill: Increased synthesis of the heme-free β^{GH} globin chain and subunit exchange with a free α-chain pool. J. Clin. Invest. *50*:388, 1971.
Rieder, R. F.: Translation of β-globin mRNA in β-thalassemia and the S and C hemoglobinopathies. J. Clin. Invest. *51*:364, 1972.
Rieder, R. F.: Globin chain synthesis in Hb D (Punjab)-β-thalassemia. Blood *47*:113, 1976.
Rieder, R. F., and Bradley, T. B.: Hemoglobin Gun Hill: An unstable protein associated with chronic hemolysis. Blood *32*:355, 1968.
Rieder, R. F., and James, G. W., III: Imbalance in alpha and beta globin synthesis associated with a hemoglobinopathy. J. Clin. Invest. *54*:948, 1974.
Rieder, R. F., and Weatherall, D. J.: Studies on hemoglobin biosynthesis: asynchronous synthesis of hemoglobin A and hemoglobin A_2 by erythrocyte precursors. J. Clin. Invest. *44*:42, 1965.
Rieder, R. F., Zinkman, W. H., and Holtzman, N. A.: Hemoglobin Zürich: Clinical, chemical and kinetic studies. Am. J. Med. *39*:4, 1965.
Rieder, R. F., Oski, F. A., and Clegg, J. B.: Hemoglobin Philly (β35 Tyrosine→Phenylalanine): Studies in the molecular pathology of hemoglobin. J. Clin. Invest. *48*:1627, 1969.
Rieder, R. F., Wolf, D. J., Clegg, J. B., et al.: Hemoglobin Bushwick, β74 (E18) Gly→Val: Rapid postsynthetic destruction of an unstable hemoglobin. Blood *44*:946, 1974.
Rieder, R. F., Wolf, D. J., Clegg, J. B., et al.: Rapid postsynthetic destruction of unstable haemoglobin Bushwick. Nature *254*:725, 1975.
Rieder, R. F., Woodbury, D. H., and Rucknagel, D. L.: The interaction of α-thalassaemia and haemoglobin G Philadelphia. Br. J. Haematol. *32*:159, 1976.
Riegel, K., Versmold, H., Windhorst, H., et al.: Thyroxine and red cell 2,3-diphosphoglycerate in the newborn period. Klin. Wochenschr. *51*:138, 1973.
Rifkind, R. A.: Heinz body anemia: an ultrastructural study. II. Red cell sequestration and destruction. Blood *26*:433, 1965.
Rifkind, R. A., and Danon, D.: Heinz body anemia—an ultrastructural study: I. Heinz body formation. Blood *25*:885, 1965.
Rigas, D. A., and Koler, R. D.: Decreased erythrocyte survival in hemoglobin H disease as a result of the abnormal properties of hemoglobin H: the benefit of splenectomy. Blood *18*:1, 1961.
Riggs, A.: Mechanism of the enhancement of the Bohr effect in mammalian hemoglobins by diphosphoglycerate. Proc. Natl. Acad. Sci. USA *68*:2062, 1971.
Riggs, A., and Gibson, Q. H.: Oxygen equilibria and kinetics of isolated subunits from hemoglobin Kansas. Proc. Natl. Acad. Sci. U.S.A. *70*:1718, 1973.
Riggs, T. E., Shafer, A. W., and Guenter, C. A.: Acute changes in oxyhemoglobin affinity; effects on oxygen transport and utilization. J. Clin. Invest. *52*:2660, 1973.
Ringelhann, B.: Immunodeficiency in sickle-cell anemia. N. Engl. J. Med. *289*:326, 1973.
Ringelhann, B., and Konotey-Ahulu, F. I. D.: Immunological studies and sickle cell crises in Ghana. Afr. J. Med. Sci. *4*:17, 1973.
Ringelhann, B., Konotey-Ahulu, F. I. D., Talapatra, N. C., et al.: Haemoglobin K Woolwich ($\alpha_2\beta_2{}^{132}$ Lysine→Glutamine) in Ghana. Acta Haematol. (Basel) *45*:250, 1971.
Roberts, A. V., Weatherall, D. J., and Clegg, J. B.: The synthesis of human hemoglobin A_2 during erythroid maturation. Biochem. Biophys. Res. Commun. *47*:81, 1972.
Roberts, A. V., Clegg, J. B., Weatherall, D. J., et al.: Synthesis *in vitro* of anti-Lepore haemoglobin. Nature [New Biol.] *245*:23, 1973.
Robinson, M. G., and Halpern, C.: Infections, Escherichia coli and sickle cell anemia. JAMA *230*:1145, 1974.
Robinson, M. G., and Watson, R. J.: Pneumococcal meningitis in sickle-cell anemia. N. Engl. J. Med. *274*:1006, 1966.
Rodriguez, J. M., and Shahidi, N. T.: Erythrocyte 2,3-diphosphoglycerate in adaptive red-cell–volume deficiency. N. Engl. J. Med. *285*:479, 1971.
Rørth, M.: Hemoglobin interactions and red cell metabolism. Ser. Haematol. *5*:82, 1972.
Rørth, M., and Nygaard, S. F.: In Rørth, M., and Astrup, P. (eds.): Oxygen Affinity of

Hemoglobin and Red Cell Acid-Base Status. Copenhagen, Munksgaard, 1972, p. 599.

Rørth, M., Nygaard, S. F., and Parving, H. H.: Red cell metabolism and oxygen affinity of healthy individuals during exposure to high altitude. In Brewer, G. (ed.): Second International Conference on Red Cell Metabolism and Function. New York, Plenum Press, 1972, p. 361.

Rosa, J., Audart, J. C., Pagnier, J., et al.: A new abnormal hemoglobin: $\alpha_2{}^{112\ \mathrm{His}\rightarrow\mathrm{Gly}}\beta_2$ Hb Dakar. XII Congress of the International Society of Hematology, New York, The Society, 1968, p. 72.

Rosa, J., Labie, D., Wajcman, H., et al.: Haemoglobin I Toulouse: β66 (E10) Lys→Glu: A new abnormal haemoglobin with a mutation localized on the E10 porphyrin surrounding zone. Nature *223*:190, 1969.

Rosa, R., Gaillardon, J., and Rosa, J.: Diphosphoglycerate mutase and 2,3-diphosphoglycerate phosphatase activities of red cells: comparative electrophoretic study. Biochem. Biophys. Res. Commun, *51*:536, 1973.

Rosa, R., Audit, I., and Rosa, J.: Evidence for three enzymatic activities in one electrophoretic band of 3-phosphoglycerate mutase from red cells. Biochemie *57*:1059, 1975.

Rose, I. A.: The state of magnesium in cells as estimated from the adenylate kinase equilibrium. Proc. Natl. Acad. Sci. USA *61*:1079, 1968.

Rose, I. A., and Warms, J. V. B.: Control of red cell glycolysis: The cause of triose phosphate accumulation. J. Biol. Chem. *245*:4009, 1970.

Rose, Z. B.: The purification and properties of diphosphoglycerate mutase from human erythrocytes. J. Biol. Chem. *243*:4810, 1968.

Rose, Z. B.: Effects of salts and pH on the rate of erythrocyte diphosphoglycerate mutase. Arch. Biochem. Biophys. *158*:903, 1973.

Rose, Z. B., and Liebowitz, J.: 2,3-Diphosphoglycerate phosphatase from human erythrocytes. J. Biol. Chem. *245*:3232, 1970a.

Rose, Z. B., and Liebowitz, J.: Direct determination of 2,3-diphosphoglycerate. Anal. Biochem. *35*:177, 1970b.

Rosemeyer, M. A., and Huehns, E. R.: On the mechanism of the dissociation of haemoglobin. J. Mol. Biol. *25*:253, 1967.

Rosenthal, A., and Mesrobian, A.: The relationship between angiography, intraerythrocytic pH and hemoglobin oxygen equilibrium. Invest. Radiol. *10*:140, 1975.

Rosenthal, A., Litwin, S. B., and Laver, M. B.: Effect of contrast media used in angiocardiography on hemoglobin-oxygen equilibrium. Invest. Radiol. *8*:191, 1973.

Rosenzweig, A. I., Heywood, J. D., Motulsky, A. G., et al.: Hemoglobin H as an acquired defect of alpha-chain synthesis: report of two cases. Acta Haematol. (Basel) *39*:91, 1968.

Ross, J., Aviv, H., Soolnick, E., and Leder, P.: *In vitro* synthesis of DNA complementary to purified rabbit globin mRNA. Proc. Natl. Acad. Sci. USA *69*:264, 1972a.

Ross, J., Ikawa, Y., and Leder, P.: Globin mRNA induction during erythroid differentiation of cultured leukemic cells. Proc. Natl. Acad. Sci. USA *69*:3620, 1972b.

Ross, J., Gielen, J., Packman, S., et al.: Globin gene expression in cultured erythroleukemic cells. J. Mol. Biol. *87*:697, 1974.

Rossi-Bernardi, L., and Roughton, F. J. W.: The specific influence of carbon dioxide and carbamate compounds on the buffer power and Bohr effects in human haemoglobin solutions. J. Physiol. (London) *189*:1, 1967.

Rossi-Bernardi, L., Roughton, F. J. W., et al.: The effect of organic phosphates on the binding of CO_2 to human hemoglobin and CO_2 transport in the circulating blood. In Rørth, M., and Astrup, P. (eds.): Oxygen Affinity of Hemoglobin and Red Cell Acid-Base Status. Copenhagen, Munksgaard, 1972, p. 225.

Rossi-Bernardi, L., Luzzana, M., Samaja, M., et al.: The functional properties of sickle cell blood. FEBS Lett. *59*:15, 1975.

Rossi-Fanelli, A., and Antonini, E.: Oxygen equilibrium of haemoglobin from Thunnus thynnus. Nature *186*:895, 1960.

Rossi-Fanelli, A., Antonini, G., and Caputo, A.: Studies on the structure of hemoglobin. Biochim. Biophys. Acta *30*:608, 1958a.

Rossi-Fanelli, A., Antonini, E., and Povoledo, D.: Further study on myoglobin II. Chemical and biochemical properties of a new type of myoglobin in molluscs. In Neuberger, A. (ed.): Symposium on Protein Structure. London, Methuen, 1958b, p. 144.

Rossi-Fanelli, A., Antonini, E., and Caputo, A.: Studies on the relations between molecular and functional properties of hemoglobin. I. The effect of salts on the molecular weight of human hemoglobin. J. Biol. Chem. *236*:391, 1961.

Roth, E. F., Nagel, R. L., Bookchin, R. M., and Grayzel, A. L.: Nitrogen mustard: an "in vitro" inhibitor of erythrocyte sickling. Biochem. Biophys. Res. Commun. *48*:612, 1972.

Roth, E. F., Jr., Nagel, R. L., Bookchin, R. M., et al.: The effects of nitrogen and sulfur mustards on hemoglobin S and intact red cells. In Hercules, J. I., Schechter, A. N., Eaton, W. A., et al. (eds.): Proceedings of First National Symposium on Sickle Cell Disease, Washington, D.C. DHEW Pub. No. 75–723 (NIH), Bethesda, Md., 1974, p. 41.

Rotter, R., Luttgens, W. F., Peterson, W. L., et al.: Splenic infarction in sicklemia during airplane flight: pathogenesis, hemoglobin analysis and clinical features of six cases. Ann. Intern. Med. *44*:257, 1956.

Rowley, P. T., and Kosciolek, B.: Distinction between two types of beta-thalassemia by inducibility of the cell-free synthesis of beta-chains by non-thalassemic soluble fraction. Nature [New Biol.] *239*:234, 1972.

Rucknagel, D. L.: The genetics of sickle cell anemia and related syndromes. Arch. Intern. Med. *133*:595, 1974.

Rucknagel, D. L., and Rising, J. A.: A heterozygote for Hb_{β}^{S}, Hb_{β}^{C}, and $Hb_{\alpha}^{G\,Philadelphia}$ in a family presenting evidence for heterogeneity of hemoglobin alpha chain loci. Am. J. Med. *59*:53, 1975.

Rucknagel, D. L., and Winter, W. P.: Duplication of structural genes for hemoglobin α and β chains in man. Ann. NY Acad. Sci. *241*:80, 1974.

Rucknagel, D. L., Spencer, H. H., and Brandt, N. J.: Hemoglobin Ann Arbor, a complex alpha chain abnormality. Abstracts, XII Congress of the International Society of Hematology, New York 1968. New York, The Society, 1968, p. 56.

Ruiz-Carrillo, A., Beato, M., Schutz, G., et al.: Cell-free translation of the globin message within polydisperse high-molecular-weight ribonucleic acid of avian erythrocytes. Proc. Natl. Acad. Sci. USA *70*:3641, 1973.

Russell, M. O., Goldberg, H. I., Friedman, S., et al.: Reversal of cerebral arterial changes in sickle cell anemia with prolonged transfusion therapy. In Hercules, J. I., Schechter, A. N., Eaton, W. A., et al. (eds.): Proceedings of First National Symposium on Sickle Cell Disease, Washington, D.C. DHEW Pub. No. 75–723 (NIH), Bethesda, Md., 1974, p. 77.

Russell, M. O., Goldberg, H. I., Reis, L., et al.: Transfusion therapy for cerebrovascular abnormalities in sickle cell disease. J. Pediatr. *88*:382, 1976.

Russo, G., and Mollica, F.: Sickle-cell haemoglobin and two types of thalassaemia in the same family. Acta Haematol. (Basel) *28*:329, 1962.

Ryan, S. J., and Goldberg, M. F.: Anterior segment ischemia following scleral buckling in sickle cell hemoglobinopathy. Am. J. Ophthalmol. *72*:35, 1971.

Salden, M., and Bloemendal, H.: Polyamines can replace the dialyzable component from crude reticulocyte initiation factors. Biochem. Biophys. Res. Commun. *68*:157, 1976.

Salden, M., Bisseling, T., Berns, A., and Bloemendal, H.: Requirement of a dialyzable component from crude initiation factors for the translation of viral and eukaryotic messenger RNA. Biochem. Biophys. Res. Commun. *65*:317, 1975.

Salhany, J. M.: The deoxygenation kinetics of hemoglobin Rainier ($\alpha_2\beta_2{}^{145\,Tyr \rightarrow Cys}$). Biochem. Biophys. Res. Commun. *47*:784, 1972.

Salhany, J. M., Keitt, A. S., and Eliot, R. S.: The rate of deoxygenation of red blood cells. Effect of intracellular 2,3-diphosphoglycerate and pH. FEBS Lett. *16*:257, 1971.

Salhany, J. M., Mathers, D. H., and Eliot, R. S.: The deoxygenation kinetics of hemoglobin partially saturated with carbon monoxide. J. Biol. Chem. *247*:6985, 1972.

Salhany, J. M., Osawa, S., and Shulman, R. G.: Spectral-kinetic heterogeneity in reactions of nitrosyl hemoglobin. Proc. Natl. Acad. Sci. USA *71*:3359, 1974.

Salhany, J. M., Ogawa, S., and Shulman, R. G.: Correlation between quaternary structure and ligand dissociation kinetics for fully liganded hemoglobin. Biochemistry *14*:2180, 1975.

Salvaggio, J. E., Arnold, C. A., and Banov, C. H.: Long-term anticoagulation in sickle-cell disease: a clinical study. N. Engl. J. Med. *269*:182, 1963.

Sampson, J., Mathews, B., Osborn, M., et al.: Hemoglobin messenger RNA translation in cell free systems from rat and mouse liver and Landschutz ascites cells. Biochemistry *11*:3636, 1972.

Sansone, G., and Pik, C.: Familial haemolytic anaemia with erythrocyte inclusion bodies, bilifuscinuria and abnormal haemoglobin (haemoglobin Galliera Genova). Br. J. Haematol. *11*:511, 1965.

Sansone, G., Carrell, R. W., and Lehmann, H.: Haemoglobin Genova: β28 (B10) Leucine → Proline. Nature *214*:877, 1967.

Sasaki, R., Ikura, K., Sugimoto, E., and Chiba, H.: Purification of biphosphoglyceromutase, 2,3 biphosphoglycerate phosphatase and phosphoglyceromutase from human erythrocytes. Europ. J. Biochem. *50*:581, 1975.

Scherrer, K.: Messenger RNA in eukaryotic cells: the life history of duck globin messenger RNA. Acta Endocrinol. *74*(Suppl. 180):95, 1973.

Schlitt, L. E., and Keitel, H. G.: Renal manifestations of sickle cell disease. A review. Am. J. Med. Sci. *239*:773, 1960.

Schmid, R., Williams, G. Z., and Clemens, T., Jr.: Familial hemolytic anemia with spontaneous erythrocyte inclusion bodies. Proceedings of VI Congress of the International Society of Hematology, Boston, 1956. New York, Grune & Stratton, 1958.

Schmid, R., Brecher, G., and Clemens, T.: Familial hemolytic anemia with erythrocyte inclusion bodies and a defect in pigment metabolism. Blood *14*:991, 1959.

Schmidt-Nielsen, K.: How Animals Work. London, Cambridge University Press, 1972.

Schmidt-Nielsen, K., and Larimer, J. L.: Oxygen dissociation curves of mammalian blood in relation to body size. Am. J. Physiol. *195*:424, 1958.

Schmidt-Nielsen, K., and Taylor, C. R.: Red blood cells: why or why not? Science *162*:274, 1968.

Schneider, R. G., Alperin, J. B., Beale, D., and Lehmann, H.: Hemoglobin I in an American Negro family: structural and hematologic studies. J. Lab. Clin. Med. *68*:940, 1966.

Schneider, R. G., Ueda, S., Alperin, J. B., et al.: Hemoglobin Sabine beta 91 (F7) Leu → Pro. An unstable variant causing severe anemia with inclusion bodies. N. Engl. J. Med. *280*:739, 1969.

Schneider, R. G., Takeda, I,, Gustavson, L. P., and Alperin, J. B.: Intraerythrocytic precipitations of haemoglobins S and C. Nature [New Biol.] *235*:88, 1972.

Schneider, R. G., Atkins, R. J., Hosty, T. S., et al.: Haemoglobin Titusville: α94 Asp → Asn. A new haemoglobin with a lowered affinity for oxygen. Biochim. Biophys. Acta *400*:365, 1975.

Schneiderman, L. J., Junga, I. G., and Fawley, D. E.: Effects of phosphate and nonphosphate buffers on thermolability of unstable haemoglobins. Nature *225*:1041, 1970.

Schnitzer, B., Rucknagel, D. L., Spencer, H. H., and Aikawa, M.: Erythrocytes: Pits and vacuoles as seen with transmission and scanning electron microscopy. Science *173*:251, 1971.

Schokker, R. C., Went, L. N., and Bok, J.: A new genetic variant of beta-thalassemia. Nature *209*:44, 1966.

Scholander, P. F.: Oxygen transport through hemoglobin solutions. Science *131*:585, 1960.

Schroeder, W. A., Cua, J. T., Matsuda, G., and Fenninger, W. D.: Hemoglobin F_I, an acetyl-containing hemoglobin. Biochim. Biophys. Acta *63*:532, 1962.

Schroeder, W. A., Shelton, J. R., Shelton, J. B., et al.: The amino acid sequence of the α chain of human fetal hemoglobin. Biochemistry *2*:1353, 1963.

Schroeder, W. A., Huisman, T. J. H., Shelton, J. R., et al.: Evidence for multiple structural genes for γ chain of human fetal hemoglobin. Proc. Natl. Acad. Sci. USA *60*:537, 1968.

Schroeder, W. A., Shelton, J. R., Shelton, J. B., et al.: World-wide occurrence of nonallelic genes for the γ chain of human foetal haemoglobin in newborns. Nature [New Biol.] *240*:273, 1972.

Schroeder, W. A., Bannister, W. H., Grech, J. L., et al.: Nonsynchronized suppression of postnatal activity in nonallelic genes which synthesize the Gγ chain in human foetal haemoglobin. Nature [New Biol.] *244*:89, 1973.

Schulman, H. M.: Evidence supporting a physiological role for the hemin-controlled translational repressor of globin synthesis in reticulocytes. Biochim. Biophys. Acta *414*:161, 1975.
Schumacher, H. R., Andres, R., and McLaughlin, G.: Arthropathy in sickle-cell disease. Ann. Intern. Med. *78*:203, 1973.
Schwartz, A. D., and Pearson, H. A.: Impaired antibody response to intravenous immunization in sickle cell anemia. Pediatr. Res. *6*:145, 1972.
Schwartz, E.: The silent carrier of beta-thalassemia. N. Engl. J. Med. *281*:1327, 1969.
Schwartz, E.: Heterozygous beta thalassemia: balanced globin synthesis in bone marrow cells. Science *167*:1513, 1970.
Schwartz, E., and Atwater, J.: α-Thalassemia in the American Negro. J. Clin. Invest. *51*:412, 1972.
Schwartz, E., and McElfresh, A. E.: Treatment of painful crises of sickle cell disease: a double-blind study. J. Pediatr. *64*:132, 1964.
Seakins, M., Gibbs, W. N., Milner, P. F., and Bertles, J. F.: Erythrocyte Hb-S concentration; an important factor in the low oxygen affinity of blood in sickle cell anemia. J. Clin. Invest. *52*:422, 1973.
Searle, J. F.: Anaesthesia and sickle-cell haemoglobin. Br. J. Anaesth. *44*:1335, 1972.
Seeler, R. A.: Deaths in children with sickle cell anemia. Clin. Pediatr. (Philadelphia) *11*:634, 1972.
Seeler, R. A.: Intensive transfusion therapy for priapism in boys with sickle cell anemia. J. Urol. *110*:360, 1973.
Seeler, R. A., and Shwiaki, M. Z.: Acute splenic sequestration crisis (ASSC) in young children with sickle cell anemia. Clinical observations in 20 episodes in 14 children. Clin. Pediatr. (Philadelphia) *11*:701, 1972.
Seeler, R. A., Metzger, W., and Mufson, M. A.: Diplococcus pneumoniae infections in children with sickle cell anemia. Am. J. Dis. Child. *123*:8, 1972.
Seid-Akhavan, M., Winter, W. P., et al.: Hemoglobin Wayne: a frameshift variant occurring in two distinct forms. Blood *40*:927, 1972.
Seid-Akhavan, M., Winter, W. P., Abramson, R. K., et al.: Hemoglobin Wayne: A frameshift mutation detected in human hemoglobin alpha chains. Proc. Natl. Acad. Sci. USA *73*:882, 1976.
Serjeant, G. R.: Sickle cell anemia: clinical features in adulthood and old age. In Abramson, H., Bertles, J. F., and Wethers, D. L. (eds.): Sickle Cell Disease—Diagnosis, Management, Education and Research. St. Louis, The C. V. Mosby Co., 1973, p. 252.
Serjeant, G. R.: Leg ulceration in sickle cell anemia. Arch. Intern. Med. *133*:690, 1974.
Serjeant, G. R., and Ashcroft, M. T.: Shortening of the digits in sickle cell anaemia—A sequela of the hand-foot syndrome. Trop. Geogr. Med. *23*:341, 1971.
Serjeant, G. R., Richards, R., Barbor, P. R., et al.: Relatively benign sickle-cell anaemia in 60 patients aged over 30 in the West Indies. Br. Med. J. *3*:86, 1968.
Serjeant, G. R., Galloway, R. E., and Gueri, M. C.: Oral zinc sulfate in sickle cell ulcers. Lancet *2*:891, 1970.
Serjeant, G. R., Petch, M. C., and Serjeant, B. E.: The in vivo sickle phenomenon: a reappraisal. J. Lab. Clin. Med. *81*:850, 1973.
Shaeffer, J. R.: Evidence for soluble α chains as intermediates in hemoglobin synthesis in the rabbit reticulocyte. Biochem. Biophys. Res. Commun. *28*:647, 1967.
Shaeffer, J. R.: Structure and synthesis of the unstable hemoglobin Sabine (alpha 2 beta 2-91 Leu → Pro). J. Biol. Chem. *248*:7473, 1973.
Shaeffer, J. R., Trostle, P. K., and Evans, R. F.: Rabbit hemoglobin biosynthesis: Use of human hemoglobin chains to study molecule completion. Science *158*:488, 1967.
Shaeffer, J. R., Trostle, P. K., and Evans, R. F.: Inhibition of the biosynthetic completion of rabbit hemoglobin by isolated human hemoglobin chains. J. Biol. Chem. *244*:4284, 1969.
Shaeffer, J. R., Desimone, J., and Kleve, L. J.: Hemoglobin synthesis studies of a family with alpha-thalassemia trait and sickle cell trait. Biochem. Genet. *13*:783, 1975a.
Shaeffer, J. R., Langley, M. A., DeSimone, J., and Kleve, L. J.: Patterns of hemoglobin assembly in reticulocytes of sickle cell trait individuals. J. Biol. Chem. *250*:8630, 1975b.
Shaeffer, J. R., Kleve, L. J.; and DeSimone, J.: β^S chain turnover in reticulocytes of sickle trait individuals with high or low concentrations of haemoglobin S. Br. J. Haematol. *32*:365, 1976.

Shafritz, D., and Anderson, W.: Factor dependent binding of methionyl-tRNAs to reticulocyte ribosomes. Nature *227*:918, 1970.

Shappell, S. D., Murray, J. A., Nasser, M. G., et al.: Acute change in hemoglobin affinity for oxygen during angina pectoris. N. Engl. J. Med. *282*:1219, 1970.

Sharma, V. S., Noble, R. W., and Ranney, H. M.: Structure-function relationship in Hemoglobin Köln (β98 Val → Met). J. Mol. Biol. *82*:139, 1974.

Shchory, M., and Ramot, B.: Globin chain synthesis in the marrow and reticulocytes of beta thalassemia, hemoglobin H disease and beta-delta thalassemia. Blood *40*:105, 1972.

Shchory, M., and Weatherall, D. J.: Haemoglobin synthesis in human fetal liver maintained in short-term tissue culture. Br. J. Haematol. *30*:9, 1975.

Shearman, J. J., Hamlyn, P. H., and Gould, H. J.: Molecular weights of separated rabbit α- and β-globin messenger RNAs. FEBS Lett. *47*:171, 1974.

Sheiness, D., and Darnell, J. E.: Polyadenylic acid segment in mRNA becomes shorter with age. Nature [New Biol.] *241*:265, 1973.

Sheldon, G. F., Plazak, L. F., Watkins, G. M., et al.: Inorganic phosphate and the oxyhemoglobin dissociation curve. Surg. Forum *22*:81, 1971.

Shen, S. C., Fleming, E. M., and Castle, W. B.: Studies on the destruction of red blood cells. V. Irreversibly sickled erythrocytes: The experimental production *in vitro*. Blood *4*:498, 1949.

Shepard, M. K., Weatherall, D. J., and Conley, C. L.: Semi-quantitative estimation of the distribution of fetal hemoglobin in red cell populations. Bull. Johns Hopkins Hosp. *110*:293, 1962.

Sherman, I. J.: The sickling phenomenon, with special reference to differentiation of sickle cell anemia from the sickle cell trait. Bull. Johns Hopkins Hosp. *67*:309, 1940.

Shibata, S., Miyaji, T., Iuchi, I., et al.: Substitution of tyrosine for histidine (87) in the α chain of hemoglobin M_{Iwate}. Acta Haematol. Jap. *27*:13, 1964.

Shibata, S., Miyaji, T., Iuchi, I., et al.: Hemoglobins M of the Japanese. Bull. Yamaguchi Med. Sch. *14*:141, 1967a.

Shibata, S., Miyaji, T., Karita, K., et al.: A new type of hereditary nigremia discovered in Akita—hemoglobin M Hyde Park disease. Proc. Jap. Acad. *43*:65, 1967b.

Shohet, S. B., Nathan, D. G., and Karnovsky, M. L.: Stages in the incorporation of fatty acids into red blood cells. J. Clin. Invest. *47*:1096, 1968.

Shulman, S., Bartlett, J., Clyde, W. A., et al.: The unusual severity of mycoplasmal pneumonia in children with sickle-cell disease. N. Engl. J. Med. *287*:164, 1972.

Silken, A. B.: Pharmacologic manipulation of human erythrocyte 2,3-diphosphoglycerate levels by prednisone administration. Pediatr. Res. *9*:61, 1975.

Simon, S. R., and Konigsberg, W. H.: Chemical modification of hemoglobins: A study of conformation restraint by internal bridging. Proc. Natl. Acad. Sci. USA *56*:749, 1966.

Singer, K.: Pure (homozygous) hemoglobin C disease. Blood *9*:1023, 1954.

Singer, K.: Hereditary hemolytic disorders associated with abnormal hemoglobins. Am. J. Med. *18*:633, 1955.

Singer, K., and Singer, L.: The gelling phenomenon of sickle cell hemoglobin: its biological and diagnostic significance. Blood *8*:1008, 1953.

Sippel, A. E., Stavrianopoulos, J. G., Schutz, G., and Feigelson, P.: Translational properties of rabbit globin mRNA after specific removal of poly (A) with ribonuclease H. Proc. Natl. Acad. Sci. USA *71*:4635, 1974.

Slater, L. M., Muir, W. A., and Weed, R. I.: Influence of splenectomy on insoluble hemoglobin inclusion bodies in β-thalassemic erythrocytes. Blood *31*:766, 1968.

Smith, C. H., Erlandson, M. E., Stern, G., and Hilgartner, M. W.: Postsplenectomy infection in Cooley's anemia. N. Engl. J. Med. *266*:737, 1962.

Smith, C. H., Erlandson, M. E., Stern, G., and Hilgartner, M. W.: Postsplenectomy infection in Cooley's anemia. Ann. NY Acad. Sci. *119*:748, 1964.

Smith, D. H., Clegg, J. B., Weatherall, D. J., et al.: Hereditary persistence of foetal haemoglobin associated with a $\gamma\beta$ fusion variant, haemoglobin Kenya. Nature [New Biol.] *246*:184, 1973.

Smith, D. W. E.: Reticulocyte transfer RNA and hemoglobin synthesis. Science *190*:529, 1975.

Smith, D. W. E., and McNamara, A. L.: Specialization of rabbit reticulocyte tRNA content for hemoglobin synthesis. Science *171*:577, 1971.

Smith, E., Rosenblatt, P., and Bedo, A. V.: Sickle cell anemia crisis: report on seven patients treated with priscoline. J. Pediatr. *43*:655, 1953.

Smith, E. W., and Krevans, J. R.: Clinical manifestations of hemoglobin C disorders. Bull. Johns Hopkins Hosp. *104*:17, 1959.

Smith, E. W., and Torbert, J. V.: Two abnormal hemoglobins with evidence for a new genetic locus for hemoglobin formation. Bull. Johns Hopkins Hosp. *102*:38, 1958.

Smith, L. L., Barton, B. P., and Huisman, T. H. J.: Subunit dissociation of the unstable hemoglobin Bibba ($\alpha_2^{136\ \mathrm{Pro}}$ (H19)β_2). J. Biol. Chem. *245*:2185, 1970.

Smith, R. S.: Iron excretion in thalassaemia major after administration of chelating agents. Br. Med. J. *2*:1577, 1962.

Smith, R. S.: Chelating agents in the diagnosis and treatment of iron overload in thalassemia. Ann. NY Acad. Sci. *119*:776, 1964.

Smits, H. L., Oski, F. A., and Brody, J. I.: The hemolytic crisis of sickle cell disease: the role of glucose-6-phosphate dehydrogenase deficiency. J. Pediatr. *74*:544, 1969.

Smolin, M. F., Zanjani, E. D., Hoffman, R., and Wasserman, L. R.: Mechanism of androgen action on erythropoiesis. Clin. Res. *23*:583A, 1975.

Snyder, L. M., and Reddy, W. J.: The effect of 3,5,3-triiodothyronine on red cell 2,3-diphosphoglyceric acid. Clin. Res. *18*:416, 1970a.

Snyder, L. M., and Reddy, W. J.: Mechanism of action of thyroid hormones on erythrocyte 2,3-diphosphoglyceric acid synthesis. J. Clin. Invest. *49*:1993, 1970b.

Sofroniadou, K., Kaltsova, A., Loukopoulos, D., et al.: Hemoglobin "Athens": an alpha-chain variant with unusual properties. Abstracts, XII Congress of the International Society of Hematology, New York. N. Y., The Society, 1968, p. 56.

Sofroniadou, K., Wood, W. G., Nute, P. E., and Stamatoyannopoulos, G.: Globin chain synthesis in the Greek type ($^A\gamma$) of hereditary persistence of foetal haemoglobin. Br. J. Haematol. *29*:137, 1975.

Soreq, H., Nudel, U., Salomon, R., et al.: In vitro translation of polyadenylate acid-free rabbit globin messenger RNA. J. Mol. Biol. *88*:233, 1974.

Spaet, T. H., Alway, R. H., and Ward, G.: Homozygous type "C" hemoglobin. Pediatrics *12*:483, 1953.

Spohr, G., Imaizumi, T., Stewart, A., and Scherrer, K.: Identification of free cytoplasmic globin mRNA of duck erythroblasts by hybridization to anti-messenger DNA and by cell-free protein synthesis. FEBS Lett. *28*:165, 1972.

Spohr, G., Imaizumi, T., and Scherrer, K.: Synthesis and processing of nuclear precursor-messenger RNA in avian erythroblasts and HeLa cells. Proc. Natl. Acad. Sci. USA *71*:5009, 1974.

Sproule, B. J., Halden, E. R., and Miller, W. F.: A study of cardiopulmonary alterations in patients with sickle cell disease and its variants. J. Clin. Invest. *37*:486, 1958.

Srivastava, S. K., Van Loon, C., and Beutler, E.: Characterization of a previously unidentified hemoglobin fraction. Biochim. Biophys. Acta *278*:617, 1972.

Staal, G. E., and Koster, J. F.: Influence of 2,3-diphosphoglycerate on phosphofructokinase of human erythrocytes? FEBS Lett. *23*:29, 1972.

Stamatoyannopoulos, G.: Gamma-thalassaemia. Lancet *2*:192, 1971.

Stamatoyannopoulos, G.: The molecular basis of hemoglobin disease. Ann. Rev. Genet. *6*:47, 1972.

Stamatoyannopoulos, G., Fessas, P., and Papayannopoulou, T.: F-thalassemia: a study of thirty-one families with simple heterozygotes and combinations of F-thalassemia with A_2-thalassemia. Am. J. Med. *47*:194, 1969a.

Stamatoyannopoulos, G., Parer, J. T., and Finch, C. A.: Physiologic implications of a hemoglobin with decreased oxygen affinity (Hemoglobin Seattle). N. Engl. J. Med. *281*:915, 1969b.

Stamatoyannopoulos, G., Bellingham, A. J., Lenfant, C., and Finch, C. A.: Abnormal hemoglobins with high and low oxygen affinity. Ann. Rev. Med. *22*:221, 1971.

Stamatoyannopoulos, G., Nute, P. E., Adamson, J. W., et al.: Hemoglobin Olympia (β20 Valine→Methionine): An electrophoretically silent variant associated with high oxygen affinity and erythrocytosis. J. Clin. Invest. *52*:342, 1973.

Stamatoyannopoulos, G., Woodson, R., Papayannopoulou, T., et al.: Inclusion body β-thalassemia trait. N. Engl. J. Med. *290*:939, 1974.

Stamatoyannopoulos, G., Wood, W. G., Papayannopoulou, T., et al.: A new form of hereditary persistence of fetal hemoglobin in Blacks and its association with sickle cell trait. Blood *46*:683, 1975.

Statius van Eps, L. W., Schouten, H., La Porte-Wijsman, L. W., and Struyker Boudier, A. M.: The influence of red blood cell transfusions on the hyposthenuria and renal hemodynamics of sickle cell anemia. Clin. Chim. Acta *17*:449, 1967.

Statius van Eps, L. W., Pinedo-Veels, C., DeVries, G. H., et al.: Nature of concentrating defect in sickle-cell nephropathy. Lancet *1*:450, 1970.

Stavem, P., Strömme, J., Lorkin, P. A., et al.: Haemoglobin M Saskatoon with slight constant haemolysis, markedly increased by sulfonamides. Scand. J. Haematol. 9:566, 1972.

Steadman, J. H., Yates, A., and Huehns, E. R.: Idiopathic Heinz body anaemia: Hb Bristol (β67[E11]Val→Asp). Br. J. Haematol. *18*:435, 1970.

Steggles, A. W., Wilson, G. N., Kantor, J. A., et al.: Cell-free transcription of mammalian chromatin: transcription of globin messenger RNA sequences from bone-marrow chromatin with mammalian RNA polymerase. Proc. Natl. Acad. Sci. USA *71*:1219, 1974.

Stein, R. E., and Urbaniak, J. R.: Sickle cell disease and the tourniquet. Is there a risk? J. Bone Joint Surg. *57*:1027, 1975.

Steinberg, M. H., and Dreiling, B. J.: Glucose-6-phosphate dehydrogenase deficiency in sickle cell anemia. Ann. Intern. Med. *80*:217, 1974.

Steinberg, M. H., Dreiling, B. J., Morrison, F. S., et al.: Mild sickle cell disease. JAMA *224*:317, 1973.

Steinberg, M. H., Adams, J. G., and Dreiling, B. J.: Alpha-thalassemia in adults with sickle-cell trait. In Hercules, J. I., Schechter, A. N., Eaton, W. A., et al. (eds.): Proceedings of First National Symposium on Sickle Cell Disease, Washington, D.C. DHEW Pub. No. 75–723 (NIH), Bethesda, Md., 1974, p. 259.

Steiner, M., Baldini, M., and Dameshek, W.: Enzymatic defects of heme synthesis in thalassemia. Ann. NY Acad. Sci. *119*:548, 1964.

Stetson, C. A., Jr.: The state of hemoglobin in sickled erythrocytes. J. Exp. Med. *123*:431, 1966.

Stockell, A., Perutz, M. F., Muirhead, H., and Glauser, S. C.: A comparison of adult and foetal horse haemoglobins. J. Mol. Biol. *3*:112, 1961.

Stockman, J. A., Nigro, M. A., Mishkin, M. M., and Oski, F. A.: Occlusion of large cerebral vessels in sickle cell anemia. N. Engl. J. Med. *287*:846, 1972.

Stokes, G. G.: On the reduction and oxidation of the colouring matter of the blood. Proc. Roy. Soc. Lond. *13*:355, 1864.

Stout, C., Holland, C. K., and Bird, R. M.: Hemoglobin D in an Oklahoma family. Arch. Intern. Med. *114*:296, 1964.

Sturgeon, P., Itano, H. A., and Bergren, W. R.: Clinical manifestations of inherited abnormal hemoglobins. II. Interaction of hemoglobin E and thalassemia trait. Blood *10*:396, 1955.

Sundin, O. H., and Williams, R. C.: Acceleration of gelation of hemoglobin S by erythrocyte membrane preparations. Fed. Proc. *35*:1524, 1976.

Suzuki, H., and Itano, H. A.: Delayed removal of N-terminal methionine from nascent globin chains in sickle-cell anemia reticulocytes. Proc. Natl. Acad. Sci. USA *70*:2059, 1973a.

Suzuki, H., and Itano, H. A.: Quantitative differences between N-terminal methionyl nascent globin chains of human and rabbit reticulocytes. Nature [New Biol.] *246*:107, 1973b.

Suzuki, T., Hayashi, A., Yamamura, Y., et al.: Functional abnormality of hemoglobin M_{Osaka}. Biochem. Biophys. Res. Commun. *19*:691, 1965.

Suzuki, T., Hayashi, A., Shimizu, A., and Yamamura, Y.: The oxygen equilibrium of hemoglobin $M_{Saskatoon}$. Biochim. Biophys. Acta *127*:280, 1966.

Svedberg, T., and Fahraeus, R.: A new method for the determination of the molecular weight of the proteins. J. Am. Chem. Soc. *48*:430, 1926.

Taketa, F., Mauk, A. G., and Lessard, J. L.: β chain amino termini of the cat hemoglobins and the response to 2,3-diphosphoglycerate and adenosine triphosphate. J. Biol. Chem. *246*:4471, 1971.

Taketa, F., Huang, Y. P., Libnock, J. A., et al.: Hemoglobin Wood (β97 [FG4]) His→Leu, A new high-oxygen-affinity hemoglobin associated with familial erythrocytosis. Biochim. Biophys. Acta *400*:348, 1975.

Tatsis, B., Dosik, H., Rieder, R., et al.: Hemoglobin Hasharon: severe hemolytic anemia and hypersplenism associated with a mildly unstable hemoglobin. Birth Defects *8*:25, 1972.

Tattersall, R. B., Pyke, D. A., Ranney, H. M., and Bruckheimer, S. M.: Hemoglobin components in diabetes mellitus. Studies in identical twins. N. Engl. J. Med. *293*:1171, 1975.

Tautz, C., and Kleihauer, E.; Gibt es ein fetales Hämoglobin beim Schwein? II. Analysen des Globins. Res. Exp. Med. (Berlin) *159*:44, 1972.

Tavill, A. S., Grayzel, A. I., London, I. M., et al.: The role of heme in the synthesis and assembly of hemoglobin. J. Biol. Chem. *243*:4987, 1968.

Tavill, A. S., Vanderhoff, G. A., and London, I. M.: The control of hemoglobin synthesis: A comparison of the role of heme in rabbit bone marrow and reticulocytes. J. Biol. Chem. *247*:366, 1972.

Taylor, J. M., Dozy, A., Kan, Y. W., et al.: Genetic lesion in homozygous α thalassaemia (hydrops foetalis). Nature *251*:392, 1974.

Teichman, N. L.: Ueber die Crystallisation der organischen Bestandtheile des Bluts. Z. Ration. Med. (N.S.) *3*:374, 1853.

Temple, G., and Lodish, H. F.: Competition between α and β globin messenger RNA. Biochem. Biophys. Res. Commun. *63*:971, 1975.

Tenhunen, R., Marver, H. S., and Schmid, R.: The enzymatic conversion of heme to bilirubin by microsomal heme oxygenase. Proc. Natl. Acad. Sci. USA *61*:748, 1968.

Terada, M., Cantor, L., Metafora, S., et al.: Globin messenger RNA activity in erythroid precursor cells and the effect of erythropoietin. Proc. Natl. Acad. Sci. USA *69*:3575, 1972.

Terry, D. W., Motulsky, A. G., and Rath, C. E.: Homozygous hemoglobin C: a new hereditary hemolytic disease. N. Engl. J. Med. *251*:365, 1954.

Thomas, E. D., Storb, R., Clift, R. A., et al.: Bone-marrow transplantation. N. Engl. J. Med. *292*:832 and 895, 1975.

Thompson, R. B., Warrington, R., Odom, J., and Bell, W. N.: Interaction between genes for delta thalassaemia and hereditary persistence of foetal haemoglobin. Acta Genet. Stat. Med. *15*:190, 1965a.

Thompson, R. B., Odom, J., and Bell, W. N.: Hb-S, beta thalassaemia, and Hb (β_2) in a family with evidence of a crossover between beta and delta loci. Acta Genet. Stat. Med. *15*:371, 1965b.

Thurmon, T. F., Boyer, S. H., Crosby, E. F., et al.: Hemoglobin switching in nonanemic sheep. III. Evidence for presumptive identity between the A $\rightarrow$ C factor and erythropoietin. Blood *36*:598, 1970.

Todd, D., Lai, M. C. S., and Braga, C. A.: Thalassaemia and hydrops foetalis—family studies. Br. Med. J. *3*:347, 1967.

Todd, D., Lai, M. C. S., Beaven, G. H., et al.: The abnormal haemoglobins in homozygous α-thalassaemia. Br. J. Haematol. *19*:27, 1970.

Tolstoschev, P., Mitchell, J., Lanyon, G., et al.: Presence of gene for β-globin in homozygous β^0 thalassaemia. Nature *259*:95, 1976.

Tomada, Y.: Demonstration of foetal erythrocyte by immunofluorescent staining. Nature *202*:910, 1964.

Tomita, S., and Riggs, A.: Studies of the interaction of 2,3-diphosphoglycerate and carbon dioxide with hemoglobins from mouse, man and elephant. J. Biol. Chem. *246*:547, 1971.

Torlontano, G., Tata, A., and Camagna, A.: A rapid screening test for thalassaemic trait. Acta Haematol. (Basel) *48*:234, 1972.

Torrance, J. D.: The role of fructose in restoration of organic phosphate compounds in outdated bank blood. J. Lab. Clin. Med. *82*:489, 1973.

Torrance, J. D.: Diphosphoglycerate mutase assay: the effect of pyruvate, lactate dehydrogenase and thyroid hormone on the assay. Clin. Chim. Acta *50*:103, 1974.

Torrance, J. D., and Bartlett, G. R.: Altitude hypoxia and erythrocyte phosphates. Biochim. Biophys. Acta *215*:409, 1970.

Torrance, J. D., Jacobs, P., Restrepo, A., et al.: Intraerythrocytic adaptation to anemia. N. Engl. J. Med. *283*:165, 1970.

Tosteson, D. C., Carlsen, E., and Dunham, E. T.: The effects of sickling on ion transport. I. Effect of sickling on potassium transport. J. Gen. Physiol. *39*:31, 1956.

Trabuchet, G., Dahmane, M., Pagnier, J., et al.: Hb J Mexico in Algeria: arguments for an heterogeneous distribution of α genes. FEBS Lett. *61*:156, 1976.

Travis, S. F., Sugarman, H. J., Ruberg, R. L., et al.: Alterations of red-cell glycolytic intermediates and oxygen transport as a consequence of hypophosphatemia in patients receiving intravenous hyperalimentation. N. Engl. J. Med. *285*:763, 1971.

Trivelli, L. A., Ranney, H. M., and Lai, H.: Hemoglobin components in patients with diabetes mellitus. N. Engl. J. Med. *284*:353, 1971.

Tso, S. C.: Red cell survival studies in haemoglobin H disease using [^{51}Cr] chromate and [^{32}P] di-isopropyl phosphofluoridate. Br. J. Haematol. *23*:621, 1972.

Tuchinda, S., Rucknagel, D. L., Minnich, V., et al.: The coexistence of the genes for hemoglobin E and α thalassemia in Thais, with resultant suppression of hemoglobin E synthesis. Am. J. Hum. Genet. *16*:311, 1964.

Tyuma, I., and Shimizu, K.: Different response to organic phosphates of human fetal and adult hemoglobins. Arch. Biochem. Biophys. *129*:404, 1969.

Tyuma, I., Benesch, R. E., and Benesch, R.: The preparation and properties of the isolated alpha and beta subunits of Hemoglobin A. Biochemistry *5*:2957, 1966.

Tyuma, I., Shimizu, K., and Imai, K.: Effect of 2,3-diphosphoglycerate on the cooperativity in oxygen binding of human adult hemoglobin. Biochem. Biophys. Res. Commun. *43*:423, 1971.

Udem, L., Ranney, H. M., Bunn, H. F., and Pisciotta, A.: Some observations on the properties of hemoglobin M-Milwaukee-1. J. Mol. Biol. *48*:489, 1970.

Valeri, C. R., and Fortier, N. L.: Red-cell 2,3-diphosphoglycerate and creatine levels in patients with red-cell mass deficits or with cardiopulmonary insufficiency. N. Engl. J. Med. *281*:1452, 1969.

Valeri, C. R., and Hirsch, N. M.: Restoration in vivo of erythrocyte adenosine triphosphate, 2,3-diphosphoglycerate, potassium ion and sodium ion concentrations following the transfusion of acid-citrate-dextrose–stored human red blood cells. J. Lab. Clin. Med. *73*:722, 1969.

Valtis, D. J., and Kennedy, A. C.: Defective gas-transport function of stored red blood cells. Lancet *1*:119, 1954.

Van Enk, A., Lang, A., White, J. M., and Lehmann, H.: Benign obstetric history in women with sickle-cell anaemia associated with α-thalassaemia. Br. Med. J. *4*:524, 1972.

Van Vliet, G., and Huisman, T. H. J.: Changes in the haemoglobin types of sheep as a response to anaemia. Biochem. J. *93*:410, 1964.

Varat, M. A., Adolph, R. J., and Fowler, N. O.: Cardiovascular effects of anemia. Am. Heart J. *83*:415, 1972.

Veismold, H., Kohne, E., Riegel, K., et al.: Oxygen carrying functions of blood in hereditary methemoglobinemia: ambivalent effects of 2,3-diphosphoglycerate. In Gerlach, E., Moser, K., Deutsch, E., et al. (eds.): Erythrocytes, Thrombocytes, Leukocytes. Stuttgart, 1973, pp. 171–174. (Recent Advances in Membrane and Metabolic Research, 2nd International Symposium, Vienna, 1972.)

Vella, F., and Lehmann, H.: Haemoglobin D Punjab (D Los Angeles). J. Med. Genet. *11*:341, 1974.

Vella, F., Labossiere, A., Wiltshire, B., et al.: The occurrence of hemoglobins E and M Saskatoon in central Canada. Am. J. Clin. Pathol. *60*:314, 1973.

Vella, F., Kamuzora, H., Lehmann, H., et al.: A second family with hemoglobin M Saskatoon in Saskatchewan. Clin. Biochem. *7*:186, 1974.

Verdier, F., Fay, M., and Korobaeff, M.: Mésure de l'affinite de l'hémoglobine pour l'oxygène. Application aux malades atteints d'angine de poitrine avec coronarographie normale étude de dix cas. Nouv. Presse Méd. *4*:1550, 1975.

Verma, I. M., Temple, G. F., Fan, H., and Baltimore, D.: *In vitro* synthesis of DNA complementary to rabbit reticulocyte 10S RNA. Nature [New Biol.] *235*:163, 1972.

Versmold, H., Horn, K., Windthorst, H., and Riegel, K. P.: The rapid postnatal increase of red cell 2,3-diphosphoglycerate: its relation to plasma thyroxine. Respir. Physiol. *18*:26, 1973.

Vokonas, P. S., Cohn, P. F., Klein, M. D., et al.: Hemoglobin affinity for oxygen in the anginal syndrome with normal coronary arteriograms. J. Clin. Invest. *54*:409, 1974.

Waddell, W. J., and Bates, R. G.: Intracellular pH. Physiol. Rev. *49*:285, 1969.

Wade, L. J., and Stevenson, L. D.: Necrosis of the bone marrow with fat embolism in sickle cell anemia. Am. J. Clin. Pathol. *17*:47, 1941.

Wajcman, H., Byckova, V., Haidas, S., et al.: Consequences of heme loss in unstable hemoglobins: a study of hemoglobin Köln. FEBS Lett. *13*:145, 1971.

Wajcman, H., Belkhodja, O., and Labie, D.: Hb Setif: G1(94) α Asp → Tyr. A new α chain hemoglobin variant with substitution of the residue involved in hydrogen bond between unlike subunits. FEBS Lett. *27*:298, 1972.

Wajcman, H., Labie, D., and Schapira, G.: Two new hemoglobin variants with deletion: Hemoglobin Tours (Thr β87 [F3] deleted) and hemoglobin St. Antoine ([Gly→Leu β74–75] [E18–19] deleted). Consequences for oxygen affinity and protein stability. Biochim. Biophys. Acta *295*:495, 1973a.

Wajcman, H., Leroux, A., and Labie, D.: Functional properties of hemoglobin Hammersmith. Biochimie *55*:119, 1973b.

Waks, M., and Beychok, S.: Induced conformational state in human apohemoglobin on binding of haptoglobin 1–1. Effect of added heme as a probe of frozen structures. Biochemistry *13*:15, 1974.

Waks, M., Yip, Y. K., and Beychok, S.: Influence of prosthetic groups on protein folding and subunit assembly. Recombination of separated human alpha- and beta-globin chains with heme and alloplex interactions of globin chains with heme-containing subunits. J. Biol. Chem. *248*:6462, 1973.

Waldeck, F.: Ein mikrophotometrisches Verfahren zur Aufnahme der Sauerstoffbindungskurve von einzelnen Erythrocyten. Pfluegers Arch. *295*:1, 1967.

Walker, B. R., and Alexander, F.: Uric acid excretion in sickle cell anemia. JAMA *215*:255, 1971.

Waltemath, C. L.: Oxygen uptake, transport and tissue utilization. Anesth. Analg. (Cleveland) *49*:184, 1970.

Wapnick, A. A., Lynch, S. R., Charlton, R. W., et al.: The effect of ascorbic acid deficiency on desferrioxamine-induced urinary iron excretion. Br. J. Haematol. *17*:563, 1969.

Ward, J., and Smith, A. L.: Hemophilus influenzae bacteremia in children with sickle cell disease. J. Pediatr. *88*:261, 1976.

Wasi, C., Wasi, P., and Thongcharoen, P.: Serum-immunoglobulin levels in thalassaemia and the effect of splenectomy. Lancet *2*:237, 1971.

Wasi, P.: The alpha thalassaemia genes. J. Med. Assoc. Thai. *53*:677, 1970.

Wasi, P.: Streptococcal infection leading to cardiac and renal involvement in thalassaemia. Lancet *1*:949, 1971.

Wasi, P.: Is the human globin α-chain locus duplicated? Br. J. Haematol. *24*:267, 1973.

Wasi, P., Na-Nakorn, S., and Suingdumrong, A.: Hemoglobin H disease in Thailand: a genetical study. Nature *204*:907, 1964.

Wasi, P., Disthasongchan, P., and Na-Nakorn, S.: The effect of iron deficiency on the levels of hemoglobins A_2 and E. J. Lab. Clin. Med. *71*:85, 1968.

Wasi, P., Na-Nakorn, S., Pootrakul, S., et al.: Alpha- and beta-thalassemia in Thailand. Ann. NY Acad. Sci. *165*:60, 1969.

Watson, J. D.: Molecular Biology of the Gene. 2nd ed. Reading, Mass., W. A. Benjamin, 1970.

Watson-Williams, E. J.: Sickle-cell crisis treated with Rheomacrodex. Lancet *1*:1053, 1963.

Watson-Williams, E. J., Beale, D., Irvine, D., and Lehmann, H.: A new haemoglobin, D-Ibadan (β87 threonine→lysine), producing no sickle cell/haemoglobin D disease with haemoglobin S. Nature *205*:1273, 1965.

Waxman, H., and Rabinovitz, M.: Control of reticulocyte polyribosome content and hemoglobin synthesis by heme. Biochim. Biophys. Acta *129*:369, 1966.

Waxman, H., Freedman, M., and Rabinovitz, M.: Studies with Fe^{59} labelled hemin on the control of polyribosome formation in rabbit reticulocytes. Biochim. Biophys. Acta *145*:353, 1967.

Weatherall, D. J.: Abnormal haemoglobins in the neonatal period and their relationship to thalassaemia. Br. J. Haematol. *9*:265, 1963.

Weatherall, D. J.: Biochemical phenotypes of thalassemia in the American Negro population. Ann. NY Acad. Sci. *119*:450, 1964a.

Weatherall, D. J.: Hemoglobin J (Baltimore) coexisting in a family with hemoglobin S. Bull. Johns Hopkins Hosp. *114*:1, 1964b.

Weatherall, D. J.: Recent advances in the haemoglobinopathies with special reference to the first months of life. Proc. Roy. Soc. Med. *65*:747, 1972.

Weatherall, D. J., and Clegg, J. B.: The Thalassaemia Syndromes. 2 ed. Oxford, Blackwell Scientific Publications, 1972.

Weatherall, D. J., and Clegg, J. B.: Hereditary persistence of fetal haemoglobin. Br. J. Haematol. *29*:191, 1975.

Weatherall, D. J., Clegg, J. B., and Naughton, M. A.: Globin synthesis in thalassemia: an *in vitro* study. Nature *208*:1061, 1965.

Weatherall, D. J., Edwards, J. A., and Donohoe, W. T. A.: Haemoglobin and red cell enzyme changes in juvenile myeloid leukaemia. Br. Med. J. *1*:679, 1968.

Weatherall, D. J., Clegg, J. B., Na-Nakorn, S., and Wasi, P.: The pattern of disordered haemoglobin synthesis in homozygous and heterozygous β-thalassaemia. Br. J. Haematol. *16*:251, 1969a.

Weatherall, D. J., Clegg, J. B., Blankson, J., and McNeil, J. R.: A new sickling disorder resulting from interaction of the genes for haemoglobin S and α-thalassaemia. Br. J. Haematol. *17*:517, 1969b.

Weatherall, D. J., Clegg, J. B., and Wong, H. B.: The haemoglobin constitution of infants with the haemoglobin Bart's hydrops foetalis syndrome. Br. J. Haematol. *18*:357, 1970.

Weatherall, D. J., Clegg, J. B., and Knox-Macaulay, A. H. M.: A genetically determined disorder with features of both thalassaemia and congenital dyserythropoietic anaemia. Br. J. Haematol. *24*:681, 1973.

Weatherall, D. J., Pembrey, M. E., and Pritchard, J.: Fetal haemoglobin. Clin. Haematol. *3*:467, 1974.

Weatherall, D. J., Cartner, R., Clegg, J. B., et al.: A form of hereditary persistence of foetal haemoglobin characterized by uneven cellular distribution of haemoglobin F and the production of haemoglobins A and A_2 in homozygotes. Br. J. Haematol. *29*:205, 1975a.

Weatherall, D. J., Clegg, J. B., Wood, W. G., et al.: Foetal erythropoiesis in human leukaemia. Nature *257*:710, 1975b.

Weed, R. I., LaCelle, P. L., and Merrill, E. W.: Metabolic dependence of red cell deformability. J. Clin. Invest. *48*:795, 1969.

Wennberg, E., and Weiss, L.: Splenic erythroclasia: an electronic microscopic study of hemoglobin H disease. Blood *31*:778, 1968.

Wheby, M. S., Thorup, O. A., and Leavell, B. S.: Homozygous hemoglobin C disease in siblings: further comments on intra-erythrocytic crystals. Blood *11*:266, 1956.

White, J. C., Ellis, M., Coleman, P. N., et al.: An unstable haemoglobin associated with cases of leukaemia. Br. J. Haematol. *6*:171, 1960.

White, J. G.: The fine structure of sickled hemoglobin in situ. Blood *31*:561, 1968.

White, J. M.: The synthesis of abnormal haemoglobins. Ser. Haematol. *4*:116, 1971.

White, J. M.: The synthesis of abnormal hemoglobins. Biochimie *54*:657, 1972.

White, J. M.: The unstable haemoglobin disorders. Clin. Haematol. *3*:333, 1974.

White, J. M., and Ali, M.: Globin synthesis in sideroblastic anemia. II. The effect of pyridoxine, δ amino-levulinic acid and heme *in vitro*. Br. J. Haematol. *24*:481, 1973.

White, J. M., and Brain, M. C.: Defective synthesis of an unstable haemoglobin Köln (β^{98}Val → Met). Br. J. Haematol. *18*:195, 1970.

White, J. M., and Dacie, J. V.: In vitro synthesis of Hb Hammersmith (CD1 Phe → Ser). Nature *225*:860, 1970.

White, J. M., and Dacie, J. V.: The unstable hemoglobins—molecular and clinical features. Progr. Hematol. 7:69, 1971.

White, J. M., and Harvey, D. R.: Defective synthesis of α and β globin chains in lead poisoning. Nature *236*:71, 1972.

White, J. M., and Hoffbrand, A. U.: Haem deficiency and chain synthesis. Nature *248*:88, 1974.

White, J. M., Brain, M. C., Lorkin, P. A., et al.: Mild "unstable haemoglobin haemolytic anaemia" caused by haemoglobin Shepherds Bush (β74 [E18] Gly→Asp). Nature *225*:939, 1970.

White, J. M., Brain, M. D., and Ali, M.: Globin synthesis in sideroblastic anaemia. I. α and β peptide chain synthesis. Br. J. Haematol. *20*:263, 1971.

White, J. M., Lang, A., Larkin, P. A., et al.: Synthesis of haemoglobin Lepore. Nature [New Biol.] *235*:208, 1972a.

White, J. M., Lang, A., and Lehmann, H.: Compensation of β chain synthesis by the single β chain gene in Hb Lepore trait. Nature [New Biol.] *240*:271, 1972b.

White, J. M., Szur, L., Gillies, I. D. S., et al.: Familial polycythaemia caused by a new haemoglobin variant: Hb Heathrow, β103 (G5) phenylalanine → leucine. Br. Med. J. *3*:665, 1973.

Williams, R. C.: Concerted formation of the gel of hemoglobin S. Proc. Natl. Acad. Sci. USA *70*:1506, 1973.

Williamson, J. R.: General features of metabolic control as applied to the erythrocyte. In Brewer, G. (ed.): Red Cell Metabolism and Function. New York, Plenum Press, 1970, p. 117. (Adv. Exp. Med. Biol., Vol. 6.)

Williamson, R.: The protein moieties of animal messenger ribonucleoproteins. FEBS Lett. *37*:1, 1973.

Williamson, R., Drewienkiewicz, C. E., and Paul, J.: Globin messenger sequences in high molecular weight RNA from embryonic mouse liver. Nature [New Biol.] *241*:66, 1973.

Williamson, R., Crossley, J., and Humphries, S.: Translation of mouse globin messenger ribonucleic acid from which the poly (adenylic acid) sequence has been removed. Biochemistry *13*:703, 1974.

Wilson, D., and Dintzis, H.: Protein chain initiation in rabbit reticulocytes. Proc. Natl. Acad. Sci. USA *66*:1282, 1970.

Wilson, J. B., Edwards, W. C., McDaniel, M., et al.: The structure of sheep hemoglobins. II. The amino acid composition of the tryptic peptides of the non-alpha chains of hemoglobins A, B, C and F. Arch. Biochem. Biophys. *115*:385, 1966.

Wilson, M. G., Schroeder, W. A., Graves, D. A., and Kach, V. D.: Hemoglobin variations in D-trisomy syndrome. N. Engl. J. Med. *277*:953, 1967.

Wilson, W. W., Luzzana, M. R., Penniston, J. T., and Johnson, C. S., Jr.: Pregelation aggregation of sickle cell hemoglobin. Proc. Natl. Acad. Sci. USA *71*:1260, 1974.

Wiltshire, B. G., Clark, K. G., Lorkin, P. A., et al.: Haemoglobin Denmark Hill 95 (G2) Pro → Ala, a variant with unusual electrophoretic and oxygen-binding properties. Biochim. Biophys. Acta *278*:459, 1972.

Winkelstein, J. A., and Drachman, R. H.: Deficiency of pneumococcal serum opsonizing activity in sickle cell disease. N. Engl. J. Med. *279*:459, 1968.

Winslow, R. M., Swenberg, M.-L., Gross, E., et al.: Hemoglobin McKees Rocks ($\alpha_2\beta_2{}^{145\ \mathrm{Tyr}\rightarrow\mathrm{Term}}$) A human "nonsense" mutation leading to a shortened β-chain. J. Clin. Invest. *57*:772, 1976.

Winterbourn, C. C., and Carrell, R. W.: Characterization of Heinz bodies in unstable haemoglobin haemolytic anaemia. Nature *240*:150, 1972.

Winterbourn, C. C., and Carrell, R. W.: The attachment of Heinz bodies to the red cell membrane. Br. J. Haematol. *25*:585, 1973.

Winterbourn, C. C., and Carell, R. W.: Studies of hemoglobin denaturation and Heinz body formation in the unstable hemoglobins. J. Clin. Invest. *54*:678, 1974.

Winterhalter, K. H.: The sequence of linkage between the prosthetic groups and the polypeptide chains of hemoglobin. Nature *211*:932, 1966.

Winterhalter, K. H., and Colosimo, A.: Chromatographic isolation and characterization of isolated chains from hemoglobin after regeneration of sulfhydryl groups. Biochemistry *10*:621, 1971.

Winterhalter, K. H., and Deranleau, D. A.: The structure of a hemoglobin carrying only two hemes. Biochemistry *6*:3136, 1967.

Winterhalter, K. H., and Glatthaar, B.: Intermediates of hemoglobin and their relation to biosynthesis. Ser. Haematol. *4*:84, 1971.

Winterhalter, K. H., and Wüthrich, K.: Structural investigations of modified haemoglobins by nuclear magnetic resonance spectroscopy. J. Mol. Biol. *63*:477, 1972.

Winterhalter, K. H., Amiconi, G., and Antonini, E.: Functional properties of a hemoglobin carrying heme only on α chains. Biochemistry *7*:2228, 1968.

Winterhalter, K. H., Heywood, J., Huehns, E., and Finch, C. A.: The free globin in human erythrocytes. Br. J. Haematol. *16*:523, 1969.

Winterhalter, K. H., Ioppolo, C., and Antonini, E.: Distribution of heme in systems containing heme-free and heme-bound hemoglobin chains. Biochemistry *10*:3790, 1971.

Wishner, B. C., and Love, W. E.: Crystals of deoxy sickle cell hemoglobin. In Hercules, J. I., Schechter, A. N., Eaton, W. A., et al. (eds.): Proceedings of First National Symposium on Sickle Cell Disease, Washington, D.C. DHEW Pub. No. 75–723 (NIH), Bethesda, Md., 1974, p. 85.

Wishner, B. C., Ward, K. B., Lattman, E. E., and Love, W. E.: Crystal structure of sickle-cell deoxyhemoglobin at 5 Å resolution. J. Mol. Biol. *98*:179, 1975.

Wishner, B. C., Hanson, J. C., Ringle, W. M., and Love, W. E.: Crystal structure of sickle cell deoxyhemoglobin. In Waterman, M., and Cottam, L. (eds.): Molecular and Cellular Aspects of Sickle Cell Disease. In press, 1976.

Wittenberg, J. B.: Myoglobin-facilitated diffusion of oxygen. J. Gen. Physiol. *49*:57 (Part 2), 1965.

Wolf, J. L., Mason, R. G., and Honig, G. R.: Regulation of hemoglobin β-chain synthesis in bone marrow erythroid cells by α chains. Proc. Natl. Acad. Sci. USA *70*:3405, 1973.

Wolff, J. A., and Luke, K. H.: Management of thalassemia: a comparative program. Ann. NY Acad. Sci. *165*:423, 1969.

Wolman, I. J.: Transfusion therapy in Cooley's anemia: growth and health as related to long-range hemoglobin levels, a progress report. Ann. NY Acad. Sci. *119*:736, 1964.

Wolman, I. J., and Ortolani, M.: Some clinical features of Cooley's anemia patients as related to transfusion schedules. Ann. NY Acad. Sci. *165*:407, 1969.

Wong, S. C., and Huisman, T. H. J.: Further evidence for non-linkage of the Hb α and Hb β structural loci in man. Clin. Chim. Acta *38*:473, 1972.

Wood, L., and Beutler, E.: The effect of ascorbate and dihydroxyacetone on the 2,3-diphosphoglycerate and ATP levels of stored human red cells. Transfusion *14*:272, 1974.

Wood, W. G., and Stamatoyannopoulos, G.: Globin synthesis in fractionated normoblasts of β-thalassemia heterozygotes. J. Clin. Invest. *55*:567, 1975.

Wood, W. G., and Weatherall, D. J.: Haemoglobin synthesis during human foetal development. Nature *244*:162, 1973.

Wood, W. G., Stamatoyannopoulos, G., Lim, G., and Nute, P. E.: F-cells in the adult: Normal values and levels in individuals with hereditary and acquired elevations of Hb F. Blood *46*:671, 1975.

Woodson, R. D., Torrance, J. D., Shappell, S. D., and Lenfant, C.: The effect of cardiac disease on hemoglobin-oxygen binding. J. Clin. Invest. *49*:1349, 1970.

Woodson, R. D., Wranne, B., and Detter, J. C.: Effect of increased blood oxygen affinity on work performance of rats. J. Clin. Invest. *52*:2717, 1973.

Woodson, R. D., Heywood, J. D., and Lenfant, C.: Oxygen transport in hemoglobin Köln. Effect of increased oxygen affinity in absence of compensatory erythrocytosis. Arch. Intern. Med. *134*:711, 1974.

Wranne, B., Woodson, R. D., and Detter, J. C.: Bohr effect: interaction between H^+, CO_2 and 2,3-DPG in fresh and stored blood. J. Appl. Physiol. *32*:749, 1972.

Wyatt, J. P., and Orrahood, M. D.: Massive fat embolism following marrow infarction in sickle cell anemia. Arch. Pathol. *53*:233, 1952.

Wyman, J.: Linked functions and reciprocal effects in hemoglobin: a second look. Adv. Protein Chem. *19*:223, 1964.

Wyman, J., and Allen, D. W.: The problem of the heme interactions in hemoglobin and the basis of the Bohr effect. J. Polymer. Sci. *7*:499, 1951.

Yamaoka, K., Cottman, G. L., and Waterman, M. R.: Spin-label studies at F9(93)β of deoxyhemoglobin S aggregation. Biochem. Biophys. Res. Commun. *58*:1058, 1974.

Yataganas, X., and Fessas, P.: The pattern of hemoglobin precipitation in thalassemia and its significance. Ann. NY Acad. Sci. *165*:270, 1969.

Yip, L. C., and Balis, M. E.: Inhibitory effects of 2,3-DPG on enzymes of purine nucleotide metabolism. Biochem. Biophys. Res. Commun. *63*:722, 1975.

Yoffey, J. M.: The stem cell problem in the fetus. Isr. J. Med. Sci. *7*:825, 1971.

Yoshida, A., and Lin, W.: Amino-terminal formylmethionine– and amino-terminal-methionine–cleaving enzymes in rabbit. J. Biol. Chem. *247*:952, 1972.

Yoshida, A., Watanabe, S., and Morris, J.: Initiation of rabbit hemoglobin synthesis: Methionine and formylmethionine at the N-terminal. Proc. Natl. Acad. Sci. USA *67*:1600, 1970.

Young, J. A., Lichtman, M. A., and Cohen, J.: Reduced red cell 2,3-diphosphoglycerate and adenosine triphosphate hypophosphatemia and increased hemoglobin-oxygen affinity after cardiac surgery. Circulation *47*:1313, 1973.

Zak, S. J., Brimhall, B., Jones, R. T., and Kaplan, M. E.: Hemoglobin Andrew-Minneapolis $\alpha_2{}^{A}\beta_2{}^{144\,Lys\rightarrow Asn}$: a new high-oxygen-affinity mutant human hemoglobin. Blood *44*:543, 1974.

Zalusky, R., Ross, J., and Katz, J. H.: Dissociation and exchange of α chains in an unstable haemoglobin. Proceedings of XIII Congress of the International Society of Hematology, Munich, 1970.

Zanjani, E. D., Mann, L. I., Burlington, H., et al.: Evidence for a physiologic role of erythropoietin in fetal erythropoiesis. Blood *44*:285, 1974a.

Zanjani, E. D., Peterson, E. N., Gordon, A. S., and Wasserman, L. R.: Erythropoietin production in the fetus: the role of the kidney and maternal anemia. J. Lab. Clin. Med. *83*:281, 1974b.

Zarkowsky, H. S., and Hochmuth, R. M.: Sickling times of individual erythrocytes at zero PO_2. J. Clin. Invest. *56*:1023, 1975.

Zimmon, D. S.: Changing oxyhemoglobin dissociation curve in hepatic encephalopathy. Clin. Res. *20*:469, 1972.

Zipp, A., James, T. L., Kuntz, I. D., et al.: Water proton magnetic resonance studies of normal and sickle erythrocytes: temperature and volume dependence. Biochim. Biophys. Acta *428*:291, 1976.

Zito, R., Antonini, E., and Wyman, J.: The effect of oxygenation on the rate of digestion of human hemoglobins by carboxypeptidases. J. Biol. Chem. *239*:1804, 1964.

Zucker, W., and Schulman, H.: The synthesis of globin dimers by a reticulocyte cell-free system. Biochim. Biophys. Acta *138*:400, 1967.

Zucker, W., and Schulman, H.: Stimulation of globin-chain initiation by hemin in the reticulocyte cell-free system. Proc. Natl. Acad. Sci. USA *59*:582, 1968.

INDEX

Note: Page numbers in *italics* refer to illustrations; those followed by (t) refer to tables; those followed by *f* refer to footnotes.